Robert K. Silverman, MD, FACOG

Professor and Chair
Department of Obstetrics and Gynecology
SUNY Upstate Medical University
Syracuse, New York

Obesity Medicine
Management of Obesity in Women's Health Care

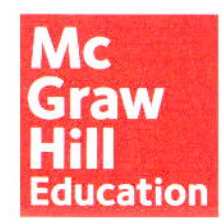

New York   Chicago   San Francisco   Athens   London   Madrid   Mexico City
Milan   New Delhi   Singapore   Sydney   Toronto

Obesity Medicine: Management of Obesity in Women's Health Care

Copyright © 2017 by McGraw-Hill Education, Inc. All rights reserved. Printed in China. Except as permitted under the United States Copyright Act of 1976, no part of this publication may be reproduced or distributed in any form or by any means, or stored in a data base or retrieval system, without the prior written permission of the publisher.

1 2 3 4 5 6 7 8 9   DSS   22 21 20 19 18 17

MHID 0-07-184351-5
ISBN 978-0-07-184351-5

Notice

Medicine is an ever-changing science. As new research and clinical experience broaden our knowledge, changes in treatment and drug therapy are required. The authors and the publisher of this work have checked with sources believed to be reliable in their efforts to provide information that is complete and generally in accord with the standards accepted at the time of publication. However, in view of the possibility of human error and changes in medical sciences, neither the editors nor the publisher nor any other party who has been involved in the preparation or publication of this work warrants that the information contained herein is in every respect accurate or complete, and they disclaim all responsibility for any errors or omissions or for the results obtained from use of the information contained in this work. Readers are encouraged to confirm the information contained herein with other sources. For example and in particular, readers are advised to check the product information sheet included in the package of each drug they plan to administer to be certain that the information contained in this work is accurate and that changes have not been made in the recommended dose or in the contraindications for administration. This recommendation is of particular importance in connection with new or infrequently used drugs.

This book was set in Utopia by Cenveo® Publisher Services.
The editors were Andrew Moyer and Regina Y. Brown.
The production supervisor was Richard Ruzycka.
The cover designer was Randomatix.
Production management was provided by Sonam Arora, Cenveo Publisher Services.
RR Donnelley was printer and binder.

This book is printed on acid-free paper.

Catalog-in-Publication Data is on file for this title at the Library of Congress.

McGraw-Hill books are available at special quantity discounts to use as premiums and sales promotions, or for use in corporate training programs. To contact a representative please visit the Contact Us pages at www.mhprofessional.com.

Contents

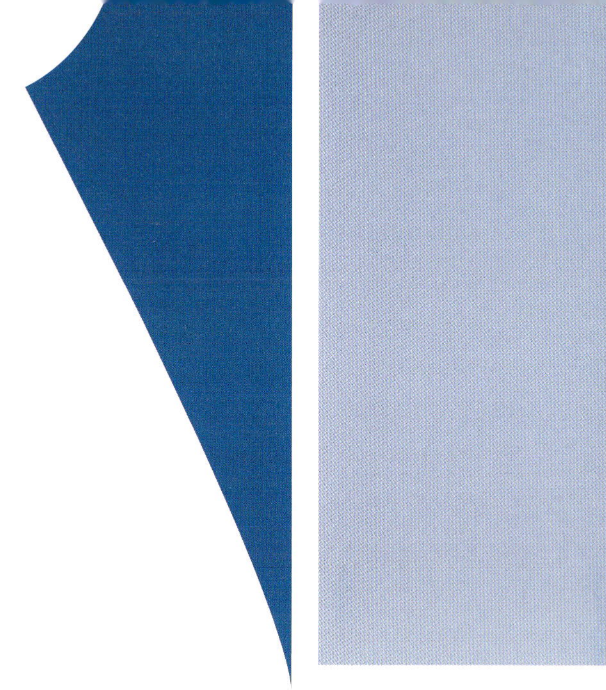

Contributors

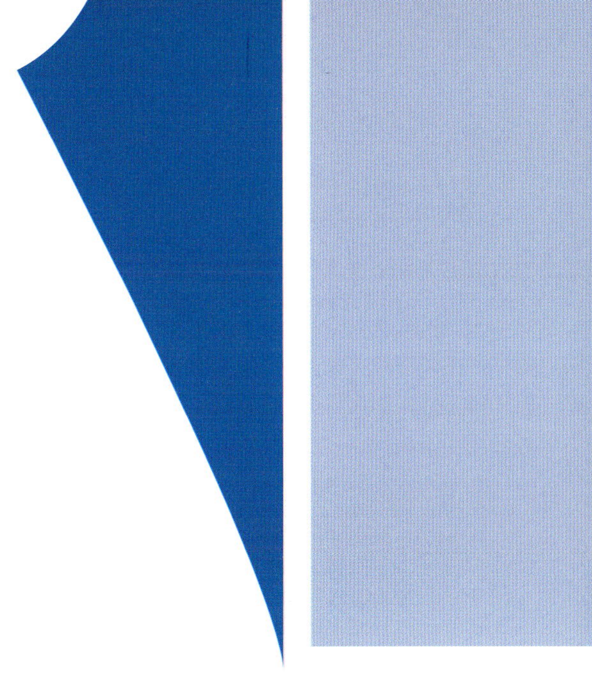

Ravi Adhikary, MD
Assistant Professor
Department of Radiology
SUNY Upstate Medical University
Syracuse, New York

Rinki G. Agarwal, MD
Assistant Professor
Medial Director of Gynecology Oncology Program
Department of Obstetrics and Gynecology
SUNY Upstate Medical University
Syracuse, New York

Scott P. Albert, MD
Assistant Professor
Division Chief Breast Care Center
Division Chief Endocrine (Thyroid) Surgery
Medial Director Breast Cancer Program
Department of Surgery
SUNY Upstate Medical University
Syracuse, New York

Norman F. Angell, MD, PhD, MBA
Department of Obstetrics and Gynecology
North Central Bronx Hospital
Bronx, New York

Stephen J. Bacak, Fellow, DO, MPH
Division of Maternal-Fetal Medicine
University of Rochester Medical Center
Rochester, New York

Shawky Z. A. Badawy, MD
Professor
Department of Obstetrics and Gynecology
Professor of Pathology
Division Chief of Reproductive Endocrinology and
    Infertility
SUNY Upstate Medical University
Syracuse, New York

Vanessa M. Barnabci, MD, PhD
Professor and Chairman
Department of Obstetrics and Gynecology
University at Buffalo School of Medicine and
    Biomedical Sciences
Buffalo, New York

Sherry Blumenthal, MD
Womencare OB/GYN
Associate Surgeon
Abington Memorial Hospital
Abington, Pennsylvania
Clinical Assistant Professor
Temple University of Medicine
Philadelphia, Pennsylvania

Alan D. Bolnick, MD
Department of Obstetrics and Gynecology
Women's and Children Hospital of Buffalo
Wayne State University School of Medicine
Detroit, Michigan

Gizelda T. B. Casella, MD, PhD
Department of Rehabilitation
Syracuse Veterans Affairs Medical Center
Syracuse, New York
Department of Physical Medicine and Rehabilitation
SUNY Upstate Medical University
Syracuse, New York

Jayne R. Charlamb, MD, FACOG, IBCLC
Associate Professor
Department of Obstetrics and Gynecology
Associate Professor of Medicine
Associate Professor of Pediatrics
SUNY Upstate Medical University
Syracuse, New York

Niamh Condon, DO
Division of Maternal Fetal Medicine
Pinnacle Health System
Harrisburg, Pennsylvania

Robert N. Cooney, MD
Professor and Chair
Department of Surgery
SUNY Upstate Medical University
Syracuse, New York

Thomas H. Dennison, PhD
Professor of Practice in Public Administration
  and International Affairs
Director, Program in Health Services Management
  and Policy
Director, Lerner Center for Public Health Promotion
  Professor of Public Health, SUNY Upstate Medical
  University
Senior Research Associate, Center for Policy Research
The Maxwell School
Syracuse University
Syracuse, New York

John Donnelly, MD
Department of Pediatrics and Internal Medicine
Christiana Care Health System
Newark, Delaware

John Epling, MD
Professor and Chair
Department of Family Medicine
Professor of Public Health Preventative Medicine
SUNY Upstate Medical University
Syracuse, New York

John J. Folk, MD, FACOG
Associate Professor
Division Maternal Fetal Medicine
Department of Obstetrics and Gynecology
Division of Pulmonary and Critical Care Medicine
Department of Medicine
SUNY Upstate Medical University
Syracuse, New York

Anil Ghimire, MD
Assistant Professor
Department of Medicine
SUNY Upstate Medical University
Syracuse, New York

Michael Iannuzzi, MD
Professor and Chair
Department of Internal Medicine
SUNY Upstate Medical University
Syracuse, New York

Jeffrey R. Johnson, MD
Chairman
Department of Obstetrics and Gynecology
Maternal-Fetal Medicine
Wentworth-Douglass Hospital
Dover, New Hampshire

Leah Kaufman, MD, FACOG
Associate Professor and Vice Chair
Department of Obstetrics and Gynecology
SUNY Upstate Medical University
Syracuse, New York

Satinder Kaur, MD
Assistant Professor
Department of Obstetrics and Gynecology
Wayne State University School of Medicine
Detroit, Michigan

Rae-Ellen W. Kavey, MD, MPH
University of Rochester Medical Center
Rochester, New York

Kara C. Kort, MD
Department of Surgery
St. Joseph's Hospital Health Center
Syracuse, New York

David Landsberg, MD, FACP, FCCP
Associate Professor and Chief of Medicine
Clinical Associate Professor of Emergency Medicine
Crouse Hospital
Syracuse, New York

Sandra D. Lane, PhD, MPH
Laura J. and L. Douglas Meredith Professor
Professor of Public Health and Anthropology
Syracuse University
Syracuse, New York
Research Professor
Department of Obstetrics and Gynecology
SUNY Upstate Medical University
Syracuse, New York

Robert Roger Lebel, MD, FACMG
Professor in Pediatrics
Professor of Medicine
Professor of Obstetrics and Gynecology
Professor of Pathology
Chief and Director of Medical Genetics
SUNY Upstate Medical University
Syracuse, New York

Shaveta Malik, MD
Clinical Assistant Professor
Department of Obstetrics and Gynecology
University at Buffalo School of Medicine and
    Biomedical Sciences
Buffalo, New York

Federico G. Mariona, MD, FACOG, FACS
Division of Maternal Fetal Medicine
Wayne State University School of Medicine
Detroit, Michigan
Michigan Perinatal Associates
Dearborn, Michigan

Renee E. Mestad, MD, MSCI
Assistant Professor
Division Chief General Obstetrics and Gynecology
Department of Obstetrics and Gynecology
SUNY Upstate Medical University
Syracuse, New York

Lillian Msambichaka, MD
Department of Pediatrics and Internal Medicine
Christiana Care Health System
Newark, Delaware

Unzila Ali Nayeri, MD
Assistant Professor
Division of Maternal-Fetal Medicine
SUNY Upstate Medical University
Syracuse, New York

Deborah L. Pollack, PhD
Clinical Psychologist
SUNY Upstate Medical University
Syracuse, New York

Elizabeth E. Puscheck, MD
Professor
Division Director Reproductive Endocrinology and
    Infertility
Department of Obstetrics and Gynecology
Wayne State University School of Medicine
Detroit, Michigan

Benjamin Silverman, MD
Department of Pediatrics and Internal Medicine
Christiana Care Health System
Newark, Delaware

Amy R. Slutzky, PhD, MLIS
Health Sciences Library
SUNY Upstate Medical University
Syracuse, New York

Alexandra C. Spadola, MD
Associate Professor
Department of Obstetrics and Gynecology
Division of Maternal-Fetal Medicine
SUNY Upstate Medical University
Syracuse, New York

Parikshith Sumathi, MD
Assistant Professor
Department of Anesthesiology/Pain Medicine
SUNY Upstate Medical University
Syracuse, New York

Eddie H. M. Sze, MD
Professor of Obstetrics and Gynecology
Director of Urogynecology and Pelvic Reconstructive
 Surgery
Director of Women's Center/University OB/GYN
 Associates
Division of Urogynecology
Department of Obstetrics and Gynecology
SUNY Upstate Medical University
Syracuse, New York

Maida Taylor, MD, MPH, FACOG
Department of Obstetrics, Gynecology, and
 Reproductive Sciences
University of California San Francisco
San Francisco, California

P. Sebastian Thomas, MD
Professor and Chair
Department of Anesthesiology
SUNY Upstate Medical University
Syracuse, New York

Brian Thompson, MD
Assistant Professor
Department of Obstetrics and Gynecology
Assistant Dean for Diversity
SUNY Upstate Medical University
Syracuse, New York

Loralei L. Thornburg, MD
James R. Woods, Jr. Professor of Obstetrics and
 Gynecology
Associate Professor of Obstetrics and Gynecology
Director of Division of Maternal-Fetal Medicine
Program Director of Maternal-Fetal Medicine
 Fellowship
University of Rochester Medical Center
Rochester, New York

Margaret A. Turk, MD
Professor
Department of Physical Medicine and Rehabilitation
Pediatrics
SUNY Upstate Medical University
Syracuse, New York

Serdar H. Ural, MD, FACOG
Professor and Director
Division of Maternal Fetal Medicine
The Pennsylvania State University College of Medicine
Hershey, Pennsylvania

Zevidah Vickery, MD, MSCI
Assistant Professor
Department of Obstetrics and Gynecology
SUNY Upstate Medical University
Syracuse, New York

Preface

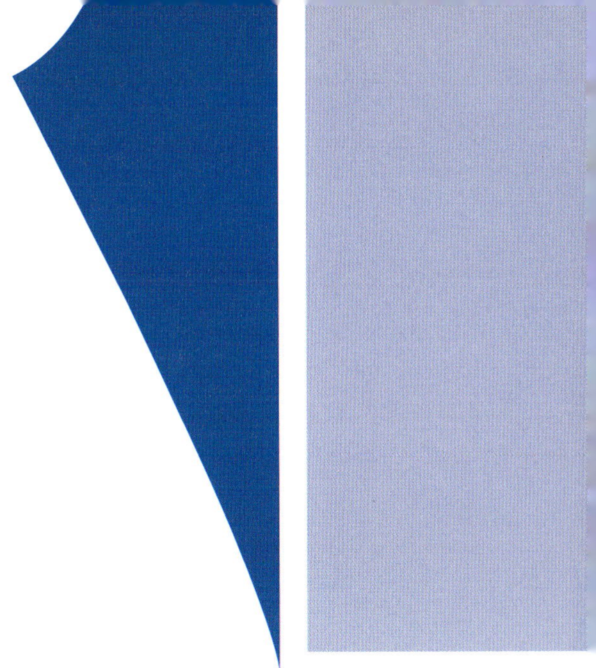

The study of obesity and obesity-related comorbidities continues to increase in scope. The recognition that obesity contributes to significant health care costs has come to the forefront of medicine in all specialties. Journals across most disciplines have hundreds of articles published each year on research related to obesity and obesity-related illnesses. The economic cost of obesity continues to rise and with it mounting concern that health care providers and facilities will be affected both financially and in regard to access to care. The realization that obesity has such a dramatic impact on our society has come slowly to most individuals.

The need for a better informed public, improved access to education, and better understanding of the stressors obesity places on individuals and institutions has highlighted the need for consolidated resources. Few medical schools spend more than a few hours or, at best, isolated single lectures on obesity as part of their curriculum. This is in contrast to the reality that obesity will affect all health care providers in their careers. Few physicians are prepared to discuss the myriad issues related to obesity other than in a passing fashion.

Few resources exist for health care providers that compile a summarization of research and recommendations for care for patients with obesity. There needs to be increased emphasis on these issues in health care education for all types of providers. This book will serve as a resource for any level provider to further investigate major topics that their patients with obesity will encounter. It represents a consolidation of information into one source; until now, this central source has been lacking for women's health care.

The field of obesity medicine continues to rapidly evolve. Any practitioner involved in women's health care should be able to use this book as a resource to improve their knowledge base and to help counsel patients and their families. This text should serve as stimulus to future investigators to carry out research in treatment and management of obesity in women's health care.

Robert K. Silverman, MD
SUNY–Upstate Medical University
Syracuse, New York

Dedication and Acknowledgments

No project of this magnitude could be developed without the help of many individuals. From Alyssa Fried at McGraw-Hill to my administrative assistants, Christine Rydelek and Sunny Falcone, my appreciation has no bounds. My wife, Carol, has endured my endless conversations on obesity and its impact on the health care system. My sons, Ben and Andrew, have seen their father obsessed with a topic that at times must have seemed overwhelming. I hope this book will serve as a resource for providers in all areas of medicine and allow them to gain understanding of the complexity of the issues and the need for expenditures of significant resources in the future.

Robert K. Silverman, MD

Introduction

Biological and Genetic Determinants of Obesity

CHAPTER 1

Mani Yahyavi, MD

Yakov Rubinchik, MD

Robert Roger Lebel, MD, FACMG

INTRODUCTION
SINGLE-GENE CONDITIONS
COPY NUMBER VARIANTS
GWAS AND THE DISCOVERY OF *FTO*

EPIGENETIC FACTORS
BEHAVIORAL GENETICS
CONCLUSION

INTRODUCTION

The prevalence of obesity has increased dramatically in recent decades. Increased body habitus correlates with enhanced availability of low-cost, high-calorie foods. A mismatch in caloric intake and energy expenditure leads to excess body fat accumulation. There are, however, interindividual differences in susceptibility to obesity with exposure to the same obesogenic environment. It is likely that this variability in metabolism, energy storage, or neural hormonal components affecting behavior has genetic, epigenetic, or genomic components.

Gregor Johann Mendel discovered the laws of heredity that bear his name[1] by combining diligent observation, prudent choice of experimental organism, and mental discipline. These allowed him to discern and then explain patterns consistent with unitary particulate determinative factors governing discrete phenotypic traits (genes). This insight is an example of Pascal's dictum that "chance favors the prepared mind."[2] Unitary genetic traits such as sickle cell disease are the delight of educators, who employ them to convey foundational concepts in biology with elegant simplicity: one gene, one protein, one phenotype. This, of course, allows for oversimplification. By contrast, complex traits such as intelligence involve the interaction of multiple genes with various environmental influences. Readers of this text will likely have encountered Mendelian genetics. However, anyone whose genetics learning occurred more than a decade ago may reference and update their vocabulary of new concepts in genomics by referencing various genetics textbooks.[3,4]

SINGLE-GENE CONDITIONS

The first single-gene mutation associated with obesity was identified in 1994 by positional cloning of the ob/ob mouse strain. The mutation was mapped to the leptin (*lep*) gene, which encodes a 16-kDa secreted hormone produced primarily by white adipose tissue.[5] Subsequently, a mutation in the leptin receptor gene (*lepr*) was identified in another obese strain of mice. The leptin receptor is primarily expressed in the hypothalamus, and this hormonal signaling pathway plays an important role in regulation of food intake in both strains of mice. As it eventually became clear, the same is true in humans. Rare homozygous mutations and polymorphisms in both the *LEP* and *LEPR* genes have been identified in patients with severe forms of early-onset obesity and hyperphagia[6] (see Sidebar 1-1). Leptin deficiency also manifests with reduced insulinlike growth factor 1 (IGF-1) levels, elevated insulin levels, hypothalamic hypothyroidism, impaired growth hormone secretion, and hypogonadotropic hypogonadism. Replacement of leptin by administration of the exogenous peptide has shown remarkable reversal of obesity in patients with homozygous mutations in *LEP*.[7]

Further research into the leptin signaling pathway elucidated other genes involved in energy homeostasis. Proopiomelanocortin (*POMC*) has its expression positively regulated by leptin. Loss-of-function (LOF) mutations in *POMC* are notable for early-onset hyperphagia and obesity, adrenal insufficiency, pale skin, and red hair.[8] It is produced by the arcuate nucleus of the hypothalamus[9] and is cleaved to produce alpha-melanocyte-stimulating hormone (α-MSH), a ligand that acts on the melanocortin 4 receptor (MC4R), a seven-transmembrane G-protein-linked receptor that is also expressed in the hypothalamus. MC4R likely transmits the signals from the leptin pathway to downstream effectors through the paraventricular nucleus of the hypothalamus.[10] Both autosomal recessive and dominant LOF mutations in *MC4R*

SIDEBAR 1-1　Leptin Insufficiency

Hassan, the first child of healthy first cousins, was born at term weighing 3680 g. He presented to the clinic at 2.5 years of age weighing 34 kg (>99.9th percentile) with a height of 93.5 cm (69th percentile) and a BMI of 38.6 (>99.9th percentile). The parents reported food-seeking behavior and hyperphagia. Given the high clinical suspicion of a disturbance in the satiety signal in the CNS, serum levels of leptin were measured and found to be elevated.[76] Current recommendations for measuring serum leptin for children with rapid weight gain in the first months of life[77] have been supported by low or absent levels of leptin in previously described cases[78–81]; this patient had high levels of the hormone.

Sequencing of both the leptin receptor (*LEPR*) and ligand (*LEP*) genes was performed, demonstrating a novel homozygous mutation in *LEP*. The c.298G→T transversion with its amino acid change (p.D100Y) was not observed in screening of 720 ethnically similar children and was not listed on dbSNP (Single-Nucleotide Polymorphism Database) or other databases. Protein-modeling studies localized the mutation to the binding pocket, suggesting inability of the mutant ligand to bind to the receptor. The mutated gene was cloned; both in vitro and in vivo experiments confirmed it to be nonfunctional.

Treatment options were discussed, and the patient was started on 0.03 mg of subcutaneous metreleptin per kilogram of lean body weight per day. Rapid changes in eating behavior, calorie intake, and weight loss followed. This patient has congenital leptin deficiency due to biologically inactive leptin associated with high circulating hormone levels. This case further illustrates that elevated or even normal levels of the hormone do not rule out disease-causing mutations in the gene encoding leptin, and the correct diagnosis may be awaiting discovery.

SIDEBAR 1-2   Bardet-Biedl Syndrome

The pregnancy for Toni was uneventful, but at birth she was noted to have extra fingers; these were removed surgically, and for the next year no one had any concern about her. However, learning disabilities were eventually appreciated, and she received therapies leading up to school, where an individualized education plan (IEP) includes a comprehensive program to help her reach her best potential. She is approaching puberty, and it has been found that she is losing her eyesight to retinitis pigmentosa.

There are well over 100 genetic syndromes that include obesity as a feature; one of these is due to leptin deficiency, and another is caused by a defect in the leptin receptor (see Sidebar 1-1). Many of the syndromes are also characterized by other anatomic anomalies. When the affected individual also has polydactyly, learning disability, hypogonadism, and retinitis pigmentosa, the diagnosis is probably Bardet-Biedl syndrome, which usually is inherited as an autosomal recessive (Online Mendelian Inheritance in Man [OMIM] #209900), due to mutations in the *BBS1* gene located on chromosome 11q13.2.

However, approximately 20 other genes are also associated with Bardet-Biedl syndrome. Some of these are associated with lists of features, which differ somewhat from the classic constellation described. If it is possible to document exactly which genetic changes underpin Toni's clinical diagnosis of Bardet-Biedl syndrome, that information can be applied to new pregnancies in the family, allowing pregnancies to go forward unaffected by this condition. This syndrome is an excellent example of genetic heterogeneity and variable expression.

have been found,[11] and they are strongly associated with obesity (Sidebar 1-2).[12] Population studies show that pathogenic *MC4R* mutations account for approximately 2% of childhood and adult obesity cases.[13,14]

PCSK1 codes for proprotein convertase subtilisin/kexin type 1,[15] an integral component of the post-translational proteolytic processing of POMC.[16,17] Mutations in the *PCSK1* (also known as *PC1*) gene have been identified in patients with severe childhood obesity, abnormal glucose homeostasis, reduced plasma insulin with elevated proinsulin levels, hypogonadotropic hypogonadism, and hypocortisolemia. Even carriers of mutations causing partial *PCSK1* deficiency have a significantly higher risk of obesity.[18]

SIM1 is one of the effectors of MC4R in controlling energy homeostasis and has been shown to have an essential role in embryonic neurogenesis within the ventral neurogenic region in *Drosophila*.[19] LOF mutations in *SIM1* have been characterized in mouse models and identified in humans, resulting in severe hyperphagia and obesity, developmental delays, short extremities, and hypotonia.[20-22] Functional studies of hyperphagic obesity in *Sim1*-deficient mice suggest a role in the leptin-melanocortin-oxytocin pathway and that postnatal central nervous system (CNS) deficiency of *Sim1* is sufficient to cause hyperphagic obesity.[23]

Brain-derived neurotrophic factor (BDNF) is another effector that regulates eating behavior and energy balance downstream of MC4R.[24] Knockout studies in mice demonstrated obesity and hyperactivity. LOF mutation in one copy of the gene was found in a girl with hyperphagia, early-onset obesity, cognitive impairment, and hyperactivity. A missense variant in the BDNF receptor encoded by *NTRK2* has also been reported in a boy with severe obesity and memory impairment.[25]

Adiponectin (encoded by the *ADIPOQ* gene) is a hormone secreted by adipose tissue that modulates metabolic processes, including glucose regulation and fatty acid breakdown.[26] It is associated with both obesity and diabetes mellitus type 2 (DMT2), where it has notably reduced expression levels.[27] Similarly, proline-to-alanine substitution at position 12 in the peroxisome proliferator-activated receptor gamma (*PPAR*) gene is associated with both obesity and DMT2.[28,29]

GPR120 (also known as *O3FAR1*) encodes a G-protein-coupled receptor for unsaturated long-chain free fatty acids that plays a critical role in energy homeostasis by obesity, glucose intolerance, fatty liver with decreased adipocyte differentiation, and lipogenesis. Furthermore, a deleterious arginine-to-histidine mutation at position 270 inhibits *GPR120* signaling in obese subjects.[30] As a lipid sensor, *GRP120* provides a link between physiological response and the environment, in particular providing insights to the mechanism by which an obesogenic, high-calorie, fatty diet may contribute to obesity and associated complications like fatty liver. Such environment-sensitive genes provide particular interest in translational research as potential drug targets for prevention or treatment of obesity.[31]

COPY NUMBER VARIANTS

Regions of genetic material may be lost or duplicated in one individual compared to others, with no apparent phenotypic consequence. Such changes (*microdeletions* or *microduplications*) are called *copy number variants (CNVs)*. They may involve many tens of thousands of nucleotides, such that the loss or gain would seem intuitively to have important phenotypic consequence, but does not. Knowledge of the human genome has evolved rapidly over the last decade. We now have a large catalog of CNVs that are known to have no phenotypic importance, but we also have another list of deletions and duplications that are well established to have causative relationship to more or less well-defined adverse phenotypes. There is also a third list of changes that appear to imply pathology but have not as yet been documented as such in the literature.

That third group is cause for consternation in the clinical setting, where theoretical importance does not suffice to explain an adverse phenotype or to enlighten the family in terms of optimum management or long-term prognosis. The role of CNVs in causing adverse phenotypes is coming into focus gradually; there is evidence that apparently unimportant CNVs might become important if an individual has more than one of them.[32] Testing for genomic changes (comparative genomic hybridization, or chromosome microarray) is now a routine clinical approach to the evaluation of individuals with intellectual disability, autism spectrum, or multiple anatomic anomalies.[33,34] Studying the genome in greater depth, with whole-exome analysis (next-generation DNA sequencing), is used only in the most complex cases, but as the cost of this approach falls, it is likely to replace microarray in the future.[35] Such testing sometimes allows for predictive or preventive measures.[36]

A portion of a chromosome may be missing or extra, with more or less serious consequence. Some are well known, such as cri-du-chat syndrome, which is associated with missing part of the short arm of number 5; or Wolf-Hirshhorn syndrome, which is associated with missing a portion of the short arm of number 4. Prader-Willi syndrome usually involves missing a portion of the long arm of number 15 (see Sidebar 1-3), while Williams syndrome is found with a missing part of the long arm of number 7. The 22q11 deletion syndrome involves loss of that segment and goes by several names (DiGeorge syndrome, Shprintzen syndrome, velocardiofacial syndrome).

The CNVs are considered either common variants with frequencies greater than 5% or rare variants with frequencies less than 1% in the general population. Several structural variants have also been found to have associations with obesity. One such association is the common CNV on chromosome 10q11.22 that encompasses the pancreatic polypeptide receptor 1 (*PPYR1*) gene, with low copy numbers and deletions observed in individuals with increased body mass index (BMI).[37] Another common CNV on 11q11, encompassing olfactory receptor genes *OR4P4, OR4S2*, and *OR4C6*, has a deletion allele that is associated with extreme early-onset obesity.[38] Large meta-analysis studies have demonstrated deletions associated with increased BMI near the hypothalamic-expressed neuronal growth regulator 1 (*NEGR1*) gene, while a 21-kb CNV was also mapped upstream of *GPRC5B* with a nonrisk deletion allele.[39] Further studies of *GPRC5B* in deficient mice found protection from diet-induced obesity and highlight its role as a major node in adipose signaling systems that link diet-induced obesity to DMT2.[40]

Large deletions in 16p11.2 have been shown to result in a 43-fold increase in the risk of morbid obesity.[41] Interestingly, reciprocal duplications at this locus have been found to demonstrate a mirror effect on phenotype, with an 8-fold increase in the risk of being underweight.[42] *SH2B1* is the common gene to all 16p11.2 deletions, and genome-wide association studies (GWAS) have revealed single-nucleotide polymorphisms (SNPs) within *SH2B1* that are associated with BMI.[43] Functional studies in knockout mice show disrupted leptin and insulin signaling that supports the role of this gene in energy homeostasis regulation.[44] In addition, LOF mutations in *SH2B1* have been associated with aggressive and maladaptive behaviors.[45]

GWAS AND THE DISCOVERY OF *FTO*

Many genes have been implicated in monofactorial forms of obesity, and a large number of polymorphisms with smaller effect size associated with adiposity have been discovered through GWAS. Although monogenic forms of obesity are rare, they are often severe with a large effect size, having clinical importance in screening and early intervention. The complex contribution of polygenic variants and epigenetics may not currently have significant clinical utility, but researchers are finding applications for risk and outcome prediction to enhance clinical decision-making that eventually will be integrated into clinical practice. Research in this field has enhanced our understanding of the pathophysiology of obesity and is rapidly evolving with advances in sequencing technologies toward the promise of new therapeutics and personalized medicine.

Polygenic (or common) obesity is the result of the combined contribution of multiple genetic variants in the setting of environmental risk factors. The candidate gene study of the genetics of obesity in mice and humans has provided great insights into the mechanism of energy homeostasis. Yet, this approach has been limited to known pathways with strong monogenic components because we see what we know and expect to see in complex situations. The advent of GWAS in part addresses this issue due to its global capability and power in screening for novel loci of association without requiring a priori knowledge of the biological mechanism.

Many new loci and pathways in obesity have been discovered via GWAS. One of the most notable genes discovered this way is the fat mass and obesity-associated *FTO* gene, which harbors one of the first common variants found to be strongly correlated with obesity in humans.[46] The cluster of SNPs in *FTO* was discovered in 2007 during GWAS for DMT2 by the Wellcome Trust Case Control Consortium.[47] Once the data were corrected for BMI, it was realized that the associated phenotype was obesity rather than DMT2.[48] Multiple studies in both children and adults of different ancestries have validated these findings.[49-51]

Although rare variants in the monogenic forms of obesity have greater effect size, *FTO* variants remain those with the most robust association with common obesity due to their high frequency in the population.[52] The SNP rs9939609 shows the strongest association with BMI in Caucasians, where the A allele is associated with increased BMI versus the protective T allele.[53] SNP rs3751812 has been found to capture obesity association in subjects of both African and European ancestry.[54] Other studies confirmed these obesogenic variants in Asian subjects.[55] Secondary associations have been investigated for diseases such as DMT2 with a predominantly obesogenic population. One recent meta-analysis of 5 studies investigating the link between *FTO* SNPs and polycystic ovary syndrome (PCOS) susceptibility concluded that rs9939609 in East Asians is associated with PCOS risk independent of BMI.[56]

Functional studies of the role of genes such as *FTO* in energy intake regulation are needed to determine a causal contribution. *FTO* is highly expressed in human hypothalamus, pituitary, and adrenal glands, suggesting a potential role in the hypothalamic-pituitary-adrenal (HPA) axis governing energy balance.[57] *FTO* expression has been found significantly upregulated in the arcuate nucleus of rats after food deprivation, and it is negatively correlated with the expression of orexogenic Galanin-like-peptide (GALP), which is involved in the stimulation of food intake.[58] Increased expression is associated with energy intake regulation but not feeding reward.[59] Functional studies have shown *FTO* product localizes to the cellular nucleus, consistent with a potential role in nucleic acid demethylation and regulation of gene expression.[60]

There is evidence suggesting that *FTO* may act during the early stages of life on tissue remodeling and epigenetic modifications when energy homeostasis is first established. Epigenetic changes in *FTO* expression have been noted when the fetal energy supply is above (maternal obesity) or below (placental insufficiency) physiological needs.[61] Such modifications would be predicted to promote higher energy intake and storage in key organs regulating energy homeostasis and support a role for *FTO* during organogenesis in the early programming of energy balance and metabolic regulation.

EPIGENETIC FACTORS

Changes in the nucleotide sequence of a gene may have no effect, slight effect, or dramatic effect on the function of the final protein product. Once any change in the nucleotide sequence has taken place, it is conserved in the cells that descend from the cell in which it occurred. Whether a variant or a mutation, change in the DNA sequence is permanent. There is, however, also a mechanism for *temporary* changes in the information. Low molecular weight moieties, most often methyl groups, can be covalently bound to nucleotides in a process known as imprinting. This renders the information encoded in the gene unreadable; however, imprinting is reversible, so that an apparently useless gene might become readable again after another generation. These changes are called *epigenetic* changes, defined as inheritable and reversible phenomena that affect gene expression without altering the underlying base pair sequence. Epigenomics is the study of genome-wide epigenetic modifications, and insight regarding this layer of complexity is providing us with clues regarding the connection of genetic predisposition and environmental exposure to generate a phenotype.

Epigenomic data have provided substantial evidence of epigenetic changes in obese subjects. Such changes can be inherited or acquired in utero and throughout development. Environmental factors such as diet and exposure to bioactive compounds highlight the ability of epigenetic cellular responses to the nutritional status of the environment through the regulation of gene expression and activity by mechanisms such as DNA methylation, histone tail modifications, and chromatin remodeling.

Prader-Willi syndrome (see Sidebar 1-3) is the classic example of a heritable imprinting disorder that is caused by genetic and epigenetic errors in the region of chromosome 15q11-q13. The paternal copy in this region is deleted, while the maternal copy is inactivated by methylation to produce a unique phenotype that differs from the alternate deletion on the maternal copy that produces what is known as Angelman syndrome. In a recent study of *Drosophila*, chromatin changes in the father's sperm were found to transmit an obesogenic phenotype. The role of chromatin-modifying proteins such as Su(var) were characterized, and further analysis of adipose tissues from both mice and humans showed that deficits in the orthologous chromatin-modifying proteins were associated with obesity.[62] This study highlights that the epigenetic responses to the environment may be inherited from one generation to the next.

It is important to note that several endocrine-modulating chemicals with the ability to modify epigenetic markers have been identified that are associated obesity. These substances, such as monobenzyl, monoethylhexyl phthalates and bisphenol A (BPA) are found in plastics and may be ingested or absorbed through the skin.[63] Maternal exposure to several such chemical substances during pregnancy has been found to be associated with increased BMI in offspring.[64] These substances may also distress neural circuits that regulate feeding behavior, in particular the dopaminergic reward system discussed in this text, to increase the risk of obesity.[65] Both the European Union and Canada have banned the use of BPA in baby bottles, and proper guidance by the obstetrician to avoid such toxins is important.

Hallmarks of obesity are an enhanced proinflammatory status and observation of the rise in adipokines such as leptin and cytokines, in particular tumor necrosis factor alpha (TNF-α). It was postulated that epigenetic regulation of gene expression could be used as obesogenic biomarkers. Further studies of *TNF* and *LEP* promoter methylation levels in adipose tissue demonstrated a greater response to a low-calorie diet in the lower methylation level group for both genes, supporting the potential predictive utility of these epigenetic biomarkers.[66] This was one of the first examples of using epigenetic markers as early predictors of metabolic risks and advancing toward epigenetic-based personalized interventions. Advancements in epigenomic techniques such as ChIP-Seq (chromatin immunoprecipitation sequencing), whole-genome sequencing, and microarray assays for methylation have since allowed for epigenome-wide association studies, the exploration of DNA methylation patterns describing a multitude of epigenomic phenomena and their complex interactions.[67]

BEHAVIORAL GENETICS

Investigators in the field of behavior genetics seek to elucidate deterministic factors underlying behavioral patterns that predispose individuals to obesity. Understanding how genetic variations can affect eating habits that lead to obesity should enhance empathy for certain individuals who continually struggle with weight control. Such insights may help clinicians appropriately encourage and guide patients in understanding their circumstances and the difficulty of achieving auspicious nutritional behaviors. Nutritional choices involve decisions on both the material of food and the quantity that an individual elects to eat.

Satiety plays an important role in how much food someone chooses to eat because if a person does not feel full, it is likely that eating will continue beyond what is nutritionally required for survival and lead to fat storage of the calories and potentially to obesity. There are likely many genetic polymorphisms that play a role in satiety, as has been suggested in a recent study of pediatric twin subjects. In this cross-sectional observational study, 28 common obesity-related SNPs were identified and chosen to create a Polygenic Risk Score (PRS), while the satiety response of the children was measured using the Child Eating Behavior Questionnaire.[68] The study showed that the higher the PRS of a child, the less satiety response was shown. It is to be expected that adults will have similar genetic influences on satiety and behavior. Another study employed 8 genes involved in or related to the leptin-melanocortin pathway in the regulation of satiety and risk of developing obesity, showing similar associations between high-risk alleles of these genes and increased BMI.[69]

Dopamine plays an important role in the reward system of the brain and modulates individual interactions with the environment to ideally benefit the organism. It is no surprise that we find that the consumption of food activates the dopaminergic reward circuitry, yet the level of activation varies with the nature of the nutrient. Unfortunately, the types of food that have been found to cause the greatest increase in dopamine release are rich in fats and sugars.[70] In addition, this greater spike in dopamine release enforces the consumption of greater quantities of such obesogenic foods. In a recent study, 29 individuals who ranged from healthy to obese were given milk shakes high in sugar and fat, then monitored for functional magnetic resonance (fMRI) activity of the DS dopamine type 2/3 receptor (D2R/D3R).[71] The results showed that there was a positive correlation between BMI and D2R/D3R availability, showing a connection between the consumption of food high in fat and sugar and the release of dopamine.

Reward deficiency syndrome has recently been described: Genetic and epigenetic changes lead to hypodopaminergic functional disturbances in the reward circuitry of the brain.[72] This results in abnormal craving behavior. Further evidence for the connection between the ingestion of certain foods and dopamine release includes the observation that carbohydrate binging stimulates the brain's production of and utilization of dopamine, the proximal location of enkephalinergic neurons in the mesolimbic system to glucose receptors, highly concentrated glucose releases dopamine through the activation of calcium, and a significant correlation between the dopamine metabolite homovanillic acid in the CSF and blood glucose levels. In addition, many of the brain circuits involved in the release of dopamine due to ingestion of certain foods have been proven to be the same as the circuits involved in psychoactive drug addiction.

The neuromedin U (NMU) receptor is found in the paraventricular nucleus (PVN) of the hypothalamus (PVN). In a recent study, investigators found that when *nmur2* knockout rats were fed a (45%) fat-rich diet in comparison to the standard chow, they consumed greater quantities of food, at a greater pace, and significantly gained more body weight.[73] The rats also demonstrated a strong preference for and greater binge-type food consumption of the high-fat diet. The study showed that *nmur2* signaling in the PVN plays a role in the quantity of high-fat foods eaten as well as preference for high-fat foods without changing the quantity of non-high-fat food eaten. The study has not been replicated in humans, but the NMU receptor is present in the PVN of humans and may play a role in some people choosing to eat an excessive high-fat diet, leading to obesity.

Genetic variations in *FTO* show one of the strongest genetic determinants of body weight as well and have been linked with impaired neural processing of food stimuli. Recent research has provided data implicating interactions between ghrelin and *FTO*.[74] The hormone ghrelin has been suggested to be the molecular mediator of *FTO* on feeding behavior. One study reported widespread differences between *FTO* risk allele carriers in homeostatic and reward-processing neural networks and responsiveness to circulating acyl-ghrelin within brain regions that regulate appetite, reward processing, and incentive motivation. Furthermore, this study demonstrated differences of fMRI signal activation in the *FTO* genotyped subjects to images of high versus low-calorie food at fasted versus satiated nutritional status 60 minutes postprandial. Another study observed similar fMRI signals in individuals with the *FTO* genotype rs8050136 on neural processing of food-related stimuli 30 minutes after glucose ingestion.[75] These studies indicate that individuals who carry the *FTO* risk allele are more likely to overeat and be obese because they have less postprandial activity in the prefrontal cortex, which plays a major role in the inhibitory control of eating.

The field of behavioral genetics relative to consumption patterns leading to obesity is relatively new (Sidebar 1-4). Implementation of techniques such as fMRI have been fruitful, but at this time, there are limited neuropharmacological interventions to help treat obesity. There may be medications as well as gene testing in the near future that will help with controlling what kind of foods and how much food individuals choose to eat. In the absence of direct interventions, it can also be helpful to explain to patients the biological reasons why they may be making poor dietary decisions, overeating, and having difficulty in creating better eating habits. The patients should be encouraged to avoid foods high in fat and carbohydrates and to eat slowly to allow for the neuroendocrine response of satiety to take place. Behavioral genetic knowledge of obesity should help the physician be more empathetic toward some individuals who struggle in making decisions to avoid becoming obese or to lose weight if they are already obese.

CONCLUSION

Research into the genetic underpinning of obesity through family studies and animal models has identified a multitude of genes associated with monogenetic forms of obesity and the integral role of neurological appetite regulation through the leptin-melanocortin pathway. With the advent of GWAS, many more novel common genetic variants were uncovered that contribute to the pathogenesis of polygenic obesity. Furthermore, the identification of rare CNVs of large effect size and advances in epigenetics are enhancing our understanding of the biological complexities of obesity. Yet, the transition from association to causality remains a challenge for polygenic and complex diseases. With advances in sequencing technology and data analysis, along with functional studies, we may better characterize the role of individual genes and their variants, increasing our understanding of the pathogenetic mechanisms.

Lifestyle modifications, in particular diet and exercise, are crucial in weight control, irrespective of an individual's genetic profile. Emotional stress and depression, in conjunction with external socioeconomic factors, may predispose an individual toward overeating, yet there are certainly genetic contributions that formulate the difference in the desire and eating drive between people. Even the failure of behavioral interventions may be due to genetic dysregulation of neuronal circuits. The genetically predisposed individual must exercise a greater conscious effort to lose the excess weight. In addition, the neuroendocrine and metabolic adaptions to an obese homeostasis become increasingly difficult to surmount. The inherent appetite-regulating factors, such as impaired satiety, that predispose one to obesity may be identified, and focused pharmacological and behavioral modification tools can be personalized to the neurobiological status of the individual.

Currently, molecular characterization of syndromic and monofactorial forms of obesity is possible and crucial for intervention in cases of severe early-onset obesity. One promising application of obesity genetics research is in risk prediction of bariatric surgery outcomes. Studies have found SNPs in *FTO* that appear to confer significant differences in postoperative weight reduction based on the genetic profiles. Other genes, such as *MC4R*, have been studied in their risk prediction for therapeutic obesity surgeries. A potential application of this research is detailed in a clinical scenario in this chapter (see Sidebar 1-5). Advances in sequencing technology and data synthesis are expanding our understanding of the genetic and biological basis of multifactorial disorders such as obesity and ultimately permitting personalization of future therapeutic approaches.

REFERENCES

1. Mendel G. Versuche über Pflanzen-Hybriden. *Verhandlung Nat Forsch Verein Brunn*. 1866;4:3–47. [English translation: Stern C, Sherwood ER, eds. *The Origin of Genetics*. San Francisco: Freeman; 1966.]

2. Lebel RR, Spranger JW. Chance favors the prepared mind: a brief moral biography of Gregor Johann Mendel (7/22/1822–1/6/1884). *Proc Greenwood Genet Center*. 2008;27:3–5.

3. Jorde LB, Carey JC, Bamshad MJ. *Medical Genetics*. 4th ed. St. Louis, MO: Mosby; 2009.

4. Turnpenny PD, Ellard S. *Emery's Elements of Medical Genetics*. 11th ed. Edinburgh: Churchill Livingstone; 2011.

5. Zhang Y, Proenca R, Maffei M, et al. Positional cloning of the mouse obese gene and its human homologue. *Nature*. 1994 Dec 1;372(6505):425–432.

6. Montague CT, Farooqi IS, Whitehead JP, et al. Congenital leptin deficiency is associated with severe early-onset obesity in humans. *Nature*. 1997 Jun 26; 387(6636):903–908.

7. Farooqi IS, Matarese G, Lord GM, et al. Beneficial effects of leptin on obesity, T cell hyporesponsiveness, and neuroendocrine/metabolic dysfunction of human congenital leptin deficiency. *J Clin Invest*. 2002;110(8):1093–1103. doi:10.1172/JCI15693.

8. Krude H, Gruters A. Implications of proopiomelanocortin (*POMC*) mutations in humans: the *POMC* deficiency syndrome. *Trends Endocrinol Metab*. 2002;11:15–22.

9. Pritchard LE, Turnbull AV, White A. Pro-opiomelanocortin processing in the hypothalamus: impact on melanocortin signalling and obesity. *J Endocrinol*. 2002;172:411–421.

10. Challis BG, Pritchard LE, Creemers JW, et al. A missense mutation disrupting a dibasic prohormone processing site in pro-opiomelanocortin (POMC)

increases susceptibility to early-onset obesity through a novel molecular mechanism. *Hum Mol Genet.* 2002 Aug 15;11(17):1997–2004.

11. Farooqi IS, Yeo GSH, Keogh JM, et al. Dominant and recessive inheritance of morbid obesity associated with melanocortin 4 receptor deficiency. *J Clin Invest.* 2000;106(2):271–279.

12. Farooqi IS, Keogh JM, Yeo GS, et al. Clinical spectrum of obesity and mutations in the melanocortin 4 receptor gene. *N Engl J Med.* 2003 Mar 20;348(12):1085–1095.

13. Lubrano-Berthelier C, Dubern B, Lacorte JM, et al. Melanocortin 4 receptor mutations in a large cohort of severely obese adults: prevalence, functional classification, genotype-phenotype relationship, and lack of association with binge eating. *J Clin Endocrinol Metab.* 2006 May;91(5):1811–1818. Epub 2006 Feb 28.

14. Stutzmann F, Tan K, Vatin V, et al. Prevalence of melanocortin-4 receptor deficiency in Europeans and their age-dependent penetrance in multigenerational pedigrees. *Diabetes.* 2008;57(9):2511–2518. doi:10.2337/db08-0153.

15. Jackson RS, Creemers JW, Ohagi S, et al. Obesity and impaired prohormone processing associated with mutations in the human prohormone convertase 1 gene. *Nat Genet.* 1997 Jul;16(3):303–306.

16. Farooqi IS, Volders K, Stanhope R, et al. Hyperphagia and early-onset obesity due to a novel homozygous missense mutation in prohormone convertase 1/3. *J Clin Endocrinol Metab.* 2007;92:3369–3373.

17. O'Rahilly S, Gray H, Humphreys PJ, et al. Brief report: impaired processing of prohormones associated with abnormalities of glucose homeostasis and adrenal function. *N Engl J Med.* 1995;333:1386–1390.

18. Creemers JWM, Choquet H, Stijnen P, et al. Heterozygous mutations causing partial prohormone convertase 1 deficiency contribute to human obesity. *Diabetes.* 2012;61(2):383–390. doi:10.2337/db11-0305.

19. Crews ST, Thomas JB, Goodman CS. The *Drosophila* single-minded gene encodes a nuclear protein with sequence similarity to the per gene product. *Cell.* 1995;52:143–151.

20. Michaud JL, Boucher F, Melnyk A, et al. Sim1 haploinsufficiency causes hyperphagia, obesity and reduction of the paraventricular nucleus of the hypothalamus. *Hum Mol Genet.* 2001 Jul 1;10(14):1465–1473.

21. Holder JL, Butte NF, Zinn AR. Profound obesity associated with a balanced translocation that disrupts the *SIM1* gene. *Hum Mol Genet.* 2000;9:101–108.

22. Holder JL Jr, Zhang L, Kublaoui BM, et al. Sim1 gene dosage modulates the homeostatic feeding response to increased dietary fat in mice. *Am J Physiol Endocrinol Metab.* 2004 Jul;287(1):E105–E113. Epub 2004 Feb 24.

23. Tolson KP, Gemelli T, Gautron L, et al. Postnatal Sim1 deficiency causes hyperphagic obesity and reduced Mc4r and oxytocin expression. *J Neurosci.* 2010;30:3803–3812.

24. Xu B, Goulding EH, Zang K, et al. Brain-derived neurotrophic factor regulates energy balance downstream of melanocortin-4 receptor. *Nat Neurosci.* 2003;6(7):736–742. doi:10.1038/nn1073.

25. Yeo GS1, Connie Hung CC, Rochford J, et al. A de novo mutation affecting human TrkB associated with severe obesity and developmental delay. *Nat Neurosci.* 2004;7:1187–1189.

26. Díez J, Iglesias P. The role of the novel adipocyte-derived hormone adiponectin in human disease. *Eur J Endocrinol.* 2003;148(3):293–300. doi:10.1530/eje.0.1480293.

27. Ukkola O, Santaniemi M. Adiponectin: a link between excess adiposity and associated comorbidities. *J Mol Med.* 2002;80:696–702.

28. Deeb SS, Fajas L, Nemoto M, et al. A Pro12Ala substitution in PPARgamma2 associated with decreased receptor activity, lower body mass index and improved insulin sensitivity. *Nat Genet.* 1998 Nov;20(3):284–287.

29. Altshuler D, Hirschhorn JN, Klannemark M, et al. The common PPARgamma Pro12Ala polymorphism is associated with decreased risk of type 2 diabetes. *Nat Genet.* 2000;26:76–80.

30. Ichimura A, Hirasawa A, Poulain-Godefroy O, et al. Dysfunction of lipid sensor GPR120 leads to obesity in both mouse and human. *Nature.* 2012;483:350–354.

31. Hara T, Hirasawa A, Ichimura A, et al. Free fatty acid receptors FFAR1 and GPR120 as novel therapeutic targets for metabolic disorders. *J Pharm Sci.* 2011;100:3594–3601.

32. Girirajan S, Rosenfeld JA, Coe BP, et al. Phenotypic heterogeneity of genomic disorders and rare copy-number variants. *N Engl J Med.* 2012;367(14):1321–1331. doi:10.1056/NEJMoa1200395.

33. Riggs ER, Wain KE, Riethmaier D, et al. Chromosomal microarray impacts clinical management. *Clin Genet.* 2014;85(2):147–153.

34. Henderson LB, Applegate CD, Wohler E, et al. The impact of chromosomal microarray analysis on medical management: a retrospective analysis. *Genet Med.* 2014;16(9):657–664.

35. Worthey EA, Mayer AN, Syverson GD, et al. Making a definitive diagnosis: successful clinical application of whole exome sequencing in a child with intractable inflammatory bowel disease. *Genet Med.* 2011;13:255–262.

36. Phan-Hug F, Beckmann JS, Jacquemont S. Genetic testing in patients with obesity. *Best Pract Res Clin Endocrinol Metab.* 2011;26(2):133–143.

37. Sha B, Yang T, Zhao L, et al. Genome-wide association study suggested copy number variation may be associated with body mass index in the Chinese population.

J Hum Genet. 2009;54(4):199–202. doi:10.1038/jhg.2009.10.

38. Jarick I, Vogel CI, Scherag S, et al. Novel common copy number variation for early onset extreme obesity on chromosome 11q11 identified by a genome-wide analysis. *Hum Mol Genet.* 2011;20:840–852.

39. Speliotes EK, Willer CJ, Berndt SI, et al. Association analyses of 249,796 individuals reveal 18 new loci associated with body mass index. *Nat Genet.* 2010;42:937–948.

40. Kim YJ, Sano T, Nabetani T, et al. GPRC5B activates obesity-associated inflammatory signaling in adipocytes. *Sci Signal.* 2012 Nov 20;5(251):ra85. doi:10.1126/scisignal.2003149.

41. Walters RG, Jacquemont S, Valsesia A, et al. A novel highly-penetrant form of obesity due to microdeletions on chromosome 16p11.2. *Nature.* 2010;463(7281):671–675. doi:10.1038/nature08727.

42. Jacquemont S, Reymond A, Zufferey F, et al. Mirror extreme BMI phenotypes associated with gene dosage at the chromosome 16p11.2 locus. *Nature.* 2011;478(7367):97–102. doi:10.1038/nature10406.

43. Speliotes EK, Willer CJ, Berndt SI, et al. Association analyses of 249,796 individuals reveal 18 new loci associated with body mass index. *Nat Genet.* 2010;42(11):937–948. doi:10.1038/ng.686.

44. Ren D, Zhou Y, Morris D, Li M, Li Z, Rui L. Neuronal SH2B1 is essential for controlling energy and glucose homeostasis. *J Clin Invest.* 2007;117(2):397–406. doi:10.1172/JCI29417.

45. Doche ME, Bochukova EG, Su H-W, et al. Human *SH2B1* mutations are associated with maladaptive behaviors and obesity. *J Clin Invest.* 2012;122(12):4732–4736. doi:10.1172/JCI62696.

46. Frayling TM, Timpson NJ, Weedon MN, et al. A common variant in the *FTO* gene is associated with body mass index and predisposes to childhood and adult obesity. *Science (New York, NY).* 2007;316(5826):889–894. doi:10.1126/science.1141634.

47. The Wellcome Trust Case Control Consortium. Genome-wide association study of 14,000 cases of seven common diseases and 3000 shared controls. *Nature.* 2007;447(7145):661–678. doi:10.1038/nature05911.

48. Zeggini E, Weedon MN, Lindgren CM, et al. Multiple type 2 diabetes susceptibility genes following genome-wide association scan in UK samples. *Science (New York, NY).* 2007;316(5829):1336–1341. doi:10.1126/science.1142364.

49. Dina C, Meyre D, Gallina S, et al. Variation in FTO contributes to childhood obesity and severe adult obesity. *Nat Genet.* 2007;39(6):724–726. doi:10.1038/ng2048.

50. Paternoster L, Evans DM, Aagaard Nohr E, et al. Genome-wide population-based association study of extremely overweight young adults—the GOYA study. Awadalla P, ed. *PLoS ONE.* 2011;6(9):e24303. doi:10.1371/journal.pone.0024303.

51. Scuteri A, Sanna S, Chen W-M, et al. Genome-wide association scan shows genetic variants in the *FTO* gene are associated with obesity-related traits. Barsh G, ed. *PLoS Genet.* 2007;3(7):e115. doi:10.1371/journal.pgen.0030115.

52. Loos RJF, Yeo GSH. The bigger picture of *FTO*—the first GWAS-identified obesity gene. *Nat Rev Endocrinol.* 2014;10(1):51–61. doi:10.1038/nrendo.2013.227.

53. Hinney A, Nguyen TT, Scherag A, et al. Genome wide association (GWA) study for early onset extreme obesity supports the role of fat mass and obesity associated gene *(FTO)* variants. Kronenberg F, ed. *PLoS ONE.* 2007;2(12):e1361. doi:10.1371/journal.pone.0001361.

54. Grant SFA, Li M, Bradfield JP, et al. Association analysis of the *FTO* gene with obesity in children of Caucasian and African ancestry reveals a common tagging SNP. Maedler K, ed. *PLoS ONE.* 2008;3(3):e1746. doi:10.1371/journal.pone.0001746.

55. Dorajoo R, Blakemore AIF, Sim X, et al. Replication of 13 obesity loci among Singaporean Chinese, Malay and Asian-Indian populations. *Int J Obesity.* 2011;36(1):159–163. doi:10.1038/ijo.2011.86.

56. Cai X, Liu C, Mou S. Association between fat mass-and-obesity-associated (FTO) gene polymorphism and polycystic ovary syndrome: a meta-analysis. Franks S, ed. *PLoS ONE.* 2014;9(1):e86972. doi:10.1371/journal.pone.0086972.

57. Su AI, Wiltshire T, Batalov S, et al. A gene atlas of the mouse and human protein-encoding transcriptomes. *Proc Natl Acad Sci U S A.* 2004;101(16):6062–6067. doi:10.1073/pnas.0400782101.

58. Fredriksson R, Hägglund M, Olszewski PK, et al. The obesity gene, *FTO*, is of ancient origin, upregulated during food deprivation and expressed in neurons of feeding-related nuclei of the brain. *Endocrinology.* 2008;149(5):2062–2071.

59. Olszewski PK, Fredriksson R, Olszewska AM, et al. Hypothalamic FTO is associated with the regulation of energy intake not feeding reward. *BMC Neurosci.* 2009;10:129. doi:10.1186/1471-2202-10-129.

60. Gerken T, Girard CA, Tung Y-CL, et al. The obesity-associated *FTO* gene encodes a 2-oxoglutarate–dependent nucleic acid demethylase. *Science (New York, NY).* 2007;318(5855):1469–1472. doi:10.1126/science.1151710.

61. Gulati P, Yeo GSH. The biology of FTO: from nucleic acid demethylase to amino acid sensor. *Diabetologia.* 2013;56(10):2113–2121. doi:10.1007/s00125-013-2999-5.

62. Ost A, Lempradl A, Casas E, et al. Paternal diet defines off-spring chromatin state and intergenerational obesity. *Cell.* 2014;159:1352–1364.

63. Janesick A, Blumberg B. Endocrine disrupting chemicals and the developmental programming of adipogenesis and obesity. *Birth Defects Res C Embryo Today.* 2011;93(1):34–50. doi:10.1002/bdrc.20197.

64. Newbold RR. Impact of environmental endocrine disrupting chemicals on the development of obesity. *Hormones (Athens).* 2010;9:206–217.

65. Rezg R, El-Fazaa S, Gharbi N, Mornagui B. Bisphenol A and human chronic diseases: current evidences, possible mechanisms, and future perspectives. *Environ Int.* 2014;64:83–90. doi:10.1016/j.envint.2013.12.007.

66. Cordero P, Campion J, Milagro FI, et al. Leptin and TNF-alpha promoter methylation levels measured by MSP could predict the response to a low-calorie diet. *J Physiol Biochem.* 2011;67(3):463–470. doi:10.1007/s13105-011-0084-4.

67. Martínez JA, Milagro FI, Claycombe KJ, Schalinske KL. Epigenetics in adipose tissue, obesity, weight loss, and diabetes. *Adv Nutr.* 2014;5(1):71–81. doi:10.3945/an.113.004705.

68. Llewellyn CH, Trzaskowski M, van Jaarsveld CHM, Plomin R, Wardle J. Satiety mechanisms in genetic risk of obesity. *JAMA Pediatr.* 2014;168(4):338–344. doi:10.1001/jamapediatrics.2013.4944.

69. Wang Y, Wang A, Donovan SM, Teran-Garcia M. Individual genetic variations related to satiety and appetite control increase risk of obesity in preschool-age children in the STRONG Kids Program. *Hum Hered.* 2013;75(2–4):152–159. doi:10.1159/000353880.

70. Cruz JD, Coke T, Karagiorgis T, et al. c-Fos induction in mesotelencephalic dopamine pathway projection targets and dorsal striatum following oral intake of sugars and fats in rats. *Brain Res Bull.* 2015;111:9–19. doi:10.1016/j.brainresbull.2014.11.002.

71. Cosgrove KP, Veldhuizen MG, Sandiego CM, Morris ED, Small DM. Opposing relationships of BMI with BOLD and dopamine D2/3 receptor binding potential in the dorsal striatum. *Synapse.* 2015;69(4):195–202.

72. Blum K, Thanos PK, Gold MS. Dopamine and glucose, obesity, and reward deficiency syndrome. *Front Psychol.* 2014;5:919. doi:10.3389/fpsyg.2014.00919.

73. Benzon CR, Johnson SB, McCue DL, Li D, Green TA, Hommel JD. Neuromedin U receptor 2 knockdown in the paraventricular nucleus modifies behavioral responses to obesogenic high-fat food and leads to increased body weight. *Neuroscience.* 2014;258:270–279. doi:10.1016/j.neuroscience.2013.11.023.

74. Karra E, O'Daly OG, Choudhury AI, et al. A link between FTO, ghrelin, and impaired brain food-cue responsivity. *J Clin Invest.* 2013;123(8):3539–3551. doi:10.1172/JCI44403.

75. Heni M, Kullmann S, Veit R, et al. Variation in the obesity risk gene *FTO* determines the postprandial cerebral processing of food stimuli in the prefrontal cortex. *Mol Metab.* 2014;3(2):109–113. doi:10.1016/j.molmet.2013.11.009.

76. Wabitsch M, Funcke JB, Lennerz B, et al. Biologically inactive leptin and early-onset extreme obesity. *N Engl J Med.* 2015;372(1):48–54. doi:10.1056/NEJMoa1406653. PubMed PMID: 25551525.

77. Farooqi IS. The severely obese patient—a genetic work-up. *Nat Clin Pract Endocrinol Metab.* 2006;2(3):172–177. doi:10.1038/ncpendmet0137.

78. Montague CT, Farooqi IS, Whitehead JP, et al. Congenital leptin deficiency is associated with severe early-onset obesity in humans. *Nature.* 1997;387:903–908.

79. Strobel A, Issad T, Camoin L, Ozata M, Strosberg AD. A leptin missense mutation associated with hypogonadism and morbid obesity. *Nat Genet.* 1998;18(3):213–215. doi:10.1038/ng0398-213.

80. Fatima W, Shahid A, Imran M, et al. Leptin deficiency and leptin gene mutations in obese children from Pakistan. *Int J Pediatr Obes.* 2011;6:419–27.

81. Fischer-Posovszky P, Schnurbein JV, Moepps B, et al. A new missense mutation in the leptin gene causes mild obesity and hypogonadism without affecting T cell responsiveness. *J Clin Endocrinol Metab.* 2010;95(6):2836–2840. doi:10.1210/jc.2009-2466.

82. Butler AA, O'Rourke RW. Bariatric surgery in the era of personalized medicine. *Gastroenterology.* 2013;144(3). doi:10.1053/ j.gastro.2013.01.027.

83. Sarzynski MA, Jacobson P, Rankinen T, et al. Associations of markers in 11 obesity candidate genes with maximal weight loss and weight regain in the SOS bariatric surgery cases. *Int J Obes.* 2010;35(5):676–683. doi:10.1038/ijo.2010.166.

84. Hatoum IJ, Stylopoulos N, Vanhoose AM, et al. Melanocortin-4 receptor signaling is required for weight loss after gastric bypass surgery. *J Clin Endocrinol Metab.* 2012;97(6):E1023–E1031. doi:10.1210/jc.2011-3432.

85. Zechner JF, Mirshahi UL, Satapati S, et al. Weight-independent effects of Roux-en-Y gastric bypass on glucose homeostasis via melanocortin-4 receptors in mice and humans. *Gastroenterology.* 2013;144(3):10. doi:1053/j.gastro.2012.11.022.

86. Wang G-J, Tomasi D, Volkow ND, et al. Effect of combined naltrexone and bupropion therapy on the brain's reactivity to food cues. *Int J Obes.* 2014;38(5):682–688. doi:10.1038/ijo.2013.145.

Economic Costs of Obesity

Thomas H. Dennison, PhD

INTRODUCTION

This chapter provides an overview of the economic costs of obesity in the United States with a particular focus on the costs of obesity related to women's health care. The chapter begins by briefly introducing the relationship of obesity with health problems that often result in increased costs. Costs, both direct and indirect, are defined, and overall costs associated with obesity are reviewed. The chapter then largely addresses the costs of obesity related to women's health care, particularly obstetrical and gyne-cological services.

ECONOMIC COSTS OF OBESITY

Costs of obesity and its comorbidities are both direct and indirect. Direct costs include the medical care interventions to treat morbidity associated with obesity. Indirect costs include costs that are secondary to obesity, increases in premature mortality, reduction in productivity, and increases in insurance costs.

Direct Costs

Direct costs include direct patient care services, such as outpatient and inpatient health services, laboratory and radiological tests, and drug therapy. Obese individuals incur, on average, annual medical care expenditures of $732 higher than individuals of normal weight.[1] A systematic review of the direct costs of obesity found that obese individuals have medical costs approximately 30% higher than their normal-weight

""

peers.[2] Annual spending due to obesity has been estimated at 9.1% of annual medical spending in the United States.[3] A more recent study, which employed Medical Expenditure Panel Survey (MEPS) data, estimated that medical care associated with obesity is 20.6% of U.S. health care expenditures.[4] It is estimated that Medicare and Medicaid are responsible for approximately 42% of this spending.[3]

Indirect Costs

Indirect costs, which are more difficult to measure than direct costs, can be defined as resources forgone as a result of a health condition and fall into various categories. Indirect costs include higher disability insurance premiums, decreased labor market productivity, and premature mortality. Published research findings offer a wide range of estimates for the total indirect costs of obesity; direct comparison of results across studies is difficult due to a set of methodological issues, including the date of measurement, representativeness of the sample, and scope of measurement.[5]

Indirect costs include the value of lost work; days missed from work are a cost to both employees (in lost wages) and employers (in work not completed). Obese employees miss more days from work due to short-term absences, long-term disability, and premature death than nonobese employees.[6] The cost of absenteeism for obese and morbidly obese was estimated at $4.2 billion each year.[7] These individuals may also work at less than full capacity (also known as presenteeism). The costs of absenteeism and presenteeism resulting from obesity among full-time employees based on 2006 MEPS data were estimated at $73.1 billion annually, with roughly two-thirds of those costs associated with approximately one-third of employees with a body mass index (BMI) over 35. Wang et al.[8] estimated that absenteeism and presenteeism associated with a high BMI result in a loss of between 1.7 and 3 million productive person-years in working US adults. The probability of total employer costs increasing partly due to disability, workers' compensation claims, and days of work lost increases for individuals with a BMI of 25 and higher.[9]

Indirect costs also include costs of insurance. Employers pay higher life insurance premiums and pay out more for workers' compensation for employees who are obese than for employees who are not.[10]

Obesity is associated with premature mortality. Obesity and overweight in adulthood are associated with large decreases in life expectancy and increases in early mortality, similar to the decreases related to smoking.[11] Not only is overall life expectancy decreased, but also quality of life is diminished. A number of studies found that obesity impairs health-related quality of life (HRQL), and that higher degrees of obesity are associated with greater impairment.[12] Groessel et al.[13] found that for every 20 people living 1 year with obesity the result is the loss of 1 quality-adjusted life-year (QALY), translating into nearly 3 million QALYs lost each year in the United States.

COST OF OBESITY ASSOCIATED WITH WOMEN'S HEALTH CARE

The health of women is negatively affected by obesity. Obese women (and men) are dramatically at risk for diabetes, which is associated with higher risk of cardiovascular diseases. Low-back pain, knee osteoarthritis, and depression may also be linked to obesity in women.[14] Overweight and obese individuals are also at higher risk for developing hypertension.[15]

Women, compared to men, suffer a disproportionate burden of disease, and cost, associated with obesity,[4] particularly from lower HRQL and late-life mortality.[16] For the purposes of this chapter, however, the discussion focuses on the direct, rather than indirect, costs of provision of care associated with women's health.

Obesity in Pregnancy

In the United States, more than one-half of pregnant women are overweight or obese, putting them at higher risk of a number of complications of pregnancy, including gestational diabetes mellitus, hypertension, preeclampsia, cesarean delivery, and postpartum weight retention. In addition, obese women are more prone to intrapartum, operative, and postoperative complications.[17] These conditions result in increased use of health care services, including longer stay, more use of ancillary testing, more medications, and increased use of ambulatory services, particularly physician visits.[18] Pathi, Esen, and Hildreth[19] found that morbidly obese women had higher rates of use of ultrasound scans, more antenatal visits, and a longer stay in the hospital and that the baby of an obese mother is 10 times more likely to be admitted to the special care baby unit. Galtier-Dereure, Boegner, and Bringer[20] found that women with a BMI over 29, compared to normal-weight controls, had a longer hospital stay of 4.3 days, on average, often due to more frequent cesarean deliveries and postoperative endometritis.

While the increased use of health care services in overweight and obese pregnant women has been documented, relatively few data exist that clearly show the increased costs of obesity in pregnancy in the United States. A retrospective study done in 1995 in France found that the cost of prenatal care in overweight women was higher than their normal-weight peers by a factor of approximately 5–16 times, depending on the level of obesity.[21] A study in Scotland that looked at the relationship of increased maternal BMI and increased risk of minor complications (including symphysis pubis dysfunction, chest infection, heartburn, and carpal tunnel syndrome) during pregnancy found an increase in the cost of health care interventions, including outpatient visits and medication to treat these conditions in women with higher BMIs.[22]

A later study by Dennison et al.[23] found again that there is an increased cost associated between maternal BMI and increased health service costs. In a sample in the United States of all hospitalizations for pregnant women for which obesity was coded as a secondary diagnosis, charges were $1805 higher than for other stays.[24] These findings were echoed by Watson et al.,[25] who found higher costs of hospitalization for women who were overweight and obese (as well as for women who were underweight) in Australia. A study of women in Wales found, after adjusting for maternal age, parity, comorbidity, and ethnicity, mean total costs were 23% higher among overweight women and 37% higher among obese women.[26]

Consequences for Offspring of Obese Mothers

The problem does not stop with the obese pregnant woman; children of obese women are at increased risk of prematurity, stillbirth, injury during childbirth, and childhood obesity. Children who are breastfed are less likely to develop obesity in later life, but maternal obesity is also associated with a decreased intention to breastfeed, decreased initiation of breastfeeding, and decreased duration of breastfeeding.[14] Childhood obesity has been estimated to add $19,000 to the cost of care over the lifetime,[27] resulting in costs of over $14 billion in the United States.[28]

A Spanish study found that offspring born from obese women are more prone to the development of health issues over the life span, including obesity, type 2 diabetes, cardiovascular disease, and cancer.[29] A study in Australia found that children of mothers classified as obese had an increased risk of hospitalization for all causes of a factor of 1.5 over the first 5 years of life.[30]

Other Women's Health Concerns and Obesity

Obesity is also associated with an increased risk of certain cancers in women, specifically postmenopausal breast, endometrial, cervical, and perhaps ovarian cancer.[14] There is an association between obesity and fertility. Obesity, particularly abdominal obesity, is associated with metabolic syndrome and is strongly related to polycystic ovary syndrome.[31] A study done in the Netherlands found being overweight resulted in an increase in cost per pregnancy and a decreased number of pregnancies for women undergoing fertility treatment,[32] although these findings were not replicated in a study done in the United Kingdom.[33]

SUMMARY

It is clear that overweight and obesity are associated with higher levels of morbidity in women (and in men). The overall cost of obesity has been researched and documented. The implications of overweight and obesity in women have also been widely studied, particularly in pregnancy. Overweight and obesity have also been implicated in poorer health status in other areas of women's health, and the negative impact on offspring of obese women has been shown. It is clear that there are economic costs associated with these negative outcomes.

However, relatively little work has been published that quantifies the actual costs of overweight and obesity on women's health concerns in the United States. Studies in other similar countries have shown higher costs of direct care for both ambulatory and inpatient care. And, there is some limited evidence from work done in the United States. It is nevertheless clear that the issues of overweight and obesity contribute to poorer health status and higher costs in caring for women.

FUTURE RESEARCH DIRECTIONS

While it is evident that overweight and obesity contribute to diminished health status and higher spending levels, the costs particular to gynecological and obstetrical services are not well documented in the United States. Clearer and more direct evidence describing the health status and economic impact of overweight and obese women, particularly in pregnancy, coupled with findings in the literature about interventions that have been shown to help with weight management, would support forwarding policies to incorporate (and fund) efforts to address the problem.

REFERENCES

1. Bhattacharya J, Bundorf MK. The incidence of the healthcare costs of obesity. *J Health Econ.* 2009;28(3):649–658.
2. Withrow D, Alter DA. The economic burden of obesity worldwide: a systematic review of the direct costs of obesity. *Obes Rev.* 2010;(12):131–141.
3. Finkelstein EA, DiBonaventura M, Burgess S, Hale B. The cost of obesity in the workplace. *J Occup Environ Med.* 2010;52(10):971–976.
4. Cawley J, Meyerhoefer C. The medical care costs of obesity: an instrumental variables approach. *J Health Econ.* 2012;(31):219–230.

5. Hammond R, Levine R. The economic impact of obesity in the United States. *Diabetes Metab Syndr Obes.* 2010;(3):285–295.

6. Colditz GA. Economic costs of obesity. *Am J Clin Nutr.* 1992;(55):503S–507S.

7. Cawley J, Rizzo JA, Haas K. Occupation-specific absenteeism costs associated with obesity and morbid obesity. *J Occup Environ Med.* 2007;49(12):1317–1324.

8. Wang YC, McPherson K, Marsh T, Gortmaker SL, Brown M. Health and economic burden of the projected obesity trends in the USA and the UK. *Lancet.* 2011;378(9793):815–825.

9. Van Nuys K, Globe D, Ng-Mak D, Cheung H, Sullivan J, Goldman D. The association between employee obesity and employer costs: evidence from a panel of US employers. *Am J Health Promot.* 2014;28(5):277–285.

10. Trogdon JG, Finkelstein EA, Hylands T, Dellea PS, Kamal-Bahl SJ. Indirect costs of obesity: a review of the current literature. *Obes Rev.* 2008;9:489–500.

11. Peeters A, Barendregt J, Willekens F, Mackenbach J, Al Mamun A, Boneux L. Obesity in adulthood and its consequences for life expectancy: a life-table analysis. *Ann Intern Med.* 2003;138:24–32.

12. Fontaine K, Barofsky I. Obesity and health-related quality of life. *Obes Rev.* 2001;2:173–182.

13. Groessel EJ, Kaplan RM, Barrett-Connor E, Ganiats TG. Body mass index and quality of well-being in a community of older adults. *Am J Prev Med.* 2004;26(2):126–129.

14. Kulie T, Slattengren DO, Redmer J, Counts H, Eglash A, Schrager S. Obesity and women's health: an evidence based review. *J Am Board Fam Med.* 2011,24.75–05.

15. Plaisted CS, Istfan NW. Metabolic abnormalities of obesity. In: Blackburn GL, Kanders BS, eds. *Obesity Pathophysiology, Psychology and Treatment.* Boston: Chapman & Hall; 1994:80.

16. Muenning P, Lubetkin E, Haomiao J, Franks P. Gender and the burden of disease attributable to Obesity. *Am J Public Health.* 2006;96(9):1662–1668.

17. American College of Obstetricians and Gynecologists. *Obesity in Pregnancy.* Washington, DC: American College of Obstetricians and Gynecologists; January 2013. Committee Opinion Number 549.

18. Chu S, Bachman D, Callaghan W, et al. Association between obesity during pregnancy and increased use of health care. *N Engl J Med.* 2008;358(14):1444–1453.

19. Pathi A, Esen U, Hildreth A. A comparison of complications of pregnancy and delivery in morbidly obese and non-obese women. *J Obstet Gynaecol.* 2006;26(6):527–530.

20. Galtier-Dereure F, Boegner C, Bringer J. Obesity and pregnancy: complications and cost. *Am J Clin Nutr.* 2000;(71):1242S–1248S.

21. Galtier-Dereure F, Montepeyroux F, Boulot P, Bringer J, Janiol C. Weight excess before pregnancy: complications and cost. *Int J Obes Rel Metab Disord.* 1995;19:443–448.

22. Denison F, Norrie G, Graham B, Lynch J, Harper N, Reynolds R. Increased maternal BMI is associated with an increased risk of minor complications during pregnancy with consequent cost implications. *BJOG.* 2009;116(11):1467–1472.

23. Dennison FC, Norwood P, Bhattacharya S, et al. Association between maternal body mass index during pregnancy, short term morbidity and increased health service costs: a population based study. *BJOG.* 2014;121:72–82.

24. Trasande L, Lee M, Liu Y, Weitzman M, Savitz D. Incremental charges, costs, and length of stay associated with obesity as a secondary diagnosis among pregnant women. *Med Care.* 2009;47(10):1046–1052.

25. Watson M, Howell S, Johnston T, Callaway L, Khor SL, Cornes S. Pre-pregnancy BMI: costs associated with maternal underweight and obesity in Queensland. *Aust N Z J Obstet Gynecol.* 2013;53(3):243–249.

26. Morgan KL, Rahman MA, Macey S, et al. Obesity in pregnancy: a retrospective prevalence-based study on health service utilisation and costs on the NHS. *BMJ Open.* 2014;4(2):e003983.

27. Finkelstein EA, Graham WC, Malhotra R. Lifetime direct medical costs of childhood obesity. *Pediatrics.* 2014;133(5):854–862.

28. Trasande L, Liu Y, Fryer G, et al. Effects of childhood obesity on hospital care and costs, 1999–2005. *Health Aff* (Millwood). 2009;28(1):w751–w760, 2009.

29. Galliano D, Bellver J. Female obesity: short and long term consequences on the offspring. *Gynecol Endocrinol.* 2013;29(7):626–631.

30. Cameron CM, Shibl R, McClure RJ, Ng SK, Hills AP. Maternal pregravid body mass index and child hospital admissions in the first 5 years of life: results from an Australian birth cohort. *Int J Obes.* 2014;38(10):1268–1274.

31. Hu FB. Overweight and obesity in women: health risks and consequences. *J Womens Health.* 2003;12(2):163–172.

32. Koning AM, Kuchenbecker WK, Groen H, et al. Economic consequences of overweight and obesity in infertility: a framework for evaluating the costs and outcomes of fertility care. *Hum Reprod Update.* 2010;16(3):246–254.

33. Maheshwari A, Scotland G, Bell J, McTavish A, Hamilton M, Bhattacharya S. The direct health services costs of providing assisted reproduction services in overweight or obese women: a retrospective cross-sectional analysis. *Hum Reprod.* 2009;24(3):633–639.

Pregnancy and Obesity in Social Context

Sandra D. Lane, PhD, MPH

CHAPTER 3

INTRODUCTION
SOCIAL DETERMINANTS OF OBESITY AMONG
   PREGNANT WOMEN

STIGMA AND OBESITY IN PREGNANCY
WHAT ABOUT PERSONAL RESPONSIBILITY?

INTRODUCTION

The American College of Obstetricians and Gynecologists (ACOG) noted that the dramatic increase in obesity in the United States in the later part of the 20th century is reflected among childbearing women.[1] The National Health and Nutrition Examination Survey of obesity among adults, conducted in 2011 to 2012, found that 36.1% of adult women were obese; among African American women, the figure reached 56.6%, and among Hispanic women, it was 44.4%.[2] Those alarming statistics not only have important clinical significance but also reflect social, political, and ecological trends that provide the context to and contribute as risk factors to poor pregnancy outcomes.

In this chapter, I use two social science conceptual paradigms to understand obesity in pregnancy: social determinants and stigma. The chapter reviews published studies, national-level data, as well as studies and data from Syracuse, New York, conducted by my colleagues and me.

SOCIAL DETERMINANTS OF OBESITY AMONG PREGNANT WOMEN

The most useful definition of social determinants of health is that of the World Health Organization: "the causes of the causes."[3] Social determinants, in this model, are political, societal, and ecological risk factors that increase the likelihood of disease. They can be distinguished from clinical causes of ill health, in that clinical causes address immediate biological etiologies, whereas social determinants address a broader context of risk that takes place at an earlier phase in the condition. In the case of obesity, for example, the Centers for Disease Control and Prevention succinctly stated the clinical etiologies as "eating too many calories and not getting enough physical activity."[4] The social determinants approach, looking at the broader context in which obesity occurs, takes into account the factors that lead to poor diet or inadequate exercise or even altered metabolism. Understanding those social factors helps to explain why disadvantaged populations experience greater obesity and with it obesity-related health conditions.

A growing literature considers the influence of food deserts on health and obesity. Food deserts are geographical areas with few or no retail sources of fresh produce, low-fat dairy, or other healthful food.[5] In many US cities, urban renewal led to the displacement of low-income residents, movement of wealthier people to the suburbs, and closing of neighborhood food markets. What food outlets remain in many communities are corner stores mostly selling lottery tickets, cigarettes, and malt liquor, as well as fast food franchises.[6]

In Syracuse, New York, our research team found food deserts to be significantly associated with intrauterine growth restriction (IUGR).[7] Women residing during pregnancy in census tracts without access to full-service grocery markets had nearly four times the rate of IUGR, compared with those living in areas with greater access to healthy food and controlling for both race and Medicaid insurance as a proxy for poverty. In a subsequent analysis, which included all Syracuse births for a 2.25-year period among woman delivering at the largest birth hospital, the zip codes in which women with the highest proportion of obesity (>27% vs. <21%) lived were also the locations of food deserts.

The absence of healthy food does not mean an intake of fewer calories. Instead, residents of impoverished inner cities with food deserts often make up for the lack of fresh produce with prepared food, which is loaded with sodium, refined carbohydrates, unhealthy fat, and preservatives.[8] In a teaching exercise with medical students at Upstate Medical University, we paired the students with adult patients with chronic disease and asked the students to shop for food with their patients. One of the student teams reported that their patient, who was obese and had type 2 diabetes, with poor circulation and renal complications, shopped for food at the local dollar store. The dollar store sold boxed and canned prepared food, but no fresh produce. The paradox of an overabundance of total calories, combined with malnutrition of micronutrients, may explain the finding that obese women have higher rates of neural tube defects because a major risk factor for neural tube defects is inadequate folic acid intake in the months prior to conception.[9]

Neighborhood violence is a second social determinant of obesity in pregnant women. Violent neighborhoods make it unsafe to walk for exercise and make parents reluctant to have their children play outside.[6] A study conducted in Dallas, Texas, reported that women who perceived their neighborhood environment unfavorably, a measure that included sidewalks, housing quality, and violence, had higher waist circumferences and BMIs.[10] Similarly, a study on prepregnancy BMIs among Latinas in Phoenix, Arizona, concluded that the neighborhood physical and social characteristics, including safety and motor vehicle traffic, provided conditions that increased the likelihood of obesity.[11]

A third social determinant of obesity among pregnant women relates to the ingestion of specific substances. While it is true that no one factor has caused the dramatic rise in obesity, numerous authors argued that sweetened soda ingestion, and the intake of other sugar-sweetened beverages, accounts for a disproportionate amount of the recent population-wide BMI increase.[12–16] Endocrinologist and pediatrician

Robert Lustig pointed to the contemporary habit of consuming sweetened drinks as a key factor in promoting obesity.[17] Daily consumption of highly sweetened liquid is unusual in human diets historically and cross culturally. Many cultures prepare special highly sweetened foods, usually for celebratory feasts, but such treats usually also contain protein, fat, and fiber, nutrients that slow the metabolic uptake of the sugar, honey, or fructose in the food. They are also consumed in discrete servings, in contrast to sweetened drinks, which may be sipped throughout the day. In contrast, Lustig claimed that our "obesogenic" environment of sugar-laden fast food and highly sweetened drinks leads to insulin and leptin resistance, blunting satiety and decreasing physical activity.[18]

The Centers for Disease Control and Prevention assessed the price increase of a variety of foods between 1982 and 2002. Costs of fruits and vegetables rose by 258% during that period, whereas the cost of sweetened soft drinks only increased by 26%.[19] The reason that soft drinks remained cheaper than healthy alternatives is that the United States subsidizes corn growers, between 1985 and 2013 totaling $84.4 billion.[20] Corn subsidies allow high-fructose corn syrup to be marketed more cheaply than would be the case without subsidies, resulting in ever-larger servings.[21] In 1995, for example, a serving of soda came to 7 ounces, whereas our contemporary "big gulps" reach 40 ounces or more.[19] Consumption of sweetened soda tripled in the past two decades. A recent study found that over 27% of New York City adult residents consumed 12 ounces of sweetened soda daily, the equivalent of 10 teaspoons of sugar.[15]

Faculty at Upstate Medical University conducted a pilot study of the ingestion of sweetened soda and other beverages among pregnant women.[22] In our review of MEDLINE studies, we could not identify any other such studies. The study's initial findings were that many women drank fewer sweetened beverages than prior to pregnancy, often because such drinks worsened their reflux, and some women consumed large quantities, even liters of soda. The study's recommendation was that antenatal care providers, and nutritionists providing education to pregnant women, ask about their clients' consumption of sweetened beverages.

A fourth social determinant of obesity, the psychosocial stress associated with exposure to racism, has been identified as a potential risk factor for elevated visceral fat deposition.[23-26] The hypothesized biological pathway for stress to lead to abdominal obesity is via elevated cortisol, which in turn increases fat deposition and appetite. Research among Afro Caribbean women found their perceived stress due to internalized racism to be significantly associated with waist circumference and with elevated salivary cortisol.[27] Two additional studies found self-reported discrimination to be a risk factor for adiposity.[28] The deleterious effects of such exposure to discrimination have been identified as a risk factor to explain the disproportionate amount of cardiac disease among African Americans.[29] Visceral abdominal fat (VAF) is itself a risk factor for poor glucose control during pregnancy.[30] A study that measured the depth of VAF among pregnant women at 11 and 14 weeks' gestation, which they subsequently compared with the women's 2-hour glucose tolerance tests at 16 and 22 weeks, found VAF to account for 42% of the variance in insulin resistance.

Obesity itself may be a social determinant of elevated teen pregnancy, via the mechanism of early puberty.[6] Increased body weight among prepubescent girls appears to be a driving factor in the alarming drop in the age of menarche during the 20th century.[31] Prior to the modern era, growing girls in many cultures endured periodic food shortage due to drought, crop failures, or even the yearly cycle in which stored food was consumed sparingly during the winter prior to modern food storage and refrigeration. Female food intake in many traditional societies was also limited by cultural beliefs that restricted their access to certain foods or that religiously prescribed fasts.[32,33] Without antibiotics and vaccines, children suffered lingering illnesses with attendant anorexia, diarrhea, and months of growth interruption. The advent of puberty, in those conditions, fell late into the teen years. Philippine Island hunter-gatherer girls, for example, living in similar premodern conditions in the 1980s when they were studied,[34] began menstruating at age 17. In France in 1840, the average age of menarche was over 15 years, dropping by 2000 to 12.6 years.[35]

Evolutionary scientists still disagree on the precise factors contributing to this preternatural sexual maturation, but most credit some aspect of the present-day food abundance and increased body weight. Frisch,[36] in 1993, claimed in her "critical fat hypothesis" that human females needed a precise set point of fat deposits to ovulate. Later studies concluded that there is no precise set point of body weight or percentage of body fat that leads to the first menstruation in all populations.[37]

Nevertheless, body weight,[38] fat deposition, and the specific area of fat deposition[39] have all been demonstrated to precede first menstruation. For example, a longitudinal cohort study of Chinese girls that began at age 8.5 compared three groups: underweight, normal weight, and obese.[40] The obese girls experienced earlier breast maturation (measured as breast II development) and menarche than the other two groups. A study in New Zealand found increased adiposity to be associated with earlier menarche and decreased insulin sensitivity.[41] Another study, looking at nationwide cross-sectional data from the United States, remarked on the consistent finding that girls with higher BMIs reached puberty earlier.[42] The authors of that study, reviewing rodent studies on puberty and fat suggested that rising leptin may be the key trigger precipitating the onset of puberty. So, childhood obesity that leads to earlier puberty results in a longer period of time at which the young girls are fertile. Recent studies of adolescent brain development showed that the understanding of the consequences of their behavior, predicting risks, and controlling emotions develops during the teen years.[43] Early pubertal sexual maturity, in our modern era, now often precedes sufficient cognitive development to make wise choices regarding sexuality and reproduction.

STIGMA AND OBESITY IN PREGNANCY

In *Stigma: Notes on the Management of Spoiled Identity*, Erving Goffman described stigma as an attribute that is deeply discrediting to the possessor.[44] Goffman drew the word *stigma* from tattoos, scars, or facial injuries that marked criminals among the early Greeks. Such marks characterized the bearer as having a moral failing. The mark was thus discrediting, not because it marred the bearer's physical appearance, but because of its social meaning.

Obesity in contemporary society is similarly stigmatizing. Araújo, Pena, and Freitas described social attitudes toward obesity as "a 'moral panic' that robs obese individuals of 'social acceptance.'"[45] A review of the scientific literature on public attitudes toward obesity "documented harmful weight-based stereotypes that overweight and obese individuals are lazy, weak-willed, unsuccessful, unintelligent, lack self-discipline, have poor willpower, and are noncompliant with weight-loss treatment."[46]

Women, in particular, face social censure for increased body size, a circumstance in popular culture called "fat shaming."[47,48] A European telephone-based social survey found that women received greater numbers of negative remarks from strangers regarding their obesity than men.[49] Fifty overweight and obese women participated in a study in which they documented every weight-related interaction; the women recorded 1077 such humiliating experiences in 1 week.[50] Leading bioethicist Daniel Callahan, in the *Hastings Center Report*, called for increased social disapproval and governmental coercion as a strategy to reduce obesity, an intervention he termed "stigmatization lite."[51]

Exposure to such stigmatizing stereotypes, however, may lead to lowered self-esteem and shame. Medical students who were overweight or obese were found to have elevated anxiety, depression, and drug use, compared with their underweight or normal-weight peers.[52] A review of 23 studies examining the link between weight stigma and health behavior found that obese individuals subjected to negative comments and actions were less likely to follow clinical recommendations, engaged in more drug and alcohol abuse, and had greater anxiety.[53] Callahan's call for increasing the stigmatization of obesity not only may fail as an inducement to weight loss but also may cause considerable harm.

Physicians, nurses, and other health care providers share many of the negative attitudes toward obesity held by the general public. Studies of clinicians from Europe and the United States have documented bias toward their obese patients.[54,55] A part of this bias emerges from the difficulties health care professionals face in caring for obese patients. Many have expressed to researchers the frustrations they have encountered in trying to help their patients adopt healthier behaviors and lose weight. Some providers also exhibit less-conscious bias toward their obese patients. One study that enrolled 399 physicians from a variety of specialties found that 40% held negative bias toward obese patients.[56] A study among physician assistant students, using a psychometric measure call the Fat Phobia Scale, demonstrated that 13.6% of the students had strongly negative views of the obese.[57] A study that audio recorded and then analyzed the conversations of 39 primary care providers and their 208 patients found that although the physicians gave similar advice to patients of all BMI levels, they "demonstrated less emotional rapport" with the obese patients.[58]

Pregnancy is arguably one of the most important life events when trust between health care providers and patients can make a substantial difference in the health of the mother and the lifelong health of her child. The importance of this trust, and the mother's follow-through with healthy behavior, means that any issues that decrease effective provider-patient communication can be particularly serious. Avoiding negative attitudes and bias toward obese pregnant patients is so important that the Committee on Ethics of ACOG issued a 2014 opinion on the need for sensitive and respectful care of such patients.[59] Yet, a poll of obstetrical practices in South Florida found that 15 refused to accept new patients who weighed over 200 to 250 lb.[60]

A study among pregnant women and health care students in Queensland, Australia, documented that women with higher BMIs reported that they felt the quality of care was lower than a control group of patients with a lower BMI.[61] The medical and midwifery students in this study were presented with hypothetical pregnant patients, with the only difference being the BMI of each fictive patient; the students exhibited less-positive attitudes toward the descriptions of patients with higher BMIs.

WHAT ABOUT PERSONAL RESPONSIBILITY?

I have taught groups of medical, nursing, physician assistant, public health, and social work students, as well as obstetrical/gynecological and psychiatric residents. Because of my academic and research background in anthropology and epidemiology, my teaching addresses the social, cultural, and environmental factors influencing health. Social determinants of health and stigma are common components of my lectures. In every class, one or more students raise the question: What about personal responsibility? I imagine that on examining the material presented previously, some readers similarly want to ask the same question.

Individual health behavior—taking personal responsibility for our health—is critically important. Eating nutritious food, exercising, wearing seat belts or bicycle helmets, and avoiding cigarette smoking all depend on individual decisions to enact good health behavior. Environmental, cultural, and social influences are often equally important. Consider the situation of automobile safety prior to seat belts, airbags, and drunk-driving legislation. In the mid-1960s, prior to Ralph Nader's efforts to promote legislation to mandate car seat belts, airbags, and other mechanical improvements, catastrophic auto injuries were blamed on poor driving.[62] It was true that better drivers had fewer accidents, just like today.

Those of us who survived childhood without major windshield head injuries in those pre-1960 days owe thanks to our parents' careful driving. In contemporary cars, with safer brakes, airbags, and seat belts and with stronger laws against impaired driving, major injury is less likely during accidents.[63] It took Congress enacting laws to force the automobile companies to make cars safer and laws to make seat belt use mandatory. Most of those changes did not involve personal health behavior; rather, they took collective political action. But, individual responsibility in driving remains critically important, as any parent whose teenager has learned to drive can attest.

That situation is similar to our alarming epidemic of obesity. The increase in average BMI in the United States, and in many countries worldwide, beginning in the late 20th century is so widespread that changes in individual behavior can only be part of the cause. Some of the environmental factors promoting weight gain in childhood are themselves positive. Who would want to return to the era when measles, mumps, rubella, and other childhood diseases for which we have effective vaccinations regularly interrupted the growth and weight gain of children? Some of the environmental factors that may be promoting obesity can be resolved with legislative efforts. For example, using tax dollars to subsidize corn production and the subsequent less-costly sale of high-fructose corn syrup may be an environmental promoter of obesity. Taking sweetened soda out of schools,[64] as many school districts have done, is at least temporally associated with a slight decrease in childhood obesity,[65] although we cannot say with the available evidence how much difference this one step has made. Making environmental and policy changes to reduce the likelihood of obesity will not negate the importance of good health behavior, but it may complement positive behavioral changes.

When the Institute of Medicine (IOM) produced the report *Unequal Treatment*, documenting the inequalities in health care of people of color in the United States, many health care providers strongly objected to the notion that they would treat patients of different backgrounds differently.[66] Yet, that landmark report did document substantial health care disparities by race and ethnicity, even among patients with equal health insurance. Since that report was released, a wealth of research and program development has sought to eliminate health disparities. The review presented in this chapter on bias against obese patients indicates that obese patients may face similar health care inequalities to those faced by patients of color prior to the IOM report.

While social determinants and stigma are not traditional clinical areas of focus, they may greatly influence the incidence of obesity and the medical care of obese pregnant women. Many of the social and environmental factors promoting obesity make it difficult for women, especially those living in poverty, to maintain a healthy weight. Obstetricians and other clinicians who seek to assist their patients to choose nutritious food and to exercise may become frustrated in their efforts. The paucity of retail sources of healthy food in inner-city food deserts, the expense of fresh produce compared to salt- and sugar-laden prepared food, and the danger of walking for exercise in violent neighborhoods limit the extent to which many patients can follow through with their providers' advice to eat fewer calories and exercise more. To address those obstacles, we may need to move beyond viewing obesity as solely an issue of individual behavior and make community-wide changes that promote healthy eating and physical activity.

Weight stigma itself may result in less-adequate health care for obese women and for pregnant women may negatively affect the health of their infants. This is a critical area for further study. Obesity as a source of discrimination in health care settings could be addressed much as racial and ethnic health disparities have been. Bringing awareness to this potential health inequity may be critical to improving the outcomes for the increasing number of obese childbearing women.

REFERENCES

1. Obesity in pregnancy. Committee Opinion No. 549. American College of Obstetricians and Gynecologists. *Obstet Gynecol*. 2013;121:213–217.

2. *National Health and Nutrition Examination Survey, 2011–2012.* http://americannutritionassociation.org/newsletter/usda-defines-food-deserts.

3. Solar O, Irwin A. *A Conceptual Framework for Action on the Social Determinants of Health.* Geneva, Switzerland: World Health Organization. Social Determinants of Health Discussion, Paper 2 (Policy and Practice).

4. Centers for Disease Control and Prevention. Childhood obesity causes and consequences. http://www.cdc.gov/obesity/childhood/causes.html. Last reviewed April 27, 2012. Last updated June 19, 2015. Accessed September 1, 2015.

5. American Nutrition Association, "USDA Defines food deserts," *Nutrition Digest,* 38(2):1. http://americannutritionassociation.org/newsletter/usda-defines-food-deserts.

6. Lane SD. *Why Are Our Babies Dying? Pregnancy, Birth and Death in America.* Boulder, CO: Paradigm; 2008.

7. Lane SD, Keefe RH, Rubinstein RA, et al. Structural violence, urban retail food markets, and low birth weight. *Health Place.* 2008;14(3):415–423.

8. Food Research and Action Center. *Food Insecurity and Obesity: Understanding the Connections.* Washington, DC: Food Research and Action Center; Spring 2011.

9. Wang M, Wang ZP, Gao LJ, Gong R, Sun XH, Zhao ZT. Maternal body mass index and the association between folic acid supplements and neural tube defects. *Acta Paediatr.* 2013 Sep;102(9):908–913.

10. Powell-Wiley TM, Ayers CR, de Lemos JA, et al. Relationship between perceptions about neighborhood environment and prevalent obesity: data from

the Dallas Heart Study. *Obesity (Silver Spring)*. 2013 Jan;21(1):E14–E21.

11. Smith LL, Larkey LK, Roe DJ, Bucho-Gonzalez JA, Saboda K, Ainsworth BE. Self-reported physical activity patterns among low-income Latina women in Arizona. *Womens Health Issues*. 2014 May–Jun;24(3):e353–e361.

12. Park S, McGuire LC, Galuska DA. Regional differences in sugar-sweetened beverage intake among US adults. *J Acad Nutr Diet*. 2015 Jul 28. pii: S2212-2672(15)00661-9.

13. Almeida J, Duncan DT, Sonneville KR. Obesogenic behaviors among adolescents: the role of generation and time in the United States. *Ethn Dis*. 2015 Winter;25(1):58–64.

14. Rosenkoetter E, Loman DG. Self-efficacy and self-reported dietary behaviors in adolescents at an urban school with no competitive foods. *J Sch Nurs*. 2015 Oct;31(5):345–352.

15. Kumar GS, Pan L, Park S, et al. Centers for Disease Control and Prevention. Sugar-sweetened beverage consumption among adults—18 states, 2012. *MMWR Morb Mortal Wkly Rep*. 2014 Aug 15;63(32):686–690.

16. Park S, Pan L, Sherry B, Blanck HM. Consumption of sugar-sweetened beverages among US adults in 6 states: Behavioral Risk Factor Surveillance System, 2011. *Prev Chronic Dis*. 2014 Apr 24;11:E65.

17. Lustig RH. Fructose: it's "alcohol without the buzz." *Adv Nutr*. 2013 Mar 1;4(2):226–235.

18. Lustig R. *Obesity Before Birth: Maternal and Prenatal Influences on the Offspring*. New York: Springer; 2010.

19. Sturm R. Childhood obesity—what we can learn from existing data on societal trends, part 2. *Prev Chronic Dis*. 2005 Apr. http://www.cdc.gov/pcd/issues/2005/.

20. EWG Farm Subsidies. Corn subsidies in the United States totaled $84.4 billion from 1995–2012. http://farm.ewg.org/progdetail.php?fips=00000&progcode=corn. Accessed September 1, 2015.

21. Fields S. The fat of the land: do agricultural subsidies foster poor health? *Environ Health Perspect*. 2004;112(14):A820–A823.

22. Mestad R, Campbell J, Lane SD. Sweetened soda intake among pregnant women. Presentation at: Ob/Gyn Grand Rounds, Upstate Medical University, Syracuse, NY, October 21, 2011.

23. Brondolo E, Love EE, Pencille M, Schoenthaler A, Ogedegbe G. Racism and hypertension: a review of the empirical evidence and implications for clinical practice. *Am J Hypertens*. 2011 May;24(5):518–529.

24. Cooper R. The role of genetic and environmental factors in cardiovascular disease in African Americans. *Am J Med Sci*. 1999 Mar;317(3):208–213.

25. Hayman LW Jr, McIntyre RB, Abbey A. The bad taste of social ostracism: the effects of exclusion on the eating behaviors of African-American women. *Psychol Health*. 2015;30(5):518–533.

26. Mwendwa DT, Gholson G, Sims RC, et al. Coping with perceived racism: a significant factor in the development of obesity in African American women? *J Natl Med Assoc*. 2011 Jul;103(7):602–608.

27. Cozier YC, Wise LA, Palmer JR, Rosenberg L. Perceived racism in relation to weight change in the black women's health study. *Ann Epidemiol*. 2009;19(6):379–387. doi:10.1016/j.annepidem.2009.01.008.

28. Hickson DA, Lewis TT, Liu JL, et al. The Associations of Multiple Dimensions of Discrimination and Abdominal Fat in African American Adults: The Jackson Heart Study. *Ann Behav Med*. 2012 Feb;43(1):4–14. doi:10.1007/s12160-011-9334.

29. Albert MA, Williams DR. Invited commentary: discrimination—an emerging target for reducing risk of cardiovascular disease? *Am J Epidemiol*. 2011 Jun 1; 173(11):1240–1243.

30. De Souza LR, Kogan E, Berger H, et al. Abdominal adiposity and insulin resistance in early pregnancy. *J Obstet Gynaecol Can*. 2014 Nov;36(11):969–975.

31. Biro FM, Khoury P, Morrison JA. Influence of obesity on timing of puberty. *Int J Androl*. 2006 Feb;29(1):272–277.

32. Simoons F. *Eat Not This Flesh: Food Avoidances From Pre-history to the Present*. 2nd ed. Madison: University of Wisconsin Press; 1994.

33. Spielmann KA. A review: dietary restrictions on hunter-gatherer women and the implications for fertility and infant mortality. *Hum Ecol*. 1989 Sep;17(3):321–345.

34. Goodman MJ, Estioko-Griffin A, Griffin PB, Grove JS. Menarche, pregnancy, birth spacing and menopause among the Agta women foragers of Cagayan province, Luzon, the Philippines. *Ann Hum Biol*. 1985 Mar–Apr;12(2):169–177.

35. Sharp G. Changing biology: Age at first menstruation," *Sociological Images,* September 19, 2008. https://thesocietypages.org/socimages/2008/09/19/changing-biology-age-at-first-menstruation/.

36. Frisch RE. Critical fat. *Science*. 1993 Aug 27;261 (5125):1103–1104.

37. Sherar LB, Baxter-Jones AD, Mirwald RL. The relationship between body composition and onset of menarche. *Ann Hum Biol*. 2007 Nov–Dec;34(6):673–677.

38. Dunger DB, Ahmed ML, Ong KK. Effects of obesity on growth and puberty. *Best Pract Res Clin Endocrinol Metab*. 2005 Sep;19(3):375–390.

39. Lassek WD, Gaulin SJ. Brief communication: menarche is related to fat distribution. *Am J Phys Anthropol*. 2007 Aug;133(4):1147–1151.

40. Zhai L, Liu J, Zhao J, et al. Association of obesity with onset of puberty and sex hormones in Chinese girls: a 4-year longitudinal study. *PLoS ONE*. 2015 Aug 6; 10(8):e0134656.

41. Wilson DA, Derraik JG, Rowe DL, Hofman PL, Cutfield WS. Earlier menarche is associated with lower insulin sensitivity and increased adiposity in young adult women. *PLoS ONE*. 2015 Jun 10;10(6):e0128427.

42. Kaplowitz PB. Link between body fat and the timing of puberty. *Pediatrics*. 2008 Feb;121(Suppl 3):S208–S217. doi:10.1542/peds.2007-1813F.

43. Spielberg JM, Galarce EM, Ladouceur CD, et al. Adolescent development of inhibition as a function of SES and gender: Converging evidence from behavior and fMRI. *Hum Brain Mapp*. 2015 Aug;36(8):3194–3203. doi:10.1002/hbm.22838.

44. Goffman E. *Stigma: Notes on the Management of Spoiled Identity*. Englewood Cliffs, NJ: Prentice-Hall; 1963.

45. Araújo KL, Pena PG, Freitas MD. Suffering and prejudice: paths taken by obese nutritionists seeking weight loss. *Cien Saude Colet*. 2015 Sep;20(9):2787–2796.

46. Puhl RM, Heuer CA. Obesity stigma: important considerations for public health. *Am J Public Health*. 2010;100(6):1019–1028, p. 1019.

47. Brown H. *Body of Truth: How Science, History, and Culture Drive Our Obsession With Weight—and What We Can Do About It*. Boston: Da Capo Lifelong Books; 2015.

48. Layne J. Seven things that you might not think are fat shaming that definitely are. *Bustle*. https://www.bustle.com/articles/109182-7-things-you-might-not-think-are-fat-shaming-that-definitely-are. September 8, 2015.

49. Sikorski C, Spahlholz J, Hartlev M, Riedel-Heller SG. Weight-based discrimination: an ubiquitary phenomenon? *Int J Obes (Lond)*. 2015 Aug 27. doi:10.1038/ijo.2015.165.

50. Seacat JD, Dougal SC, Roy D. A daily diary assessment of female weight stigmatization. *J Health Psychol*. 2016;21(2):228–240. Epub 2014 Mar 18.

51. Callahan D. Obesity: chasing an elusive epidemic. *Hastings Cent Rep*. 2013 Jan–Feb;43(1):34–40.

52. Phelan SM, Burgess DJ, Puhl R, et al. The adverse effect of weight stigma on the well-being of medical students with overweight or obesity: findings from a national survey. *J Gen Intern Med*. 2015 Sep;30(9):1251–1258. doi:10.1007/s11606-015-3266-x.

53. Papadopoulos S, Brennan L. Correlates of weight stigma in adults with overweight and obesity: a systematic literature review. *Obesity (Silver Spring)*. 2015 Sep;23(9):1743–1760. doi:10.1002/oby.21187.

54. Jochemsen-van der Leeuw HG, van Dijk N, Wieringa-de Waard M. Attitudes towards obesity treatment in GP training practices: a focus group study. *Fam Pract*. 2011 Aug;28(4):422–429.

55. Lynch HF. Discrimination at the doctor's office. *N Engl J Med*. 2013 May 2;368(18):1668–1670.

56. Jay M, Kalet A, Ark T, et al. Physicians' attitudes about obesity and their associations with competency and specialty: a cross-sectional study. *BMC Health Serv Res*. 2009 Jun 24;9:106. doi:10.1186/1472-6963-9-106.

57. Wolf C. Physician assistant students' attitudes about obesity and obese individuals. *J Physician Assist Educ*. 2010;21(4):37–40.

58. Gudzune KA, Beach MC, Roter DL, Cooper LA. Physicians build less rapport with obese patients. *Obesity (Silver Spring)*. 2013 Oct;21(10):2146–2152.

59. Ethical issues in the care of the obese woman. Committee Opinion No. 600. American College of Obstetricians and Gynecologists. *Obstet Gynecol*. 2014;123:1388–1393.

60. LaMendola B. Some ob-gyns in South Florida turn away overweight women. *Sun Sentinel*, May 16, 2011.

61. Mulherin K, Miller YD, Barlow FK, Diedrichs PC, Thompson R. Weight stigma in maternity care: women's experiences and care providers' attitudes. *BMC Pregnancy Childbirth*. 2013 Jan 22;13:19. doi:10.1186/1471-2393-13-19.

62. Nader, R. *Unsafe at Any Speed: The Designed-In Dangers of the American Automobile*. New York: Grossman; 1965.

63. US Department of Transportation. *2013 Motor Vehicle Crashes: Overview*. Washington, DC: US Department of Transportation; December 2014.

64. Terry-McElrath YM, O'Malley PM, Johnston LD. School soft drink availability and consumption among US secondary students. *Am J Prev Med*. 2013 Jun;44(6):573–582.

65. Centers for Disease Control and Prevention. Progress on childhood obesity. *CDC Vital Signs*. August 2013, p. 1. http://www.cdc.gov/VitalSigns/pdf/2013-08-vitalsigns.pdf.

66. Betancourt JR, Maina AW. The Institute of Medicine report "Unequal Treatment": implications for academic health centers. *Mt Sinai J Med*. 2004 Oct;71(5):314–321.

General

The Obese Adolescent Female

Rae-Ellen W. Kavey, MD, MPH

ADOLESCENT OBESITY: PREVALENCE AND IMPORTANCE

The prevalence of obesity in childhood and adolescence has increased dramatically in the United States and in all developed countries since the early 1970s. Throughout childhood, obesity is defined as a body mass index (BMI) at or above the 95th percentile for age and sex using standard Centers for Disease Control and Prevention (CDC) growth curves; overweight is defined as BMI greater than the 85th to the 94th percentile. From National Health and Nutrition Examination Surveys (NHANES) data, the prevalence of obesity in 12- to 19-year-olds was 6.1% in 1971–1974 and

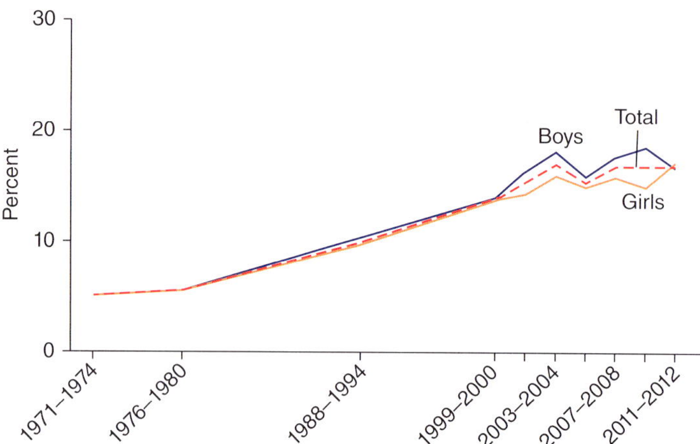

FIGURE 4-1. Trends in obesity among children and adolescents aged 2–19 years, by sex: United States, selected years 1971–1974 throughout 2011–2012. (From Fryar CD, Carroll MD, Ogden CL. *Prevalence of Overweight and Obesity Among Children and Adolescents: United States, 1963–1965 Through 2011–2012.* Atlanta, GA: National Center for Health Statistics; September 2014. Retrieved December 19, 2014. www.cdc.gov/nchs/data/hestat/obesity_child_11_12/obesity_child_11_12.pdf).

increased serially at each evaluation to 20.5% in 2011–2012 (Figure 4-1).[1] Overall, 23.9 million American children (32% of boys and 31.6% of girls) have a BMI at or above the 85th percentile and are classified as overweight or obese.[2]

There are major discrepancies in obesity prevalence by sex, by racial and ethnic group, and by socioeconomic status (SES). From NHANES 2011–2012, 18.3% of non-Hispanic white male adolescents and 20.9% of non-Hispanic white female adolescents were obese compared with 21.4% of non-Hispanic black males and 22.7% of non-Hispanic black females, 23.9% of Hispanic males and 21.3% of Hispanic females, and 14.8% of Asian males and 7.3% of Asian females.[1] Using parental education as an SES standard, data from NHANES and from the National Survey of Children's Health show that, since 2002, obesity rates have declined to less than 10% in adolescents whose parents have at least a 4-year college degree, close to the prevalence in 1970; this compares with a prevalence of 20%–25% in adolescents whose parents have at most a high school education.[3]

The severity of obesity has also been increasing exponentially over time. Severe obesity is defined as BMI greater than 120% of the 95th percentile for age/sex or an absolute BMI greater than 35 kg/m^2. From NHANES data, the prevalence of severe obesity is 5%–7% in males and 4%–6% in females.[4] This is the fastest-growing subcategory of obesity in children and adolescents, in males and females, and in all racial/ethnic groups.[5]

Taken together, these statistics provide overwhelming evidence that obesity is an important problem for those who provide health care to adolescent females. In addition, obesity tracks strongly from childhood into adulthood, with an overall predicted prevalence of about 70%.[4] In the Bogalusa Heart Study, of those with severe obesity at 12 years of age, 100% were obese as adults; 65% were morbidly obese, with BMI above 40 kg/m^2.[6] Obesity is directly associated with risk factors for cardiovascular disease (CVD), including adverse levels of lipids and blood pressure (BP); metabolic risks, including severe insulin resistance and glucose intolerance; plus inflammation.[7–10] Severe obesity is even more strongly linked to increased cardiovascular risk. Investigators from the Bogalusa Heart Study quantified cardiovascular and metabolic risk factors, including dyslipidemia, hypertension, and hyperinsulinemia, in children 5 to 17 years of age. Among children with a BMI greater than the 95th percentile, 70%, 39%, and 18% had 1, 2, or 3 or more CVD risk factors, respectively. Contrast this with children with a BMI above the 99th percentile, with 84%, 59%, and 33% having 1, 2, or

3 or more identified CVD risk factors, respectively.[6] Obese adolescents are clearly at high risk for CVD.

Evidence for the impact of obesity and its associated constellation of risk factors on the heart and coronary vasculature of obese adolescents comes from many sources. Noninvasive imaging demonstrates that obesity in adolescence predicts abnormalities of left ventricular (LV) hypertrophy and function, plus increased carotid thickness and stiffness in adult life.[11-13] These are known precursors of clinical CVD. Pathologic studies link obesity and CVD risk factors associated with obesity directly to the presence of early atherosclerosis in the coronary arteries and aorta in adolescents and young adults who died suddenly and unexpectedly.[14,15] There are now longitudinal studies linking adolescent obesity to coronary heart disease events in adult life. In the Princeton Lipid Research Follow-Up Study, obese adolescents with insulin resistance and dyslipidemia developed clinical CVD events at 28-year follow-up when compared with subjects without this risk constellation in adolescence.[16]

Identification and management of obesity are important issues for all those who provide care to adolescent females. Adolescence is a time when health habits are formed and risk behaviors like poor diet, physical inactivity, and cigarette smoking are often initiated. Primary care physicians are well positioned to provide important health guidance in this critical time period. The US Preventive Services Task Force provides evidence-based guidelines for adolescent health care in which screening for obesity is specifically recommended.[17] Guidance for identification and management of obesity in adolescents is provided in the 2011 National Heart, Lung, and Blood Institute (NHLBI) Expert Panel Guidelines for Cardiovascular Health (Table 4-1).[18] The first step is calculation and recording of BMI, with defined steps for specific management of elevated BMI and for identification of associated cardiovascular risks. All of this information is of special importance to those providing gynecologic and obstetric care to adolescents because the initial reproductive health visit is recommended to take place between 13 and 17 years of age.[19] An analysis of adolescent health care visits revealed that the gynecologist is identified as the primary physician for 36% of older female adolescents, so screening for obesity, dyslipidemia, hypertension, insulin resistance, and type 2 diabetes will often need to occur in this setting.[20]

ADOLESCENT OBESITY AND MENARCHE

Puberty is the complex process by which children develop secondary sexual characteristics and reproductive competence. The series of biologic changes that characterize the process involves complex neural and endocrinologic interactions that are described in terms of sequence and timing. Beginning in 1962, Tanner defined 5 specific stages of breast and pubic hair development in girls; these remain the cornerstone for describing pubertal development.[21,22] The Tanner stages are shown in Table 4-2, Table 4-3, and Figure 4-2.

There has been a well-documented decrease in the age of puberty (defined as the onset of menarche), from 16 to 17 years in the late 19th century to approximately 13 years of age by the middle of the 20th century, attributed to improved health and nutrition.[23] In the United States, by 1970 there was a further decline to just under 13 years of age.[24] Over the last 40 years, a gradual decrease has continued, so that white girls in the United States experience their first menstrual periods at 12.6 years, African

TABLE 4-1 NHLBI Guideline Recommendations for Management of Adolescent (12–21 Years) Patients with Overweight and Obesity[a]

Grades reflect the findings of the evidence review.
Recommendations reflect the consensus opinion of the Expert Panel.

Identify adolescents at increased risk for obesity because of parental obesity, change in physical activity +/− excess gain in BMI for focused diet/physical activity education × 6 m *BMI/BMI percentile stable → reinforce current program, 6-month follow-up* *Increasing BMI/BMI percentile → RD counseling for energy-balanced diet, intensified physical activity × 3 months*	Grade B *Recommend*
BMI 85th to 95th percentile: Excess weight gain prevention with adolescent as change agent for energy-balanced CHILD 1 diet, reinforced physical activity recommendations × 6 months *Improvement in BMI percentile → continue current program* *Increasing BMI percentile → RD counseling for energy-balanced weight control diet, intensified physical activity, 3-month follow-up*	Grade B *Recommend*
BMI ≥ 95th percentile: Specific assessment for comorbidities[b]:	Grade B *Strongly recommend*
BMI ≥ 95th percentile with no comorbidities: Office-based weight loss plan: Family-centered with adolescent as change agent for behavior modification counseling, RD counseling for (−) energy-balanced diet, Rx for increased MVPA, decreased sedentary time × 6 months *Improvement in BMI/BMI percentile → continue current program* *No improvement in BMI/ BMI percentile → referral to comprehensive multidisciplinary weight loss program with peers × 6 months* *If no improvement in BMI/BMI percentile→ consider initiation of medication under care of experienced MD × 6–12 months*	Grade B *Strongly recommend*
BMI ≥ 95th percentile with comorbidities or BMI > 35 kg/m²: Refer to comprehensive lifestyle weight loss program for intensive management × 6–12 months *Improvement in BMI/BMI percentile → continue present program* *No improvement in BMI/BMI percentile → consider initiation of weight loss medication under care of experienced clinician × 6–12 months* *BMI far above 35 kg/m² and comorbidities unresponsive to lifestyle therapy for > 1 year, consider bariatric surgery/referral to center with experience/expertise in these procedures*	Grade A *Strongly recommend*

Abbreviations: MVPA, moderate-to-vigorous physical activity; RD, registered dietician.
[a]From National Heart, Lung, and Blood Institute, National Institutes of Health.
[b]**Comorbidities: Hypertension, dyslipidemia, T2DM.**

TABLE 4-2 Tanner Stages of Breast Development[a]

Tanner 1	Prepubertal. No glandular tissue. Areola follows skin contours of the chest.
Tanner 2	Breast bud stage with small area of surrounding glandular tissue. Areola begins to widen.
Tanner 3	Further enlargement of breast and areola. Breast begins to become elevated, and gland tissue extends beyond the areolar borders. Areola continues to enlarge but remains in contour with surrounding breast.
Tanner 4	Increased breast size and elevation. Areola and papilla form a secondary mound above contour of surrounding breast.
Tanner 5	Mature stage. Breast reaches adult size. Areola returns to contour of surrounding breast with projection of papilla only.

[a]Retrieved from NIH-NICHD website, January 15, 2015.

TABLE 4-3   Tanner Stages of Pubic Hair Development[a]

Tanner 1	Prepubertal. No pubic hair.
Tanner 2	Sparse growth of long, downy hair with slight pigmentation along labia majora.
Tanner 3	Darker, coarser, and curly hair, spreading sparsely over pubis.
Tanner 4	Adult-type dark, coarse, curly hair across pubis but with no extension to medial surface of thighs.
Tanner 5	Horizontal extension of pubic hair onto medial surface of thighs.

[a]Retrieved from NIH-NICHD website, January 15, 2015.

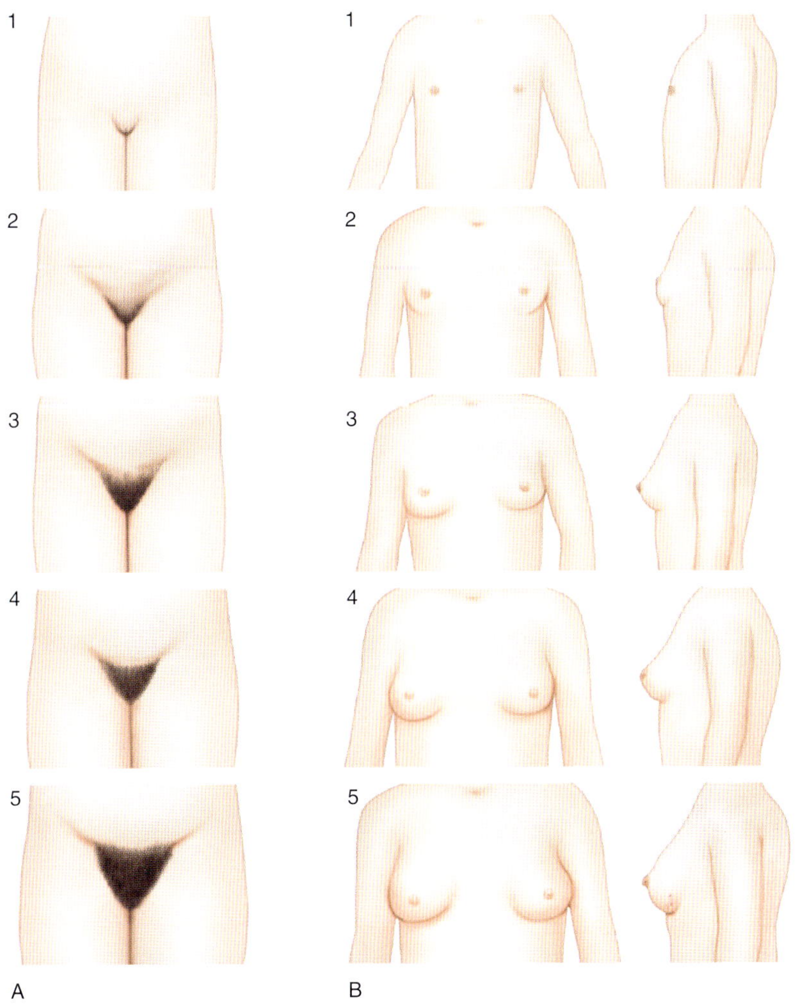

FIGURE 4-2. Tanner stages in females. (Retrieved from NIH-NICHD website, https://www.cdc.gov/nchs/data/nhanes/nhanes3/cdrom/nchs/manuals/phys.pdf, January 15, 2015.)

American girls at 12.1 years, and Latinas at 12.2 years.[25] Earlier age at menarche has been strongly linked to obesity in multiple epidemiologic studies.[26] For example, in a longitudinal, multisite cohort study, white and black girls recruited at 9 years of age were divided into 3 groups based on age at menarche. The girls with earliest menarche had significantly higher mean BMI than the midonset girls, who had higher mean BMI than the late-onset group.[27] In the Bogalusa Heart Study, serial cross-sectional studies performed in 6- to 17-year-old girls showed that earlier age at menarche correlated significantly with increasing BMI.[28]

In addition to the decrease in the age of menarche, there has been an even greater decline in the age at initiation of breast development. A longitudinal multisite study of more than a thousand girls followed from 6 to 8 years of age showed that at 7 years of age, 10.4% of white girls, 23.4% of black girls, and 14.9% of Hispanic girls had attained Tanner stage 2 or greater breast development.[29,30] Adiposity in early childhood has been shown to precede early breast development, with elevated age-normalized BMI at 3 years of age and increased velocity of BMI change from 3 to 7 years of age each significantly correlated with earlier breast development.[31] Ascertainment of the Tanner stage of breast development can be complicated by the presence of obesity because fat tissue can be mistaken for breast tissue. This has been specifically addressed in longitudinal studies by use of palpation for glandular tissue rather than inspection alone or by use of the Tanner-described characteristics of areolar development.[26,30] These methods should be used by clinicians in assessing pubertal stage in obese girls.

Puberty is known to be associated with a reduction in insulin sensitivity in all adolescents. The fall in insulin sensitivity during puberty is associated with a compensatory increase in insulin secretion.[32,33] This hyperinsulinemic pattern is exaggerated in obese adolescents. In adults, the combination of insulin resistance with obesity is characteristic of the metabolic syndrome and frequently presages development of overt type 2 diabetes. In the Bogalusa Heart Study, serial cross-sectional surveys showed that early menarche was associated with higher BMI and fasting insulin levels in childhood and adolescence and with higher fasting glucose (FG) levels in young adulthood.[34]

The mechanisms that underlie the association between childhood obesity and earlier pubarche are unclear. One potential explanation is related to leptin, a hormone produced by adipocytes that regulates appetite. Leptin levels are elevated in obese children, and there is a high correlation between leptin levels and BMI.[35] Both cross-sectional and longitudinal studies indicated a marked rise in serum leptin concentrations preceding changes in luteinizing hormone (LH) and estradiol, the hormones that initiate puberty.[36] Higher leptin levels are significantly associated with lower age at menarche.[37] A threshold level of leptin is thought to be necessary for puberty to progress, so elevated levels of leptin associated with obesity may function as a permissive factor allowing early initiation of puberty.[38]

New research suggests that a combination of obesity-related hormonal disturbances together with inflammation, known to be increased in obese individuals, could explain the observed relationship between obesity and the declining age of puberty in girls. Sex hormone–binding globulin (SHBG) binds to the sex hormones androgen and estrogen. SHBG levels are initially high in childhood but decline significantly before puberty; this is thought to potentially be a critical factor in pubertal initiation. In a recently released longitudinal study, SHBG levels correlated inversely with BMI and insulin and positively with the inflammatory marker C-reactive protein. Obese girls had lower SHBG levels at 5 years of age, reached Tanner stage 2 earlier, and had earlier LH secretion and earlier menarche.[39]

Other studies suggest that environmental chemicals are important in the etiology of early puberty. We are exposed to many estrogenically active chemicals, so-called xenoestrogens, in the course of everyday life. These include phthalates, parabens, and phenols, which are components in consumer products such as plastics, detergents, pharmaceuticals, and cosmetics. Findings from NHANES showed that the most common phthalates, parabens and phenols, are detectable in the urine of more than 90% of Americans.[40] A small study identified phthalate esters in the serum of Puerto Rican girls with premature breast development; this study was not controlled for BMI.[41] Postmenopausal women with high serum levels of phthalates and phenols were found to have elevated breast density, a marker for risk of breast cancer, on mammography.[42] Further research is warranted to evaluate the relative roles of obesity and estrogenically active chemicals in endocrine disruption, including premature thelarche.

Regardless of the specific etiology, obesity-related early puberty has important health implications. Several large studies have shown an increased incidence of psychosocial problems, including depression, anxiety, and risk-taking behaviors.[43] Early development of breast tissue and early puberty are also known to be risk factors for breast cancer, presumably because of the prolonged exposure to estrogen. A meta-analysis showed that breast cancer risk increases by 5% for each year younger at menarche.[44] Younger age at breast development was shown to independently increase the risk of breast cancer in a recent cohort study.[45] Finally, obesity-related early puberty predicts adult obesity and all of its important comorbidities: hypertension, dyslipidemia, diabetes, and premature atherosclerotic disease.[43,46]

OBESITY AND POLYCYSTIC OVARY SYNDROME IN ADOLESCENCE

Polycystic ovary syndrome (PCOS) is the most common endocrine disorder in women. Originally described in adult females with infertility and hyperandrogenism, the diagnosis has now broadened to include a heterogeneous group of disorders. There is a strong familial basis, but no single underlying genetic abnormality has been defined, suggesting that PCOS develops from a combination of heritable and environmental factors, among which obesity is prominent. Adult females with PCOS present with varying phenotypes in different clinical settings based on their symptoms (acne, hirsutism, or hair loss to dermatology; infertility to obstetrics; and irregular periods to gynecology), so there needs to be a high index of suspicion to correctly identify all cases. The most recent evidence-based guideline, published in 2013, recommends using the presence of 2 of these 3 criteria as diagnostic:

1. Androgen excess, diagnosed clinically or biochemically;
2. Ovulatory dysfunction, either oligo- or anovulation;
3. Polycystic ovaries on ultrasound using defined criteria.

These factors are described in detail in Table 4-4. The expert panel who developed these guidelines also recommended a change in name because the presence of polycystic ovaries is not a requirement for diagnosis.[47]

TABLE 4-4 Proposed Diagnostic Criteria for PCOS in Adults

Category	Abnormality	Criteria
Androgen status	Clinical hyperandrogenism	Hirsutism, male pattern; acne; androgenic alopecia.
	Biochemical hyperandrogenism	Elevated total, bioavailable, or free serum testosterone.
Menstrual history	Oligo- or anovulation	Frequent bleeding at < 21-day intervals or infrequent bleeding at > 35-day intervals. Midluteal progesterone can be used to verify anovulation.
Ovarian appearance	Polycystic ovaries on ultrasound	Unilateral presence of ≥ 12 follicles 2–9 mm in diameter ± ovarian volume > 10 mL without a cyst or dominant follicle.

Polycystic ovary syndrome is commonly associated with obesity (present in 50% of patients) and with insulin resistance; impaired glucose tolerance and overt type 2 diabetes are also well described, reported in up to 38% of women with PCOS. Evidence is inconclusive that this constellation of risk factors, when associated with hyperandrogenism in PCOS, increases risk for premature atherosclerotic disease beyond the risk associated with the baseline constellation.

The diagnosis of PCOS in adolescence is challenging because the normal physiology of adolescence mimics many PCOS features. Oligomenorrhea is common after menarche during normal puberty, as is acne, considered a sign of hyperandrogenism in adults. Multifollicular ovarian morphology, a normal pubertal appearance, can be interpreted as polycystic ovaries on ultrasound evaluation.[48] Insulin resistance is also a normal feature of the pubertal transition. The diagnosis of PCOS can be especially challenging in obese adolescents because girls with BMI greater than the 95th percentile for age have been consistently shown to have significantly higher levels of insulin and testosterone than normal-weight girls at the same pubertal stage.[49] Finally, adolescent girls with PCOS have an increased risk of the metabolic syndrome associated with increasing androgen levels, independent of obesity and insulin resistance.[48]

Current guidelines suggest consideration of PCOS in adolescent girls with persistent oligomenorrhea, particularly when there is a positive family history of PCOS. In this setting, the presence of clinical signs of androgen excess or biochemical evidence of hyperandrogenism can be used to make the diagnosis in the absence of other causes for androgen excess.[47] Demonstration of androgen excess can be difficult because of variability in testosterone levels by assay and by lab norms and because there are asymptomatic women with mild androgen excess. A plasma-free testosterone level above the normal adult range is the best single indicator of androgen excess. Anovulatory symptoms plus polycystic ovary morphology on ultrasound are not sufficient to make a diagnosis of PCOS in adolescents as multifollicular ovarian morphology is a normal feature in adolescence. Other causes to be excluded include thyroid dysfunction, hyperprolactinemia, nonclassical congenital adrenal hyperplasia, and Cushing's syndrome.[47] Some have proposed that the heterogeneity of clinical and biochemical factors in women with PCOS can be explained by the action of early-onset obesity in genetically susceptible individuals.[50] Further research is needed to clarify a potential early role for obesity-mediated hyperandrogenism in the genesis of PCOS in susceptible peripubertal girls.

Once the diagnosis of PCOS is made, current guidelines recommend an oral glucose tolerance test (OGTT) to screen for impaired glucose tolerance, with rescreening every 3–5 years.[47] Comprehensive cardiovascular and metabolic risk screening would also include a fasting lipid profile, BP evaluation and measurement of hepatic function. As treatment, hormonal contraceptives are recommended as the first-line approach for menstrual abnormalities, hirsutism, and acne. Lifestyle therapy is recommended as the primary approach to obesity and insulin resistance, with addition of metformin if there is impaired glucose tolerance or type 2 diabetes mellitus (T2DM).[47] Recent research suggests that severe insulin resistance is characteristic of PCOS in obese adolescent females and that metformin should always be considered in this setting.[51]

PREGNANCY IN THE OBESE ADOLESCENT

Childbearing in the teenage years has been declining steadily since 1960. In the most recent report from the National Division of Vital Statistics, published in 2014, the birth rate of 26.6 births per 1000 teenagers aged 15 to 19 years is less than half the 1991 rate.[52] The birth rate has also declined for 15- to 17-year-olds and for all racial and ethnic groups (Figure 4-3). There have been similar steady declines in the rates of pregnancies and abortions in teenaged females across all racial and ethnic groups.[53]

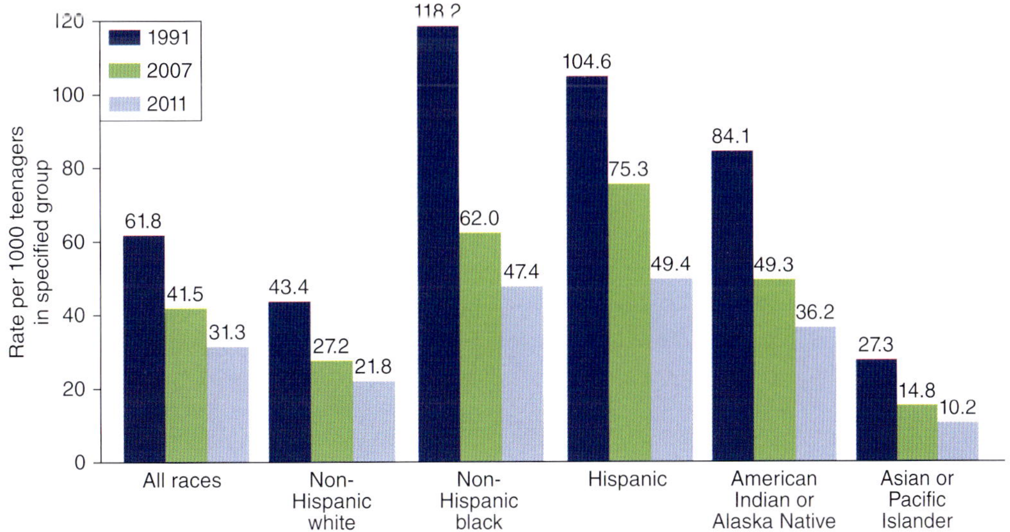

FIGURE 4-3. Birth rates for teenagers aged 15–19, by race/ethnic origin: United States, 1991, 2007, and 2011. (From Martin JA, Hamilton BE, Ventura SJ. *Births: Final Data for 2012.* Hyattsville, MD: National Center for Health Statistics; 2013. http://www.cdc.gov/nchs/data/databriefs/db123.pdf; Retrieved January 22, 2015.)

Unfortunately, when babies are born to teenaged mothers, they have a significantly increased risk for a variety of poor pregnancy outcomes, with highest risks in the youngest mothers. From 2012 data, 9.6% of babies born to 15- to 17-year-old mothers had low birth weight compared with 9.2% of babies born to 18- to 19-year-old mothers and 7.9% to mothers over 20 years of age.[53] Preterm birth rates are significantly higher for young teenaged mothers: In this instance, 14.7% of babies are born prematurely to 15- to 17-year-olds compared with 12.6% to 18- to 19-year-olds and 11.4% to mothers over 20. Low birth weight and premature birth are associated with greater risk for illness, developmental delays, and death in the first year of life. In 2010, the infant mortality rate averaged 9 per 1000 live births for mothers 15–19 years of age compared with 5.87 per 1000 for women aged 20 and over.

Pregnancy in the obese adolescent occurs in this high-risk context with significant additional obesity-related risk to maternal and fetal health. In adults, maternal obesity is associated with significantly increased risk for pregnancy complications, including preeclampsia, hypertension, gestational diabetes, miscarriage, preterm delivery, cesarean delivery, and stillbirth.[54,55] Obesity during pregnancy is also associated with increased use of health care and physician services and longer hospital stays for delivery. Studies in pregnant obese adolescents confirmed these same risks, with a higher prevalence of maternal hypertension, gestational diabetes, preeclampsia, cesarean delivery, and early stillbirth.[56]

Obesity has important health consequences for mothers after delivery. Adolescent females with high prepregnancy BMI and with excessive gestational weight gain are at known risk for postpartum weight retention and subsequent sustained obesity. From NHANES data, teen birth is a significant independent predictor of overweight and obesity later in life.[57] Gestational diabetes mellitus (GDM), strongly linked to prepartum BMI and excessive weight gain in pregnancy, also predicts development of type 2 diabetes: Approximately 50% of obese women with GDM will develop type 2 diabetes in the first decade postpregnancy.[58] In epidemiologic studies, history of GDM is also associated with increased risk of developing the metabolic syndrome and excess heart disease risk.[59] In the longitudinal Coronary Artery Risk Development in Young Adults (CARDIA) study, women were followed prospectively from a baseline age of 18–30 years and underwent carotid artery imaging 20 years later as a noninvasive measure of atherosclerosis. Women with GDM history had significantly greater carotid intima media thickness compared with women without GDM. The difference was attenuated but still significant when prepregnancy BMI was included in the analysis.[60] These increased risks for type 2 diabetes, metabolic syndrome, and CVD are even more serious when pregnancy occurs in an obese teenager because the metabolic insults occur earlier in life and the duration of risk exposure is extended.

Obesity in pregnancy is also associated with increased risks for offspring, independent of pregnancy complications. As noted, there is a higher incidence of premature birth and low birth weight, and these are associated with significantly greater risk for illness, developmental delay, and death in the first year of life.[52–55] Infants born to obese mothers have an increased risk for obesity developing in childhood and persisting into adult life. This relationship was even stronger when GDM was present.[61,62]

Maternal obesity is significantly linked to congenital anomalies in offspring, including congenital heart disease and neural tube defects, with increasing risk with increasing adiposity.[63] Overweight and obese women who lose weight before pregnancy have been shown to have healthier pregnancies. The American Congress of Obstetricians and Gynecologists has developed specific recommendations for management of pregnancy in obese women.[64] These include preconception assessment and counseling about the maternal and fetal risks associated with obesity in pregnancy and referral to a weight reduction program. At the initial prenatal visit, measurement of height, weight, and BMI is recommended to inform appropriate gestational weight gain for the obstetrician and the patient. Nutritional counseling should be made available and regular exercise recommended. Anesthesia consultation is recommended before labor because of the increased problems with pain management during labor and anesthesia should cesarean section be necessary. There are specific recommendations to reduce the risk for wound breakdown, infections and venous thromboembolism after cesarean section. Finally, weight reduction counseling should be continued postpartum and before any attempt at another pregnancy. All of these recommendations apply equally to the pregnant, obese adolescent. In addition, the America Academy of Pediatrics (AAP) has developed recommendations for a teen-friendly clinic setting to provide comprehensive reproductive health care while addressing the unique biologic, cognitive, and psychosocial needs of adolescents.[65]

OBESITY COMORBIDITIES IN THE ADOLESCENT: PREVALENCE, DIAGNOSIS, MANAGEMENT

Obesity in adolescence is strongly associated with a range of serious comorbidities, including hypertension, dyslipidemia, insulin resistance/prediabetes, nonalcoholic fatty liver disease (NAFLD), bone and joint problems, sleep apnea, and social/psychological problems. Looking at just the risk factors for CVD, 70% of obese youth aged 5 to 17 years have at least 1 risk factor.[6] Obesity has important long-term health effects, including CVD and stroke, type 2 diabetes, and cancer. In fact, current adolescent overweight is forecast to increase future adult obesity by 5% to 15% by 2035, resulting in more than 100,000 excess prevalent cases of CVD.[66] In this section, the most important comorbidities associated with obesity in adolescence are reviewed, and diagnosis and topic-specific management strategies are outlined. An overall approach to management of obesity in adolescents ends the section.

Hypertension
Prevalence and Significance
Blood pressure levels that define hypertension in adults are clear, derived from outcome data demonstrating increased risk for CVD when systolic BP exceeds 140 mm Hg and diastolic BP exceeds 90 mm Hg. Hypertension in children and adolescents is more difficult to define because outcome data are largely unavailable and BP is strongly correlated with age, gender, and body size. This has resulted in tables of normative BP values based on age, sex, and height.[67] Using these tables, hypertension in adolescents is defined as systolic or diastolic BP greater than the 95th percentile for age, sex, and height on at least 3 separate occasions. Prehypertension is defined as BP readings greater than 120/80 mm Hg but less than the 95th percentile on 3 separate occasions.

Using this definition, the overall prevalence of hypertension in adolescence averages 3.5%, but it is substantially higher in obese adolescents. In a study of high school students, the prevalence of hypertension and prehypertension combined was 30% in adolescent boys and 23% to 30% in adolescent girls, depending on ethnicity.[68] From a long-term follow-up study, individuals who were obese at a mean age of 12 years had quadruple the risk of hypertension as adults at a mean age of 33 years.[69] Obesity is the largest single risk factor for hypertension in childhood and is a strong predictor of hypertension in adulthood.

Pathophysiology of Obesity-Related Hypertension

The mechanisms by which obesity contributes to the development of hypertension are multiple, complex, and, as yet, incompletely understood. Sodium retention is believed by many to be the common pathway leading to obesity-related hypertension.[70]

1. *Hyperinsulinemia*: Hyperinsulinemia, often seen with abdominal obesity, can result in chronic sodium retention by direct effects on the renal tubules and indirectly through stimulation of the sympathetic nervous system (SNS) and augmentation of aldosterone secretion. Insulin is also believed to be the signal that links dietary intake and nutritional status to SNS activity; multiple studies have reported increased SNS activity in obese individuals. Increased vascular resistance has been shown to correlate directly with fasting insulin levels and to improve with weight loss.

2. *Hyperuricemia*: Hypertension is commonly seen in association with hyperuricemia, and this may be primary or related to hyperinsulinemia. In adolescents with essential hypertension, almost 90% were reported to have increased uric acid levels compared with only 30% of adolescents with secondary hypertension and no normotensive controls. In a randomized, double-blind, placebo-controlled, crossover trial of allopurinol in children with newly diagnosed essential hypertension, there was a significant reduction in BP associated with reduction of uric acid levels.[70]

3. *Vascular stiffness*: Increased measures of vascular stiffness are reported in obese adolescents; these may be primary and therefore contributory to pressure increase or may be secondary to established hypertension. Findings include increased carotid intima media thickness (cIMT) and reduced forearm blood flow response to ischemia with increased minimum vascular resistance. Increased cIMT has been shown to occur with obesity alone and to a greater extent with obesity and hypertension. Increased vascular resistance has been shown to correlate directly with fasting insulin levels and to improve with weight loss.

4. *Renin-angiotensin-aldosterone system*: Stimulation of the renin-angiotensin-aldosterone system (RAAS) is also believed to contribute to the development of hypertension in obese individuals. The RAAS is an important modulator of efferent glomerular arteriolar tone and of tubular reabsorption of sodium. Obese adolescents have been shown to have significantly higher supine and upright aldosterone levels with no difference in plasma renin levels. In obese adolescents, a given increment in plasma renin activity produced a greater change in aldosterone levels than in nonobese patients, and weight loss resulted in a significant decrease in plasma aldosterone.

Diagnosis of Hypertension in Obese Children and Adolescents

The Fourth Report on Childhood Blood Pressure from the NHLBI[67] recommended that BP be measured routinely at all health care encounters in children aged 3 years and older. Without appropriate measurement and interpretation, increased BP cannot be recognized and necessary treatment strategies cannot be implemented. There are several important issues to consider in the measurement of BP in this age group, especially use of the appropriate cuff size. This requires special care in obese adolescents with large arms. The cuff bladder should have a width that covers approximately two-thirds of the upper arm and a length that encircles at least 80% of the upper arm. Use of a cuff that is too small artificially raises the BP. Ideally, BP should be measured by auscultation, using a mercury sphygmomanometer. An automated oscillometric device is acceptable for initial measurement, but elevated readings should be confirmed by auscultation. Three separate readings should be made and averaged after a 10-minute rest period.

Once an accurate BP measurement is obtained, interpretation requires use of the normative tables, which provide BP percentiles derived from population studies of healthy children. As described previously, high BP is defined as systolic or diastolic BP at or above the 95th percentile based on sex, age, and height percentile on at least 3 separate occasions. Prehypertension is defined as systolic or diastolic BP between the 90th and the 95th percentile for sex, age, and height. However, during and after puberty, the 90th percentile is higher than the adult definition of prehypertension (120/80 mm Hg), so, in this age range, BPs higher than 120/80 mm Hg and lower than the 95th percentile are diagnosed as prehypertension. The complete normative BP tables are available with percentile values in the Fourth Report.[67]

White-coat hypertension is a concern in children and adolescents. This form of hypertension occurs when BPs are increased in a clinic or office setting but are normal at home; this is especially common in adolescent females. Using 24-hour ambulatory BP monitoring or home BP measurements, white-coat hypertension can be evaluated in adolescents with consistent high BP readings on repeated clinic measurements. White-coat hypertension is at least as common among obese adolescents as it is in nonobese adolescents, so ambulatory BP monitoring is an important way to confirm the diagnosis of hypertension, especially if drug treatment is being considered. Normal standards have been established for pediatric ambulatory BP.[71]

Secondary hypertension is rare in adolescents and usually manifests with severe BP elevation so that it can be distinguished clinically from the moderate BP elevations seen with primary hypertension. To exclude renal disease, the most common cause of secondary hypertension in adolescents, standard laboratory evaluation for hypertension includes checking blood urea nitrogen and creatinine levels, urinalysis, and a complete blood cell count (CBC).

Assessment for evidence of LV hypertrophy as evidence of target organ damage should be performed if a diagnosis of hypertension is made. Echocardiographic determination of LV mass is based on standard measurements indexed for body size using height to the 2.7 power. This method has been shown to most closely account for lean body mass, excluding the effects of obesity. Increased LV mass has been reported in obese children and in children with untreated hypertension. Outcome-based standards for LV mass are not available for children. A conservative cut point for the presence of increased LV mass is 51 $g/m^{2.7}$; this is higher than the 99th percentile throughout childhood and adolescence, and in adults, this level has been shown to be associated with increased cardiovascular morbidity.

Treatment of Hypertension in Obese Adolescents

Weight loss is the cornerstone of hypertensive management in obese adolescents and has been consistently shown to lower BP in multiple studies. Maximal decreases in BP have been achieved when a weight loss program combined diet change with physical conditioning. Several recent studies have addressed the role of diet specifically as it relates to BP. A meta-analysis of the effect of reducing salt intake on BP in children and adolescents found that a modest reduction in salt intake did decrease systolic and diastolic BP in normotensive children. In adults, the Dietary Approaches to Stop Hypertension (DASH) intervention trial showed that a diet high in fruits and vegetables, low-fat or fat-free dairy products, whole grains, fish, poultry, beans, seeds, and nuts and low in salt, sodium, sweets, added sugars, fats, and red meat substantially reduced both systolic and diastolic BP among hypertensive and normotensive individuals. Sustained adherence to a DASH-style diet has been shown to be associated with lower risk of coronary heart disease and stroke on long-term follow-up. A randomized controlled trial (RCT) of the DASH diet was assessed in 57 adolescents with prehypertension or hypertension. At 3-month follow-up, the DASH group had a significantly greater decrease in systolic BP associated with higher intake of fruits, low-fat dairy products, potassium, and magnesium and a lower intake of total fat compared with the usual care group. Further information about this approach is provided in the weight management section at the end of this chapter.

When diet, exercise, and behavior counseling are not effective in reducing weight and controlling BP, drug therapy to support weight loss can be considered. Drug treatment of obesity to manage hypertension has not been specifically studied, but pharmacologic treatment of obesity has been investigated in a small number of RCTs in adolescents. For male and female adolescents with severe increase of BMI and insulin resistance, including females with PCOS, the addition of metformin to a comprehensive multidisciplinary weight loss program significantly reduced weight and BMI and improved insulin resistance and lipid levels at 4- to 6-month follow-up. In randomized trials in severely obese adolescents, the addition of orlistat or sibutramine to a comprehensive multidisciplinary weight loss program improved weight loss, BMI, BP, and measures of metabolic risk at 12-month follow-up. However, tachycardia was reported as an adverse event in significantly more patients treated with sibutramine, and this drug is no longer recommended for use in adolescents. Finally, small case series of adolescents with severe obesity who had failed weight management indicated that bariatric surgery in conjunction with a comprehensive multidisciplinary weight loss program can improve weight loss, BP, insulin resistance, and glucose tolerance.[70]

PHARMACOLOGIC TREATMENT OF HYPERTENSION—There has never been a natural history study of untreated primary hypertension in the pediatric age group, so the long-term consequences of untreated hypertension in an asymptomatic, otherwise-healthy adolescent are unknown. However, long-term follow-up of more than 4000 children followed for a mean of 23 years demonstrated that individuals with persistently elevated BP from adolescence into adult life had significantly increased cIMT, known to correlate with incident cardiovascular events.[72] There is an almost-complete lack of data on the long-term effects of antihypertensive medications initiated in childhood. Because of this incomplete evidence, use of pharmacologic therapy in adolescents is limited to the following indications: (1) symptomatic hypertension; (2) secondary hypertension;

(3) evidence of hypertensive target organ damage; (4) hypertension plus diabetes (types 1 and 2); or (5) persistent hypertension despite nonpharmacologic measures.

There are some subpopulations of children for which the benefits of pharmacologic treatment are reasonably clearly established, making the decision to prescribe drug therapy more likely to produce a clinical benefit. Chief among these are children with chronic kidney disease (CKD), for whom it has been shown that lower BP reduces the rate of CKD progression. In addition, one small study has shown that pharmacologic treatment can reduce LV mass index and microalbuminuria in obese children and adolescents with primary hypertension. However, in other groups of children, a conservative approach still seems warranted given the lack of evidence of benefit and concern over possible adverse medication effects unique to the pediatric age group.

ANTIHYPERTENSIVE MEDICATIONS IN THE ADOLESCENT—Although many individual antihypertensive compounds have now been studied in the pediatric and adolescent age groups, no studies comparing different agents have been conducted. Therefore, it is unknown whether one class of agent is better than another in children and adolescents. Without evidence-based guidance for choice of drug, any single class of agent is recommended as acceptable for use in children and adolescents. Choice of initial medication should be tailored to the patient's underlying pathophysiology and the presence of concurrent conditions. Most antihypertensive medications used in children and adolescents do have accepted dose ranges based on body weight as outlined the Fourth Report.[67] A stepped-care approach is recommended, with initiation of a single agent at the lowest recommended dose as the first step. BP response to dose increases to the highest recommended level should be carefully monitored before addition of a second agent. This allows for individualization of therapy according to the needs of the patient and facilitates detection of adverse effects before drug doses are increased or new agents added. Drugs prescribed for use in children and adolescents should have pediatric labeling approved by the Food and Drug Administration and should be indicated for pediatric use.

LONG-TERM USE OF ANTIHYPERTENSIVE MEDICATIONS IN CHILDREN AND ADOLESCENTS—As In adults, antihypertensive therapy in children and adolescents must be monitored closely both for efficacy and for potential adverse effects. BP should be measured in the office every 2 to 4 weeks until good control is achieved. For children with uncomplicated primary hypertension and no hypertensive target organ damage, goal BP should be less than the 95th percentile for age, gender, and height, whereas for children with secondary hypertension, diabetes, or hypertensive target organ damage, goal BP should be less than the 90th percentile for age, gender, and height. These goals are consistent with current recommendations for therapy for hypertension in adults and also parallel the prescribing practices of many pediatric nephrologists. Once control is achieved, office BP measurement every 3 to 4 months is appropriate. Home BP measurement or ambulatory BP monitoring can also be incorporated into the treatment plan to optimize achievement of goal BP. Periodic laboratory monitoring may also be required, particularly if a diuretic or agent affecting the renin-angiotensin system is prescribed or if the hypertensive child or adolescent has underlying renal disease as the cause of the hypertension. Female adolescents should be counseled regarding the need to use an effective method of contraception if treatment with an angiotensin-converting enzyme (ACE) inhibitor or angiotensin receptor blocker (ARB) is indicated.

Adherence to treatment is an important long-term issue in the treatment of hypertension in children and adolescents because most patients are asymptomatic, and compliance is difficult in this situation. This situation is particularly difficult in adolescents, who do not like to be perceived as different from their peers and in whom parental influence is reduced. If BP control can be achieved with a single drug taken once a day, the likelihood of compliance is increased, and this should be taken into consideration when the initial agent is chosen. The adverse effect profile of the medication may also affect adherence; newer agents such as long-acting calcium channel blockers and agents affecting the renin-angiotensin system have lower rates of adverse effects than older agents, such as β-adrenergic blockers, and may therefore be preferable.

A small number of hypertensive children and adolescents, specifically those obese patients who make significant progress with lifestyle modification, may be candidates for withdrawal of therapy after a period of sustained BP control. Parents may be especially interested in attempting this goal to avoid an indefinite period of drug therapy beginning at a young age. Home and ambulatory BP monitoring and assessment for resolution of hypertensive target organ damage are necessary if withdrawal of medications is considered.

Dyslipidemia

Prevalence and Significance

Evaluation of lipid abnormalities in pediatrics has traditionally focused on the identification of children and adolescents with severe elevation in total cholesterol (TC) and low-density lipoprotein cholesterol (LDL-C) levels, usually in the context of heterozygous familial hypercholesterolemia (FH). This lipid pattern occurs in approximately 1 in 500 individuals and is inherited as an autosomal dominant characteristic. It is not associated with obesity. Children with FH have severely elevated TC and LDL-C levels from birth and are at established high risk for premature CVD.

By contrast, the pediatric obesity epidemic has resulted in a large population of children and adolescents with abnormal lipid levels: those with secondary combined dyslipidemia (CD). The CD pattern associated with obesity consists of elevated triglycerides (TGs) and non-HDL-C, decreased high-density lipoprotein cholesterol (HDL-C), and top normal to mildly elevated LDL-C. Normal TG levels in adolescents 10–18 years of age are less than 130 mg/dL, and HDL-C averages 55 mg/dL in females and 45 mg/dL in males (Table 4-5). In the dyslipidemia associated with obesity, TG levels are usually between 150 and 400 mg/dL, and HDL-C is less than 40 mg/dL.[73] NHANES data indicate this pattern is highly prevalent, present in more than 40% of adolescents with BMI greater than the 95th percentile. Insulin resistance, another common feature in obese children and adolescents, contributes significantly to development of CD by enhancing hepatic delivery of nonesterified free fatty acids for TG production. Analysis by nuclear magnetic resonance (NMR) spectroscopy showed that the CD pattern is represented at the lipid subpopulation level as both an increase in small, dense LDL and in overall LDL particle (LDL-P) number plus a reduction in total HDL-C and in large HDL particles (HDL-Ps). High LDL-P and especially elevated small, dense LDL-Ps facilitate LDL entrapment in the arterial subendothelial matrix, and reduced large HDL-Ps decrease cholesterol efflux; thus, this is a highly

TABLE 4-5 Acceptable, Borderline, and High Plasma Lipid, Lipoprotein, and Apolipoprotein Concentrations (mg/dL) for Children and Adolescents[a,b]

Note: Values given are in milligrams per deciliter; to convert to SI units, divide the results for TC, LDL-C, HDLC, and non-HDL-C by 38.6; for TG, divide by 88.6.

Category	Acceptable	Borderline	High[c]
TC	<170	170–199	≥200
LDL-C	<110	110–129	≥130
Non-HDL-C	<120	120–144	≥145
TG			
0–9 years	<75	75–99	≥100
10–19 years	<90	90–129	≥130

Category	Acceptable	Borderline	Low[c]
HDL-C	>45	40–45	<40

[a]From Reference 1.
[b]Values for plasma lipid and lipoprotein levels are from the National Cholesterol Education Program (NCEP) Expert Panel on Cholesterol Levels in Children. Non-HDL-C values from the Bogalusa Heart Study are equivalent to the NCEP Pediatric Panel cut points for LDL-C.
[c]The cut points for high and borderline high represent approximately the 95th and 75th percentiles, respectively. Low cut points for HDL-C represent approximately the 10th percentile.

atherogenic phenotype. The CD pattern seen with traditional lipid profile analysis identifies the atherogenic pattern seen with NMR analysis.

Pathophysiology of Combined Dyslipidemia of Obesity

Evidence from autopsy studies and subclinical vascular testing demonstrates the strong relationship between CD and accelerated atherosclerosis.[73] Combined dyslipidemia is the most common lipid pattern seen with clinical CVD. In the Framingham Offspring Study, CD on standard lipid profile has been shown to identify elevated small LDL-P on NMR spectroscopy and to predict early clinical CVD events. In the long-term Princeton Follow-up Study, elevated TG and TG/HDL-C ratio at 12 years of age predicted clinical CVD events at late follow-up 3 to 4 decades later. This is the first childhood lipid parameter shown to be associated with clinical CVD events. In both the Pathobiological Determinants of Atherosclerosis in Youth Study and the Bogalusa Heart Study, high non-HDL-C, high TGs, and low HDL-C were strongly associated with autopsy evidence of premature atherosclerosis. Subclinical vascular changes measured noninvasively have also been shown to be related to CD: High TGs and low HDL in youth are independent predictors of increased cIMT and vascular stiffness. A report from the longitudinal Young Finns study revealed that, at 21-year follow-up, subjects with the CD pattern beginning in childhood had significantly increased cIMT compared with normolipidemic controls, even after adjustment for other risk factors; cIMT was further increased when the dyslipidemia occurred in the context of the metabolic syndrome. Thus, the CD pattern seen with obesity in childhood and adolescence predicts vascular dysfunction in young adulthood and early clinical events in adult life.

Diagnosis of Combined Dyslipidemia

In children and adolescents with overweight and obesity, the NHLBI guidelines recommend lipid screening when BMI greater than the 85th percentile is first identified.[18] The relevant section of the screening algorithm from the guidelines is shown in Table 4-6. The initial screening test can be nonfasting or fasting. In the nonfasting condition, TC and HDL-C are measured; both are stable in the nonfasting state. These measures allow calculation of non-HDL-C from TC – HDL-C. Non-HDL-C is a measure of all of the atherogenic components of circulating lipids and lipoproteins. Non-HDL-C is a significant predictor of the presence of atherosclerosis at autopsy, as powerful as any other lipoprotein cholesterol measure in children and adolescents. For children, adolescents, and adults, non-HDL-C is more predictive of persistent dyslipidemia and therefore atherosclerosis and future events than TC, LDL-C, or HDL-C alone. Alternatively, a fasting lipid profile can be used for screening.

Normative values for all of the lipid components are shown in Table 4-5 and abnormal levels requiring intervention are shown in the algorithm in Table 4-6. Routine lipid screening is not recommended for those aged 12 to 16 years because of significantly decreased sensitivity and specificity for predicting adult LDL-C levels and significantly increased false-negative results in this age group. However, selective screening to identify abnormal lipid levels requiring intervention is recommended for obese adolescents. When dyslipidemia is diagnosed, careful assessment to identify coexisting factors that exponentiate risk for accelerated atherosclerosis is recommended.

Management of Combined Dyslipidemia

Treatment for CD of obesity is primarily lifestyle change; this is often highly effective in the short term.[18] The focus is on lowering TGs with a resultant, reciprocal increase in HDL-C. CD has been shown to be responsive to changes in weight status, diet composition, and activity. Most important, in obese children, adolescents, and adults, even small amounts of weight loss are associated with significant decreases in TG levels and increases in HDL-C levels. Even without weight loss, exercise training is associated with a significant decrease in TG levels and an increase in HDL-C, with reversion to baseline when subjects became less active. A diet that limits both simple carbohydrate intake and calories has been shown to effectively address both CD and obesity in children, adolescents, and adults.[18,74]

Based on this evidence, a diet low in simple carbohydrates and sugar is recommended for adolescents with CD; the principles of this kind of diet are shown in Table 4-7. A regular exercise schedule is also recommended, consistent with activity recommendations for all healthy adolescents (Table 4-8). This approach has been shown to effectively address CD in obese adolescents.[74] However, no data are available currently evaluating the NMR or vascular response to lifestyle change in CD in adolescents and there are no studies of long-term lifestyle change.

Drug Therapy for Combined Dyslipidemia

In the rare child with CD and severe hypertriglyceridemia for whom diet and exercise interventions are insufficient, there are medication options that can be considered.[18] If TG levels are above 500 mg/dL at initial or follow-up visits, drug therapy should be

TABLE 4-6 NHLBI Guideline Recommendations for Lipid Assessment in Adolescents[a]

Grades reflect the findings of the evidence review.
Recommendation levels reflect the consensus opinion of the expert panel.

9–11 years	Universal screening	Grade B Strongly recommend
	→Measure nonfasting lipid profile (LP): Calculate non-HDL-C: Non-HDL–C =TC – HDL-C[a] If non-HDL-C ≥ 145 mg/dL, HDL-C < 40 mg/dL → Measure fasting LP: If LDL-C ≥ 130 mg/dL, non-HDL-C ≥ 145 mg/dL, HDL-C < 40 mg/dL, TG ≥ 100 mg/dL if < 10 years, ≥ 130 mg/dL if ≥ 10 years → Repeat FLP after 2 weeks but within 3 months, average results: If average LDL-C ≥ 130 → LDL algorithm If average TG ≥ 100 < 10 years; ≥ 130 ≥ 10 years ± non-HDL-C ≥ 145 ± HDL-C < 40 → Combined dyslipidemia/TG algorithm *OR* **→Measure fasting LP**: If LDL-C ≥ 130 mg/dL, non-HDL-C ≥ 145 mg/dL, HDL-C < 40 mg/dL, TG ≥ 100 mg/dL if < 10 years, ≥ 130 mg/dL if ≥ 10 years → Repeat FLP after 2 weeks but within 3 months, average results: If average LDL-C ≥ 130 → LDL algorithm If average TG ≥ 100 < 10 years; ≥ 130 ≥ 10 years ± non-HDL-C ≥ 145 ± HDL-C < 40 → Combined dyslipidemia/TG algorithm (Figure 4-4)	
11–19 years	No routine screening	Grade B Recommend
	New knowledge of	Grade B Strongly recommend
	• Parent, grandparent, aunt/uncle, or sibling with MI, angina, stroke, CABG/ stent/angioplasty, sudden death < 55 years in males, < 65 years in females • Parent with TC ≥ 240 mg/dL or known dyslipidemia • Patient has diabetes, hypertension, BMI ≥ 85th percentile, or smokes cigarettes • Patient has a moderate- or high-risk medical condition **→ Measure fasting LP:** If LDL-C ≥ 130, non-HDL-C ≥ 145, HDL-C < 40, TG ≥ 100 < 10 years; ≥ 130 ≥ 10 years → Repeat FLP after > 2 weeks, < 3 months, average results: If average LDL-C ≥ 130 → LDL algorithm If average TG ≥ 100 < 10 years; ≥ 130 ≥ 10 years +/– non-HDL-C ≥ 145+ HDL-C < 40 → Combined dyslipidemia/TG algorithm (Figure 4-4)	

Abbreviations: CABG, coronary artery bypass graft; MI, myocardial infarction.
[a]From National Heart, Lung, and Blood Institute, National Institutes of Health.

considered because these patients are at risk for pancreatitis. The TG level and the timing for consideration of more advanced therapy if baseline levels are less than 500 mg/dL are outlined in the algorithm from the NHLBI guidelines (Figure 4-4). The statin medications have been studied in adults with CD and have been shown to reduce total LDL-P numbers and to selectively decrease small, dense LDL. One trial in children with FH showed similar results, with a significant decrease in total LDL-P number and in small, dense LDL concentration.[18]

Omega-3 fish oil supplements, described as effective treatment for hypertriglyceridemia in adults, have not been shown to be effective in adolescents. In adults, fibrates have been used to lower TG levels, and a small series in children demonstrated effective reductions in TG levels and an associated increase in HDL-C levels.[18] Finally, niacin has been used extensively in adults, but there is limited experience in children, with a single series demonstrating a high rate of side effects. The use of any medication in youths with CD should be undertaken with the assistance of a lipid specialist.

Insulin Resistance, Metabolic Syndrome, and Type 2 Diabetes

Insulin Resistance: Prevalence and Pathophysiology

Pubertal insulin resistance is physiologic, beginning with pubertal initiation and resolving by the end of puberty. There is an approximately 50% decrease in insulin

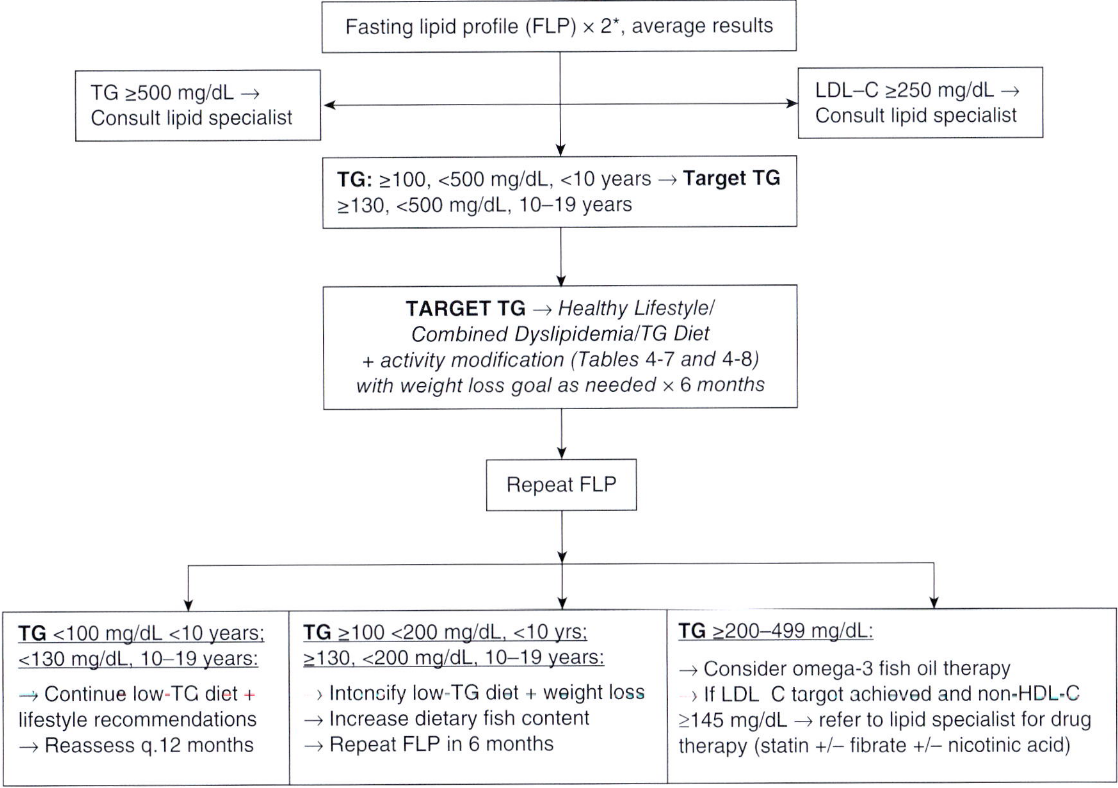

FIGURE 4-4. NHLBI guideline recommendations for management of combined dyslipidemia/high triglycerides. (From National Heart, Lung, and Blood Institute, National Institutes of Health.)

sensitivity during puberty, associated with a compensatory doubling of insulin secretion and maintenance of glucose homeostasis. In normal-weight individuals, insulin sensitivity returns to baseline levels by Tanner stage 5. The pattern of insulin resistance is exaggerated in obese adolescents and persists after puberty is complete. In the Bogalusa Heart Study, serial cross-sectional surveys showed that higher BMI was associated with higher fasting insulin levels in childhood and adolescence and with higher FG levels in young adulthood.[34] Understanding of nonphysiologic insulin resistance in adolescents is still evolving, but it is known to be strongly associated with hypertension, CD, and NAFLD, all components of the metabolic syndrome. As described previously, insulin resistance is also associated with obesity, hyperandrogenism, and ovulatory dysfunction in PCOS.[49]

Metabolic Syndrome: Prevalence and Pathophysiology

The combination of insulin resistance with obesity in adults is characteristic of the metabolic syndrome and frequently presages T2DM. Strong evidence supports obesity, especially central obesity, as the predominant correlate of the metabolic syndrome.[75] In adults, the metabolic syndrome is defined as 3 or more of the following components: elevated waist circumference as a measure of visceral fat, elevated TG levels, reduced HDL-C, elevated BP, or impaired FG. Recently, NAFLD has been designated as the hepatic component of the metabolic syndrome.

In the United States, the metabolic syndrome is reported in 34%–39% of adults, including 7% of men and 6% of women in the 20- to 30-year-old age group. There is as yet no agreed-on definition for the metabolic syndrome in childhood, but analysis of cross-sectional data from NHANES (1988–1994) showed an overall 4.2% prevalence of the metabolic syndrome cluster among adolescents aged 12 to 19 years. The syndrome cluster was present in 28.7% of obese adolescents compared with 0.1% of those with a BMI below the 85th percentile. As age and the degree of obesity increase, the prevalence of the metabolic syndrome cluster increases, reported in 38.7% of moderately obese (mean BMI 33.4 kg/m^2) and 49.7% of severely obese (mean BMI 40.6 kg/m^2) adolescents. While there is continued debate about the definition of the metabolic syndrome in children and adolescents, there is strong consensus that the combination of obesity, insulin resistance, CD, and hypertension is a powerful predictor of cardiometabolic risk measured as subclinical vascular dysfunction and clinical CVD.

Type 2 Diabetes Mellitus: Prevalence and Pathophysiology

In adults, insulin resistance in the context of the metabolic syndrome frequently precedes development of overt T2DM. Initially, the pancreas compensates for insulin resistance by increasing insulin production, and glucose levels remain normal. However, as this capacity decreases, hyperglycemia and then overt diabetes develop. The progression from insulin resistance to T2DM has been documented in children and adults.[75] The initial transition is marked by impaired glucose tolerance, with FG levels between 100 and 126 mg/dL. The diagnosis of diabetes is made when fasting plasma glucose (FPG) is 126 mg/dL or greater; when post-OGTT challenge plasma glucose is greater than 200 mg/dl; or when there are symptoms of diabetes and a casual plasma glucose of 200 mg/dL or greater. There is usually a strong family history of T2DM in adolescents who develop this diagnosis, with 45% to 80% of patients having at least one parent with T2DM and 74% to 100% having a first- or second-degree relative with this diagnosis. Previously considered a disease of adults, T2DM is now increasingly common in adolescents. A recent case ascertainment study in the United States found that the prevalence of T2DM was 0.46 per 1000 individuals in 2009, highest in black and Hispanic youth, and a 31% increase from 2001.[76] There was an accompanying increase in the prevalence of type 1 diabetes mellitus.

DIAGNOSIS—In adolescents with insulin resistance, insulin levels are high, but glucose measures are all normal. Screening for insulin resistance is not recommended because it is a physiologic condition in adolescents. Nonetheless, recognition of progressive or severe obesity should prompt consideration of evaluation for impaired glucose tolerance. Routine screening for impaired glucose tolerance with a FPG is recommended in overweight children more than 10 years of age with 2 of the following additional factors: family history of T2DM in first- or second-degree relative; high-risk racial/ethnic background (Native American, African American, Latino, Asian American, Pacific Islander); or signs of insulin resistance or conditions associated with insulin resistance (acanthosis nigricans, hypertension, dyslipidemia, or PCOS)[18] (Table 4-9). This screening should be repeated every 2 years.

TABLE 4-9	American Diabetes Association Screening Recommendations for T2DM in Childhood

Overweight, defined by BMI ≥ 85th percentile for age and gender
Plus any two of the following risk factors:
- Family history of T2DM in first- or second-degree relative
- Race/ethnicity (Native American, African American, Latino, Asian American, Pacific Islander)
- Signs of insulin resistance or conditions associated with insulin resistance (acanthosis nigricans, hypertension, dyslipidemia, or polycystic ovary syndrome)

Screening procedure:
Age of initiation: ≥10 years, or at onset of puberty, if puberty occurs at a younger age
Frequency: Every 2 years
Test: Fasting plasma glucose

Normal FG is less than 100 mg/dL, and impaired FG is 100–125 mg/dL; this is described as prediabetes. If prediabetes is detected, screening should be repeated every 6 months as these adolescents are at high risk for development of diabetes. If FG exceeds 126 mg/dL, a provisional diagnosis of diabetes is made, and further evaluation is needed. There is no recommended screening for the metabolic syndrome, but evaluation for components of this syndrome complex in obese adolescents is recommended as described previously in this section.

The diagnosis of diabetes is made when FPG is 126 mg/dL or greater; post-OGTT plasma glucose is greater than 200 mg/dL; there are symptoms of hyperglycemia and a random plasma glucose of 200 mg/dL or greater; or hemoglobin A_{1c} (HbA_{1c}) is more than 6.5%. In general, the benign clinical picture, context of obesity, and signs of insulin resistance allow ready distinction between T1DM and T2DM. However, there is overlap between these diagnoses, so measurement of insulin levels and diabetes autoantibody testing should be considered. Most patients with early T2DM are asymptomatic without the symptoms of polydipsia, polyuria, and weight loss that characterize T1DM or other rare forms of diabetes. A small number of adolescents with T2DM may present acutely with ketoacidosis and require urgent management, but this is rare. More commonly, the diagnosis is made after screening in a high-risk adolescent.

MANAGEMENT—No specific management of insulin resistance is needed, but lifestyle recommendations to prevent progression to T2DM and screening for impaired FG, hypertension, and dyslipidemia are recommended, as described previously. By contrast, management of T2DM is well defined, with recent evidence-based guidelines from the AAP focusing on glycemic control with normal FG and HbA_{1c}, improved insulin sensitivity, and identification and treatment of comorbidities.[77]

The guideline emphasizes joint management of patients by primary care providers and pediatric endocrinologists, with engagement of the adolescent and family in the care process. Initial treatment combines lifestyle change with medication. The lifestyle approach addresses weight loss with a diet very similar to that recommended for management of CD and hypertension, with portion control, elimination of sugar-sweetened beverages, and substitution of complex carbohydrates for simple carbohydrates. Overall recommendations for weight management in obese adolescents are provided at the end of this chapter. Increased activity is also specifically recommended. A 13-week randomized trial of supervised aerobic activity compared low-dose (20-min/d) to high-dose (40-min/d) supervised activity to usual activity in sedentary, obese children.[78] The main outcome measures were postintervention T2DM risk assessed by insulin resistance from OGTT, aerobic fitness, percentage body fat via dual-energy x-ray absorptiometry and visceral fat via magnetic resonance. The study found that either 20 or 40 min/d of aerobic training significantly improved fitness and demonstrated dose-response benefits for insulin resistance and general and visceral adiposity regardless of sex or race. This is consistent with the AAP guideline, which also recommends limitation of nonacademic "screen time" to less than 2 hours per day.

Simultaneous initiation of drug therapy is also recommended.[77] In the unusual situation where the adolescent is ketotic or presents with ketoacidosis, where random plasma glucose levels exceed 250 mg/dL or HbA_{1c} is greater than 9% or where the distinction between T1DM and T2DM is unclear, initiation of insulin under the care of an endocrinologist is recommended. For the vast majority of asymptomatic adolescents, the first-line recommended agent is metformin, which decreases hepatic glucose production, decreases intestinal absorption of glucose, and improves insulin sensitivity by increasing peripheral glucose uptake and utilization. Metformin is an oral agent that is relatively easy to use as it does not produce hypoglycemia in patients with T2DM. It also has proven potential for weight loss or weight neutrality. Specific recommendations for use of metformin and for monitoring of blood glucose and HbA_{1c} are provided in the guideline.

Explicit screening for diabetic comorbidities is recommended.[77] Hypertension and CD are each common, present in about 65% of adolescents with established T2DM. If detected, aggressive treatment of hypertension and CD is recommended per guidelines from the American Heart Association.[79] Retinopathy is also relatively common, recorded in about 10% of individuals with T2DM diagnosed before 30 years of age. Initial comprehensive ophthalmological exam is recommended in all patients. Nephropathy is also a significant comorbidity, so screening for microalbuminuria at presentation and then annually is recommended. If microalbuminuria is found to be persistent, initiation of prophylactic ACE inhibitor therapy is recommended. Finally, depression is a significant comorbidity whose detection is likely dependent on observation by the family and the primary care provider.

Nonalcoholic Fatty Liver Disease

Prevalence and Significance

Nonalcoholic fatty liver disease is the most common chronic liver disease in children, adolescents, and adults.[80] It was first described in the 1980s and is defined as hepatic fat infiltration in more than 5% of hepatocytes on liver biopsy with no evidence of hepatocellular injury and no history of alcohol intake. NAFLD is strongly associated with obesity, affecting at least 38% of obese adolescents in autopsy series and about 50% of obese adolescents in epidemiologic surveys. The exact prevalence is unknown because of lack of screening guidelines and underrecognition secondary to the requirement for invasive liver biopsy for definitive diagnosis. NAFLD may progress to nonalcoholic steatohepatitis (NASH) and rarely to advanced fibrosis and cirrhosis, but this is extremely rare before adult life. From biopsy series, the prevalence of NAFLD increases significantly with age.

There are racial and ethnic disparities with the prevalence of NAFLD, which is highest in Hispanics and Asians and lowest in African Americans. Beyond racial and ethnic characteristics, there is a strong genetic predisposition, with multiple gene polymorphisms identified as significant. Recently, there has been a growing body of evidence specifically implicating sedentary lifestyle, high-fructose diet, and altered gut microbiome in the genesis of NAFLD. NAFLD is frequent in patients with PCOS, confirming a relevant clinical association between these 2 conditions.[81]

Overall, the current state of the evidence indicates that the etiology of NAFLD is complex, resulting from environmental exposures on a genetically susceptible background with multiple independent modifiers. With the current obesity epidemic, this is clearly an important comorbidity in obese adolescent females.

Pathophysiology

Hepatic fat deposition usually occurs in the context of generalized obesity but reflects much more strongly the presence of increased visceral adiposity. In obese children and adolescents, sequential increase in waist circumference is associated with progressive increase in odds ratio for prediction of ultrasound-detected hepatic steatosis. NAFLD is strongly associated with insulin resistance and all of the components of the metabolic syndrome cluster; in a study of adolescents with biopsy-proven NAFLD, 80% had biochemical evidence of insulin resistance. Fat accumulation in the liver is a significant, obesity-independent predictor of T2DM.[82]

In the liver, insulin resistance leads to overproduction of glucose and very LDLs. This leads to mild hyperglycemia and, further, compensatory hyperinsulinemia and hypertriglyceridemia with secondary HDL lowering. At least 60% of patients with NAFLD have hypertriglyceridemia, and half have low HDL-C. In adolescents with NAFLD confirmed by magnetic resonance imaging (NMR), NMR analysis shows the classic atherogenic dyslipidemic pattern characterized by increased concentrations of small, dense LDL and decreased large HDL.[83] The diagnosis of NAFLD is also significantly associated with markers of systemic inflammation known to be associated with accelerated atherosclerosis.

Currently, NAFLD is considered to be the hepatic component of the metabolic syndrome and has been shown to be a strong independent predictor of CVD in adults. In children and adolescents, NAFLD is strongly associated with pathologic evidence of atherosclerosis at autopsy and with ultrasound vascular markers associated with atherosclerosis.[84]

Diagnosis

The diagnosis of NAFLD requires demonstration of hepatic steatosis by imaging or histology with no history of significant alcohol consumption, no competing etiologies for hepatic steatosis, and no coexisting causes for chronic liver disease. Demonstration of abnormal histology requires liver biopsy with hepatic fat infiltration in more than 5% of hepatocytes; noninvasive imaging techniques are suboptimal. To date, there are no evidence-based guidelines for diagnosis of NAFLD. Consensus guidelines recommend physical exam for hepatomegaly, measurement of waist circumference to assess visceral adiposity, and evaluation for signs of insulin resistance in obese children and adolescents, but there are no general guidelines for screening.[85] Consideration should be given to screening adolescent females with PCOS for NAFLD.

Liver function tests are the most commonly used indirect marker of NAFLD, with consensus that alanine aminotransferase (ALT) or aspartate aminotransferase (AST) levels above 50 U/L in male or female adolescents are abnormal and require further evaluation. An ALT level above 200 U/L is considered evidence of severe NAFLD. Serum levels of alkaline phosphatase and gamma-glutamyltransferase (GGT) can also be mildly elevated, so complete liver function testing is recommended plus evaluation of CBC, electrolytes, serum urea nitrogen (BUN), coagulation profile, international normalized ratio (INR), ferritin, and uric acid. To assess for associated metabolic abnormalities, measurements of fasting lipid profile and glucose and insulin levels are recommended, as well as HbA_{1c} and OGTT. To exclude other causes of liver dysfunction, testing for hepatitis, Wilson disease, hypothyroidism, cystic fibrosis, celiac disease, α_1-antitrypsin deficiency, metabolic diseases, and autoimmune disease should be considered.

Liver ultrasound is the most commonly used imaging modality, providing a reasonable estimate of the degree of hepatic steatosis. Ultrasonography scores strongly correlate with the presence and extent of hepatic fat demonstrated at liver biopsy, but ultrasound is insensitive when the liver contains less than 33% fat or when the BMI exceeds 40 kg/m^2. Overall, the sensitivity of hepatic ultrasound is reported to range from 60% to 94%, with a specificity of 84% to 100%. Computed tomography (CT) is more sensitive but is rarely used because of radiation exposure. MRI has the greatest accuracy to determine hepatic fat content but is rarely used clinically because of its high cost. Various techniques are used to predict more severe hepatic involvement with fibrosis, but these are not usually applicable in the adolescent in whom NAFLD is being evaluated. Consideration of liver biopsy is recommended when liver function tests are abnormal and ultrasound evaluation is inconclusive. It is hoped ongoing research will identify and validate clinical techniques for diagnosis of NAFLD in the near future.

Management

Weight management is the primary therapy for NAFLD, but exercise therapy has been shown to be effective even in the absence of weight loss. Limited reports suggest that lifestyle change can be effective in this setting.[86] There are no validated medications for treatment of NAFLD. There has been one RCT of high-dose vitamin E versus metformin versus placebo in 173 children and adolescents with biopsy-proven NASH with no benefit in lowering ALT. However, secondary analysis showed that treatment with vitamin E twice daily for 96 weeks was associated with significantly greater improvement in histological findings.[87] An ongoing RCT of probiotics may yield useful results in the future.

COMPREHENSIVE APPROACH TO WEIGHT MANAGEMENT IN ADOLESCENTS WITH OBESITY-RELATED COMORBIDITIES

As described in the previous sections, weight loss has been shown to be effective primary therapy for each of the described obesity-related comorbidities. A comprehensive but straightforward weight management approach that can be initiated in the pediatric, gynecologic, family practice, or subspecialty setting is needed, and a suggested plan is described here. The process begins with calculation of appropriate

TABLE 4-10 Estimated Energy Requirements (in Kilocalories [kcal]) for Adolescents by Gender and Age Group at Three Levels of Physical Activity[a]

Gender	Age (years)	*Sedentary*[b]	*Moderately Active*[c]	*Active*[d]
			Activity Level[b,c,d]	
Female	9–13	1600	1600–2000	1800–2200
	14–18	1800	2000	2400
	19–30	2000	2000–2200	2400
Male	9–13	1800	1800–2200	2000 2600
	14–18	2200	2400–2800	2800–3200
	19–30	2400	2600–2800	3000

[a]These levels are based on estimated energy requirements from the Institute of Medicine (IOM) *Dietary Reference Intakes* macronutrients report (2002), calculated by gender, age, and activity level for reference-size individuals. *Reference size*, as determined by the IOM, is based on median height and weight for ages up to age 18 years and median height and weight for that height to give a body mass index of 21.5 for adult females and 22.5 for adult males.
[b]A sedentary activity level in childhood, as in adults, means a lifestyle that includes only the light physical activity associated with typical day-to-day life.
[c]Moderately active in childhood means a lifestyle that includes some physical activity, equivalent to an adult walking about 1.5 to 3 miles per day at 3 to 4 miles per hour, in addition to the light physical activity associated with typical day-to-day life.
[d]Active means a lifestyle that includes more physical activity, equivalent to an adult walking more than 3 miles per day at 3 to 4 miles per hour, in addition to the light physical activity associated with typical day-to-day life.
[e]The calorie ranges shown recognize the needs of different ages within the group. For growing children and adolescents, more calories are needed at older ages.

energy intake for age, gender, and activity level of the adolescent using Table 4-10. Then, a diet low in simple carbohydrates, sugar, and added salt is recommended. For all dietary change in children and adolescents, initial family based training with a registered dietitian has been shown to be the most effective way to both begin and sustain change.

As part of the NHLBI guidelines, the DASH diet was modified for use in childhood. This simple diet plan is rich in fruits and vegetables, low-fat or fat-free dairy products, whole grains, fish, poultry, beans, seeds, and nuts and low in sweets and added sugars, fats, and red meat (Table 4-11).[18] A diet composition like this is effective for management of hypertension and CD and reflects the guideline recommendations for adolescents with T2DM.[77]

A regular exercise schedule is also strongly recommended. As described in the T2DM section, a RCT in obese children showed that a regular exercise schedule with 20 or 40 minutes of aerobic exercise 5 days per week significantly improved fitness and demonstrated dose-response benefits for insulin resistance and general and visceral adiposity.[78] This was supervised exercise, and to allow for variations in compliance in the typically unsupervised setting, an hour of moderate-to-vigorous activity is recommended every day of the week. Application of these simple recommendations with infrequent monitoring has been associated with weight loss and improvement in comorbidities in obese adolescents.[68,74] When this approach is unsuccessful, referral to a multidisciplinary weight loss program is recommended.[18]

TABLE 4-11 DASH-Style Eating Plan: Servings per Day by Food Group and Total Energy Intake

Food Group	1200 Calories	1400 Calories	1600 Calories	1800 Calories	2000 Calories	2600 Calories	Serving Sizes	Examples and Notes	Significance of Food Group to DASH Eating Plan
Grains[a]	4–5	5–6	6	6	6–8	10–11	1 slice bread 1 oz dry cereal[b] ½ cup cooked rice, pasta, or cereal[b]	Whole-wheat bread and rolls, whole-wheat pasta, English muffin, pita bread, bagel, cereals, grits, oatmeal, brown rice, unsalted pretzels and popcorn	Major sources of energy and fiber.
Vegetables	3–4	3–4	3–4	4–5	4–5	5–6	1 cup raw leafy vegetable ½ cup cut-up raw or cooked vegetable ½ cup vegetable juice	Broccoli, carrots, collards, green beans, green peas, kale, lima beans, potatoes, spinach, squash, sweet potatoes, tomatoes	Rich sources of potassium, magnesium, and fiber.
Fruits	3–4	4	4	4–5	4–5	5–6	1 medium fruit ¼ cup dried fruit ½ cup fresh, frozen, or canned fruit ½ cup fruit juice	Apples, apricots, bananas, dates, grapes, oranges, grapefruit, grapefruit juice, mangoes, melons, peaches, pineapples, raisins, strawberries, tangerines	Important sources of potassium, magnesium, and fiber.
Fat-free or low-fat milk and milk products	2–3	2–3	2–3	2–3	2–3	3	1 cup milk or yogurt 1½ oz cheese	Fat-free milk or buttermilk; fat-free, low-fat, or reduced-fat cheese; fat-free/low-fat regular or frozen yogurt	Major sources of calcium and protein.
Lean meats, poultry, and fish	3 or less	3–4 or less	3–4 or less	6 or less	6 or less	6 or less	1 oz cooked meats, poultry, or fish 1 egg[c]	Select only lean; trim away visible fats; broil, roast, or poach; remove skin from poultry	Rich sources of protein and magnesium.
Nuts, seeds, and legumes	3 per week	3 per week	3–4 per week	4 per week	4–5 per week	1	1/3 cup or 1½ oz nuts 2 tbsp peanut butter 2 tbsp or ½ oz seeds ½ cup cooked legumes (dried beans, peas)	Almonds, filberts, mixed nuts, peanuts, walnuts, sunflower seeds, peanut butter, kidney beans, lentils, split peas	Rich sources of energy, magnesium, protein, and fiber.

Food Group						Serving Sizes	Examples and Notes	Significance to the DASH Eating Plan
Fats and oils	1	1	2	2–3	2–3	3	1 tsp soft margarine 1 tsp vegetable oil 1 tbsp mayonnaise 2 tbsp salad dressing	Soft margarine, vegetable oil (canola, corn, olive, safflower), low-fat mayonnaise, light salad dressing	DASH study had 27% of calories as fat, including fat in or added to foods.
Sweets and added sugars	3 or less per week	3 or less per week	3 or less per week	5 or less per week	5 or less per week	≤2	1 tbsp sugar 1 tbsp jelly or jam ½ cup sorbet, gelatin dessert 1 cup lemonade	Fruit-flavored gelatin, fruit punch, hard candy, jelly, maple syrup, sorbet and ices, sugar	Sweets should be low in fat.

Abbreviations: oz = ounce; tbsp = tablespoon; tsp = teaspoon.
[a]Whole grains are recommended for most grain servings as a good source of fiber and nutrients.
[b]Serving sizes vary between ½ cup and 1¼ cups, depending on cereal type. Check product's Nutrition Facts label.
[c]Because eggs are high in cholesterol, limit egg yolk intake to no more than 4 per week; 2 egg whites have the same protein content as 1 oz meat. Fat content changes serving amount for fats and oils. For example, 1 tbsp regular salad dressing = 1 serving; 1 tbsp low-fat dressing = ½ serving; 1 tbsp fat-free dressing = zero servings.

REFERENCES

1. Ogden CL, Carroll MD, Kit BK, et al. Prevalence of childhood and adult obesity in the United States, 2011–2012. *JAMA*. 2014;311(8):806–814.

2. Go AS, Mozaffarian D, Roger VL, et al. Heart disease and stroke statistics—2014 update: a report from the American Heart Association. *Circulation*. 2014;129(3):e28–e292.

3. Frederick CB, Snellman K, Putnam RD. Increasing disparities in adolescent obesity. *Proc Natl Acad Sci U S A*. 2014;111(4):1338–1342.

4. Kelly AS, Barlow SE, Rao G, et al. Severe obesity in children and adolescents: identification, associated health risks and treatment approaches. A scientific statement from the American Heart Association. *Circulation*. 2013;128:1689–1712.

5. Skelton JA, Cook SR, Auinger P, et al. Prevalence and trends of severe obesity among US children and adolescents. *Acad Pediatr*. 2009;9:322–329.

6. Freedman DS, Mei Z, Srinivasan SR, et al. Cardiovascular risk factors and excess adiposity among overweight children and adolescents: the Bogalusa Heart Study. *J Pediatr*. 2007;150:12–17.

7. Morrison JA, Barton BA, Biro FM, et al. Overweight, fat patterning, and cardiovascular disease risk factors in black and white boys. *J Pediatr*. 1999;135:451–457.

8. Muntner P, He J, Cutler JA, et al. Trends in blood pressure among children and adolescents. *JAMA*. 2004;291:2107–2113.

9. Arslanian S, Suprasongsin C. Insulin sensitivity, lipids, and body composition in childhood: is "syndrome X" present? *J Clin Endocrinol Metab*. 1996;81:1058–1062.

10. Sinaiko AR, Steinberger J, Moran A, et al. Relation of body mass index and insulin resistance to cardiovascular risk factors, inflammatory factors, and oxidative stress during adolescence. *Circulation*. 2005;111:1985–1991.

11. Toprak A, Wang H, Chen W, et al. Relation of childhood risk factors to left ventricular hypertrophy (eccentric or concentric) in relatively young adulthood (from the Bogalusa Heart Study). *Am J Cardiol*. 2008;101:1621–1625.

12. Juonala M, Viikari JS, Kähönen M, et al. Life-time risk factors and progression of carotid atherosclerosis in young adults: the Cardiovascular Risk in Young Finns study. *Eur Heart J*. 2010;31:1745–1751.

13. Freedman DS, Patel DA, Srinivasan SR, et al. The contribution of childhood obesity to adult carotid intima-media thickness: the Bogalusa Heart Study. *Int J Obes (Lond)*. 2008;32:749–756.

14. Berenson GS, Srinivasan SR, Bao W, et al. Association between multiple cardiovascular risk factors and atherosclerosis in children and young adults: the Bogalusa Heart Study. *N Engl J Med*. 1998:338:1650–1656.

15. McGill HC Jr, McMahan CA, Zieske AW, et al. Association of coronary heart disease risk factors with microscopic qualities of coronary atherosclerosis in youth. *Circulation*. 2000;102:374–379.

16. Morrison JA, Friedman LA, Gray-McGuire C. Metabolic syndrome in childhood predicts adult cardiovascular disease 25 years later: the Princeton Lipid Research Clinics Follow-up Study. *Pediatrics*. 2007;120:340–345.

17. Ham P, Allen C. Adolescent health screening and counseling. *Am Fam Physician*. 2012;86(12):1109–1116.

18. NHLBI Expert Panel on Integrated Guidelines for Cardiovascular Health and Risk Reduction in Children and Adolescents: summary report. *Pediatrics*. 2011;(Suppl 5):S1–S48.

19. American College of Obstetricians and Gynecologists. *Primary and Preventive Care for Female Adolescents. Guidelines for Adolescent Care*. 2nd ed. Washington, DC: American College of Obstetricians and Gynecologists; 2011:25–42.

20. Rand CM, Shone LP, Albertin C, et al. National health care visit patterns of adolescents: implications for delivery of new adolescent vaccines. *Arch Pediatr Adolesc Med*. 2007;161(3):252–259.

21. Tanner JM. *Growth at Adolescence*. 2nd ed. Oxford, UK: Blackwell Scientific; 1962:36–39.

22. Marshall WA, Tanner JM. Variations in patterns of pubertal changes in girls. *Arch Dis Child*. 1969;44(235):291–303.

23. Wyshak G, Frisch RE. Evidence for a secular trend in age of menarche. *N Engl J Med*. 1982;306:1033–1035.

24. Biro FM, Greenspan LC, Galvez MP. Puberty in girls of the 21st century. *J Pediatr* Adolesc Gynecol. 2012 Oct;25(5):289–94.

25. Biro, FM, Khoury P, Morrison JA. Influence of obesity on timing of puberty. *Int J Androl*. 2006;26:272–277.

26. Kaplowicz P. Link between body fat and the timing of puberty. *Pediatrics*. 2008;121(Suppl 3):S208–S217.

27. Biro FM, McMahahon RP, Striegel-Moore R, et al. Impact of pubertal timing on growth in black and white female adolescents: the National heart, Lung and Blood Institute Growth and health study. *J Pediatr*. 2001;138(5):636–643.

28. Wattigney WA, Srinivasan SR, Chen W, et al. Secular trend of earlier onset of menarche with increasing obesity in black and white girls: the Bogalusa Heart Study. *Ethnicity Dis*. 1999;9:181–189.

29. Biro FM, Galvez MP, Greenspan LC, et al. Pubertal assessment and baseline characteristics in a mixed longitudinal study of girls. *Pediatrics*. 2010;126:583–589.

30. Biro FM, Greenspan LC, Galvez MP, et al. Onset of breast development in a longitudinal cohort.

Pediatrics. 2013 Dec;132(6):1019–1027. doi:10.1542/peds.2012–3773. Epub 2013 Nov 4.

31. Lee JM, Appugliese D, Kaciroti N, et al. Weight status in young girls and the onset of puberty. *Pediatrics.* 2007;119(3):e624.

32. Caprio S, Plewe G, Diamond MP, et al. Increased insulin secretion in puberty: a compensatory response to reductions in insulin sensitivity. *J Pediatr.* 1989;114:963–967.

33. Caprio S, Tamborlane WV. Effect of puberty on insulin action and secretion. *Semin Reprod Endocrinol.* 1994;12:90–96.

34. Frontini MG, Srinivasan SR, Berenson GS. Longitudinal changes in risk variables underlying metabolic syndrome X from childhood to young adulthood in female subjects with a history of early menarche: the Bogalusa Heart Study. *Int J Obes Relat Metab Disord.* 2003;27(11):1398–1404.

35. Hassink SG, Sheslow DV, de Lancey E, et al. Serum leptin in children with obesity: relationship to gender and development. *Pediatrics.* 1996;98(2 pt 1):201–203.

36. Garcia-Mayor RV, Andrade A, Rios M, et al. Serum leptin levels in normal children: relationship to age, gender, body mass index, pituitary gonadal hormones and pubertal stage. *J Clin Endocrinol Metab.* 1997;82(9):2849–2855.

37. Matkovic V, Ilich JZ, Skugor M, et al. Leptin is inversely related to age at menarche in human females. *J Clin Endocrinol Metab.* 1997;82(10):3239–3245.

38. Shalitin S, Phillip M. Role of obesity and leptin in the pubertal process and pubertal growth. *Int J Obesity.* 2003;27:869–874.

39. Pinkney J, Streeter A, Hosking J, et al. Adiposity, chronic inflammation and the pubertal decline in sex hormone-binding globulin in children: evidence for associations with the timing of puberty. *J Clin Endocrinol Metab.* 2014;99(9):3224–3232.

40. Calafat AM, Ye X, Wong LY, Bishop AM, Needham LL. Urinary concentrations of four parabens in the US population: NHANES 2005-2006. *Environ Health Perspect.* 2010;118:679–685.

41. Colon I, Caro D, Bourdony CJ, et al. Identification of phthalate esters in the serum of young Puerto Rican girls with premature breast development. *Environ Health Perspect.* 2000;108:895–900.

42. Sprague BL, Trentham-Dietz A, Hedman C, et al. Circulating serum xenoestrogens and mammographic breast density. *Breast Cancer Res.* 2013;15:R45–R53.

43. Golub MS, Collman GW, Foster PMD, et al. Public health implications of altered pubertal timing. *Pediatrics.* 2008;121(Suppl 3):S218–S230.

44. Collaborative Group on Hormonal Factors in Breast Cancer. Menarche, menopause, and breast cancer risk: individual participant meta-analysis, including 118,964 women with breast cancer from 117 epidemiological studies. *Lancet Oncol.* 2012;13(11):1141–1151.

45. Bodicoat DH, Schoemaker MJ, Jones ME, et al. Timing of pubertal stages and breast cancer risk: the Breakthrough Generations Study. *Breast Cancer Res.* 2014 Feb 4;16(1):R18.

46. Prentice P, Viner RM. Pubertal timing and adult obesity and cardiometabolic risk in men and women: a systematic review and meta-analysis. *Int J Obes.* 2013;37:1036–1043.

47. Legro RS, Arslanian SA, Ehrmann DA, et al. Diagnosis and treatment of polycystic ovary syndrome: an endocrine society clinical practice guideline. *J Clin Endocrinol Metab.* 2013;98:4565–4592.

48. Burgert TS. PCOS in adolescence: diagnostic dilemmas and management considerations. In: Pal L, ed. *Polycystic Ovary Syndrome. Current and Emerging Concepts.* New York. Springer Science and Business Media; 2014:245–264.

49. Apter D, Butzow T, Laughlin GA, et al. Metabolic features of polycystic ovary syndrome in adolescent girls with hyperandrogenism. *J Clin Endocrinol Metab.* 1995;80(10):2966–2973.

50. McCartney CR, Prendegast KA, Chhabra S, et al. The association of obesity and hyperandrogenemia during the pubertal transition in girls: obesity as a potential factor in the genesis of postpubertal hyperandrogenism. *J Clin Endocrinol Metab.* 2006;91:1714–1722.

51. Cree Green M, Diniz Behn C. Hepatic and adipose insulin resistance in polycystic ovarian syndrome. Presented at the Pediatric Academic Societies Annual Scientific Sessions; May 2014; Vancouver, BC, Canada.

52. Ventura SJ, Hamilton BE, Mathews TJ. National and state patterns of teen births in the United States, 1940-2013. *Natl Vital Stat Rep.* 2014;63(4):1–33.

53. Kost K, Henshaw S. *US Teenage Pregnancies, Births and Abortions, 2010; National and State Trends by Age, Race and Ethnicity.* New York: Guttmacher Institute; 2014. http://www.guttmacher.org/pubs/USTPtrends10.pdf.

54. Gaillard R, Durmus B, Hofman B, et al. Risk factors and outcomes of maternal obesity and excessive weight gain during pregnancy. *Obesity (Silver Spring).* 2013;21(5):1046–1065.

55. Cnattinguis S, Villamor E, Johansson S, et al. Maternal obesity and risk of preterm delivery. *JAMA.* 2013;309(22):2362–2370.

56. Haeri S, Guichard I, Baker AM, et al. The effect of teenage maternal obesity on perinatal outcomes. *Obstet Gynecol.* 2009;113(2 Pt 1):300–304.

57. Chang T, Choi H, Richardson CR, et al. Implications of teen birth for overweight and obesity in adulthood. *Am J Obstet Gynecol.* 2013;110:e1–e7.

58. Bellamy L, Casas J-P, Hingorani AD, et al. Type 2 diabetes mellitus after gestational diabetes: a systematic review and meta-analysis. *Lancet.* 2009;33:1773–1779.

59. Bentley-Lewis R. Late cardiovascular consequences of gestational diabetes mellitus. *Semin Reprod Med.* 2009;27:322–329.

60. Gunderson EP, Chiang V, Pletcher MJ, et al. History of gestational diabetes mellitus and future risk of atherosclerosis in mid-life: the Coronary Artery Risk Development in Young Adults study. *J Am Heart Assoc.* 2014;3:e000490.

61. O'Reilly JR, Reynolds RM. The risk of maternal obesity to the long-term health of the offspring. *Clin Endocrinol.* 2013;78(1):9–16.

62. Kim SY, Sharma AJ, Callaghan WM. Gestational diabetes and childhood obesity: what is the link? *Curr Opin Obstet Gynecol.* 2012;24(6):376–381.

63. Watkins ML, Rasmussen SA, Honein MA, et al. Maternal obesity and risk for birth defects. *Pediatrics.* 2003;111(Suppl 1):1152–1158.

64. Committee on Obesity in Pregnancy, American Congress of Obstetricians and Gynecologists. Practice/obesity in pregnancy. http://www.acog.org/Resources-and-Publications/Committee-Opinions/Committee-on-Obstetric Committee opinion number 49, January 2013. Accessed December 20, 2014.

65. Elements of youth-friendly contraceptive and reproductive health services. In: Fisher MM, Alderman EM, Kreipe RE, Rosenfeld WD, eds. *AAP Textbook of Adolescent Health Care.* Elk Grove Village, IL: American Academy of Pediatrics; 2011;427–643.

66. Bibbins-Domingo K, Coxson P, Pletcher MJ, Lightwood J, Goldman L. Adolescent overweight and future adult coronary heart disease. *N Engl J Med.* 2007;357:2371–2379.

67. NHLBI Working Group on High Blood Pressure. The fourth report on the diagnosis, evaluation and treatment of high blood pressure in children and adolescents. *Pediatrics.* 2004;114(2 suppl 4th report):555–576.

68. Flynn JT, Falkner BE. Obesity hypertension in adolescents: epidemiology, evaluation and management. *J Clin Hypertens.* 2011;13:323–331.

69. Watson SE, Hannon TS, Eckert GJ, et al. Adult hypertension risk is more than quadrupled in obese children. AHA, High Blood Pressure Research 2013 Scientific Sessions; New Orleans, LA. Abstract 036. http://my.americanheart.org/idc/groups/ahamah-public/@wcm/@sop/@scon/documents/downloadable/ucm_455971.pdf.

70. Kavey REW, Daniels SR, Flynn JT. Management of high blood pressure in children and adolescents. *Cardiol Clin.* 2010;28:597–607.

71. Flynn JT, Daniels SR, Hayman LL, et al. Update: ambulatory BP monitoring in children and adolescents. A scientific statement from the American Heart Association. *Hypertension.* 2014;63:1116–1135.

72. Juhola J, Magnussen CG, Berenson GS, et al. Combined effects of child and adult elevated blood pressure on subclinical atherosclerosis: the International Childhood Cardiovascular Consortium. *Circulation.* 2013;128(3):217–224.

73. Cook S, Kavey RE. Dyslipidemia and pediatric obesity. *Pediatr Clin North Am.* 2011;58(6):1363–1371.

74. Pratt RE, Kavey RE, Quinzi D. Combined dyslipidemia in obese children: response to a focused lifestyle approach. *J Clin Lipidol.* 2014;8(2):181–186.

75. Steinberger J, Daniels SR, Eckel RH, et al. Progress and challenges in metabolic syndrome in children and adolescents. A scientific statement from the American Heart Association. *Circulation.* 2009;119:628–647.

76. Dabalea D, Mayer-Davis EJ, Saydah S, et al. SEARCH for Diabetes in Youth Study. Prevalence of type 1 and type 2 diabetes among children and adolescents from 2001 to 2009. *JAMA.* 2014;311(17):1778–1786.

77. Copeland KC, Silverstein J, Moore KR, et al. Management of newly diagnosed type 2 diabetes mellitus(T2DM) in children and adolescents. Clinical practice guideline from the American Academy of Pediatrics. *Pediatrics.* 2013;131(2):364–382.

78. Davis CL, Pollock NK, Waller JL, et al. Exercise dose and diabetes risk in overweight and obese children. A randomized controlled trial. *JAMA.* 2012;308(11):1103–1112.

79. Kavey RE, Allada V, Daniels SR, et al. Cardiovascular risk reduction in high-risk pediatric patients: a scientific statement from the American Heart Association. Endorsed by the American Academy of Pediatrics. *Circulation.* 2006;114(24):2710–2738.

80. Giorgio V, Prono F, Graziano F, Nobili V. Pediatric non-alcoholic fatty liver disease: old and new concepts on development, progression, metabolic insight and potential treatment targets. *BMC Pediatr.* 2013;13:40–50.

81. Cerda C, Perez-Avuso RM, Riquelme A, et al. Nonalcoholic fatty liver disease in women with polycystic ovary syndrome. *J Hepatol.* 2007;47(3):412–417.

82. Nobili V, Marcellini M, Devito R, et al. NAFLD in children: a prospective clinical pathological study and effect of lifestyle advice. *Hepatology.* 2006;44:458–465.

83. Alkhouri N, Carter-Kent C, Elias M, Feldstein AE. Atherogenic dyslipidemia and cardiovascular risk in children with nonalcoholic fatty liver disease. *Clin Lipidol.* 2011;6(3):305–314.

84. Pacifico L, Chiesa C, Anania C, et al. Nonalcoholic fatty liver disease and the heart in children and adolescents. *World J Gatroenterol.* 2014;20(27):9055–9071.

85. Vajiro P, Lenta S, Socha P, et al. Diagnosis of NAFLD in children and adolescents: position paper of the ESPGHAN Hepatology Committee. *J Pediatr Gastroenterol Nutr*. 2012;54:700–713.

86. Devore S, Lake K, Nicholas L, et al. A multidisciplinary clinical program is effective in reducing BMI and ALT in pediatric patients with NAFLD. *J Pediatr Gastroenterol Nutr*. 2010;51:E68.

87. Lavine JE, Schwimmer JB, Natta ML, et al. Effect of vitamin E or metformin for treatment of NAFLD in children and adolescents. The TONIC randomized trial. *JAMA*. 2011;304:1659–1668.

Women With Disabilities and Obesity

Gizelda T. B. Casella, MD, PhD

INTRODUCTION

Health care for people with disability is not commonly discussed in health education, particularly in medical education, despite the increasing prevalence of people with disability within the United States. Clinicians have reported discomfort in managing the health of people with disability,[1] and people with disability often report negative experiences with their health care because of the practitioners' lack of knowledge.[2] There are clear health and health care disparities noted when comparing the care people with and without disability receive.[3,4] This is especially true for women with disability.[5-7] In general, disability is associated with obesity, and women with disability represent a large proportion of those with obesity and disability.

This chapter focuses on obesity and women with disability by providing definitions and background about the scope of the problem, presenting knowledge about nutrition and exercise or physical activity needs of women with disability, describing outcomes from weight management programs and interventions, and posing recommendations for practice. It is hoped that practitioners will better appreciate the needs and issues of women with disability as they relate to healthy weight management.

SCOPE OF THE PROBLEM

Definitions

Disability holds many meanings for professionals and consumers alike. Most people identify disability by diagnosis: cerebral palsy, spinal cord injury (SCI), multiple sclerosis, macular degeneration, or rheumatoid arthritis. Disability actually describes the mismatch between an impairment (e.g., loss of function of one side of the body due to a stroke or hemiparesis) and the environment (e.g., need to climb 5 steps to access a medical appointment); changing the environment with a ramp decreases the "disability" by allowing more independence or access. The World Health Organization has successfully promoted identifying disability by function: problems with mobility, self-care, cognition, vision/hearing, and living independently.[8] There is also often reference to activities of daily living (ADL), such as bathing and dressing, instrumental activities of daily living (IADL), such as shopping and driving, and employment or ability/limitations to work when discussing disability.

The US surveys (self- or family report) are increasingly using 6 functional disability characteristics (i.e., mobility, self-care, vision, cognition, independent living) to identify disability; however there is no etiology given for that specific disability of limitation. Thus, disability statistics in the United States identify limitations for any reason, including aging, injury, mental health, chronic diseases, and other defined conditions. A current review of national disability surveys noted four survey types (national household surveys; surveys of health, disability, aging, and long-term care; surveys of youth, education, and transition; and other surveys), for a total of 40 surveys that capture some elements of disability.[9] Data can be compared among surveys because of sampling, weighting, and other analyses that differ; some surveys have been updated or modified and cannot be compared to previous years. There are few registries (inclusive of all or most people who carry a specific diagnosis) supported in the United States, and some represent rare diseases. Typically, the more common disability diagnoses (e.g., stroke, cerebral palsy, SCI, traumatic brain injury) are not represented.

Epidemiology

Most recent disability statistics (self-reported functional limitations) note that 1 in 5 adult Americans (22.2% or 53,316,677 persons) report some type of functional disability, be it limitations in vision, cognition, mobility, or self-care or ability to live independently.[10] Women reported a higher prevalence of disability (24.4%) than men (19.8% disability in general or within the 5 categories increased with increasing age). Mobility limitation or physical disability is most frequently reported, followed by cognitive disability. These latest statistics are the results of a self-report survey (Behavior Risk Factor Surveillance System or BRFSS) and do not specify reasons for disability, as is true for most US national surveys.

Analyses of survey data showed that people with disability have a high rate of overweight and obesity,[11] and the association for women is higher.[12] However, there is no ability to determine cause and effect: Is obesity the cause of the disability, or is there actually a direct association with a specific type of disability? The prevalence of obesity in disability may vary by disability type or medical condition. People with intellectual disability (ID) do appear to have a higher risk for overweight or obesity;

specifically, women with ID appear to be at even more risk.[13,14] Diabetes tends to predispose to obesity.[15] Men and women with either mental health or physical disabilities appear to have a higher risk for obesity.[8] However "disability" is defined, women appear to show increasing disability with age and obesity.[10]

People with disability consistently have a higher rate of poverty than those without disability.[16] Barriers to changing that status include lack of accessible housing and transportation, access to education, and prejudices; all items affected by these barriers are needed to maintain health and a healthy weight. Poverty can be associated with unhealthy weight, both overweight and malnutrition. For people with disability and obesity/overweight, there is a significantly greater health care utilization and cost compared to those without disability.[17]

Measurement of Healthy Weight

An area that is receiving increasing attention is how obesity is measured or defined in disability. As seen in previous chapters, body mass index (BMI) commonly quantifies obesity. However, BMI initially was developed to identify sedentary behavior; because of the ease in administering this measurement technique, it has now become the standard by which we define obesity. However, BMI requires accurate weight and height measurement, both of which may not be possible for women with mobility limitations. Accurate weights for women using wheelchairs require an accessible scale. Accurate height measurement for women with contractures or amputation of both lower limbs may not be possible. A weight adjusted for limb loss should be the weight of concern, not the actual weight. Use of BMI as the standard does not take into account metabolic changes seen in many disability types or the acute or chronic muscle wasting or premature sarcopenia seen in people with long-term disability.[18]

Body composition and percentage body fat are the keys to determining healthy weight versus overweight and obesity. Typical measures used in health care to assess the presence of obesity, such as standard weights or BMI, are therefore mere proxies for the actual determination of healthy weight. While these typical measures may be appropriate in the general population, they may not be suitable for many disability types because of muscle wasting, fatty replacement, metabolic differences, or limb loss. Body composition and healthy weight status has been well studied in people with SCI. Those with SCI have higher body fat mass than controls for the same BMI,[19] and waist circumference (WC) underestimates abdominal (visceral) fat.[20]

In-depth assessment of visceral and subcutaneous fat is likely of more importance in disability than in the general population. Numerous studies reported limitations in standard measures for obesity in the population of people with disability. Measurements that are practical and have shown promise for use in some disability populations are WC and waist-to-hip ratio (WHR). Skinfold thickness and bioelectrical impedance analysis (BIA) have provided more in-depth understanding of body composition in disability populations and can be done in clinical settings. BMI may be accurate for people with ID; WHR has been shown to be a strong predictor of cardiometabolic risks for adults with cerebral palsy.[21]

However, none of these techniques has been standardized for disability types. The Amputee Coalition of America has developed a calculation to assist with determining weight status, although it has not been validated against body composition measures.[22] Research studies consider dual-energy x-ray absorptiometry (DEXA), hydrometry, and magnetic resonance imaging (MRI) to be accurate methods to assess body fat mass in any population; however, they are too expensive, time consuming, and impractical for clinical use.

Understanding that healthy weight in most types of disability links to body composition rather than to actual weight measurement or BMI is important. As well, it is important to understand that people with disability may have additional atypical problems with weight loss. Although weight loss in people with disability, especially fat mass loss, is associated with improved mobility,[23] weight loss must be carefully monitored to avoid worsening lean mass content and bone mineral loss, which may lead to malnourishment and therefore an aggravation of disability, especially in an elderly population.[24] Weight itself may not be the best primary outcome measure to evaluate success in weight management programs, but rather decrease in body fat, increase in muscle mass, improvement in mobility,[25] or decrease in inflammatory markers that accompany metabolic syndrome. There is no clear guidance for best practices; however, serial and accurate measures using the best and most practical method should be considered. It has been demonstrated that BMI does not accurately identify healthy weight in many types of disability.[26]

Barriers to Access/Participation in Health Promotion Activities

There are many public health programs designed to engage the public in weight loss or maintenance activities. However, accessibility for people with disability is often not considered. This is true for participation not only in weight maintenance programs but also in other forms of public health programs for women with disability, such as cancer screening.[6,7,27] There are two common reasons for limited participation: attitudinal and environmental. All too often, clinicians do not consider discussion of or referral for health promotion programs, including weight management. It is important for clinicians to understand that people with disability have a different perception of health than the general population; therefore, they may be less likely to ask questions about health-promoting behaviors.[28] The clinician's negative attitude is difficult to overcome and usually relates to the clinician's training experiences and previous patient encounters.

Environmental concerns include financial or insurance support, transportation to events, social supports, universal design to allow entry to facilities, sensory adjustments (e.g., large print or braille, sign language or interpreter), and modifications of activities needed for those with focal or generalized weakness, limited range of motion, use of wheelchairs and other equipment, and limited cognitive ability.[29,30] The Americans With Disability Act provides guidance for accessibility.[31] Inaccessible facilities, lack of knowledge about modifications to meet specific needs, poor attitudes, and unfriendly environments often create insurmountable barriers to participation for many people with disability. Besides the barriers noted, there are ways to promote weight management for people with disability that begin with engaging women with disability in discussions and decisions about their health (see Table 5-1).

TABLE 5-1 Barriers and Facilitators for Adults with Disability to Engage in Formal Weight Control Programs

Barriers	*Facilitators*
Personal lack of knowledge and skills	Engaging women with disability in discussions and decisions
Fear of injury or failure	Education or knowledge about healthy behaviors
Negative attitudes by health care providers and social supports	Creative and knowledgeable professionals
Poor family healthy behaviors	Formal goal setting
Stress, including personal and in the family network	Promotion of activities by health care professionals
Personal choices	Family support and participation
Fatigue	Involvement of friends and peers in activities
Lack of initiative	Desire to be active
Limited function or capability	Models or directions for participation with adaptations
Inability to control behaviors	Making activities a part of the routine: repetition and consistency promote ongoing activities
Inaccessible facilities or resources	Accessible facilities and opportunities, with knowledgeable staff
Need for aid assistance	Policies and resources promoting participation
Economic restrictions	
Policies and procedures of facilities or programs	

NUTRITION AND DISABILITY

People with disability face many barriers to access healthy foods that help in weight management, because of both disability and socioeconomic status[32,33] (see Table 5-2). Both urban and suburban neighborhoods have limited environmental accessibility and availability of affordable foods.[34] In addition to having the needed resources, people with disability may have problems with swallowing or chewing foods, further limiting options of healthy and affordable foods.[35] Medication use may also interfere with healthy food choices; medications may promote weight gain, stimulate appetite, or have other side effects that otherwise limit nutrition. Poor fruit and vegetable intake can be associated with ADL, IADL, and lower extremity impairments,[36] and decrease

TABLE 5-2 Barriers to Access Healthy Foods

Resource	*Description*
Human/social	Physical health Mobility independence Social support/personal assistance Cognitive ability Meal planning and food prep skills Knowledge of systems
Material	Finances Transportation Time
Contextual elements	Climate Safety Physical environment Local food access

in the intake of calcium, vitamin D, magnesium, and phosphorus is associated with decreased physical performance in elderly men and women.[37] In a prospective observational study of 2160 multiethnic women aged 42–52 years, Tomey et al.[38] observed that higher cholesterol, fat, and saturated fat intake increased the likelihood of physical limitation, and that lower intake of fruits, vegetables, and fibers was associated with reports of higher functional limitation. The use of supplements may improve this scenario. Women with disability tend to have higher odds of using dietary supplements, although increase in BMI does not appear to be associated with their use.[39]

People with disability have lower fat free mass and bone mineral content and higher fat mass than those without disability.[40] While this is typically attributed to a lower level of physical activity,[41] dietary imbalance (e.g., excessive intake of dietary fatty acid and simple carbohydrates) has also been implicated.[40] Increase in protein intake may be beneficial to maintain muscle mass during planned weight loss.[43]

EXERCISE AND PHYSICAL ACTIVITY AND DISABILITY

Exercise and physical activity are important for people with and without disability to maintain health and function. People with disability can participate in many levels of exercise and can benefit from aerobic and anaerobic exercise. Improving and maintaining function is certainly important for people with many types of disability and functional limitations. Of course, there may be a need for modifications to exercise. Many exercises can be modified for weakness and contracture, and equipment can be adjusted for use. People with disability, their health care providers, and others in their support systems often assume that engaging in routine activities, especially those activities that require significant work, are "exercise." However, maintaining typical daily activities is not exercise. Therefore, education about the need for and safety of exercise is important and required before there may be any consideration of participating in an exercise program. Many people with disability starting an exercise program often report fatigue with exercise, and this can be attributed to both the disability and previous sedentary lifestyles. Inactivity has been reported to be a major contributing factor to weight gain and deteriorating aerobic capacity, muscular fitness, and independence for people with disability.[44]

People with disability who have never exercised will be at a low level of performance with the additional challenge and consequently need guidance about starting an activity or exercise program. Therefore, providers and clinicians must be aware of the benefits of exercise for people with disability, as well as the possible complications. Osteoporosis is a risk for fracture, and aggressive or assisted exercise (e.g., strenuous weight lifting or use of functional electrical stimulation or robotics) should be used with caution and initially under supervision. Lower motor neuron injury weakness will have only a limited benefit from strengthening exercises, and aggressive exercise may increase weakness. Some disability types are progressive or not stable, and understanding the variability is important. Fitness practitioners with more education about disability, who hold various professional degrees related to physical activity and fitness, and who have had experience with diverse populations demonstrate more competence in directing those types of programs.[45]

WEIGHT MANAGEMENT PROGRAMS FOR WOMEN WITH DISABIILTY

Overview

People with disability have increased challenges to participating in organized weight control programs. They are at higher risk for poverty[46] and have less access to weight loss programs,[47] health clubs, accessible equipment for people with physical limitations,[30,48] affordable transportation,[49] or other social supports.[50] The common complaints of pain, fatigue, and weakness[51] often prevent them from participating or impede clinicians from making a referral for weight management. However, weight loss programs for people with many disability types have been shown to be feasible and efficacious, although usually through small or uncontrolled studies.[52] As in most programs that study weight management, the outcomes reported are only over limited time frames.

The 2013 Guideline for Managing Overweight and Obesity in Adults[53–55] summarizes the literature based on 5 questions. When considering people with disability, the answers to these questions may not be the same as for the general population.

1. Which person with disability needs to lose weight?

   As noted, people with disability are at risk for weight gain for a multiplicity of reasons. The typical sedentary lifestyle may be directly related to the disability or may have been chosen. Underlying metabolic issues or sarcopenia must be suspected or recognized by the clinician. As has been noted, use of BMI does not adequately identify healthy weight status for most people with disability. However, serial measures of some marker or change in function or fit of equipment should initiate consideration for further evaluation and initiating a weight loss program. Monitoring a marker serially during the weight reduction program is important, although percentage body fat should be the ultimate target.[30] Health-related fitness or functional status markers may also be used. There are no known differences between men and women with disability in determining candidates for weight loss programs.

2. For individuals with disability who can benefit from weight loss, what is the optimum level of weight loss?

   Improved cardiovascular health is an ultimate goal of weight loss. This would hold true for people with and without disability.[57] The target weight loss needs to be individualized, taking into account the cause and type of disability, the severity of the metabolic syndrome, the associated mobility impairment, and the presence of weakness, contracture, or other associated condition that may limit exercise. Again, decreasing the percentage body fat is key, although there has been no specific research to determine the optimal change required. The magnitude of weight loss should take into account typical health benefits and anticipated improvements in function. There have been no differences noted between men and women with disability.

3. Which diet is the most effective for weight loss in people with disabilities?

   As long as there is a negative energy balance (expenditure is greater than intake), no particular diet has proven to have higher efficacy. Standards used for the general population likely suffice in most instances. Estimates of total energy expenditure in people with disability need to take into account age, baseline disease, the lower activity level, and metabolic status[58-61]; gender does not appear to affect estimates. Estimates of the total energy expenditure can be obtained with the help of questionnaires specifically designed for people with disabilities.[62-66]

People with disability tend to have a lower baseline energy requirement. Weight loss requires an energy deficit, in this case without worsening the lean body mass. High-protein diets may prevent lean body mass loss in patients with sarcopenic obesity.[67] Protein-energy malnutrition that occurs with significantly lower food intake is associated with risk of falls and disability in the elderly[68,69]; supplementation with proteins and vitamin D diminishes this risk of falls and may prevent further disability.[70,71] As in the general population, a good estimate of typical caloric intake can be provided by 24-hour recalls, food-frequency questionnaires, and estimated diet records[72-74] with nutritional analysis software.[75]

Adults with functional mobility impairments appear to have a higher prevalence for metabolic syndrome[51,76]; therefore, consideration of those diet programs that focus on decreasing cardiometabolic risks may be of benefit.[77,78]

4. **For people with disability, is diet or exercise the best way to lose weight?**
    A successful weight loss program should include diet, physical activity, and behavioral counseling for changes whether or not a disability is present. The program content does not appear to be dependent on gender. Possible differences in styles of communication or modifications for disability (e.g., cognition, hearing impairment) should be acknowledged. When diet is associated with physical activity, there is greater weight loss and decrease in cardiometabolic risk.[79] Physical activity involves aerobic exercises to maximize fat loss, especially in visceral adipose tissue,[80] and resistance training (anaerobic exercise) to preserve lean body mass. People with disability may require adaptations to the exercise program to accommodate their physical limitations. Counseling for behavior change should take into account disability aspects, including modifications for cognitive impairments. Mobility and financial issues may prevent people with disability from accessing face-to-face counseling and supervision of physical activity. Nutritional counseling alone has been reported as ineffective for weight management and change in cardiovascular risk for people with disability,[81] and additional counseling for problem solving, stress management, and self-efficacy. Coaching, both on site[82] and web based,[83] appears to be beneficial in achieving weight loss for persons with disability.

5. **How can people with disability maintain weight loss?**
    For the general population, Wing and Hill[84] defined successful weight loss maintenance as intentional loss of at least 10% of body weight maintained for at least 1 year. Individuals who kept their weight off for 2 years or more were more likely to succeed in keeping it off. There are no specific data related to women with disability, but there may be some lessons to generalize from the larger population, modified for disability specific issues.[85] Healthy weight management requires behavioral lifestyle changes,[86] and there may be an additional component of support needed for people with disability.

6. **Should anyone with physical disability receive bariatric surgery?**
    Bariatric surgery may be offered to people whose BMI is greater than 40 or with a BMI above 35 and associated obesity comorbidities who have failed conservative

treatment.[54] People with disability are now also being offered bariatric surgery, and there are case reports and series related to adolescents and adults with spina bifida,[87] SCI,[88,89] ID,[90] Prader-Willi syndrome,[91,92] and multiple sclerosis.[93] In general, people with disability note similar benefits, such as decreased cardiovascular risks and improved physical functioning,[94] sleep, and health perception.[95] However, similar complications are also noted, and monitoring is required to determine disability-specific issues or responses.

At present, the indications for bariatric surgery for people with disability must be individualized. Typical BMI or other criteria used to recommend bariatric surgery and long-term safety need to be established for people with disability, given their higher prevalence of nutritional and neurological impairments. Significant weight loss or change to body composition through diet, exercise, and behavioral modifications may not be realistic in this population, leaving bariatric surgery as an effective and viable option.

Specific Disability Information and Programs
Spinal Cord Injury

Weight and body composition have been fairly well studied in SCI, and the majority of subjects are men by virtue of the underlying epidemiology. However, there is some information specific to women with SCI. The WC is commonly used to follow weight status and body composition, and a measurement above 88 cm indicates that a woman with SCI has increased cardiovascular risk. BMI above 22 kg/m^2 should be considered obese for a man or woman with SCI.[96] Resting energy expenditure or caloric need averages 1042 to 1290 kcal/d for women with SCI. Dietary recommendations for people with SCI have been adapted from the US Department of Agriculture (USDA) Dietary Guidelines for Americans 2010.[97] Recommendations are to follow general guidelines, with adjusted targets for WC and BMI.

There has been success reported for people with SCI and overweight/obesity participating in a weight control program, although only over a single time period.[98] The intervention was based in education on nutrition, exercise, stress management, and group support (much like programs for people without disability) and consisted of (1) caloric restriction diet of 1200 kcal for women and 1400 kcal for men; (2) 90-minute group classes led by a dietitian once a week for 12 weeks; (3) introduction of a 30-minute exercise session at week 6 to be continued at home. After the 12-week period of intervention, there were typical improvements in cardiovascular risk profiles and function; also, there was maintenance of bone mineral content and lean mass as assessed by DEXA and stable blood hemoglobin and serum albumin. Although not studied for efficacy, the University of Alabama at Birmingham Spinal Cord Injury Model System (UAB-SCIMS) has a free web-based program, the EatRight® Weight Management Program, for people with SCI and disorders. It consists of a 12-week program that includes a workbook and a video. The EatRight Weight Management Program promotes foods with low energy density and high complex carbohydrates.[99]

Bariatric surgery has been performed in persons with paraplegia who have failed conservative treatment. Significant weight loss and improved cardiovascular risk profile was achieved.[88,89] Although improved mobility was noted in these reports, an additional report indicated improved profile and no change in functional status.[100]

Stroke

Again, there has not been an assessment of BMI or WC for determining obesity in people poststroke, and standard criteria are used. Weight loss should be pursued if BMI is 30 kg/m^2 or greater or BMI is 25 to 29.9 30 kg/m^2 with either an increased WC (>102 cm for men and >88 cm for women) or at least 2 additional cardiovascular risk factors (hypertension, diabetes mellitus, and dyslipidemia).[101]

Stroke survivors in a predominantly African American community proved effective in reducing cholesterol and weight, increasing fitness and life satisfaction, and decreasing social isolation through a 12-week intervention.[102] The intervention consisted of meeting for 3 days a week for 12 weeks of fitness and nutrition education, physical activity, and health behavior changes. The program, including transportation, was offered at no cost and provided a place to perform the exercises and a personalized program to minimize fatigue.[47] A low-fat, low-cholesterol diet with substitutions appropriate to a patient's budget and preferences were emphasized. The curriculum for the health behavior consisted of education on stroke risk factors, goal setting, stress management, and change in societal role, among others. Although actual weight and BMI improved, there was no change in WHR and skinfold thickness. There were no differences in outcomes between men and women stroke survivors.

A promising randomized controlled trial using the SystemCHANGE™ has been proposed by Plow et al.[103] to manage obesity in stroke survivors. The SystemCHANGE consists of a comprehensive weight management program combining diet, physical activity, and sleep management. The proposed diet, with an increase in fruits and vegetables and limitation of fatty foods, is based on the Guidelines for Americans 2010.[104] Physical activity will be based in a graded strength training program of major muscle groups. Education on sleep hygiene and techniques to achieve better quality sleep and adequate sleep duration are important components of the program due to the association between obesity and sleep disturbances.[105-107] This intervention will be administered through 12 face-to-face group meetings during 3 months and then 3 more months of follow-up phone calls. The control group will be individuals who will receive pamphlets with information on diet, physical activity, and sleep, along with follow-up calls.

Limb Loss

People with limb loss, especially lower limb loss, from dysvascular causes such as diabetes mellitus and peripheral vascular disease should be monitored for weight control. From a practical perspective, a person using a lower limb prosthesis must be mindful of the increased cardiac demand of walking (may be a 100%–200% increase depending on level of amputation and bilaterality) and the weight restrictions for use of high-performance components (e.g., knee and ankle/foot components, socket and suspension designs). Excess weight compounds the orthopedic and cardiovascular effects for the amputee. Reports note metabolic demands with walking increase dramatically with below-knee (transtibial) and above-knee (transfemoral) amputations. As has already been noted, accurate weight status is difficult to determine. The Amputee Coalition of America has developed a calculation for determining healthy weight measurement[22] and has resources for education about the importance of weight management. In a study of weight loss intention and barriers to dietary changes in veterans with lower limb amputations, there were few participants who engaged in a comprehensive organized program,[108] despite recognizing the need. Weight management strategies and programs should be a part of health discussions with women with limb loss.

Intellectual Disability

In a recent analysis of an ongoing longitudinal health and ID study, adults with ID, compared to the general population, have a higher prevalence of obesity and severe obesity. Being female, having Down syndrome, taking medications associated with weight gain (e.g., medications for depression, hypertension, anxiety, epilepsy, diabetes, or sleep disorder), less physical activity, and drinking large amounts of soda were associated with higher rates of obesity.[109] Therefore, women with ID should be monitored for weight status, and it appears that WC, WHR, and BMI may be used for that monitoring.

A variety of weight management and health promotion programs have been studied related to people with ID. Most employed a group education strategy about nutrition, physical activity and exercise, and lifestyle changes, all modified for cognitive limitations, for up to 7 months.[110,111] Group physical activity or exercise was also offered. For those programs showing success with changes to BMI or increase in physical activity, there was follow-up and on-site support. However, these changes may not be long lasting without continued support systems in place.

McDermott et al. noted that decreased BMI did not continue to the 1-year follow-up. In a nutrition-only focused program, in-home support for basic menu planning was needed to effect change, although long-term follow-up was not done.[112] A program solely for women with ID covered an 8-week curriculum on women's health, including weight management, and was well attended, but efficacy was not established.[113] It would appear that a modified curriculum with ongoing support and follow-up (for people with ID and their care providers) is necessary to maintain long-term lifestyle changes and decreased cardiovascular risks. Outcome measures, however, should be targeting body composition and percentage body fat.[55]

Multiple Sclerosis

Overweight and obesity have been reported in 50%–70% of persons with multiple sclerosis. Reasons for this include decreased physical activity, glucocorticoid treatment, and chronic inflammation. The majority of health promotion programs for women with multiple sclerosis focus on self-efficacy, rather than weight management.[114,115] In a study of the health beliefs of individuals with multiple sclerosis, participants focused more on physical conditioning and functioning rather than on general health conditions and recognized that overweight would result from decreased activity. Participants (84% women) believed they would benefit from physical activity and remain healthy, even in the context of their disease and progression. Those who scored high on self-efficacy and appreciation of the benefits of exercise were more likely to participate in exercise and physical activity.[116]

Across Disability Types

The majority of weight management and health promotion programs for people with disability studied have included people with many disability types, rather than focusing on a specific disability type. Important aspects of successful programs involve ongoing support, such as routine goal setting with updates, comradery with peers, group education sessions, and routine coaching by staff (see Table 5-3).

TABLE 5-3 Across Disability Weight Management Programs

Author	Disability Types	Design/Intervention	Outcome Measures	Results
Horner-Johnson et al., 2011[117]	Adults with physical, sensory, cognitive, mental health, other, multiple	$N = 95$; randomized controlled trial with wait list comparison Health Lifestyles curriculum in 2.5-day workshop and monthly 2-hour support groups	Health Promoting Lifestyle Profile II at baseline and 4, 7, and 10 months and following 9 months of support group; focus on PA, nutrition, heath responsibility, spiritual growth, stress management, interpersonal relationships	Significant improvement all subscales in intervention group; wait list group also improved after participation
Reichard et al., 2015[50]	Adults with low-income and mobility impairments	126 enrolled; 98 completed; 60 at 1-year follow-up; comparison randomized across "usual care" diet education and Stoplight Diet, both modified for disability 12 months simple regular exercise based on ability + 6 months active dieting, then 6 months diet or weight management Monthly meetings with coach for 6 months; food models for portion size Incentivized diet and BMI change first 6 months at meetings	Accurate weight/height, BMI Daily diet nutrition tracking form; 24-hour diet recall at monthly meeting; analyzed for nutrition/calories Satisfaction survey completed when leaving or completing program	Both diets resulted in weight loss Stoplight Diet with weight loss 6 and 12 months; usual care at 6 months only Food costs noted as problematic Portion control more effective than limiting portions
Rimmer et al., 2013[83]	Adults with SCI, multiple sclerosis, spinabifida (SB), cerebral palsy, stroke, lupus	$N = 102$; randomized to 3 groups: physical activity (PA) only, PA plus nutrition, and control Intervention: online tool kit and coaching First 4 months: weekly phone coaching to set goals Last 5 months: decreasing calls Monthly newsletter and personal feedback	Measured height/weight, BMI PA and Disability Interview Survey Barriers to PA Fat- and fiber-related dietary behaviors	Decreased weight and BMI in intervention groups

Although people with disability may appreciate the benefits of exercise and activity, a common concern or difficulty to overcome is the "hard work" or fatigue associated with organizing and participating in the activity.[43] An innovative approach, in which women with disability were in the majority, using a telephone and web-based coaching strategy was successful, with positive changes in biomedical markers, physical activity, and nutrition intake.[83]

RECOMMENDATIONS

Obesity is commonly seen in disability, and women in particular are at increased risk for this. Measurement of healthy weight status should relate to body composition and body fat, and for the most part BMI should not be used. Sarcopenia and the metabolic syndrome are likely common in disability, although there has not been standardization of measurements for each disability type, and further research is needed. There is no clear guidance for best practices; however, serial and accurate measures using the best and most practical method should be considered. There should be vigilance in monitoring healthy weight for women with disability.

Women with a variety of disability types can participate in exercise, although there may be guidance needed. Health maintenance programs, including education for and direction on diet, exercise, and counseling for lifestyle changes and continuation of maintenance programs, have been proven effective for improving cardiovascular risk profiles, healthy weight status, and function for men and women with disability. Key elements are similar to the general population and include modification of approaches for disability (e.g., environmental accessibility, cognitive accessibility, multiple modalities for sensory impairments) and ongoing follow-up and coaching. Maintaining support through some type of consistent coaching may result in longer-lasting participation and improvements.

REFERENCES

1. Wilkinson J, Dreyfus D, Cerreto M, Bokhour B. "Sometimes I feel overwhelmed": educational needs of the family physicians caring for people with intellectual disabilities. *Intellect Develop Disabil.* 2012;50(3):243–250.

2. Iezzoni LI, Long-Bellil LM. Training physicians about caring for persons with disabilities: "Nothing about us without us!" *Disabil Health J.* 2012;5(2):136–139.

3. Iezzoni LI, Ngo LH, Li D, et al. Treatment disparities for disabled Medicare beneficiaries with stage I non-small cell lung cancer. *Arch Phys Med Rehabil.* 2008;89:595–601.

4. Mahmoudi E, Meade MA. Disparities in access to health care among adults with physical disabilities: analysis of a representative national sample for a 10-year period. *Disabil Health J.* 2015;8:182–190.

5. McCarthy EP, Ngo LH, Roetzheim RG, et al. Disparitieis in breast cancer treatment and survival for women with disabilities. *Ann Intern Med.* 2006; 145:637–645.

6. Llewellyn G, Balandin S, Poulos A, McCarthy L. Disability and mammography screening: intangible barriers to participation. *Disabil Rehabil.* 2011;33(19–20):1755–1767.

7. Reichard A, Stolzle H, Fox MH. Health disparities among adults with physical disabilities or cognitive limitations compared to individuals with no disabilities in the United States. *Disabil Health J.* 2011;4:59–67.

8. United Nations World Health Organization (WHO) and World Bank. General health care. In: *World Report on Disability.* Geneva, Switzerland: WHO; 2011:57–92. http://www.refworld.org/docid/50854a322.html. Accessed December 9, 2015.

9. Livermore G, Whalen D, Prenovitz S, Aggarwal R, Bardos M. Disability data in national surveys. http://www.hppd.vcu.edu/documents/2012/DisabilityDatainNationalSurveysAugust2011.pdf. August 22, 2011. Accessed December 2, 2015.

10. Courtney-Long EA, Carroll DD, Zhang QC, et al. Prevalence of disability and disability type among adults—United States, 2013. *MMWR Morb Mortal Wkly Rep.* 2015, July 31;64(29):777–783.

11. An R, Andrade F, Chiu C-Y. Overweight and obesity among US adults with and without disabilities. *Prev Med Rep.* 2015;2:419–422.

12. Armour BS, Courtney-Long E, Campbell VA, Wethington HR. Estimating disability prevalence among adults by body mass index: 2003–2009 National Health Interview Survey. *Prev Chronic Dis.* 2012;9:120136.

13. deWinter CF, Bastiaanse LP, Hilgenkamp TIM, Evenhuis HM, Echteld MA. Overweight and obesity in older people with intellectual disability. *Res Dev Disabil.* 2012;33:398–405.

14. Mikulovic J, Vanhelts J, Salleron J, et al. Overweight in intellectually-disabled population: physical, behavioral and psychological characteristics. *Res Dev Disabil.* 2014;35:153–161.

15. Rimmer JH, Wang E. Obesity prevalence among a group of Chicago residents with disabilities. *Arch Phys Med Rehabil.* 2005;86(7):1461–1464.

16. Brucker DL, Houtenvillw AJ. People with disabilities in the United States. *Arch Phys Med Rehabil.* 2015;96:771–774.

17. Peterson MD, Mahmoudi E. Healthcare utilization associated with obesity and physical disability. *Am J Prev Med.* 2015;48(4):426–435.

18. Peterson MD, Gordon PM, Hurvitz EA. Chronic disease risk among adults with cerebral palsy: the role of premature sarcopenia, obesity and sedentary behavior. *Obes Rev.* 2013;14:171–182.

19. Jones LM, Legge M, Goulding A. Healthy body mass index values often underestimate body fat in men

with spinal cord injury. *Arch Phys Med Rehabil.* 2003;84(7):1068–1071.

20. Edwards LA, Bugaresti JM, Buchholz AC. Visceral adipose tissue and the ratio of visceral to subcutaneous adipose tissue are greater in adults with than in those without spinal cord injury, despite matching waist circumferences. *Am J Clin Nutr.* 2008;87(3):600–607.

21. Peterson MD, Haapala HJ, Hurvitz EA. Predictors of cardiometabolic risk among adulst with cerebral palsy. *Arch Phys Med Rehabil.* 2012;93:816–821.

22. Amputee Coalition of America. Limb Loss Resource Center. About BMI. http://www.amputee-coalition. org/limb-loss-resource-center/resources-by-topic/ healthy-living/about-bmi/. Accessed December 2, 2015.

23. Beavers KM, Miller ME, Rejeski WJ, Nicklas BJ, Kritchevsky SB. Fat mass loss predicts gain in physical function with intentional weight loss in older adults. *J Gerontol A Biol Sci Med Sci.* 2013;68(1):80–86.

24. Morley JE, von Haehling S, Anker SD, Vellas B. From sarcopenia to frailty: a road less traveled. *J Cachexia Sarcopenia Muscle.* 2014;5(1):5–8.

25. Plow MA, Moore S, Husni ME, Kirwan JP. A systematic review of behavioural techniques used in nutrition and weight loss interventions among adults with mobility-impairing neurological and musculoskeletal conditions. *Obes Rev.* 2014;15(12):945–956.

26. Wells JCK, Fewtrell MS. Measuring body composition. *Arch Dis Child.* 2006;91:612–617.

27. Smeltzer SC. Preventive health screening for brest and cervical cancer and osteoporosis in women with disabilities. *Fam Community Health.* 2006;29(Suppl 1): 35S–43S.

28. Drum CE, Horner-Johnson W, Krahn GL. Self-rated health and healthy days: examining the "disability paradox." *Disabil Health J.* 2008;1:71–78.

29. Rimmer JH, Hsieh K, Graham BC, Gerber BS, Gray-Stanley JA. Barrier removal in increasing physical activity levels in obese African American women with disabilities. *J Womens Health.* 2010;19(10):1869–1876.

30. Rimmer JH, Riley B, Wang E, Rauworth A. Accessibility of health clubs for people with mobility disabilities and visual impairments. *Am J Public Health.* 2005;95(11):2022–2028.

31. US Department of Justice, Civil Rights Division, Disability Rights Section. Accessible information exchange: meeting on a level playing field. http:// www.ada.gov/business/accessiblemtg.htm. Accessed December 2, 2015.

32. Campbell CC. Food insecurity: a nutritional outcome or a predictor variable? *J Nutr.* 1991;121(3):408–415.

33. Webber CB, Sobal J, Dollahite JS. Physical disabilities and food access among limited resource households. *Disabil Stud Q.* 2007;27(3):9–21.

34. Mojtahedi MC, Boblick P, Rimmer JH, Rowland JL, Jones RA, Braunschweig CL. Environmental barriers to and availability of healthy foods for proplr with mobility disabilities living in urban and suburban neighborhoods. *Arch Phys Med Rehabil.* 2008;89(11):2174–2179.

35. Centers for Disease Control and Prevention, National Center on Birth Defects and Developmental Disabilities. Disability and obesity. http://www. cdc.gov/ncbddd/disabilityandhealth/obesity.html. Accessed December 2, 2015.

36. Houston DK, Stevens J, Cai J, Haines PS. Dairy, fruit, and vegetable intakes and functional limitations and disability in a biracial cohort: the Atherosclerosis Risk in Communities Study. *Am J Clin Nutr.* 2005;81(2):515–522.

37. Sharkey JR, Giulianic, Haines PS, Branch LG, Busby-Whitehead J, Zohoori N. Summary measure of dietary musculoskeletal nutrient (calcium, vitamin D, magnesium, and phosphorus) intakes is associated with lower-extremity physical performance in homebound elderly men and women. *Am J Clin Nutr.* 2003;77(4): 847–856.

38. Tomey KM, et al. Dietary intake related to prevalent functional limitations in midlife women. *Am J Epidemiol.* 2008;167(8):935–943.

39. An R, Chiu CY, Andrade F. Nutrient intake and use of dietary supplements among US adults with disabilities. *Disabil Health J.* 2015;8(2):240–249.

40. Bertoli S, et al. Nutritional status and dietary patterns in disabled people. *Nutr Metab Cardiovasc Dis.* 2006;16(2):100–112.

41. Straight CR, Brady AO, Evans E. Sex-specific relationships of physical activity, body composition, and muscle quality with lower-extremity physical function in older men and women. *Menopause.* 2015;22(3):297–303.

43. Ormsbee MJ, et al. Osteosarcopenic obesity: the role of bone, muscle, and fat on health. *J Cachexia Sarcopenia Muscle.* 2014;5(3):183–192.

44. Malone LA, Baarfield JP, Brasher JD. Oerceived benefits and barriers to exercise among persons with physical disabilities orchornic health conditions within action or maintenance stages of exercise. *Disabil Health J.* 2012;5:254–260.

45. Kasser SL, Rizzo T. An exploratory study of fitness practitioner intentions toward exercise programming for individuals with multiple sclerosis. *Disabil Health J.* 2013;6:188–194.

46. Turk MA, Mudumbi SV. The United States' response to the World Report on Disability. *Am J Phys Med Rehabil.* 2014;93(1 Suppl 1):S27–S35.

47. Kinne S, Patrick DL, Doyle DL. Prevalence of secondary conditions among people with disabilities. *Am J Public Health.* 2004;94(3):443–445.

48. Arbour-Nicitopoulos KP, Ginis KA. Universal accessibility of "accessible" fitness and recreational facilities for persons with mobility disabilities. *Adapt Phys Activ Q.* 2011;28(1):1–15.

49. Rimmer JH, Wang E, Smith D. Barriers associated with exercise and community access for individuals with stroke. *J Rehabil Res Dev.* 2008;45(2):315–322.

50. Reichard A, Saunders MD, Saunders RR, et al. A comparison of two weight management programs for adults with mobility impairments. *Disabil Health J.* 2015;8(1):61–69.

51. Weil E, et al. Obesity among adults with disabling conditions. *JAMA.* 2002;288(10):1265–1268.

52. Bazzano AT, et al. The Healthy Lifestyle Change Program: a pilot of a community-based health promotion intervention for adults with developmental disabilities. *Am J Prev Med.* 2009;37(6 Suppl 1):S201–S208.

53. Jensen MD, et al. 2013 AHA/ACC/TOS guideline for the management of overweight and obesity in adults: a report of the American College of Cardiology/American Heart Association Task Force on Practice Guidelines and the Obesity Society. *Circulation.* 2014;129(25 Suppl 2):S102–S138.

54. Jensen MD, et al. 2013 AHA/ACC/TOS guideline for the management of overweight and obesity in adults: a report of the American College of Cardiology/American Heart Association Task Force on Practice Guidelines and the Obesity Society. *J Am Coll Cardiol.* 2014;63(25 Pt B):2985–3023.

55. Ryan D, Heaner M. Guidelines (2013) for managing overweight and obesity in adults. Preface to the full report. *Obesity (Silver Spring).* 2014;22(Suppl 2):S1–S3.

56. Casey AF, Rasmussen R. Reduction measures and percent body fat in individuals with intellectual disabilities: a scoping review. *Disabil Health J.* 2013;6:2–7.

57. Canadian Agency for Drugs and Technologies in Health. *Obesity Management Interventions Delivered in Primary Care for Patients with Hypertension or Cardiovascular Disease: A Review of Clinical Effectiveness.* Ottawa: Canadian Agency for Drugs and Technologies in Health; 2014.

58. Buchholz AC, McGillivray CV, Pencharz PB. Differences in resting metabolic rate between paraplegic and able-bodied subjects are explained by differences in body composition. *Am J Clin Nutr.* 2003;77(2):371–378.

59. Monroe MB, et al. Lower daily energy expenditure as measured by a respiratory chamber in subjects with spinal cord injury compared with control subjects. *Am J Clin Nutr.* 1998;68(6):1223–1227.

60. Alexander LR, et al. Resting metabolic rate in subjects with paraplegia: the effect of pressure sores. *Arch Phys Med Rehabil.* 1995;76(9):819–822.

61. Bauman WA, et al. The relationship between energy expenditure and lean tissue in monozygotic twins discordant for spinal cord injury. *J Rehabil Res Dev.* 2004;41(1):1–8.

62. de Groot S, et al. Evaluation of the physical activity scale for individuals with physical disabilities in people with spinal cord injury. *Spinal Cord.* 2010;48(7):542–547.

63. Washburn RA, et al. The physical activity scale for individuals with physical disabilities: development and evaluation. *Arch Phys Med Rehabil.* 2002;83(2):193–200.

64. Rimmer JH, Riley BB, Rubin SS. A new measure for assessing the physical activity behaviors of persons with disabilities and chronic health conditions: the Physical Activity and Disability Survey. *Am J Health Promot.* 2001;16(1):34–42.

65. van der Ploeg HP, et al. The Physical Activity Scale for Individuals With Physical Disabilities: test-retest reliability and comparison with an accelerometer. *J Phys Act Health.* 2007;4(1):96–100.

66. Latimer AE, et al. The physical activity recall assessment for people with spinal cord injury: validity. *Med Sci Sports Exerc.* 2006;38(2):208–216.

67. Li Z, Heber D. Sarcopenic obesity in the elderly and strategies for weight management. *Nutr Rev.* 2012;70(1):57–64.

68. Johnson CS. The association between nutritional risk and falls among frail elderly. *J Nutr Health Aging.* 2003;7(4):247–250.

69. Zoltick ES, et al. Dietary protein intake and subsequent falls in older men and women: the Framingham Study. *J Nutr Health Aging.* 2011;15(2):147–152.

70. Neelemaat F, et al. Short-term oral nutritional intervention with protein and vitamin D decreases falls in malnourished older adults. *J Am Geriatr Soc.* 2012;60(4):691–699.

71. Cederholm T, et al. The role of malnutrition in older persons with mobility limitations. *Curr Pharm Des.* 2014;20(19):3173–3177.

72. Beer-Borst S, Amado R. Validation of a self-administered 24-hour recall questionnaire used in a large-scale dietary survey. *Z Ernahrungswiss.* 1995;34(3):183–189.

73. Bingham SA, et al. Comparison of dietary assessment methods in nutritional epidemiology: weighed records v. 24 h recalls, food-frequency questionnaires and estimated-diet records. *Br J Nutr.* 1994;72(4):619–643.

74. De Keyzer W, et al. Relative validity of a short qualitative food frequency questionnaire for use in food consumption surveys. *Eur J Public Health.* 2013;23(5):737–742.

75. US Department of Agriculture, Healthy Meals Resource System. Nutrient analysis software approved

76. Peterson MD, et al. Obesity misclassification and the metabolic syndrome in adults with functional mobility impairments: Nutrition Examination Survey 2003–2006. *Prev Med*. 2014;60:71–76.

77. Sacks FM, et al. Effects on blood pressure of reduced dietary sodium and the Dietary Approaches to Stop Hypertension (DASH) diet. DASH-Sodium Collaborative Research Group. *N Engl J Med*. 2001;344(1): 3–10.

78. Kastorini CM, et al. The effect of Mediterranean diet on metabolic syndrome and its components: a meta-analysis of 50 studies and 534,906 individuals. *J Am Coll Cardiol*. 2011;57(11):1299–1313.

79. Dombrowski SU, Avenell A, Sniehott FF. Behavioural interventions for obese adults with additional risk factors for morbidity: systematic review of effects on behaviour, weight and disease risk factors. *Obes Facts*. 2010;3(6):377–396.

80. Ismail I, et al. A systematic review and meta-analysis of the effect of aerobic vs. resistance exercise training on visceral fat. *Obes Rev*. 2012;13(1):68–91.

81. Bertoli S, et al. Nutritional counselling in disabled people: effects on dietary patterns, body composition and cardiovascular risk factors. *Eur J Phys Rehabil Med*. 2008;44(2):149–158.

82. Bazzano AT, Zeldin AS, Diab IR, et al. WRC Project Oversight Team. The Healthy Lifestyle Change Program: a pilot of a community-based health promotion intervention for adults with developmental disabilities. *Am J Prev Med*. 2009 Dec;37(6 Suppl 1): S201–S208.

83. Rimmer JH, Wang E, Pellegrini CA, LulloC, Gerber BS. Telehealth weight management intervention for adults with physical disabilities: a randomized controlled trial. *Am J Phys Med Rehabil*. 2013;92(12):1084–1094.

84. Wing RR, Hill JO. Successful weight loss maintenance. *Annu Rev Nutr*. 2001;21:323–341.

85. Wing RR, Phelan S. Long-term weight loss maintenance. *Am J Clin Nutr*. 2005;82(1 Suppl):222S–225S.

86. Kruger J, Blanck HM, Gillespie C. Dietary practices, dining out behavior, and physical activity correlates of weight loss maintenance. *Prev Chronic Dis*. 2008;5(1):A11.

87. Miyano G, Kalra M, Inge TH. Adolescent paraplegia, morbid obesity, and pickwickian syndrome: outcome of gastric bypass surgery. *J Pediatr Surg*. 2009;44(3):e41–e44.

88. Alaedeen DI, Jasper J. Gastric bypass surgery in a paraplegic morbidly obese patient. *Obes Surg*. 2006;16(8):1107–1108.

89. Wong S, et al. Morbid obesity after spinal cord injury:an ailment not to be treated? *Eur J Clin Nutr*. 2013;67(9):998–999.

90. Heinberg LJ, Schauer PR. Intellectual disability and baratric surgery: a case study of optimization and outcome. *Surg Obes Relat Dis*. 2014;10:e105–e108.

91. Marceau P, Marceau S, Biron S, et al. Long-term experience with duodenal switch in adolescents. *Obes Surg*. 2010;20(12):1609–1616.

92. Lloret-Linares C, Faucher P, Coupaye M, et al. Camparison of body composition, basal metabolic rate and metabolic outcomes of adults with Prader Willi syndrome or lesion hypothalamic disease with primary obesity. *Int J Obes (Lond)*. 2013;37(9):1198–11203.

93. Lutrzykowski M. Bariatric surgery in morbidly obese patients in wheelchairs. *Obes Surg*. 2008;18(12):1647–1648.

94. Steele T, Cuthbertson DJ, Wilding JP. Impact of bariatric surgery on physical functioning in obese adults. *Obes Rev*. 2015;16(3):248–258.

95. Choban PS, et al. A health status assessment of the impact of weight loss following Roux-en-Y gastric bypass for clinically severe obesity. *J Am Coll Surg*. 1999;188(5):491–497.

96. Laughton GE, et al. Lowering body mass index cutoffs better identifies obese persons with spinal cord injury. *Spinal Cord*. 2009;47(10):757–762.

97. Kressler J, et al. Reducing cardiometabolic disease in spinal cord injury. *Phys Med Rehabil Clin N Am*. 2014;25(3):573–604, viii.

98. Chen Y, et al. Obesity intervention in persons with spinal cord injury. *Spinal Cord*. 2006;44(2):82–91.

99. University of Alabama Spinal Cord Injury Model System. EatRight® Weight Management Program. https://www.uab.edu/medicine/sci/uab-scims-information/eatrightr-weight-management-program. Accessed December 2, 2015.

100. Caruso D, Tower D, Goetz L. Roux-en-Y gastric bypass for intractable biliary reflux in an individual with incomplete tetraplegia. *J Spinal Cord Med*. 2015;38(4):556–558.

101. Clinical guidelines on the identification, evaluation, and treatment of overweight and obesity in adults: executive summary. Expert Panel on the Identification, Evaluation, and Treatment of Overweight in Adults. *Am J Clin Nutr*. 1998;68(4):899–917.

102. Rimmer JH, et al. Effects of a short-term health promotion intervention for a predominantly African-American group of stroke survivors. *Am J Prev Med*. 2000;18(4):332–338.

103. Plow M, et al. Randomized controlled pilot study of a SystemCHANGE weight management intervention in stroke survivors: rationale and protocol. *Trials*. 2013;14:130.

104. US Department of Health and Human Services and US Department of Agriculture, eds. *Dietary Guidelines Advisory Committee: Dietary Guidelines for Americans, 2010*. Washington, DC: US Department of Health and Human Services and US Department of Agriculture; 2010.
105. Taheri S. The link between short sleep duration and obesity: we should recommend more sleep to prevent obesity. *Arch Dis Child*. 2006;91(11):881–884.
106. Taheri S, Mignot E. Sleep well and stay slim: dream or reality? *Ann Intern Med*. 2010;153(7):475–476.
107. Nedeltcheva AV, et al. Insufficient sleep undermines dietary efforts to reduce adiposity. *Ann Intern Med*. 2010;153(7):435–441.
108. Littman AJ, McFarland LV, Thmpsons ML, et al. Weight loss intention, dietary behaviors, and barriers to dietary change in veterans with lower extremity amputations. *Disabil Health J*. 2015;8:325–335.
109. Hsieh K, Rimmer JH, Heller T. Obesity and associated factors in adults with intellectual disability. *J Intellect Disabil Res*. 2014;58(9):851–863.
110. Mann J, Zhou H, McDermott S, Poston MB. Health behavior change of adults with mental retardation:attendance in a health promotion program. *Am J Ment Retard*. 2006 Jan;111(1):62–73.
111. McDermott S, Whitner W, Thomas-Koger M, et al. An efficacy trial of "Steps to Your Health," a health promotion programme for adults with intellectual disability. *Health Educ J*. 2012;71(3):278–290.
112. Humphres K, Pepper A, Traci MA, Olson J. Nutritional intervention improves menu adequacy in group homes for adults with intellectual or developmental disabilities. *Disabil Health J*. 2009;2:136-144.
113. Lunsky Y, Straik A, Armstrong. Women Be Healthy: evaluation of a women's health curriculum for women with intellectual disabilities. *J Appl Res Intell Disabil*. 2003;16(4):247–253.
114. Stuifbergen AK, Becker H, Blozis S, Timmerman G, Kullberg V. A randomized clinical trial of a wellness intervention for women with multiple sclerosis. *Arch Phys Med Rehabil*. 2003;84:467–476.
115. Jongen PJ, Ruimschotel R, Heerings M, et al. Improved self-efficacy in persons with relapsing remitting multiple sclerosis after intensive social cognitive wellness program with participation of support partners: a 6-months observational study. *Health Qual of Life Outcomes*. 2014;12:40.
116. Kasser SL, Kosma M. Health beliefs and physical activity behaviors in adults with multiple sclerosis. *Disabil Health J*. 2012;5:261–268.
117. Horner-Johnson W, Drum CE, Abdullah N. A randomized trial of a health promotion intervention for adults with disabilities. *Disabil Health J*. 2011 Oct;4(4):254–261.

Heart Disease

CHAPTER 6

Benjamin Silverman, MD

Lilian Msambichaka, MD

John Donnelly, MD

INTRODUCTION

Cardiovascular disease (CVD) is the leading cause of death among women worldwide, causing 1 in every 4 female deaths.[1] Although 1 of 4 women in the United States has some form of CVD, only 54% of women recognize that heart disease is their number 1 killer.[2] Multiple studies have noted that women tend to have a higher mortality and morbidity from cardiovascular events compared to men. Women are less likely than men to receive aggressive or invasive treatment for heart disease compared to men.[3] There is also often a failure for both health care providers and women themselves to recognize either the underlying risks or the associated symptoms of CVD.[4] It is therefore imperative for health care providers to understand its risk factors and recommendations regarding the management of this disease.

RISK CALCULATORS

Calculation of a woman's 10-year risk of cardiovascular events is an important step in assisting women to know which modifiable risk factors could influence the risk of future disease. A 10-year risk score of CVD has become standard as an assessment tool for risk stratification. A 10-year risk of coronary heart disease (CHD) can be determined based on age, gender, and conventional risk factors, including high blood pressure (BP), dyslipidemia, glucose intolerance, and smoking.[5]

The first major model was the Framingham risk calculator. The original Framingham risk prediction algorithm to predict CHD (known as FRS-CHD) incorporated age; sex; diabetes; systolic and diastolic BPs; levels of total, low-density lipoprotein, and high-density lipoprotein cholesterol; and smoking to estimate a 10-year risk for angina, myocardial infarction (MI), or death due to CHD.[6]

Despite their prominent use, the applicability of Framingham-based algorithms to modern populations has been questioned.[7-9] Framingham-based scores are based on a homogeneous, geographically limited, Caucasian, male-dominated cohort from a prior generation when cardiovascular risk profiles and preventive pharmacotherapy were both less well developed and less used than in modern cohorts. Multiple studies in diverse populations suggest that Framingham-based risk-scoring systems may misclassify risk, particularly in women, and overestimate CHD risk.[9] In response, the Reynolds Risk Score (RRS) was developed in 2007 and included parental history of premature CHD and measurement of high-sensitivity C-reactive protein.[8] Most recently, the American Heart Association (AHA) and the American College of Cardiology (ACC) developed a new atherosclerosis cardiovascular disease (ASCVD) risk score to guide ASCVD risk-reducing therapy.[10] This new risk score uses the same traditional risk factors as the original FRSs and offers separate equations for white and African American men and women. As noted, each risk model has its limitations and therefore should be used with caution. In women, using the Reynolds score as adjunct to other risk scores may yield value for reclassification, especially for those patients who fall into the intermediate-risk category.[11]

Taking into account the tools and current guidelines as discussed, it is recommended that clinicians include a global risk assessment for all patients 20 to 79 years of age who are free from clinical ASCVD.[12,13] This risk assessment should be repeated every 4 to 6 years in persons who are found to be at low 10-year risk (<7.5%). Beginning at age 40 years, formal estimation of the absolute 10-year risk of ASCVD is recommended. Long-term or lifetime risk estimation is recommended for all persons who are between 20 and 39 years of age and for those between 40 and 59 years of age who are determined to be at low 10-year risk (<7.5%).

SCREENING ELECTROCARDIOGRAM

Directly screening for coronary artery disease with an electrocardiogram (ECG) in asymptomatic people has not been shown to be an effective tool. The US Preventive Services Task Force (USPSTF) recommends against routine screening with resting or exercise ECG for asymptomatic adults at low risk (10-year CHD risk <10%) for CHD events (evidence grade D). In addition, the task force could not find conclusive evidence that screening high- or intermediate-risk patients provided benefit.

They acknowledged that a screening ECG can find minor and clinically insignificant abnormalities that could result in further unnecessary invasive testing.

SCREENING AND TREATING RISK FACTORS

Many risk factors for CVD are modifiable by specific preventive measures. Effect of potentially modifiable risk factors associated with myocardial infarction in 52 countries, 9 potential modifiable risk factors accounted for 94% population-attributable risk of first MI in women worldwide. These risk factors include smoking, dyslipidemia, hypertension, diabetes, abdominal obesity, psychosocial factors, daily consumption of fruit and vegetables, regular alcohol consumption, and regular physical activity.[14] There are varying recommendations on screening for each of these risk factors. In addition, there is also a variable amount of evidence on the impact of treatment for some of these risk factors. In addition to these factors, there are some female-specific and nontraditional risk factors that are emerging, but with limited evidence (Table 6-1).

TABLE 6-1 Cardiovascular Risks and Screening Recommendations

	Recommendation	Grade
Blood pressure	All women age 18 and older should be screened for hypertension, defined as SBP > 140 mm Hg or DBP > 90 (2009 USPSTF recommendation). Adults aged 18–39 years with normal blood pressure and no other risk factors should be rescreened every 3–5 years. New USPSTF guidelines are expected to recommend annual screening for adults age 40 and older with additional risk factors for hypertension, including overweight or obese or African American.	A
Preeclampsia	Women with a history of preeclampsia who gave birth preterm (<37 weeks of gestation) or who have a medical history of recurrent preeclampsia should be screened annually for blood pressure, lipid disorders, and glucose intolerance.[63]	
Lipids	Women aged 45 and over should be screened for lipid disorders every 5 years if they are at increased risk for CHD.	A
	Women aged 20–45 should be screened for lipid disorders every 5 years if they are at increased risk for CHD based on risk factors.	B
Diabetes	Adults 45 years or older and all persons with risk factors regardless of age should be screened for diabetes. ADA recommends a 3-year screening interval for low-risk adults and annually for high-risk individuals. Risk factors include age, overweight or obesity, or a first-degree relative with diabetes.	B
	The USPSTF recommends screening for type 2 diabetes in asymptomatic adults with sustained blood pressure (either treated or untreated) >135/80 mm Hg.	B
Gestational diabetes	Asymptomatic pregnant women after 24 weeks of gestation should be screened for gestational diabetes.	B
Smoking	All adults should be screened for tobacco use and provided with tobacco cessation intervention. Pregnant women who smoke should be provided pregnancy-tailored counseling.	A
Obesity	The USPSTF recommends screening all adults for obesity. Clinicians should offer or refer patients with a body mass index (BMI) of 30 kg/m^2 or higher to intensive, multicomponent behavioral interventions.	B

Abbreviations: ADA, American Diabetes Association; DBP, diastolic blood pressure; SBP, systolic blood pressure.

Hypertension

Hypertension is a well-established risk factor for adverse cardiovascular outcomes, including mortality from CHD and stroke.[15-17] The lifetime risk of developing CHD is significantly higher among patients with hypertension.[12] The benefits of treating hypertension to prevent important health outcomes are well documented. For this reason, there are a number of suggestions on screening for hypertension as a means to early identification and risk factor modification. The American Congress of Obstetricians and Gynecologists (ACOG) recommends BP screening as part of women's annual health care visit.[18] The USPSTF also recommends BP screening in adults (grade A).[19] The Joint National Committee (JNC) recommends a screening interval of every 2 years for patients with BP less than 120/80 mm Hg and every year for patients with a BP of 120/80 mm Hg. Once an elevation of BP greater than 120/80 mm Hg is present, follow-up for further elevations and, ultimately, decisions on treatment will need to be discussed with the patient.

A diagnosis of hypertension requires 3 separate measures of an elevated BP done at different times. A single elevated BP would be considered "elevated BP without the diagnosis of hypertension." White-coat hypertension is the elevation of BP in a physician's office or a clinical setting but not in other settings (e.g., at home). An ambulatory BP monitor can be ordered to confirm BP trends over a 24-hour period.[20] This helps in the diagnostic process if there is any concern about persistent hypertension or inconsistent office BP numbers.

Essential hypertension is far and away the most common cause of persistent elevation of BP. Although a full review of the workup of secondary hypertension is beyond the scope of this chapter, it is important to recognize the features found on history and physical that can point in that direction. This is particularly important in the young patient without a family history of hypertension.[21] In the patient presenting with elevated BP, particular attention should be given to potential pharmaceutical causes of elevated BP, including nonsteroidal anti-inflammatory drugs (NSAIDs), hormonal contraception, licorice ingestion, sympathomimetic medications, and over-the-counter cold medications.[21]

Management for hypertension begins with therapeutic lifestyle modification. However, even under the most optimal conditions, many patients diagnosed with hypertension will need pharmacological management to optimize BP control. There have been a number of landmark trials that looked at the effect of BP management and medication choices.

Evidence for Treatment of Hypertension

The Antihypertensive and Lipid Lowering Treatment to Prevent Heart Attack Trial (ALLHAT) trial (2002) was a randomized, double-blind, multicenter trial with 33, 357 patients; 47% were women, and 35% were black. The mean age was 67, and 29 was the average body mass index (BMI).[22] It compared amlodipine to lisinopril to chlorthalidone with the primary outcome of fatal CHD and nonfatal MI. Secondary outcomes included a combination of all-cause mortality, CHD, stroke, combined coronary vascular disease, angina, coronary revascularization, peripheral arterial disease, cancer, and end-stage renal disease. Findings suggested no significant difference between the amlodipine group and the chlorthalidone group for either the primary or secondary outcomes. Subgroup analysis of women only showed no difference in the primary outcome of time to first cardiovascular event and only showed a mild protective effect of chlorthalidone against stroke. Chlorthalidone is a stronger thiazide diuretic then hydrochlorothiazide and is much less commonly used in the United States. Overall, this study was similar to the other major studies, showing that either angiotensin-converting enzyme inhibitors (ACE-Is), calcium channel blockers (CCBs), or thiazide diuretics are appropriate first-line antihypertensive agents with no difference between the primary outcome of fatal CHD and nonfatal MI.

The Anglo–Scandanvian Cardiac Outcomes Trial-Blood Pressure Lowering Arm (ASCOT-BPLA) study (2003) was a double-blind, randomized, multicenter trial of 19,257 patients; only 23% were female, 95% were Caucasian, and 37% were under age 60 with this entire group having 28.7 median BMI.[23] In the study, there was no difference between the calcium channel blocker/ACE-I arm and the β-blocker/diuretic arm when nonfatal MI plus fatal MI was the primary end point (hazard ratio [HR] 0.90, confidence internal [CI] 0.79–1.02, $p = 0.12$). The lack of significant difference was likely due to the similar change in BP in the group from 164/94 to 136/78 mm Hg after treatment. The subgroup analysis of all participants found that there was a significant protective effect for the amlodipine/ACE-I arm for all-cause mortality (HR 0.89, CI 0.81–0.99, $p = .025$); risk of development of diabetes (HR 0.70, CI 0.63–0.78, $p = < .0001$); cardiovascular mortality (HR 0.76, CI 0.65–0.89, $p = .001$); and total/nonfatal stroke (HR 0.77, CI 0.66–0.89, $p = .003$).[23] The ASCOT-BPLA study suggested that CCBs and ACE-I were superior to β-blockers/diuretics in overweight and heavier individuals in subgroup analysis. The subgroup analysis of women suggested that women had a similar reduction in overall BP with similar end point outcomes as the general study population.

The ACCOMPLISH (Avoiding cardiovascular events through combination therapy in patients living with systolic hypertension) trial (2008) was a randomized, controlled, double-blind, multicenter trial with 11,506 patients; 39.5% were women, and 31 kg/m² was the average BMI.[24] This trial compared benazepril/amlodipine to benazepril/hydrochlrorothiazide. The primary outcome singular measure was time to first cardiovascular event and included sudden death from cardiac causes, MI, stroke, coronary intervention, congestive heart failure, or resuscitation after sudden cardiac arrest. In the study, there was no significant difference between the ACE-I/CCB arm and the ACE-I/diuretic group (8.1% vs. 9.7%, respectively, with $p = .06$).[24] Similar to the subgroup results of the ASCOT-BPLA study, subgroup analysis in ACCOMPLISH showed that, in obese women, either the combination of ACE-I/CCB or ACE-I/diuretic was equally effective at reducing primary outcomes.

The effect of Antihypertensive Agents on cardiovascular events in patients with coronary disease and normal blood pressure; the CAMELOT (Comparison of Amlodipine vs. Enalapril to Limit Occurrences of Thrombosis) trial (2004), was a double-blind, randomized, multicenter trial done in the United States and Europe.[25] There were about 2000 patients in the trial; it compared amlodipine to enalapril and placebo. The primary outcome was incidence of adverse cardiovascular events. This included a composite of death, nonfatal MI, resuscitated cardiac arrest, coronary revascularization, hospitalization for angina/congestive heart failure, stroke/transient ischemic attack or new diagnosis of peripheral arterial disease. Amlodipine was found to have a significantly better result than placebo, reducing cardiovascular adverse events from 23.1% to 16.6% (HR 0.69, CI 0.54–0.88, $p = .003$) with a number needed to treat of 16 patients to prevent 1 adverse event.[25] CAMELOT also found that amlodipine was better than placebo but similar to enalapril. Critics of this study are skeptical of the results

TABLE 6-2 Hypertension Treatment Guidelines

Age 18–60, no chronic kidney disease (CKD)	Treat for BP >140/90 mm Hg for goal <140/90 mm Hg
Age >60, no CKD	Treat for BP >150/90 mm Hg for goal <150/90 mm Hg
18 and greater with CKD	Treat for BP >140/90 mm Hg for goal <140/90 mm Hg
Initial non-black population, including DM	Initiate treatment with thiazide-type diuretic, calcium channel blocker (CCB), angiotensin-converting enzyme inhibitor (ACE-I), or angiotensin receptor blocker (ARB)
General black population, including diabetes (DM)	Initial treatment with thiazide-type diuretic or CCB

Abbreviation: DM, diabetes mellitus.

because of the high dropout rate. Women and obese participants were not separately reported in this study.

Hypertension Treatment Recommendations

The current Eighth JNC (JNC8) guidelines give clear suggestions on the use of medication for the treatment of hypertension[12] (Table 6-2).

- *Age 18–29*: Initiate treatment with antihypertensives for systolic BP 140 mm Hg or greater or diastolic BP 90 mm Hg or greater. Treatment goal is BP less than 140/90 mm Hg (level of evidence E: expert opinion).
- *Age 30–59*: Initiate treatment with antihypertensives for systolic BP 140 mm Hg or greater or diastolic BP 90 mm Hg or greater. Treatment goal BP less than 140/90 mm Hg (level of evidence A for diastolic goals: multiple randomized trials).
- *Age 60 or greater*: Initiate treatment for systolic BP 150 mm Hg or greater or diastolic BP 90 mm Hg or greater. Treatment goal is BP less than 150/90 mm Hg (level of evidence A: multiple randomized trials).
- *Age 60 or greater with chronic kidney disease (CKD) or diabetes*: BP goal is less than 140/90 mm Hg (level of evidence E: expert opinion).
- *In the general non-black population*, including those with diabetes, initial antihypertensive treatment should include a thiazide-type diuretic, CCB, ACE-I, or angiotensin receptor blocker (ARB) (moderate recommendation: grade B).
- *In the general black population*, including those with diabetes, initial antihypertensive treatment should include a thiazide-type diuretic or CCB. (For the general black population, moderate recommendation: grade B; for black patients with diabetes, weak recommendation: grade C).

If the goal BPs (<150/90 mm Hg) are not reached for patients' older than 65 or are less than 140/90 mm Hg for patients aged less than 65, then the goals of treatment include the following (Table 6-3):

- If goal BP is not reached within a month of treatment, increase the dose of the initial drug or add a second drug from one of the classes in the recommendation (thiazide-type diuretic, CCB, ACE-I, or ARB). The clinician should continue to assess BP and adjust the treatment regimen until the goal BP is reached.

TABLE 6-3 Titration of Antihypertensives When BP Not at Goal[a]

BP not at goal in 1 month	Increase dose of initial drug or add second drug from a different class (thiazide-type diuretic, CCB, ACE-I or ARB)[b]
If maxed out on 2 drugs and BP not at goal	Add third antihypertensive from a separate class
If drug contraindication or on 3 drugs and BP not at goal	Add antihypertensives from other drug classes and consider referral to hypertension specialist

[a]Adapted from Eighth Joint National Committee (JNC8).
[b]Do not use ARB and ACE-I together.

- ○ If goal BP cannot be reached with 2 drugs, add and titrate a third drug from the list provided. *Do not use an ACE-I and an ARB together in the same patient.*
- If the goal BP cannot be reached using only the drugs in the recommendation because of a contraindication or the need to use more than 3 drugs to reach the goal BP, antihypertensive drugs from other classes can be used.
- Referral to a hypertension specialist may be indicated for patients in whom the goal BP cannot be attained using the previous strategy or for the management of complicated patients for whom additional clinical consultation is needed.

Certain patient populations and comorbidities could benefit from different antihypertensive choices (Table 6-4):

- The ACE-Is are generally thought to be the antihypertensives of choice for patients with mild CKD, diabetes and nephropathy, previous MI, or heart failure with ejection fraction (EF) less than 40%.[20,26-28]
- In patients with minor intolerance to ACE-Is, ARBs are generally used. However, ARBs should be *avoided* in patients who have anaphylaxis with an ACE-I.
- The β-blockers are indicated after MI and in heart failure with EF less than 40%.[28]
- Thiazide diuretics are preferred in African Americans, the elderly, and patients with heart failure and for secondary stroke prevention.[20,22,28]

Antihypertensive Side Effects

Antihypertensive medications are generally well tolerated. ACE-Is are associated with hyperkalemia and chronic dry cough.[22-25] Although seen in only 1% of patients taking ACE inhibitors, the most feared adverse event is angioedema. The β-blockers are well known for commonly causing bradycardia, fatigue, erectile dysfunction, dizziness,

TABLE 6-4 Indications for Certain Antihypertensive Classes

Use ACE-I	In mild CKD, diabetes with nephropathy, previous MI, heart failure with ejection fraction less than 40%[20,26-28]
Use ARB	In minor intolerance to ACE-I; avoid if anaphylaxis to ACE-I
Use β-blocker	After MI, heart failure with ejection fraction less than 40%[28]
Use thiazide diuretic	In African Americans, the elderly, patients with heart failure, secondary stroke prevention[20,22,28]

chest pain, dyspnea, and diarrhea.[27] CCBs can cause peripheral edema (up to about a third of all patients).[24,25] Thiazides cause hypokalemia and have been associated with sudden death at very high doses (>4 times the standard dose).[22,24]

Lipid Disorders

Screening for Dyslipidemia

Dyslipidemias are important risk factors for CHD, with the risk highest in those with a combination of risk factors. For this reason, screening and appropriate lifestyle modifications and treatment for lipid disorders are mainstays in cardiovascular event risk reductions. The US Preventive Health Task Force (USPSTF) guidelines recommend lipid screening every 5 years after age 45 years in women (but as early as age 20 if at increased risk for CVD) but does not specifically make a recommendation for screening based on obesity (grade A).[29] Obesity (BMI $\geq$ 30 kg/m^2) is one of the CHD risk factors; therefore, although no explicit recommendation is made for lipid screening in the obese population, we can infer that obesity does increase CVD, so screening should be done. ACOG as well does not recommend any single laboratory test for obese patients; the ACOG does state that screening for dyslipidemia should be based on overall health risk.[29]

Treatment of dyslipidemia to reduce cardiovascular events has been extensively studied and thus has become a mainstay of cardiac risk modification. Hyperlipidemia, once found, should initially be addressed with lifestyle management changes discussed in other parts of this chapter. Current evidence for medical management only supports the use of statins in the prevention of hyperlipidemia as a cardiovascular risk factor. The research on treatment for hyperlipidemia in the prevention of cardiovascular events is extensive, but unfortunately many of the studies had few women enrolled. Many of the studies commented on the effect on women, but conclusions need to be accepted with caution because studies are generally not powered to make strong conclusions from subgroup analysis.

Evidence for Treatment of Dyslipidemia

A number of studies have looked at the use of statins for lipid lowering in the primary prevention of cardiovascular events. Atorvastatin was found to reduce fatal CHD or nonfatal MI by 36% in one study with 10,000 patients; 1800 of the participants were women, and 28.6 was the average BMI.[26] In the subgroup analysis, a significant reduction in cardiac events remained for the patients with obesity. However, the analysis was not able to find a statistically significant reduction in events in the female subgroup.[26] The primary prevention of acute coronary events with Lovastatin in men and women with average cholesterol levels, the AFCAPS/TexCAPS trial, was stopped early for all participants after a 37% reduction in first acute major coronary events.[30] However, only 15% of the study participants were women, and the subgroup was not powered to show a significant risk reduction in cardiovascular events. In the Justification for the Use of Statins in Prevention: An Interventional Trial Evaluating Rosuvastatin (JUPITER) trial, with 38% women, rosuvastatin reduced first major cardiovascular events significantly, with an HR of 0.56, 95% CI of 0.46–0.69 ($p < .00001$) in both men and women, leading to a 44% reduction in first cardiovascular events.[31] This made the number needed to be treated to prevent 1 major cardiovascular event 95 if rosuvastatin was used for 2 years and dropped to only 45 if rosuvastatin was used for 4 years. The JUPITER subgroup analysis showed the significant effect of preventing first major coronary event for women, those with BMI over 30, and patients with metabolic syndrome.[31]

Statins are also the preferred agent for secondary prevention of CVD and have been shown to be more efficacious than diet modifications, niacin, fibrates, and cholestryamin.[32] It has also been shown that for statins to be beneficial, they must be used for at least 2 years to prevent a repeat major cardiovascular event, and there is limited benefit if used for a shorter time period.[33] In a large meta-analysis of 18 studies with about 14,000 total patients, it was shown that there was a significant risk reduction of episodes of unstable angina and need for revascularization within 12 months when statins were initiated within 14 days of a cardiovascular event such as an MI.[34]

Simvastatin has been shown to reduce MI or death from coronary disease from 17.7% to 14.4% in patients with a prior CVD equivalent.[33] The overall class of statins has been shown to be protective against coronary events, cardiac mortality, MI, and coronary interventions.[34] Yet, in women, the protective effect is not as large as in men, and there may not be an overall all-cause mortality benefit as seen in men.[34] The use of statins to reduce invasive procedures and deaths attributable to coronary events likely has a large effect on increasing quality of life for our obese female patients. Ultimately, the lack of female-specific data and data for secondary prevention of CVD with treatment of hyperlipidemia remains an area requiring further research.

Dyslipidemia Treatment Recommendations

Statin intensity can be broken down into 3 different levels: low intensity, moderate intensity, and high intensity. High-intensity statins reduce low-density lipoprotein (LDL) on average by 50%, moderate intensity reduces LDL by 30%–50%, and low intensity reduces LDL by less than 30% (Table 6-5).

- High-intensity statins are atorvastatin 20 or 40 mg and rosuvastatin 20 or 40 mg.
- Moderate-intensity statins include atorvastatin 10 or 20 mg, rosuvastatin 5 or 10 mg, simvastatin 20–40 mg, pravastatin 40 or 80 mg, lovastatin 40 mg, fluvastatin KL 80 mg, fluvastatin 40 mg twice daily, and pitavastatin 2–4 mg.
- Low-intensity statins include simvastatin 10 mg, pravastatin 10 or 20 mg, and lovastatin 20 mg.[35]

The treatment of hyperlipidemia has recently changed with the publishing of the AHA 2013 guidelines.[35] These guidelines break the primary prevention guidelines into 3 main categories (Figure 6-1):

- Individuals with an LDL greater than 190 or a triglyceride level greater than 500 should be evaluated for secondary causes.

TABLE 6-5 Statin Intensity

High intensity	Atorvastatin 20 or 40 mg, rosuvastatin 20 or 40 mg	Lowers LDL by >50%
Moderate intensity	Atorvastin 10 or 20 mg, rosuvastatin 5 or 10 mg, simvastatin 20–40 mg, pravastatin 40 or 80 mg, lovastatin 40 mg, fluvastatin KL 80 mg, fluvastatin 40 mg twice daily, and pitavastatin 2–4 mg	Lowers LDL by 30%–50%
Low intensity	Simvastatin 10 mg, pravastatin 10 or 20 mg, lovastatin 20 mg	Lowers LDL by <30%

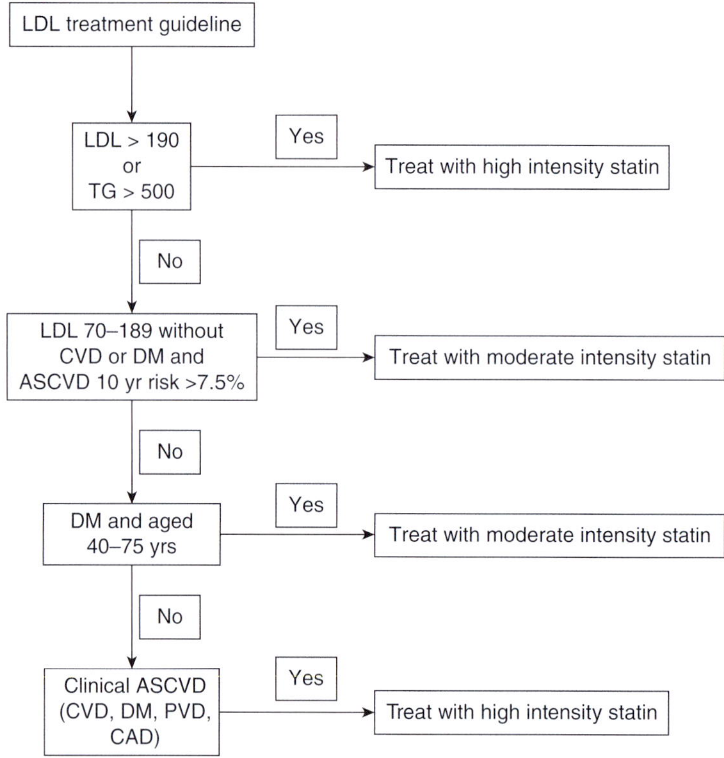

FIGURE 6-1. LDL treatment guideline. PVD, peripheral vascular disease; TG, triglyceride.

- ○ These patients should be treated with a high-intensity statin or the maximum tolerated statin dose. This has level B evidence.
- Individuals with an LDL level of 70–189 without clinical CVD or diabetes and estimated ASCVD 10-year risk greater than 7.5%.
  - ○ These patients should be treated with moderate-intensity statin therapy. This has level A evidence.
- Individuals with diabetes or CKD who are aged 40–75.
  - ○ These patients should be treated with a moderate-intensity statin if the 10-year ASCVD risk is less than 7.5%. A high-intensity statin should be used for those populations if the 10-year ASCVD risk score is greater than 7.5%. This has level A evidence.

When deciding to initiate therapy for hyperlipidemia, the preliminary workup should include a fasting lipid profile. Once medication has been started, a fasting lipid profile should be repeated in 4–12 weeks to check for medication adherence.[35] A number of medications could contribute to elevations of LDL cholesterol, including diuretics, cyclosporine, glucocorticoids, or amiodarone. Comorbid medical conditions may also have an effect on serum LDL levels. In particular, elevations of LDL can be seen in hypothyroidism, obesity, pregnancy, biliary obstruction, or nephrotic syndrome. Secondary causes of hypertriglyceridemia include medications such as oral estrogens, glucocorticoids, bile acid sequestrates, protease inhibitors, and retinoic acid. Disease states that may have elevated triglycerides include nephrotic syndrome, chronic renal failure, lipodystrophies, diabetes, hypothyroidism, obesity, and pregnancy.

Lipid Medication Side Effects

Statins have been proven to be well tolerated by most patients. However, as with all medication, adverse effects are possible. One of the common side effects of statins is elevation of alkaline transaminase (ALT) more than three times the baseline, with the prevalence being 0.42%–1.0%. In multiple studies, statins have not been shown to be significantly associated with transaminitis.[36-38] Yet, one large Cochrane study involving about 12,000 total patients showed that the relative risk (RR) of statin therapy and transaminitis was 2.49 with a CI of 1.16–5.32.[39] Overall, the risk of transaminitis is small, and for the vast majority of patients it should not be a reason to avoid statins. At this time, current guidelines do not recommend routine monitoring of hepatic transaminases.

Myopathy with an elevated creatinine kinase is another potential adverse outcome of statins. The overall prevalence is very small for myopathy, ranging from 0.11% to 0.7% in multiple studies.[30,33,39] The rate of rhabdomyolysis is also quite low at 0.05%, but there is a significant increase compared to the rate of rhabdomyolysis on placebo of 0.01%. Overall, the AHA guidelines note an excess of 0.01/100 patients. Despite the relatively low incidence of myopathy, many patients will complain of myalgia. These patients generally complain of mild muscle aches without elevation of creatinine kinase. Anecdotal reports suggest that changing the statin, reducing the intensity, or using an alternate-day dosing plan can improve complaints of myalgia.

Counterintuitively, the JUPITER trial raised concerns about the adverse effects on blood glucose from statin therapy. The study reported that new diabetes was more common in the rosuvastatin arm of the trial compared to the placebo.[31] The overall rate of excess diabetes from statins ranges from 0.2/100 patients for moderate-dose statins to 0.3/100 patients for high-intensity statins.[35] Overall, the risk of diabetes from use of a statin is much outweighed by the real benefits of protecting against MI, stroke, or ASCVD death.

Another commonly asked about potential adverse effect reported with statin use is the increased risk of breast cancer. In one trial of pravastatin, there appeared to be an increased incidence of newly diagnosed breast cancer.[39] Further studies have not shown a difference in reported rates of cancer while on statins,[33] and one study showed that there was no increased risk of breast cancer if the patient had hyperlipidemia and was on a statin (RR 1.0, CI 0.6–1.6), but that there was an increased risk of breast cancer if the patient had untreated hyperlipidemia (RR 1.6, CI 1.1–2.5).[40] When counseling patients, the current evidence does not show an increased risk of breast cancer and actually shows a potentially protective effect of statins on incidence of breast cancer.

Diabetes Mellitus

The rate of death in patients with diabetes from stroke and heart disease is about 2–4 times that of individuals without diabetes. Type 2 diabetes typically develops slowly, and progression from normal blood glucose to impaired fasting glucose (IFG) or impaired glucose tolerance (IGT) to diabetes may take a decade or longer. IFG and IGT are considered to be early stages of the disease process and are risk factors for diabetes and CVD. Because of this high predilection for cardiovascular events in patients with hyperglycemia, screening and early intervention for diabetes mellitus is an important part of cardiovascular risk reduction. However, limited data are available on prevention or delay of cardiovascular and other long-term health outcomes, including CVD events or death. No randomized, controlled trial has demonstrated a statistically significant reduction in total CVD events from tight glycemic control. The UKPDS was a prospective study with 10 years of follow up. It showed a trend toward reduced CVD events in participants randomly assigned to tight glycemic control.[41]

Smoking

Cigarette smoking is an important reversible risk factor for CHD, especially in women. Women are particularly susceptible to smoking's deleterious effects. The incidence of an MI is increased 6-fold in women who smoke at least 20 cigarettes per day compared with subjects who never smoked.[14,42] This is compared to an only 3-fold increase in incidence of MI in male smokers. The RR ratio of smokers to nonsmokers for developing atherogenic CVD is 25% higher in women than in men.[43] Although in 2013 the overall smoking rate had dropped from nearly 21 of every 100 adults (20.9%) in 2005 to nearly 18 of every 100 adults (17.8%),[1] gender-specific barriers remain a challenge. Women tend to be less successful at quitting than men. The benefits of smoking cessation at any time outweigh the health risks. Smoking cessation has been shown to reduce the risk of heart disease within 1–2 years of quitting.

Smoking Cessation Treatment

Smoking cessation is hard and requires a dedicated effort from the patient and the patient's physician. Part of the difficulty with smoking cessation is that many patients are not successful on their first attempt; it takes the majority of patients several attempts before truly achieving smoking cessation.[44]

The role of the physician is to screen patients at *every* visit for tobacco use. Then, the provider can use a tool such as the 5 *A*'s to help determine when a patient is ready to quit smoking. These 5 are ask, advise, assess, assist, and arrange.[45] Physicians should ask about tobacco use every visit, advise tobacco users to quit, assess readiness to quit, assist in helping a patient develop a smoking cessation plan, and arrange for follow-up visits for further smoking cessation counseling.

Once the plan for smoking cessation is in place, the options to help the patient quit include intensive counseling plus nicotine replacement or bupropion or exercise.[44,46,47] Quit rates are as high as 82% after 8 weeks but quickly drop to much lower rates, ranging from 21% to 27% after 6 months.[44,46,47] Intensive counseling is required usually with a dedicated nurse or smoking cessation counselor. Counseling should occur at least once weekly with the patient. One successful program that has been used is the Sister-to-Sister program, which has been successful in a variety of women's populations, including African American women living at or below the poverty line. A patient using the Sister-to-Sister program is 6 times more likely to be continuously abstinent of tobacco use at 6 months. The program includes nicotine replacement therapy, nurse-delivered behavioral group counseling weekly for 6 weeks and then at 12 and 24 weeks, and personal contact either face to face or by telephone by another health care worker in the program weekly for 24 weeks.[44]

During smoking cessation, required counseling of the patient must include counseling on the expected weight gain that occurs during smoking cessation. There has been a

TABLE 6-6 Interventions to Reduce Postsmoking Cessation Weight Gain

Chromium, ephedrine, caffeine, phenylpropanolamine	No change in weight at 12 months
Personalized weight management program	2.58 kg weight loss at 12 months
CBT	Increased weight at 6 months, no weight change when combined with bupropion
Bupropion, fluoxetine	0.38–0.87 and 0.19 kg weight loss at 12 months but not significant
Long-term exercise program	2.07 kg weight loss at 12 months
NRT	0.42 kg weight loss at 12 months but not significant
Varenicline	No weight change alone; increased weight gain by 0.51 kg when compared to bupropion

Abbreviation: CBT, cognitive-behavioral therapy.

reported 5-kg weight gain in some cases.[47] One Cochrane study examined the effects of various treatment modalities on post–smoking cessation weight gain[48] (Table 6-6):

- Pharmacologic interventions, including chromium, ephedrine, caffeine, and phenylpropanolamine, did not show a significant change in weight at 6 and 12 months post–smoking cessation.
- Personalized weight management programs led to 2.58-kg weight loss at 12 months.
- Cognitive behavioral therapy showed significant increased weight at 6 months but no change in weight gain when combined with bupropion.
- Bupropion and fluoxetine both reduced weight post–smoking cessation, leading to 0.38- to 0.87-kg and 0.19-kg weight loss, respectively. Unfortunately, neither effect was significant when analyzed.
- Long-term exercise programs lead to a 2.07-kg weight loss at 12 months post–smoking cessation.
- Nicotine replacement therapy (NRT) reduced weight gain by 0.42 kg at 12 months, but the effect was not significant.
- Varenicline did not change weight gain and, when compared to bupropion, may cause a 0.51-kg weight gain post–smoking cessation.

One way to make patients more successful with smoking cessation is to add a structured exercise program to the intensive counseling sessions. Exercise in addition to counseling and NRT will decrease the amount of weight gained compared to counseling alone and also increases the patient's success at retaining abstinence from tobacco.[46] Bupropion added to intensive behavioral counseling has been shown to help patients stay abstinent from tobacco at 12 months (23.6% vs. 8.1% with placebo, $p = .006$) and also a trend toward decreased weight gain by about 0.5 kg.[47] Nicotine replacement therapy through gum, lozenges, or patches is another potential adjunct to counseling to help with successful smoking cessation. NRT has been shown to be twice as effective as placebo in getting women to quit smoking (odds ratio [OR] 1.90, CI 1.75–2.06).[49] This effect is not seen when NRT is used for long-term maintenance of smoking cessation in women, yet has been seen in men.

For successful tobacco cessation in women, it is essential to address other comorbid substance dependence. Women who consume more than 7 alcoholic drinks weekly were more likely to relapse with their tobacco dependence than women used alcohol moderately.[50]

Although smoking is a well-known risk factor for CVD, the overall evidence for smoking cessation in women is based on multiple poor-quality studies and few randomized controlled studies. However, the standard of practice and well-known belief remain that it is essential to continue to assist patients in their attempts to quit smoking as a way to eliminate a cardiovascular risk factor.

Obesity

Obesity, defined as a BMI greater than 30, is associated with a number of risk factors for atherosclerosis, CVD, diabetes mellitus, and cardiovascular mortality.[5,51] In the Framingham Offspring Study, obesity as measured by BMI significantly and independently predicted the occurrence of CHD and CVD after adjusting for traditional risk factors.[52] The Nurses' Health Study followed 84,000 female nurses for 16 years and found that being overweight or obese was the single most important predictor of developing diabetes mellitus. After adjusting for age, family history of diabetes, smoking, exercise, and several dietary factors, the RR of diabetes mellitus was 11.2 for the 90th percentile (BMI = 29.9) versus the 10th percentile (BMI = 20.1).[53] In a large cohort study of 37,000 women in Washington State, women with a BMI greater than 35 had ORs of 2.7 and 5.4 for CAD and hypertension, respectively.[54] Abdominal obesity is more harmful in women than BMI or weight alone. It is an independent risk factor for developing CAD in both normal-weight women and overweight women.[4]

Diet and Exercise Modification

As noted, a lack of physical activity is considered a cardiac risk factor. Therefore, one of the mainstays of therapeutic lifestyle modification is counseling on increasing a women's activity level. An exercise program, defined as at least 3 times a week for 30 minutes with increased heart rate, has been shown to reduce CVD mortality. In one cross-sectional study with 10,261 patients, there was no difference between light (66% women) or moderate/vigorous (52%/46% women, respectively) exercise groups as both were associated with lower CVD mortality.[36]

A cross-sectional study with 1128 women found a trend that increased exercise correlated with decreased systolic BP, decreased fasting glucose levels, and decreased triglyceride and LDL levels.[38] This study only looked at these surrogate outcomes and did not look at actual long-term cardiac outcomes. A large meta-epidemiological study with 305 total studies and 339,274 patients studied the OR of exercise and drugs (diuretics, β-blockers, ACE-I, antiplatelets) on CVD but did not look at women or obesity separately.[55] It also included more studies comparing drug versus placebo, with none comparing exercise versus drug. In this study, there was no difference when drugs (diuretics, β-blockers, ACE-I, antiplatelets) were compared to exercise interventions (OR 0.89, 95% CI 0.76–1.04).[55]

One meta-analysis, based on 33 studies with 84,323 patients, studied pooled RR for cardiorespiratory fitness (CRF) and CVD.[56] It found that the pooled RR of low CRF and CVD was 1.47 (CI 1.35–1.61) compared to intermediate/high CRF and CVD, which was 1.07 (CI 1.01–1.13). CRF was defined as defined low, intermediate, and high CRF: less than 7.9 METs (metabolic equivalents), 7.9–10.8 METs, and 10.9 METs or more, respectively. This means for women age 40, there is a protective effect against CHD/CVD if they are able to do 7 METs of activity; for age 50, if they are able to do 6 METs of activity; and for age 60, if they are able to do 5 METs of activity.

There have been a number of studies looking at the impact of diet modification on cardiovascular risk factors. The diabetes prevention program diet showed that the combination of diet and exercise causing weight loss will prevent onset of type 2 diabetes.[57] The DASH (Dietary Approaches to Stop Hypertension) diet is considered to be a well-rounded diet rich in fruits, vegetables, and low-fat dairy products as well as decreased intake of saturated or total fat. One study with a majority of women participants has shown the DASH diet can decrease BP by an average of about 16/7.5 mm Hg when combined with exercise and decreased BP by 11/3.4 mm Hg when used alone in one study with a majority of women.[37]

Overall, the best lifestyle changes use both diet and exercise, leading to up to 8.7 kg of weight loss plus improvement of BP, especially when used in combination with intensive nutrition counseling and a supervised exercise program. Per the 2013 European Society of Hypertension and the European Society of Cardiology guidelines for hypertension, the recommended lifestyle changes that will reduce BP are[21]

- salt restriction;
- moderation of alcohol;
- high consumption of vegetables and fruits with a low-fat type of diet;
- weight reduction, then maintenance of weight reduction; and
- regular physical exercise.

Polycystic Ovary Syndrome

Although it is not on the list of major cardiac risk factors, polycystic ovary syndrome (PCOS) is associated with an increased risk of CHD in women. It is the most common endocrinopathy in women of reproductive age and is characterized by high androgens, ovulatory dysfunction, and the presence of polycystic ovaries. Women with PCOS are at increased risk for CHD because a broad range of metabolic disturbances and risk factors + for CVD affects them.[58] The Androgen Excess PCOS (AE-PCOS) Society, 2003 Rotterdam criteria, American Association of Clinical Endocrinologists, and American College of Endocrinology all recommend that women with PCOS (obese and nonobese) be screened for metabolic syndrome and CVD risk factors by the age of 30 years. It does, however, remain unclear whether screening followed by aggressive risk modification are an effective strategy in preventing CVD; long-term studies are needed to make this determination.

Menopause and Hormone Replacement Therapy

Women on average are a decade older than men when diagnosed with CHD. Many changes occur during the menopausal transition. The average US woman who reaches menopause is expected to live another 30 years. During her remaining life span, the estimated risk for a chronic medical condition is approximately 30% for CHD, 22% for dementia, 21% for stroke, 15% for hip fracture, and 11% for breast cancer.[59] Whether menopause is a risk factor itself or a marker of an increased risk state is highly debated. Women who have early menopause appear to have increased cardiac mortality.[60] Hormone replacement therapy (HRT) has been considered a potential prevention intervention for CHD. Currently, USPSTF, AHA, and ACOG all recommend against the use of HRT for primary or secondary prevention of CVD.

Family History

Although not a modifiable risk factor, family history is an independent risk factor for CHD, particularly among younger individuals with a family history of premature disease.[52,61] The importance of family history has been shown in several large cohort studies, and all showed that a positive family history is associated with greater risk of developing CHD.[52] It is important to keep family history in mind when advising patients on the need to improve the risk factors that are modifiable.

Nontraditional Risk Factors

Despite growing popularity of the use of nontraditional risk factors as screening measures, in 2009 the USPSTF stated that there is insufficient evidence to recommend these tests.[62] The risk factors they evaluated include ankle-brachial index, leukocyte count, periodontal disease, carotid intima-media thickness, coronary artery calcification score, homocysteine level, lipoprotein (a) levels, and high-sensitivity C-reactive protein (hs-CRP). The inclusion of hs-CRP in the list is particularly interesting in the face of its increasing use in risk calculators such as the Reynolds Risk Score. It is likely these "nontraditional" risk factors will have increasing studies that may eventually show utility as standard risk factors.

CONCLUSION

Cardiovascular disease does cause significant morbidity and mortality in women. There remains a paucity of studies and evidence specific to women, especially in the obese population. In general, current recommendations and guidelines originated from predominantly male studies and do not have many recommendations specific to the female or obese patient. However, these guidelines continue to serve as the starting point for a global risk assessment in women. To continue to develop gender-specific guidelines, more studies will need either to be directed toward the female patient or to have appropriate power for robust subgroup analysis. In addition, for the female patient, studies will need to incorporate both traditional and nontraditional risk factors to better inform the practitioners on the best way to reduce risk of cardiac disease in the obese female patient. For the time being, continued aggressive risk factor modification with particular attention to controlling and improving: hypertension, hyperlipidemia, diabetes mellitus, obesity, tobacco abuse, and sedentary lifestyle are likely to significantly reduce the burden of heart disease in our female patients.

REFERENCES

1. Centers for Disease Control and Prevention. Heart disease. http://www.cdc.gov/heartdisease/.
2. Mosca L, Mochari-Greenberger H, Dolor RJ, Towfighi A, Albert MA. Fifteen-year trends in awareness of heart disease in women: results of a 2012 American Heart Association national survey. *Circulation*. 2013 Mar 19;127(11):1254–1263, e1-29. doi:10.1161/CIR.0b013e318287cf2f.

3. Mehta PK, Wenger NK. Coronary heart disease in women: battle is won but the war remains. *Minerva Med*. 2007;98:459–478.

4. Weiss AM. Cardiovascular disease in women. *Prim Care*. 2009;36:73–102.

5. Preis SR, Hwang SJ, Coady S, et al. Trends in all-cause and cardiovascular disease mortality among women and men with and without diabetes mellitus in the Framingham Heart Study, 1950 to 2005. *Circulation*. 2009;119:1728–1735.

6. Wilson PW, D'Agostino RB, Levy D, et al. Prediction of coronary heart disease using risk factor categories. *Circulation*. 1998;97:1837–1847.

7. Brindle P, Emberson J, Lampe F, et al. Predictive accuracy of the Framingham coronary risk score in British men: prospective cohort study. *BMJ*. 2003;327:1267.

8. Cook NR, Paynter NP, Eaton CB, et al. Comparison of the Framingham and Reynolds Risk Scores for global cardiovascular risk prediction in the multiethnic Women's Health Initiative. *Circulation*. 2012;125:1748–1756, S1–S11.

9. Ridker PM, Buring JE, Rifai N, Cook NR. Development and validation of improved algorithms for the assessment of global cardiovascular risk in women: the Reynolds Risk Score. *JAMA*. 2007;297:611–619.

10. Goff DC, Lloyd-Jones DM, Bennett G, et al. 2013 ACC/AHA guideline on the assessment of cardiovascular risk: a report of the American College of Cardiology/American Heart Association Task Force on Practice Guidelines. *J Am Coll Cardiol*. 2014;63(25_PA): 2935–2959. doi:10.1016/j.jacc.2013.11.005.

11. Ridker PM, Buring JE, Rifai N, Cook NR. Development and validation of improved algorithms for the assessment of global cardiovascular risk in women: the Reynolds Risk Score. *JAMA*. 2007;297:611–619.

12. James PA, Oparil S, Carter BL, et al. 2014 evidence-based guideline for the management of high blood pressure in adults: report from the panel members appointed to the Eighth Joint National Committee (JNC 8). *JAMA*. 2014;311(5):507–520. doi:10.1001/jama.2013.284427.

13. National Cholesterol Education Program (NCEP) Expert Panel on Detection, Evaluation, and Treatment of High Blood Cholesterol in Adults (Adult Treatment Panel III). Third report of the National Cholesterol Education Program (NCEP) Expert Panel on Detection, Evaluation, and Treatment of High Blood Cholesterol in Adults (Adult Treatment Panel III) final report. *Circulation*. 2002;106:3143.

14. Yusuf S, Hawken S, Ounpuu S, et al. Effect of potentially modifiable risk factors associated with myocardial infarction in 52 countries (the INTERHEART study): case-control study. *Lancet*. 2004;364:937.

15. Miura K, Daviglus ML, Dyer AR, et al. Relationship of blood pressure to 25-year mortality due to coronary heart disease, cardiovascular diseases, and all causes in young adult men: the Chicago Heart Association Detection Project in Industry. *Arch Intern Med*. 2001;161:1501

16. Lewington S, Clarke R, Qizilbash N, et al. Age-specific relevance of usual blood pressure to vascular mortality: a meta-analysis of individual data for one million adults in 61 prospective studies. *Lancet* 2002;360:1903.

17. Almdal T, Scharling H, Jensen JS, Vestergaard H. The independent effect of type 2 diabetes mellitus on ischemic heart disease, stroke, and death: a population-based study of 13,000 men and women with 20 years of follow-up. *Arch Intern Med*. 2004;164:1422.

18. American Congress of Obstetricians and Gynecologists. *Well-Woman Care: Assessments and Recommendations*. Washington, DC: American Congress of Obstetricians and Gynecologists; 2013.

19. United States Preventive Services Task Force. Evidence for the reaffirmation of the US Preventive Services Task Force recommendation on screening for high blood pressure. *Ann Intern Med*. 2007;147:787–791.

20. Williams B, Poulter NR, Brown MJ, et al. British Hypertension Society guidelines for hypertension management 2004 (BHS-IV): summary. *Br Med J*. 2004;328(March):634–640.

21. Mancia G, Fagard R, Narkiewicz K, et al. 2013 ESH/ESC guidelines for the management of arterial hypertension: the Task Force for the Management of Arterial Hypertension of the European Society of Hypertension (ESH) and of the European Society of Cardiology (ESC). *Eur Heart J*. 2013;34(28):2159–2219. doi:10.1093/eurheartj/eht151.

22. The ALLHAT officers. Major outcomes in high-risk hypertensive patients randomized to or calcium channel blocker vs. diuretic. *JAMA*. 2002; 288(23):2981–2997.

23. Prevention of cardiovascular events with an antihypertensive regimen of amlodipine adding perindopril as required versus atenolol adding bendroflumethiazide as required, in the Anglo-Scandinavian Cardiac Outcomes Trial-Blood Pressure Lowering Arm (ASCOT-B). *Lancet*. 2005;366:895–906.

24. Jamerson K, Weber MA. Benzapril plus amlodipine or hydrochlorothiazide for hypertension in high-risk patients. *N Engl J Med*. 2008;359(23):2417–2428.

25. Libby P, Thompson PD, Berman L, Shi H, Buebendorf E, Topol EJ. Effect of antihypertensive agents on cardiovascular events in patients with coronary disease and normal blood pressure. *JAMA*. 2004;292(18):2217–2226.

26. Sever PS, Dahlof B, Poulter NR, et al. Prevention of coronary and stroke events with atorvastatin in hypertensive patients who have average or lower-than-average cholesterol concentrations, in the Anglo Scandinavian Cardiac Outcomes Trial-Lipid Lowering

Arm (ASCOT-LLA): a multicentre randomised controlled trial. *Lancet.* 2003;361:1149–1158.

27. Fihn SD, Gardin JM, Abrams J, et al. 2012 ACCF/AHA/ACP/AATS/PCNA/SCAI/STS guideline for the diagnosis and management of patients with stable ischemic heart disease: executive summary: a report of the American College of Cardiology Foundation/American Heart Association Task Force on Practice. *Circulation.* 2012;126(25):3097–3137. doi:10.1161/CIR.0b013e3182776f83.

28. Law MR, Morris JK, Wald NJ. Use of blood pressure lowering drugs in the prevention of cardiovascular disease: meta-analysis of 147 randomised trials in the context of expectations from prospective epidemiological studies. *BMJ.* 2009;338:b1665. doi:10.1136/bmj.b1665.

29. US Preventive Services Task Force. Final recommendation statement. Lipid disorders in adults (cholesterol, dyslipidemia): Screening, June 2008. http://www.uspreventiveservicestaskforce.org/Page/Document/RecommendationStatementFinal/lipid-disorders-in-adults-cholesterol-dyslipidemia-screening#references. Accessed March 15, 2015.

30. Downs JR, Clearfield M, Weis S, et al. Primary prevention of acute coronary events with lovastatin in men and women with average cholesterol levels. Results of AFCAPS/TexCAPS. *J Cardiothorac Vasc Anesth.* 1999;13(20):108. doi:10.1016/S1053-0770(99)90192-1.

31. Gotto AM, Kastelein JJP, Koenig W, et al. Rosuvastatin to prevent vascular events in men and women with elevated C-reactive protein. *N Engl J Med.* 2008;359(21):2195–2207.

32. Marchioli R, Maria R. The case of cholesterol lowering interventions in the Secondary Prevention of Coronary Heart Disease. *Arch Intern Med.* 1996;156:1158–1172.

33. Heart Protection Study Collaborative G. MRC/BHF heart protection study of antioxidant vitamin supplementation in 20,536 high risk individuals: a randomised placebo controlled trial. *Lancet.* 2002;360:23–33.

34. Gutierrez J, Ramirez G, Rundek T, Sacco RL. Statin therapy in the prevention of recurrent cardiovascular events. *Arch Intern Med.* 2012;172(12):909–919.

35. Stone NJ, Robinson JG, Lichtenstein AH, et al. 2013 ACC/AHA guideline on the treatment of blood cholesterol to reduce atherosclerotic cardiovascular risk in adults: a report of the American College of Cardiology/American Heart Association Task Force on Practice Guidelines. *Circulation.* 2014;129(25 Suppl 2):S1–S45. doi:10.1161/01.cir.0000437738.63853.7a.

36. Reddigan JI, Ardern CI, Riddell MC, Kuk JL. Relation of physical activity to cardiovascular disease mortality and the influence of cardiometabolic risk factors. *Am J Cardiol.* 2011;108(10):1426–1431. doi:10.1016/j.amjcard.2011.07.005.

37. Blumenthal JA, Babyak MA, Hinderliter A, et al. Effects of the DASH diet alone and in combination with exercise and weight loss on blood pressure and cardiovascular biomarkers in men and women with high blood pressure: the ENCORE study. *Arch Intern Med.* 2010;170(2):126–135. doi:10.1016/j.ycar.2011.01.119.

38. Lamonte MJ, Eisenman PA, Adams TD, Shultz BB, Ainsworth BE, Yanowitz FG. Cardiorespiratory fitness and coronary heart disease risk factors. *Circulation.* 2000;102:1623–1628.

39. Vale N, Nordmann AJ, Schwartz GG, et al. Statins for acute coronary syndrome. *Cochrane Database Syst Rev.* 2011;(9):CD006870. doi:10.1002/14651858.CD006870.pub2.

40. Kaye JA, Meier CR, Walker AM, Jick H. Statin use, hyperlipidaemia, and the risk of breast cancer. *Br J Cancer.* 2002;86(May 2001):1436–1439. doi:10.1038/sj.bjc.6600267.

41. UK Prospective Diabetes Study (UKPDS) Group. Intensive blood-glucose control with sulphonylureas or insulin compared with conventional treatment and risk of complications in patients with type 2 diabetes (UKPDS 33). *Lancet.* 1998;352:837–853. PMID: 9742976.

42. Prescott E, Hippe M, Schnohr P, et al. Smoking and risk of myocardial infarction in women and men: longitudinal population study. *BMJ.* 1998;316:1043.

43. US Department of Health and Human Services. *The Health Consequences of Smoking: A Report of the Surgeon General.* Atlanta: US Department of Health and Human Services, Centers for Disease Control and Prevention, National Center for Chronic Disease Prevention and Health Promotion, Office on Smoking and Health; 2004. www.surgeongeneral.gov/library/reports/50-years-of-progress/. 2014 20+2004. Accessed February 12, 2015.

44. Andrews JO, Felton G. The effect of a multi-component smoking cessation intervention in African American women residing in public housing. *Res Nurs Health.* 2007;30:45–60. doi:10.1002/nur.

45. Barron J, Petrilli F, Strath L, Mccaffrey R. Successful interventions for smoking in pregnancy. *MCN Am J Matern Child Nurs.* 2007;32(1):42–47.

46. Chaney SE, Sheriff S. Weight gain among women during smoking cessation. *AAOHN J.* 2008;56(3):99–105. doi:10.3928/08910162-20080301-04.

47. Levine MD, Perkins KA, Kalarchian MA, et al. Bupropion and cognitive behavioral therapy for weight-concerned women smokers. *Arch Intern Med.* 2010;170(6):543–550. doi:10.1001/archinternmed.2010.33.

48. Farley AC, Hajek P, Lycett D, Aveyard P. *Interventions for Preventing Weight Gain After Smoking Cessation [review].* Cochrane Collaboration. New York: Wiley; 2012.

49. Cepeda-Benito A, Reynoso JT, Erath S. Meta-analysis of the efficacy of nicotine replacement therapy for smoking cessation: differences between men and women. *J Consult Clin Psychol.* 2004;72(4):712–722. doi:10.1037/0022-006X.72.4.712.

50. Korhonen T, Kinnunen T, Quiles Z, Leeman RF, Terwal DM, Garvey AJ. Cardiovascular risk behavior among sedentary female smokers and smoking cessation outcomes. *Tob Induc Dis.* 2005;3(1):7–26. doi:10.1186/1617-9625--3-4.

51. Roger VL, Go AS, Lloyd-Jones DM, et al., on behalf of the American Heart Association Statistics Committee and Stroke Statistics Subcommittee. Heart disease and stroke statistics—2011 update: a report from the American Heart Association [published correction appears in *Circulation* 2011;123:e240]. *Circulation.* 2011;123(4):e18–e209.

52. Wilson PW, Bozeman SR, Burton TM, et al. Prediction of first events of coronary heart disease and stroke with consideration of adiposity. *Circulation.* 2008;118:124.

53. Carey VJ, Walters EE, Colditz GA, et al. Body fat distribution and risk of non-insulin-dependent diabetes mellitus in women. The Nurses' Health Study. *Am J Epidemiol.* 1997;145:614–619.

54. Patterson RE, Frank LL, Kristal AR, White E. A comprehensive examination of health conditions associated with obesity in older adults. *Am J Prev Med.* 2004;27:385–390.

55. Naci H, Ioannidis JP. Comparative effectiveness of exercise and drug interventions on mortality outcomes: metaepidemiological study. *BMJ.* 2013;347 (October).f5577. doi:10.1136/bmj.f5577.

56. Kodama S, Saito K, Tanaka S, et al. Cardiorespiratory fitness as a quantitative predictor of all-cause mortality and cardiovascular events in healthy men and women: a meta-analysis. *JAMA.* 2009;301(19): 2024–2035. doi:10.1001/jama.2009.681.

57. LeFevre ML. Behavioral counseling to promote a healthful diet and physical activity for cardiovascular disease prevention in adults with cardiovascular risk factors: US Preventive Services Task Force recommendation statement. *Ann Intern Med.* 2014;161(8): 587–593. doi:10.7326/M14-1796.

58. Wild RA, Carmina E, Diamanti-Kandarakis E, et al. Assessment of cardiovascular disease with polycystic ovary system: a consensus statement by the Androgen Excess and Polycystic Ovary Syndrome Society. *J Clin Endocrinol Metab.* 2010;95:2038–2049.

59. Roger VL, Go AS, Lloyd-Jones DM, et al. American Heart Association Statistics Committee and Stroke Statistics Subcommittee. Heart disease and stroke statistics—2012 update: a report from the American Heart Association. *Circulation.* 2012;125:e2–e220.

60. Mondul AM, Rodriquez C, Jacobs EJ, Caile EE. Age at natural menopause and cause-specific mortality. *Am J Epidemiol.* 2005;162(11):1089–1097.

61. Andresdottir MB, Sigurdsson G, Sigvaldason H, et al. Fifteen percent of myocardial infarctions and coronary revascularizations explained by family history unrelated to conventional risk factors. The Reykjavik Cohort Study. *Eur Heart J.* 2002;23:1655.

62. United States Preventive Services Task Force. Using nontraditional risk factors in coronary heart disease risk assessment: US Preventive Services Task Force recommendation statement. *Ann Intern Med.* 2009;151:474–482.

63. American Congress of Obstetricians and Gynecologists. High-risk factors. http://www.acog.org/About ACOG/ACOG-Departments/Annual-Womens-Health-Care/Well-Woman-Recommendations/High-Risk-Factors (preeclampsia screening). Accessed March 12, 2015.

CHAPTER 7

Asthma and Obesity

Anil Ghimire, MD

Michael Iannuzzi, MD

INTRODUCTION

Obesity alters lung function, can cause symptoms suggesting asthma, and may worsen preexisting asthma. The precise mechanisms on how obesity leads to or worsens asthma are not well elucidated. A combination of mechanical factors, adipose-released inflammatory mediators, and immune system activation appears likely responsible for the "obese-asthma" phenotype.

Pregnancy has a variable and unpredictable effect on asthma. Studies suggest maternal obesity may be a risk factor for the development of asthma in offspring.

In this chapter, we discuss the evidence linking asthma to obesity, review the proposed mechanisms, and discuss the clinical care of obese individuals with asthma (see Box 7-1 for key clinical points).

LINKING ASTHMA AND OBESITY

Asthma prevalence has increased in parallel with obesity.[1,2] Of US adults, 8% have asthma—an increase from the 1980 value of 3.1%.[2] In the bariatric surgery population with body mass index (BMI) greater than 60 kg/m^2, the asthma prevalence is estimated to be 33%.[3]

BOX 7-1 Key Clinical Points

- Obesity is a risk factor for development of asthma, but the association is weak and needs further research.
- Complex interactions between mechanical factors, inflammatory pathways, and adipokines are thought to contribute, but the exact mechanism of association is still unclear.
- Asthma in obesity lacks cellular airway inflammation.
- Obese individuals with asthma respond poorly to asthma controller medications.
- Comorbidities, especially OSA, play a significant role in clinical presentation, while GERD (although common) does not play significant role.
- Obese individuals with asthma have a poor quality of life, increased health care utilization, and increased symptoms despite lack of airway obstruction on lung function test.
- Weight loss improves symptoms and physiological derangements, but its effect on inflammation is unclear.
- Asthma in obesity has two clinical phenotypes (see Table 7-1 for details); understanding these is crucial to develop new treatment strategies in the future.
- Maternal obesity and excessive weight gain during pregnancy may increase the risk of asthma in the offspring.

Obesity is defined as BMI greater than 30 kg/m^2. While simple to calculate and commonly used, BMI is not the best measure of assessing body fat influence on respiratory diseases. BMI does not capture fat distribution patterns or assess metabolically active adipose. The android pattern (abdominal fat distribution), rather than a gynoid (gluteofemoral) pattern, is associated with higher asthma risk.[4,5] The metabolically more active ectopic fat present in muscles and viscera, as measured by computed tomography (CT) or magnetic resonance imaging (MRI), may predict asthma risk more accurately.[6]

A meta-analysis involving 333,000 adults showed a modest risk of developing asthma (odds ratio [OR] 1.5; 95% confidence interval [CI] 1.27–1.80) in overweight or obese (BMI ≥25) compared to normal-weight adults ($p < .0001$). When the analysis was restricted to obese (BMI >30), the risk doubled.[7] A positive dose-response relationship exists between obesity and asthma. Several limitations to epidemiological asthma-obesity studies exist. Many studies relied on patient-reported asthma diagnosis and so could overestimate risk by overdiagnosing asthma. Also, a U-shaped relationship between weight and risk of asthma could lead investigators to underestimate the risk. Asthma prevalence increases among individuals with either low BMI or high BMI, forming a U-shaped curve.[8] Studies that include individuals with low BMI among those with normal BMI may underestimate the obesity effect on asthma.

Studies that have assessed the effect of weight loss on asthma support the obesity and asthma association. Weight loss of at least 10% has been shown to improve lung function in obese individuals with asthma.[9] A randomized, controlled trial of bariatric surgery in patients with asthma and without asthma found significant improvement in clinical and physiological parameters. Twelve months after surgery, individuals with asthma experienced significant improvement in asthma control, quality of life, and the need for rescue β_2-agonists.[10]

Several confounding factors may be responsible for the association of asthma with obesity. For example, poor diet, lack of physical activity, and shared genes and environment may affect the incidence of both asthma and obesity independently as well as via complex interactions. In addition, patients with asthma may become overweight from the side effects of corticosteroids and lack of physical activity.

Lack of physical activity could promote asthma. Vigorous physical exercise is known to augment bronchodilation, hyperinflation, and cyclical smooth muscle stretch. Lack of these protective physiological events, in the absence of physical exercise, may lead to increased airway hyperresponsiveness (AHR) and asthma.[11]

The relationship between diet and obesity seems obvious. However, obese patients may consume no more calories than lean individuals.[12] In regard to asthma risk, types of food consumed appear more important than the total calorie intake. Lack of dietary antioxidants, such as omega-3 fatty acid, has been associated with asthma in children.[13] A high-fat diet has been shown to lead to increased airway inflammation and to impair bronchodilator recovery.[14] Obese individuals tend to have diets high in fat and low in antioxidants.[12] Despite these observations, when adjusted for diet and level of physical activity, the asthma-obesity association persists in patients who already have developed asthma. Results from prospective intervention studies, however, are conflicting.[15] Pregnancy creates a unique situation to prospectively assess the effects of dietary manipulation on the risk of asthma and obesity in children. Some cohort studies and few intervention studies suggested an advantageous effect of maternal dietary modification, especially a diet high in omega-3 polyunsaturated fatty acids (PUFAs; found in fish oil) content, on the risk of asthma in children.[16-18] Little is known about the role of maternal dietary constituents and the risk of obese asthma in the offspring. Maternal diet could alter both asthma and obesity risk by influencing fetal programming of genes in utero.

Common environmental factors and shared genes may influence the association between asthma and obesity. Studies suggested a shared genetic makeup in asthma and obesity.[19] The probability (genetic liability) of this sharing to lead to the development of asthma and obesity appears to be significantly correlated with female gender.[20] Joint asthma-obesity candidate genes, such as β_2-receptor and tumor necrosis factor alpha (TNF-α) have been identified, but not confirmed.[21] Asthma and obesity are more common in minorities and groups with low socioeconomic status. Future studies examining epigenetic mechanisms and gene-by-gene and gene-by-environment interaction are needed.

Sex Effect on Obesity and Asthma

While an asthma-obesity association has been found in both men and women, some epidemiological studies noted the association was much stronger in women. Several potential explanations for this stronger association in women exist. Studies have shown that obese women are more likely to be diagnosed with asthma as compared to obese men when they have respiratory symptoms.[22] This may be partly because women tend to seek medical care more readily for respiratory symptoms than men. This leads to misclassification when the asthma diagnosis is not verified with spirometry or challenge testing. Hormonal differences may contribute to differences in gender effect on asthma prevalence. Prepubertal boys are more often affected with asthma than prepubertal girls and the risk reverses after puberty.[23] Similarly, early menarche in school-aged obese girls increases the risk of asthma, possibly from extended estrogen exposure.[24] Women frequently report worsening of asthma symptoms around menstrual periods.[25] Multiple prospective studies of hormone replacement therapy suggested increased asthma risk in postmenopausal women (OR 1.38 to 1.57).[26-28]

Pregnancy, Asthma, and Obesity

Asthma affects 4%–6% of pregnant women. The course of asthma in pregnancy is unpredictable. One-third of pregnant women will have worsening, one-third will have no change, and one-third will have improvement in asthma symptoms during pregnancy.[29] Women with mild disease are less likely to experience problems, whereas those with severe asthma are at high risk of deterioration, especially during the period of significant weight gain in late second and third trimesters, between the 25th and the 32nd weeks of gestation. Asthma control usually reverts to the prepregnancy level within 3 months of delivery, but the severity of asthma remains consistent in subsequent pregnancies. Progesterone-mediated bronchodilation and anti-inflammatory effects of increased free cortisol might explain the improvement seen in some women.

Factors that tend to worsen asthma control are decreased functional residual capacity (FRC), increased oxidative stress, altered immune regulation in pregnancy, and increased prevalence of gastroesophageal reflux disease (GERD). Some experience worsening of symptoms because of reduction or stopping of medication secondary to fear of adverse effects to the fetus. Prepregnancy factors associated with increased risk of worsening include severe disease, poor asthma-related quality of life, and cigarette smoking.[30] Maternal obesity, after adjusting for confounders, has also been recognized as a risk factor for poor asthma control and asthma exacerbation during pregnancy.[30] Similarly, pregnant women with asthma tend to be obese compared to pregnant women without asthma.

Studies suggest an increased risk of asthma in offspring of obese pregnant women. In a population-based cohort study, pre-pregnancy birth weight and gestational weight gain were independently associated with asthma in the offspring during 7-year follow-up. This association was independent of the child's BMI.[31] Another observational study demonstrated that maternal weight gain during pregnancy can predict asthma and low lung function at 9 years of age among children who exhibited persistently elevated serum TNF-α level (lipopolysaccharide induced) at birth and 3 month.[32] A prospective randomized controlled trial of weight management in pregnancy and asthma risk in offspring is needed.

PROPOSED MECHANISMS OF ASSOCIATION

Altered Respiratory Physiology

Obesity alters respiratory function, particularly lung volumes (Figure 7-1). The effect of obesity on the respiratory system depends on the pattern of fat distribution. Central obesity (abdominal and visceral adiposity) exerts greater respiratory load than peripheral obesity (femur-gluteal adiposity) (Figure 7-2).

Functional residual capacity, the resting lung volume at the end of a tidal breath, is determined by the balance between inflationary forces due to chest wall recoil and deflationary forces due to lung parenchymal elastic recoil and collapse. Adipose tissue decreases chest wall recoil by mass loading. Increased abdominal pressure from central obesity increases the deflationary forces. Additional factors leading to a decrease in FRC include atelectasis, redistribution of blood flow, and changes in alveolar surfactant. Pregnancy further exaggerates the deflation as the size of the uterus increases in late pregnancy.

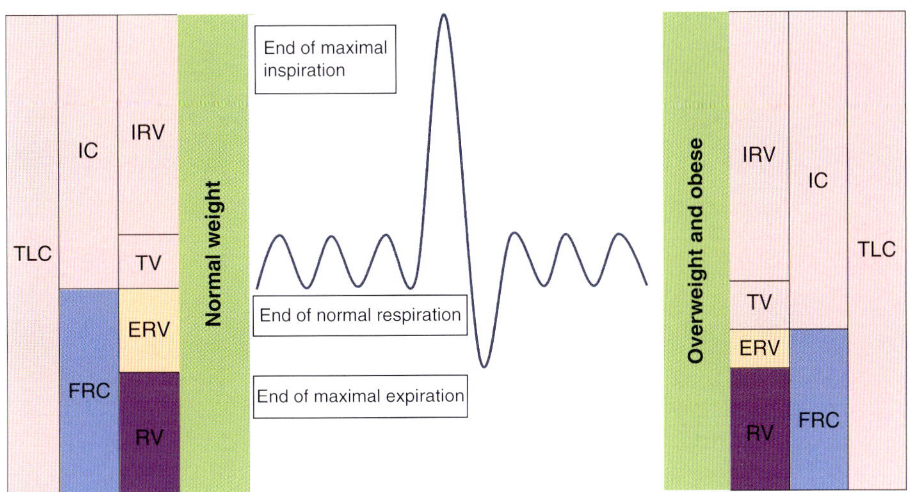

FIGURE 7-1. Lung function in normal-weight and obese individuals. ERV, expiratory reserve volume; FRC, functional residual capacity; IC, inspiratory capacity; IRV, inspiratory reserve volume; RV, residual volume; TLC, total lung capacity; TV, tidal volume.

The FRC is partitioned into two volumes (Figure 7-1): expiratory reserve volume (ERV), the air that can be forcefully exhaled after the end of a tidal breath; and residual volume (RV), the air left in the lung after the ERV has been expired. Decreased ERV out of proportion to decreased FRC is the most common finding on pulmonary function testing. Total lung capacity (TLC) is usually preserved in obesity except at extreme obesity. Diffusion capacity of the lungs for carbon monoxide (DLCO), a measure of gas transfer across the capillary surface, is normal or increased.

Airway hyperresponsiveness measured by bronchial challenge testing is the cardinal feature of asthma. Human and animal studies suggested obesity can lead to AHR.[33,34] In a study of 1725 adults with respiratory symptoms and without previous asthma diagnosis, Sood et al. showed that AHR increased with increasing BMI.[33] Surgical weight loss studies have demonstrated improvement in AHR 12 months after surgery but only in individuals with nonatopic asthma.[10] Proposed mechanisms for hyperresponsiveness in obesity are (1) increased airway smooth muscle contractility secondary to breathing at low lung volume and (2) enhanced inflammation.

Low lung volumes decrease the retractive forces on airways and decrease airway caliber. Persistent decrease in airway caliber induces changes in airway smooth muscles to shorter length and alters the actin myosin cross-bridging cycle. These changes make airway smooth muscles more reactive and contract at higher velocity.[35] Breathing at low lung volumes promotes dynamic hyperinflation and air trapping with mild bronchospasm and during tidal breathing during exertion. Hyperinflation and air trapping adds to the load that respiratory muscles need to overcome to breathe. This can give rise to an exaggerated sensation of dyspnea.

Enhanced Inflammation

Adipose tissue in obese is pro-inflammatory. CD8 T cells and macrophages are present in high numbers in the adipose tissue of obese individuals.[36,37] Inflammatory

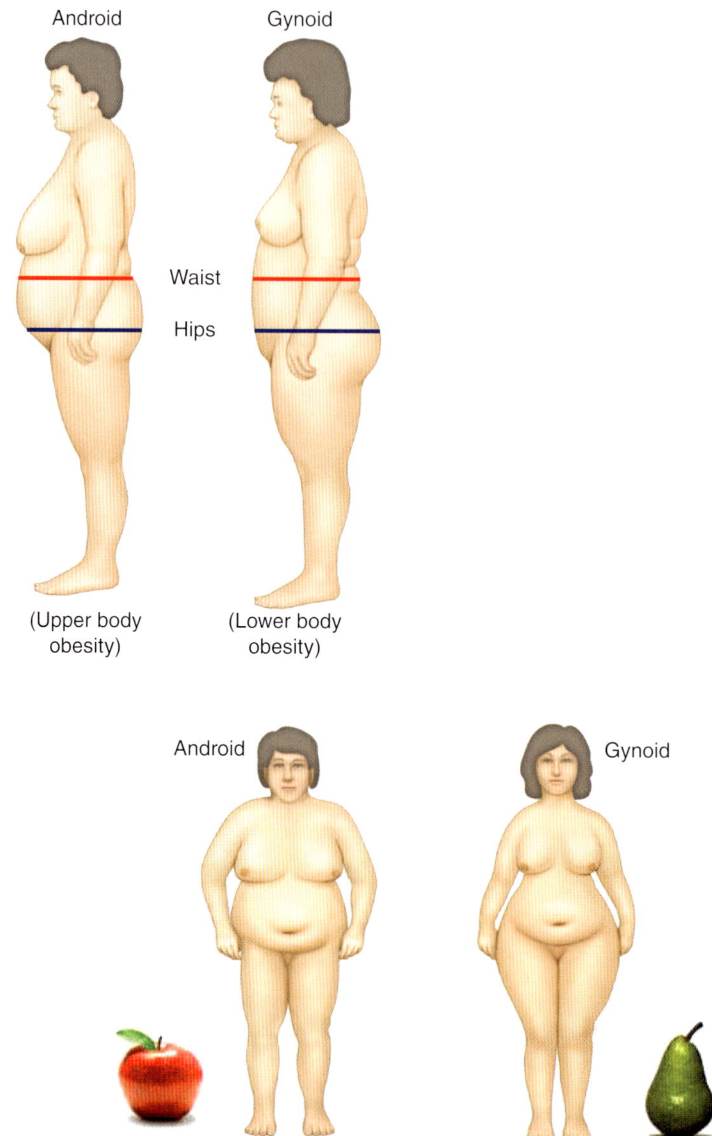

FIGURE 7-2. Body fat distribution in android and gynoid patterns.

markers such as interleukin (IL) 6 and TNF-α increase in obesity and decrease with weight loss.[38,39] The increased inflammation seen in the adipose tissue of obesity is attributed to hypoxia-induced adipocyte damage. As the adipocytes enlarge, they are pushed further away from the capillary, which leads to hypoxia and subsequent cell death.

Surprisingly, studies indicated the lack of cellular airway inflammation in obese individuals with asthma despite evidence of enhanced systemic inflammation.

Inflammatory markers in asthma, exhaled nitric oxide (eNO), and sputum eosinophils, are inversely correlated to BMI.[40,41] Obesity may affect airway inflammation by other pathways not measured by traditional markers of airway inflammation. Urinary leukotriene and 8-isoprostane, markers of oxidative stress, increase in exhaled breath condensate and urine with increasing BMI in asthma.[42,43]

Bronchoalveolar lavage (BAL) studies in obese individuals with asthma demonstrate a striking absence of eosinophils.[40,41] Evidence exists that trafficking of eosinophils from bone marrow to airways may be impaired in obesity.[44] Obese individuals with asthma have a higher number of airway submucosal eosinophils and a lower sputum eosinophil percentage compared to nonobese individuals with asthma. This discrepancy between submucosal and sputum eosinophils highlights the inadequacy of sputum as a reliable marker of airway inflammation in the study of asthma in obesity. Future studies seeking to clarify the mechanism of association between asthma and obesity need to incorporate airway wall biopsies to measure airway inflammation reliably.

Adipose tissues produce pro-inflammatory adipokine leptin and anti-inflammatory adipokine adiponectins. Blood leptin level is increased and adiponectin level is decreased in obesity.[45] Animal studies suggested that leptin infusion increases AHR in obese mice.[46] Adiponectin attenuates the effects of allergen-induced inflammation, suggesting that low levels of adiponectin in obesity may be permissive to the pro-inflammatory effects of leptins.[47] In humans, however, results are inconsistent.[48–50]

CLINICAL CARE

Currently, no specific guidelines exist for clinical care of asthma in obesity. This is an area wherein future research is needed to optimize clinical care.

Clinical Characteristics of Obese Individuals With Asthma

Obese individuals with asthma consist of two groups. The first group consists of people who have asthma and later become obese. The second group comprises people in whom asthma is the consequence of obesity. Differences between the two groups are highlighted in Table 7-1.

Obese individuals with asthma tend to have high symptom burden, poor asthma control, increased exacerbations, and increased health care utilization (hospitalization, length of stay, and medication use) compared to lean individuals with asthma.[51–53] The risk for hospitalization is nearly 5-fold higher in obese individuals with asthma. The tendency to more severe asthma, however, does not strongly correlate with physiological and inflammatory measures. Obese individuals with asthma presenting to the emergency department have a higher peak expiratory flow rate (PEFR) than normal-weight individuals with asthma and lack cellular inflammation in the airways.[53] Women tend to have poorer asthma control than men in general and in obesity. Whether this is due to increased perception of loss of asthma control in women leading to seeking medical care readily (overreporting) or a consequence of a more severe disease is unclear. Alternatively, cyclical hormonal influences around menstrual cycles can lead to poor asthma control.[29]

TABLE 7-1 Characteristics of Asthma Phenotypes in Obesity

Phenotype 1	*Phenotype 2*
Asthma precedes obesity	Obesity precedes asthma
Atopic	Nonatopic
Early onset	Late onset
Eosinophilic airway inflammation	Lack of cellular inflammation
High serum IgE	Low serum IgE
Severe airflow limitation	Less airflow limitation
Male:Female unclear	Predominantly female
Weight loss does not improve physiological and inflammatory derangements	Weight loss can restore physiological and inflammatory derangements
Resistant to steroids	Resistant to steroids
Comorbidities worsen asthma control	Comorbidities may contribute to development of asthma

Diagnosis

Asthma is diagnosed based on the presence of symptoms (cough, wheezing, shortness of breath) and objective evidence of a variable airflow obstruction or bronchial hyperresponsiveness. Symptoms of asthma are common in other respiratory illnesses, and physiologic changes from obesity itself may result in symptoms. Hence, objective measures play a particularly important role in diagnosis of asthma in obese patients. Spirometry or a methacholine challenge test is required to confirm asthma. In obese patients with asthma, spirometry usually shows no obstruction, and a methacholine challenge test is usually positive. Obstruction is defined as forced expiratory volume in 1 second (FEV_1) and forced vital capacity (FVC) ratio of less than 0.7. Obstruction, while uncommon, may be seen in some obese individuals with asthma.[54] Unlike chronic obstructive pulmonary disease (COPD), however, obstruction seen in asthma normalizes after bronchodilator administration. A negative methacholine challenge test nearly rules out the diagnosis of asthma. A positive test supports the diagnosis but may be positive in other disease conditions, such as congestive heart failure, allergic rhinitis, and COPD. In the absence of objective measurements, obese individuals presenting to emergency departments with respiratory symptoms are more likely to be misdiagnosed as having asthma than nonobese individuals.[55] This may be because, as discussed previously, physiologic changes from obesity itself may result in respiratory symptoms. In addition, obese individuals may have a greater perception of dyspnea compared to nonobese patients for the same level of spirometry. Other diagnoses to consider when evaluating an obese individual with respiratory symptoms are listed in Table 7-2.

TABLE 7-2 Differential Diagnosis of Dyspnea in the Obese

Disease Condition	*Diagnostic Workup and Management*
Vocal cord dysfunction	• Coexists with asthma or occurs separately. • Indirect laryngoscopy at time of dyspnea episode demonstrates abnormal movement of vocal cords. • Treatment is speech therapy and treatment of anxiety.
Pulmonary embolism	• Obesity is a risk factor for venous thromboembolism. • Ventilation perfusion scan or CT angiography of lung confirms the diagnosis. • Treatment is anticoagulation.
Upper airway obstruction	• Crowded upper airway anatomy in obese. • Upper airway infection leading to mucosal edema can precipitate upper airway obstruction, causing dyspnea. • Spirometry with flow volume loop may reveal obstruction.
Acute heart failure	• Severely obese demonstrate signs of left ventricular dysfunction with exercise that may precipitate acute pulmonary edema. • Chest x-ray, pro-BNP (brain natriuretic peptide), and exercise echocardiogram. • Diuresis and treatment of diastolic dysfunction.
Anxiety/panic attacks	• Anxiety or depression is common in obesity and is an important cause of health care utilization. • Screening and treating anxiety/depression.

Pharmacotherapy

Pharmacotherapy of obese individuals with asthma is similar to treatment of lean individuals with asthma as recommended by the Global Initiative for Asthma (GINA) and National Heart, Lung, and Blood Institute (NHLBI) Expert Report 3 (EPR-3) guidelines.[56,57] However, currently available medications are less effective in obese patients with asthma. Inhaled corticosteroids (ICSs) are the mainstay of treatment, but their response is attenuated. Studies have shown a reduced likelihood of achieving good control with ICS, as monotherapy or in combination with a long-acting β-agonist (LABA).[58,59] Similar poor response and an increase in exacerbation rate have been reported with theophylline. The exacerbation rate was no different for leukotriene inhibitors.[60] These findings suggest leukotriene inhibitors are an useful adjunct to ICSs in treatment of obese individuals with asthma.

The increased systemic inflammatory state associated with obesity and altered respiratory mechanics likely cause the reduced therapeutic response. Increased expression of pro-inflammatory cytokine TNF-α, which attenuates the corticosteroid-induced activation of mitogen-activated protein (MAP) kinase phosphatase 1, is thought to mediate the refractoriness of steroids.[61] Alternatively, altered respiratory mechanics causing low lung volumes result in plastic adaptation of airway smooth muscles that is unlikely to improve with anti-inflammatory agents.

Weight Loss and Dietary Modifications

Current evidence suggests a beneficial effect of weight loss. Weight loss, through dietary modifications or surgery, improves asthma control, lung function, quality of life, and medication use[62] (Figure 7-3). Results are striking with significant weight loss after bariatric surgery, but as little as 5%–10% reduction in weight using dietary modification can improve asthma control.[62,63] Besides weight loss, modification in dietary constituents can have a salutary effect in asthma control. Observational studies suggest a protective effect of a diet high in omega-3 polyunsaturated fat, as found in fish oil, in the development of asthma.[15] Similarly, a diet rich in antioxidants (fruits and vegetables), multivitamins (vitamins C, D, and E), and low in saturated fat has been reported to improve asthma control and reduce markers of inflammation in individuals with asthma.[15] Although these dietary interventions cannot be routinely recommended to all individuals with asthma, it is reasonable to encourage dietary modifications along with physical exercise for patients with poor asthma control.

Treatment of Comorbidities

Comorbidities that may cause or worsen asthma in obese individuals include obstructive sleep apnea (OSA), GERD, and depression. OSA and GERD are highly prevalent in obese populations and can contribute to poor asthma control. The high prevalence of OSA in patients with severe asthma is independent of BMI.[64] Obese patients with asthma with OSA symptoms report increased symptom burden and poor asthma control.[65] The level of asthma control correlates with the numbers of reported OSA symptoms, and witnessed apnea is the strongest predictor of poor asthma control.[66] Treatment of OSA with continuous positive airway pressure (CPAP) improves nighttime and daytime asthma symptoms.[67] Hence, screening for and treatment of OSA is important in obese individuals with asthma who have poor control of asthma.

Gastroesophageal reflux disease is common in obesity and asthma. GERD could cause asthma or worsen asthma control by reflex-mediated bronchoconstriction in response to acid in the esophagus or in the airways. Previously, GERD and asthma were thought to be causally related. Although common in obese individuals with asthma, it does not appear to be a major factor contributing to asthma control.[63] This is consistent with the finding that antireflux treatment did not provide better symptom control in patients with asthma in general.[68]

Depression is common in obesity, and the relationship is reciprocal. The association exists among overweight and obese women but only among severely obese men.[69] Similarly, depression and asthma are also correlated especially at the severe end of the disease spectrum. Studies suggest a potential causal association between the two; that is, severe asthma can lead to depression, and severe depression is a risk factor for incident asthma.[70,71] Interactions between asthma, obesity, and depression are complex and difficult to elucidate. A recent study reported increased risk (OR 2.9) of incident asthma in obese individuals with anxiety-depression.[72] Maternal stress and anxiety during pregnancy can increase the risk of asthma in children.[73] Screening and treating anxiety-depression in obese individuals could decrease asthma risk or improve asthma control. Randomized studies are required before antidepressants can be routinely recommended for obese patients with difficult-to-treat asthma.

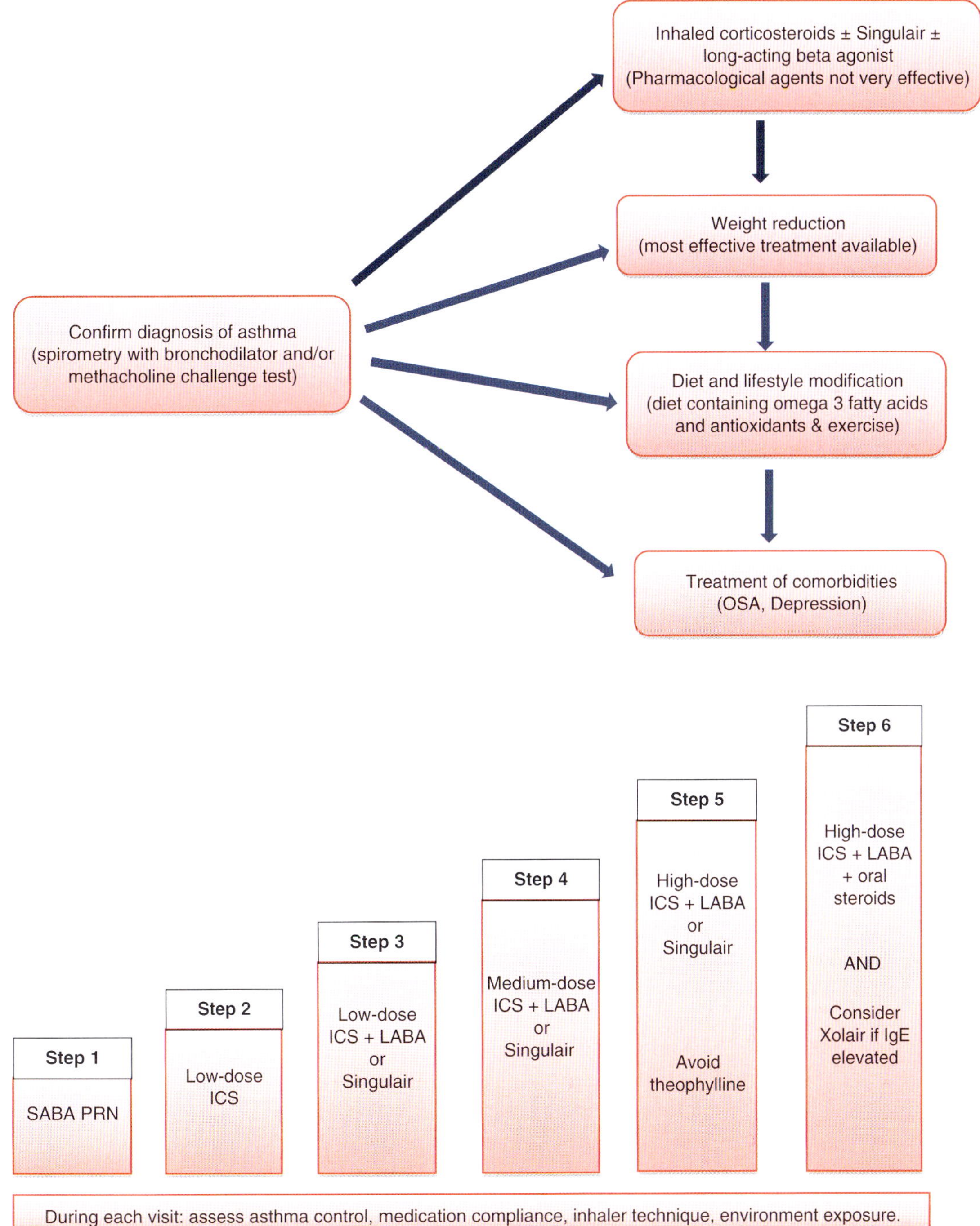

FIGURE 7-3. Treatment strategy for asthma in obese. Step-up and step-down approach to pharmacological treatment of asthma. (Adapted from NHLBI, EPR-3.) Effectiveness of this approach is unclear in obese individuals with asthma. IgE, immunoglobulin E; SABA, short-acting β-agonist.

Treatment of Pregnant Obese Women with Asthma

Maintaining good control of asthma during pregnancy is critical to prevent fetal hypoxia. A pregnant woman with well-controlled asthma should be advised to continue her medications during pregnancy. Albuterol and budesonide are the drugs of choice for acute relief and maintenance, respectively. Other inhaled corticosteroids, although not studied as extensively as budesonide, have not been found to be contraindicated. A pregnant woman whose asthma has been controlled on an ICS should continue its use in pregnancy. Salmeterol is recommended as a step-up therapy for poorly controlled asthma. Association between oral steroids and preeclampsia, preterm delivery, and low birth weight has been reported. However, it is difficult to separate the effects of drugs from the effects of asthma itself, especially in individuals with severe asthma who are prone to exacerbations that necessitate corticosteroid use.

Future Direction

The association between obesity and asthma is consistent but weak. There remain critical gaps in our current understanding of the asthma-obesity association. Future studies should distinguish between the two phenotypes of obese individuals with asthma to mitigate the role played by allergy in disease modification. A better marker of adiposity in relation to its pathogenicity in asthma is needed. Current animal models of allergic disease are inadequate to represent the complexity of obese patients with asthma. A better understanding of the biological basis for female predilection and the role played by adipokines would validate and strengthen the association. Understanding how obesity promotes AHR and renders current medications less effective is essential to advance development of new therapeutics. Clinical trials specifically targeting obese individuals with asthma are urgently needed. The role of diet modification beyond weight maintenance deserves careful exploration. Obesity during pregnancy as a potential risk factor for asthma in the offspring needs further research.

CONCLUSION

Asthma in those who are obese is increasing and is projected to become the most common asthma clinical phenotype worldwide. Obese patients with asthma consist of two groups: individuals with asthma who become obese and obese individuals who develop asthma. Asthma in the obese is characterized by lack of eosinophilic airway inflammation, poor symptom control, and relative resistance to inhaled glucocorticoids. Currently, there is no specific pharmacological treatment of obese individuals with asthma. Symptom control improves with weight loss, dietary changes, and treatment of comorbidities. Adipokines are thought to play an important role in the pathogenesis of obese individuals with asthma. Significant gaps exist in the current understanding of asthma in obesity.

REFERENCES

1. Lim SS, Vos T, Flaxman AD, et al. A comparative risk assessment of burden of disease and injury attributable to 67 risk factors and risk factor clusters in 21 regions, 1990–2010: a systematic analysis for the global burden of disease study 2010. *Lancet.* 2013;380(9859):2224–2260.
2. Akinbami OJ. *Trends in Asthma Prevalence, Health Care Use, and Mortality in the United States, 2001–2010.*

Washington, DC: US Department of Health and Human Services, Centers for Disease Control and Prevention, National Center for Health Statistics; 2012.

3. LABS Writing Group for the LABS Consortium. Relationship of body mass index with demographic and clinical characteristics in the longitudinal assessment of bariatric surgery (LABS). *Surg Obes Relat Dis.* 2008;4(4):474–480.

4. Von Behren J, Lipsett M, Horn-Ross PL, et al. Obesity, waist size and prevalence of current asthma in the California teachers study cohort. *Thorax.* 2009;64(10):889–893.

5. Romieu I, Avenel V, Leynaert B, et al. Body mass index, change in body silhouette, and risk of asthma in the E3N cohort study. *Am J Epidemiol.* 2003;158(2):165–174.

6. Sood A, Qualls C, Li R, et al. Lean mass predicts asthma better than fat mass among females. *Eur Respir J.* 2011;37(1):65–71.

7. Beuther DA, Sutherland ER. Overweight, obesity, and incident asthma: a meta-analysis of prospective epidemiologic studies. *Am J Respir Crit Care Med.* 2007;175(7):661–666.

8. Celedon JC, Palmer LJ, Litonjua AA, et al. Body mass index and asthma in adults in families of subjects with asthma in Anqing, China. *Am J Respir Crit Care Med.* 2001;164(10):1835–1840.

9. Eneli IU, Skybo T, Camargo CA Jr. Weight loss and asthma: a systematic review. *Thorax.* 2008;63(8):671–676.

10. Dixon AE, Pratley RE, Forgione PM, et al. Effects of obesity and bariatric surgery on airway hyperresponsiveness, asthma control, and inflammation. *J Allergy Clin Immunol.* 2011;128(3):508–515, e2.

11. Skloot G, Permutt S, Togias A. Airway hyperresponsiveness in asthma: a problem of limited smooth muscle relaxation with inspiration. *J Clin Invest.* 1995;96(5):2393–2403.

12. Gates JC, Huenemann RL, Brand RJ. Food choices of obese and non-obese persons. *J Am Diet Assoc.* 1975;67(4):339–343.

13. Britton JR, Pavord ID, Richards KA, et al. Dietary antioxidant vitamin intake and lung function in the general population. *Am J Respir Crit Care Med.* 1995;151(5):1383–1387.

14. Wood LG, Garg ML, Gibson PG. A high-fat challenge increases airway inflammation and impairs bronchodilator recovery in asthma. *J Allergy Clin Immunol.* 2011;127(5):1133–1140.

15. Allan K, Devereux G. Diet and asthma: nutrition implications from prevention to treatment. *J Am Diet Assoc.* 2011;111(2):258–268.

16. Lumia M, Luukkainen P, Tapanainen H, et al. Dietary fatty acid composition during pregnancy and the risk of asthma in the offspring. *Pediatr Allergy Immunol.* 2011;22(8):827–835.

17. Olsen SF, Osterdal ML, Salvig JD, et al. Fish oil intake compared with olive oil intake in late pregnancy and asthma in the offspring: 16 years of registry-based follow-up from a randomized controlled trial. *Am J Clin Nutr.* 2008;88(1):167–175.

18. Salam MT, Li Y, Langholz B, Gilliland FD. Maternal fish consumption during pregnancy and risk of early childhood asthma. *J Asthma.* 2005;42(6):513–518.

19. Hallstrand TS, Fischer ME, Wurfel MM, et al. Genetic pleiotropy between asthma and obesity in a community-based sample of twins. *J Allergy Clin Immunol.* 2005;116(6):1235–1241.

20. Thomsen S, Ulrik CS, Kyvik KO, et al. Association between obesity and asthma in a twin cohort. *Allergy.* 2007;62(10):1199–1204.

21. Melén E, Himes BE, Brehm JM, et al. Analyses of shared genetic factors between asthma and obesity in children. *J Allergy Clin Immunol.* 2010;126(3):631–637, e8.

22. Chinn S, Downs SH, Anto JM, et al. Incidence of asthma and net change in symptoms in relation to changes in obesity. *Eur Respir J.* 2006;28(4):763–771.

23. Kjellman B, Gustafsson P. Asthma from childhood to adulthood: asthma severity, allergies, sensitization, living conditions, gender influence and social consequences. *Respir Med.* 2000;94(5):454–465.

24. Al-Sahab B, Hamadeh MJ, Ardern CI, et al. Early menarche predicts incidence of asthma in early adulthood. *Am J Epidemiol.* 2011;173(1):64–70.

25. Skobeloff EM, Spivey WH, Silverman R, et al. The effect of the menstrual cycle on asthma presentations in the emergency department. *Arch Intern Med.* 1996;156(16):1837–1840.

26. Troisi RJ, Speizer FE, Willett WC, et al. Menopause, postmenopausal estrogen preparations, and the risk of adult-onset asthma. A prospective cohort study. *Am J Respir Crit Care Med.* 1995;152(4 Pt 1):1183–1188.

27. Barr RG, Wentowski CC, Grodstein F, et al. Prospective study of postmenopausal hormone use and newly diagnosed asthma and chronic obstructive pulmonary disease. *Arch Intern Med.* 2004;164(4):379–386.

28. Romieu I, Fabre A, Fournier A, et al. Postmenopausal hormone therapy and asthma onset in the E3N cohort. *Thorax.* 2010;65(4):292–297.

29. Schatz M, Harden K, Forsythe A, et al. The course of asthma during pregnancy, postpartum, and with successive pregnancies: a prospective analysis. *J Allergy Clin Immunol.* 1988;81(3):509–517.

30. Schatz M, Dombrowski MP, Wise R, et al. The relationship of asthma-specific quality of life during pregnancy to subsequent asthma and perinatal morbidity. *J Asthma.* 2010;47(1):46–50.

31. Forno E, Young OM, Kumar R, et al. Maternal obesity in pregnancy, gestational weight gain, and risk of childhood asthma. *Pediatrics*. 2014;134(2):e535–e546.

32. Halonen M, Lohman IC, Stern DA, et al. Perinatal tumor necrosis factor-α production, influenced by maternal pregnancy weight gain, predicts childhood asthma. *Am J Respir Crit Care Med*. 2013;188(1):35–41.

33. Sood A, Verhulst SJ, Varma III A, et al. Association of excess weight and degree of airway responsiveness in asthmatics and non-asthmatics. *J Asthma*. 2006;43(6):447–452.

34. Shore SA. Obesity and asthma: lessons from animal models. *J Appl Physiol (1985)*. 2007;102(2):516–528.

35. McClean MA, Matheson MJ, McKay K, et al. Low lung volume alters contractile properties of airway smooth muscle in sheep. *Eur Respir J*. 2003;22(1):50–56.

36. Weisberg SP, McCann D, Desai M, et al. Obesity is associated with macrophage accumulation in adipose tissue. *J Clin Invest*. 2003;112(12):1796–1808.

37. Rausch M, Weisberg S, Vardhana P, et al. Obesity in C57BL/6J mice is characterized by adipose tissue hypoxia and cytotoxic T-cell infiltration. *Int J Obes*. 2008;32(3):451–463.

38. Ferrante A. Obesity-induced inflammation: a metabolic dialogue in the language of inflammation. *J Intern Med*. 2007;262(4):408–414.

39. Roth CL, Kratz M, Ralston MM, et al. Changes in adipose-derived inflammatory cytokines and chemokines after successful lifestyle intervention in obese children. *Metab Clin Exp*. 2011;60(4):445–452.

40. Van Veen I, Ten Brinke A, Sterk P, et al. Airway inflammation in obese and nonobese patients with difficult-to-treat asthma. *Allergy*. 2008;63(5):570–574.

41. McLachlan CR, Poulton R, Car G, et al. Adiposity, asthma, and airway inflammation. *J Allergy Clin Immunol*. 2007;119(3):634–639.

42. Giouleka P, Papatheodorou G, Lyberopoulos P, et al. Body mass index is associated with leukotriene inflammation in asthmatics. *Eur J Clin Invest*. 2011;41(1):30–38.

43. Komakula S, Khatri S, Mermis J, et al. Body mass index is associated with reduced exhaled nitric oxide and higher exhaled 8-isoprostanes in asthmatics. *Respir Res*. 2007;8(1):32–36.

44. Desai D, Newby C, Symon FA, et al. Elevated sputum interleukin-5 and submucosal eosinophilia in obese individuals with severe asthma. *Am J Respir Crit Care Med*. 2013;188(6):657–663.

45. Maffei M, Halaas J, Ravussin E, et al. Leptin levels in human and rodent: measurement of plasma leptin and ob RNA in obese and weight-reduced subjects. *Nat Med*. 1995;1(11):1155–1161.

46. Shore SA, Schwartzman IN, Mellema MS, et al. Effect of leptin on allergic airway responses in mice. *J Allergy Clin Immunol*. 2005;115(1):103–109.

47. Shore SA, Terry RD, Flynt L, et al. Adiponectin attenuates allergen-induced airway inflammation and hyperresponsiveness in mice. *J Allergy Clin Immunol*. 2006;118(2):389–395.

48. Sood A, Ford ES, Camargo CA Jr. Association between leptin and asthma in adults. *Thorax*. 2006;61(4):300–305.

49. Sutherland TJ, Sears MR, McLachlan CR, et al. Leptin, adiponectin, and asthma: findings from a population-based cohort study. *Ann Allergy Asthma Immunol*. 2009;103(2):101–107.

50. Sood A, Qualls C, Schuyler M, et al. Low serum adiponectin predicts future risk for asthma in women. *Am J Respir Crit Care Med*. 2012;186(1):41–47.

51. Camargo CA Jr, Sutherland ER, Bailey W, et al. Effect of increased body mass index on asthma risk, impairment and response to asthma controller therapy in african americans. *Curr Med Res Opin*. 2010;26(7):1629–1635.

52. Grammer LC, Weiss KB, Pedicano JB, et al. Obesity and asthma morbidity in a community-based adult cohort in a large urban area: The Chicago Initiative to Raise Asthma Health Equity (CHIRAH). *J Asthma*. 2010;47(5):491–495.

53. Thomson CC, Clark S, Camargo CA. Body mass index and asthma severity among adults presenting to the emergency department. *Chest*. 2003;124(3):795–802.

54. Leone N, Courbon D, Thomas F, et al. Lung function impairment and metabolic syndrome: the critical role of abdominal obesity. *Am J Respir Crit Care Med*. 2009;179(6):509–516.

55. Pakhale S, Doucette S, Vandemheen K, et al. A comparison of obese and nonobese people with asthma: exploring an asthma-obesity interaction. *Chest*. 2010;137(6):1316–1323.

56. National Institutes of Health, and National Heart, Lung, and Blood Institute. "Global initiative for asthma." *Global strategy for asthma management and prevention. Revised* (2002).

57. National Heart, Lung, and Blood Institute. US Department of Health and Human Services, National Institutes of Health. *Expert panel report 3: guidelines for the diagnosis and management of asthma: full report*. 2007.

58. Peters-Golden M, Swern A, Bird SS, et al. Influence of body mass index on the response to asthma controller agents. *Eur Respir J*. 2006;27(3):495–503.

59. Boulet L, Franssen E. Influence of obesity on response to fluticasone with or without salmeterol in moderate asthma. *Respir Med*. 2007;101(11):2240–2247.

60. Dixon AE, Shade DM, Cohen RI, et al. Effect of obesity on clinical presentation and response to treatment in asthma. *J Asthma*. 2006;43(7):553–558.

61. Sutherland ER, Goleva E, Strand M, et al. Body mass and glucocorticoid response in asthma. *Am J Respir Crit Care Med*. 2008;178(7):682–687.

62. Scott H, Gibson P, Garg M, et al. Dietary restriction and exercise improve airway inflammation and clinical outcomes in overweight and obese asthma: a randomized trial. *Clin Exp Allergy.* 2013;43(1):36–49.

63. Boulet L, Turcotte H, Martin J, et al. Effect of bariatric surgery on airway response and lung function in obese subjects with asthma. *Respir Med.* 2012;106(5):651–660.

64. Julien JY, Martin JG, Ernst P, et al. Prevalence of obstructive sleep apnea–hypopnea in severe versus moderate asthma. *J Allergy Clin Immunol.* 2009; 124(2):371–376.

65. Dixon AE, Clerisme-Beaty EM, Sugar EA, et al. Effects of obstructive sleep apnea and gastroesophageal reflux disease on asthma control in obesity. *J Asthma.* 2011;48(7):707–713.

66. Teodorescu M, Consens FB, Bria WF, et al. Predictors of habitual snoring and obstructive sleep apnea risk in patients with asthma. *Chest.* 2009;135(5):1125–1132.

67. Alkhalil M, Schulman ES, Getsy J. Obstructive sleep apnea syndrome and asthma: the role of continuous positive airway pressure treatment. *Ann Allergy Asthma Immunol.* 2008;101(4):350–357.

68. American Lung Association Asthma Clinical Research Centers, Mastronarde JG, Anthonisen NR, et al. Efficacy of esomeprazole for treatment of poorly controlled asthma. *N Engl J Med.* 2009;360(15):1487–1499.

69. Luppino FS, de Wit LM, Bouvy PF, et al. Overweight, obesity, and depression: a systematic review and meta-analysis of longitudinal studies. *Arch Gen Psychiatry.* 2010;67(3):220–229.

70. Brunner WM, Schreiner PJ, Sood A, Jacobs DR Jr. Depression and risk of incident asthma in adults. The CARDIA study. *Am J Respir Crit Care Med.* 2014;189(9):1044–1051.

71. Coogan PF, Yu J, O'Connor GT, Brown TA, Palmer JR, Rosenberg L. Depressive symptoms and the incidence of adult-onset asthma in African American women. *Ann Allergy Asthma Immunol.* 2014;112(4):333–338, e1.

72. Brumpton BM, Leivseth L, Romundstad PR, et al. The joint association of anxiety, depression and obesity with incident asthma in adults: the HUNT study. *Int J Epidemiol.* 2013;42(5):1455–1463.

73. Cookson H, Granell R, Joinson C, Ben-Shlomo Y, Henderson AJ. Mothers' anxiety during pregnancy is associated with asthma in their children. *J Allergy Clin Immunol.* 2009;123(4):847–853, e11.

CHAPTER 8

Behavioral Determinants of Obesity

Deborah L. Pollack, PhD

INTRODUCTION

Behavioral determinants of obesity have been widely studied in the field of psychology, leading most to conclude that it is a complex condition that is difficult to treat with long-term success. This chapter reviews the most common theories about psychological causes of obesity, the co-occurrence of obesity and common mental disorders, and psychological treatment options for obesity and binge-eating disorder (BED). Suggestions for assessment and treatment planning are provided to help physicians determine the presence of underlying psychopathology or problematic behavior patterns and to work with their obese patients to find a program best suited to their individual psychological needs.

THE ETIOLOGY OF OBESITY: PSYCHOLOGICAL FACTORS

It is widely accepted that the etiology of obesity is multidetermined. In addition to genetic, physical, environmental, and cultural/sociological factors, psychological research has focused on individual characteristics such as personality, systems of reinforcement, cognitive processes, and developmental history, as well as the interplay of all of these factors. Decades of research have focused on the psychology of overeating and whether obese individuals differ from their nonobese counterparts in their eating behavior.[1] In the following section, the most studied theories about overeating in obesity are presented along with discussion of their current research support.

A commonly held view is that obese people are more likely to engage in *emotional eating*, using food to manage distressing or overwhelming affect. The *psychosomatic* hypothesis, first put forth by Kaplan and Kaplan[2] suggests that obese individuals likely learned as children to overeat as a way to self-soothe when anxious. Their subsequent weight gain further increases negative affect, which then leads to more overeating and obesity. The psychoanalyst Hilde Bruch[3] further hypothesized that for these individuals early developmental trauma, such as poor infant-caregiver attunement, interferes with the child's ability to distinguish between internal sensations of hunger and uncomfortable emotional states. The child therefore misinterprets emotions such as sadness and anger as hunger and will overeat to regulate these feelings.[3]

In their 2002 review, Canetti, Bachar, and Elliot[4] concluded, that for both obese and nonobese people, the presence of negative emotions (e.g., anger, sadness, boredom) leads to increased food consumption. Some research indicated that positive emotions (e.g., joy) can also increase food intake for both obese and nonobese individuals; however, the support for this conclusion is not as robust.[4] Canetti et al.[4] stated that the psychosomatic theory of obesity has received enough research support to conclude that obese individuals and dieters (obese or normal weight) are more likely to engage in emotional eating. A more recent review of binge eating and overeating in laboratory settings further supported the role of negative affect as a trigger for overeating for obese individuals, and even more strongly so for those with BED.[5]

In the late 1960s and early 1970s, Schacter argued against the psychosomatic model by developing his *externality theory* of overeating; he suggested that the sensory aspects of the food itself, such as sight, taste, and smell, lead obese people to overeat, and that perhaps differences in hypothalamic function for appetite were to blame.[6] Researchers have since challenged externality theory, positing no difference between obese and nonobese individuals' tendency to rely on internal or external factors to guide their eating behavior (Moskovich et. al., 2011; Canetti et. al., 2002).[1,4] Stroebe et al. suggested that both distressing affect and external cues seem to drive overeating for obese individuals, citing several experimental studies demonstrating how stress can trigger overeating for obese individuals, but only when the food is tasty and appealing.[7]

Nisbett developed *set point theory* as an attempt to further Schacter's hypothesis about the role of the hypothalamus in overeating.[8] According to his theory, we all have a set point for our weight, which our body will attempt to maintain by altering metabolism and eating behavior. Thus, when an obese individual loses weight through dieting, the individual's metabolism will slow, and the person will experience increased sensitivity to external cues, causing the person to overeat so that his or her body can return to its set point.[8] Although set point theory has been widely dispersed and accepted in popular culture, it has been challenged by some longitudinal studies as well as the data that obesity rates have dramatically increased over the past several decades throughout the industrialized world.[7]

Indeed, more recent neuroimaging research has suggested that it is not the hypothalamic system that drives overeating behavior, but rather neurological centers for reward and pleasure.[7] Several studies using functional magnetic resonance imaging (fMRI) technology have demonstrated that obese individuals show increased neurological reactivity regions that mediate emotional responses to food cues. There is also some evidence that weight gain decreases this receptivity, so that individuals would need to consume even more to obtain the same neurological reward experience.[7]

Another set of research on the psychological causes of obesity has focused on the role of cognition and beliefs. Herman and Mack described the *disinhibition effect* in their theory of overeating; they theorized that restrained eaters who believe that they violated their diet, whether or not they actually did, are more likely to subsequently overeat.[9] Indeed, there is strong research support demonstrating that restrained eating actually puts individuals at risk for overeating, especially in the presence of exacerbating factors such as stress, distraction, negative emotions, and depression.[1,7,10] While the state of deprivation itself may induce more intense cravings for food, this phenomenon may also be due to thoughts that occur in reaction to perceived diet violations, such as, "I've blown it now; might as well keep eating."

Stroebe et al. recently offered a *goal-conflict model* as an attempt to explain the difficulties chronic dieters have in regulating their eating.[7] These authors questioned whether set point or other physiological theories are the reason why dieters fail and tend to return to overeating patterns. Rather, they suggested that dieting is a "self-control dilemma" between two seemingly incompatible goals: food enjoyment and weight control. When dieters chronically inhibit their eating enjoyment goal, they become even more sensitive to the food-rich environment endemic to modern industrialized culture. These authors posited that intrusive thoughts about overeating tax the greater cognitive resources required to maintain a weight control goal, which ultimately leads the individual to pursue the eating enjoyment goal instead.[7]

Personality traits that correlate highly with obesity have also been extensively studied, particularly with regard to the Big 5 personality traits of neuroticism, conscientiousness, agreeableness, extraversion, and openness to experience. Researchers have found that higher levels of conscientiousness are associated with lower obesity, especially for women.[11,12] Higher levels of agreeableness have predicted higher obesity for men, and higher levels of neuroticism have been associated with lower obesity for men, but had no correlation with obesity for women.[11] Sutin et al. found that high neuroticism and low conscientiousness were associated with more weight fluctuations across one's life, and that low agreeableness and high levels of trait impulsivity were associated with higher body mass index (BMI).[12] Sutin et al. suggested that the association between personality factors and obesity are likely mediated by other factors, such as greater physiological reactivity to stress.

PSYCHIATRIC DISORDERS AND OBESITY

Binge-Eating Disorder

There is evidence to suggest that 25%–45% of obese individuals treated in weight control programs report binge eating.[13] An episode of binge eating is most commonly

TABLE 8-1 DSM-V Diagnostic Criteria for Binge Eating Disorder

To diagnose Binge Eating Disorder (BED), the individual:
1. Must engage in recurrent episodes of binge eating. A binge-eating episode is defined as eating a large amount of food (significantly more than is usual) in a discrete amount of time, such as two hours. They also must experience a sense of "lack of control" during a binge.
2. Must endorse at least three of these experiences during a binge:
   - Eating faster than normal.
   - Eating until uncomfortable.
   - Eating a large quantity of food when not hungry.
   - Eating alone due to embarrassment or shame of the amount of food consumed.
   - Feeling disgusted, depressed, or guilty following the binge.
3. Must feel distressed about their binge-eating.
4. Must binge at least once a week for three months.
5. Must not also engage in "compensatory behavior," such as purging, using laxatives, over-exercising, or severely restricting caloric intake. Such behavior would suggest the presence of bulimia nervosa or anorexia nervosa.

defined as eating a large quantity of food (much larger than what most people would eat) in a discrete amount of time. The context in which the binge occurs is important, so, for example, a reported "binge" during a holiday celebration should be interpreted as normative for that situation.[14] The episodes must also occur in a brief amount of time (typically less than 2 hours), so that although the total calories consumed may be equivalent, snacking throughout the day, or "grazing," is not considered a binge.[14] A second defining component is a subjective feeling of "loss of control" during the binge.[14] Finally, if the binge is followed by compensatory behaviors, such as purging or taking laxatives, bulimia nervosa becomes the likely diagnosis.[14]

The existence of BED as a psychiatric diagnosis is recent; in prior editions of the *Diagnostic and Statistical Manual of Mental Disorders* (*DSM*), it was included as a provisional diagnosis. BED was finally included in the latest edition of the *DSM* (*DSM-5*), published in 2013. Diagnostic criteria for the disorder are listed in Table 8-1. To meet the diagnosis of BED, patients must engage in binge-eating episodes at least once a week for 3 months or longer. These episodes must occur in a 2-hour window, and the amount consumed must be significantly greater than what is normally consumed "under similar circumstances." The binge-eating episodes must also be accompanied by a sense of lack of control. The *DSM-5* reports a 12-month prevalence of BED among US adults at a little over 2% (1.6% for females and 0.8% for males).[14]

It is important to note that not all binge eaters are obese, and not all obese people are binge eaters. It has been suggested that normal-weight binge eaters may compensate between binges by engaging in more dieting behavior than obese binge eaters.[13] Regarding the differences among obese individuals who binge eat versus obese individuals who do not, some research evidence suggests that obese binge eaters experience less perceived control over eating, more fear of weight gain, more dissatisfaction with weight, and more food and weight preoccupation.[13] Laboratory studies of binge-eating behavior (for both obese and normal-weight subjects) have demonstrated that when offered a buffet of various food options, binge eaters eat a larger quantity than their weight-matched counterparts, and they tend to choose foods that are high in sugar and fat.[13,15]

For bulimic individuals, a restrictive diet frequently precedes a binge; however, research on the antecedents of binge eating in obese individuals is not as clear.[15,16] Binge eating has been associated with weight cycling, but causality has not been determined.[15] Binge eating in obesity is also concurrent with a number of psychiatric disorders, particularly depressive disorders, panic disorders, and personality disorders,[13,15] suggesting that binge eating may be a mechanism to manage mood and anxiety for individuals with poor affect regulation. Indeed, Leehr et al.'s recent meta-analysis of laboratory studies provided strong support for the affect regulation model of binge eating for individuals with BED.[5] Finally, binge eating has also been significantly correlated with a history of physical or sexual abuse.[13]

Depression

Early research on the correlation between obesity and depression showed only weak associations; however, more recent studies have demonstrated a moderately significant link between the two, especially for women.[17] Other moderating factors include age, socioeconomic status, and race. Specifically, young Caucasian women who are of higher socioeconomic status are more likely to be depressed if obese.[18]

Much of the literature on this topic has had to grapple with a "chicken-versus-egg" type dilemma. Specifically, does depression lead to obesity, does obesity lead to depression, or are they reciprocal influences on each other? There is some evidence supporting all three pathways; however, obesity as a risk factor for depression seems to have a stronger research base, especially when high levels of body dissatisfaction are reported.[18] The role of bullying and teasing in the connection between obesity and depression has not been studied extensively; however, some studies have demonstrated that obese children and adolescents who are victims of bullying are more likely to become depressed.[18] Another moderating factor in the correlation between obesity and depression concerns the impact of decreased mobility and other physical functioning. Only a few studies have examined this relationship, but they have indicated that increased health problems and difficulties with daily functioning increased negative affect.[18]

The question of whether depression causes obesity was addressed in Blaine's meta-analysis of 16 longitudinal studies, combining 33,000 participants.[19] The results suggested that depressed individuals are significantly more likely to become obese at follow-up than their nondepressed counterparts. This effect was even greater for depressed adolescent girls, who were found to be 2.5 times more likely to become obese than their normal-weight peers over time.[19] Finally, several researchers have put forth a bidirectional hypothesis of the relationship between obesity and depression, suggesting that the chronic dieting of obese individuals and the social stigma they experience cause depression, and the lack of exercise, negative thoughts, emotional eating, and social isolation that are characteristic of depression can worsen obesity.[18,19]

Other Psychiatric Disorders

Obesity has also been found to correlate highly with other mental disorders. A New Zealand study found a strong correlation between obesity and anxiety disorders, especially posttraumatic stress disorder,[20] leading the researchers to speculate that this subgroup may be more susceptible to emotional eating to modulate anxiety. A Canadian study likewise found obesity to be positively associated with a lifetime prevalence of mood or anxiety disorders.[21] Their results further indicated that, independent of the effects of these psychiatric disorders, obese individuals are more likely to consider and attempt suicide.

There is also a high incidence of obesity for individuals with serious mental illness, such as schizophrenia.[22] Increased appetite and weight gain are common side effects of antipsychotic medication.[23] Studies have also found that those with schizophrenia have a greater tendency to engage in binge eating and night eating, and they consume more calories than non–mentally ill controls.[24] Lundgren et al. found that their sample of 22 obese patients with schizophrenia were more likely to engage in overeating behavior in response to the sensory qualities of food and were more likely to continue eating after feeling full.[22]

PSYCHOLOGICAL CONSEQUENCES OF OBESITY

Less studied than the psychological causes and correlates of obesity are the psychological consequences of living in an obese body. There is some evidence suggesting that obesity has negative consequences on self-esteem, particularly for women.[1] This seems to be worse for individuals who were teased as children and adolescents and for those with repeated failures at dieting.[1] Wardle and Cook's meta-analysis of the research on the psychological effects of obesity on children and adolescents did find moderate support for increased levels of body dissatisfaction among obese children; however, the results were weak and mixed with regard to depression and low self-esteem.[25] The authors warned professionals against the assumption that obesity causes psychological maladjustment, as many obese children seem to show resilience in the face of weight discrimination.

ASSESSMENT AND TREATMENT PLANNING

It is clear from the literature that there are numerous psychological pathways to obesity. Health care professionals are therefore cautioned against assuming typical etiological influences or even unitary causality within individual patients.[26] Rather, practitioners should adopt a sensitive and curious stance when working with obese patients to best understand the unique cognitive and emotional patterns that may be underlying their eating and exercising behavior. Health care professionals who assume a stereotypic etiology for their individual patients (e.g., that all obese patients are depressed, or emotional eaters, or nonexercisers) without directly inquiring about these habits are not only doing these patients a disservice but also may be contributing to our culture's overall weight-based discrimination.

Indeed, several studies have revealed the implicit biases that health care providers often harbor toward their obese patients. Klein et al. found their sample of 400 physicians associated obesity with poor hygiene, noncompliance, hostility, and dishonesty.[27] Similarly, Price et al. found that two-thirds of their family physician respondents stated that their obese patients lacked self-control, and 39% described them as lazy.[28] Other studies of health care professionals such as nurses and medical students yielded similar results, demonstrating that there exists substantial weight-related bias within the medical profession.[29]

This stigma within the medical field often leads to poor practice. A study of hundreds of physicians of various specialties revealed that the majority were uncomfortable discussing weight management with their obese patients, and many avoided the topic altogether.[30] Whether it is implicitly or explicitly expressed, the discrimination some obese patients feel from their medical providers can have a negative impact on their decision to seek care. Very overweight women were found to be significantly less likely to have yearly pelvic exams, especially when they reported negative body image.[31] Likewise, these researchers found that 17% of the physicians they surveyed were reluctant to perform pelvic exams on very obese women, and that number jumped to 83% when the women were also reluctant.[31] Other studies have found that obese women often delay or cancel physician appointments because of their embarrassment about their weight, fears of getting weighed, and prior negative experiences when discussing their weight with physicians.[32,33]

Mizock suggested that health care providers could reduce patients' feelings of discrimination by using the patients' preferred terminology to describe their weight (e.g., obese, overweight, large) and by focusing on the weight-related behaviors rather than the patients' weight itself.[34] Volger et al. found, in their study of 390 obese patients, that use of the term *weight* was the most desirable way to discuss their obesity, and that the term *fatness* was the least desirable.[35]

When discussing strategies for addressing a patient's obesity, it is important to keep in mind that both patients and providers are susceptible to our culture's unrealistic body-type ideal and the common misconception that, with enough diligence and perseverance, all people can mold and shape their bodies to fit that ideal. With regard to goal setting, Brownell and Wadden suggested shifting one's focus to the concept of "reasonable weight," one that will improve health and functioning but can more likely be attained by patients than an unrealistic ideal.[26] They provided a list of questions that providers can use in discussions with their patients about reasonable weight goals, including the following: "What is the largest size of clothes that you feel comfortable in, at the point you say 'I look pretty good considering where I have been'? At what weight would you wear these clothes?" and "At what weight do you believe you can live with the required changes in eating and/or exercise?" (p. 509). The authors maintained that having a reasonable weight goal will increase the likelihood that patients can achieve and maintain that goal, which in turn is likely to increase their sense of self-efficacy and reduce disappointment and feelings of failure.[26,36] In their treatment-planning discussions with patients, care providers are also encouraged to consider shifting focus to improving other physiological measures of health, such as lowered cholesterol and blood pressure. Patients can develop goals such as eating a healthier diet and increasing physical activity, and this can often improve one's health and quality of life regardless of weight loss.[36]

To date, there is no model of assessment that can accurately match patients to the type of treatment that is likely to be most beneficial[36]; however, assessing the presence of underlying psychiatric distress is important, as untreated psychopathology will likely limit patients' success with any weight loss method. There is even substantial evidence that the presence of psychiatric disorders can predict weight regain

1. Assess whether patient's weight gain is a recent occurrence or if the patient has struggled with his or her weight for many years.
    a. If recent, inquire about any stressors (e.g., loss of relationship, job, etc.; extra stress with work, school, family, etc.) that may have triggered overeating behavior.
2. Does the patient overeat as a way to cope with negative affect (e.g., anxiety, tension, stress, sadness)?
    a. If patient is experiencing anxiety or depression, inquire further about these symptoms using *DSM-V* criteria. If the patient's symptoms are significant, refer for psychological treatment.
3. Does the patient use any other behavioral strategies to cope with stress (e.g., exercising, hobbies, socializing, etc.)?
4. Do they ever binge on food?
    a. If yes, use Table 8-1 to determine whether they meet criteria for BED. If they meet criteria, begin discussing the need for specialized psychological treatment.
5. Is the patient bothered by his or her weight, and if so, why? If not, why not?
6. Has the patient ever followed a structured weight loss plan?
    a. If no, discuss options for a beginning behavioral weight loss program.
    b. If yes, inquire about why the patient believes he or she has regained the weight.
        (i) If the patient discusses using food as a way to cope with negative affect, consider referral for psychotherapy.
        (ii) If the patient does not use food to cope with negative affect, is not experiencing symptoms of a psychiatric disorder, has positive coping skills, and is otherwise physically healthy, consider referral to a body acceptance program. Continue to monitor other health indicators and encourage healthy lifestyle behaviors, such as daily exercise and healthy food choices.

following bariatric surgery.[37] Thus, a patient with BED will need a very different type of psychological treatment than a patient without any history of binge eating or emotional problems. The former will likely benefit from individual or group psychotherapy aimed at improving affect tolerance and reducing binge-eating behavior, whereas the latter may benefit more from traditional behavioral weight loss (BWL) programs or even a size acceptance model of treatment, such as Health at Every Size (HEAS).[38]

Physicians may be uncomfortable discussing a patient's obesity because they are unsure of what questions to ask to determine whether underlying psychological issues are involved with the patient's weight problems. Table 8-2 presents a brief checklist of questions to ask and topics to address during the assessment process. Figure 8-1 presents a decision tree to help ascertain what type of intervention may be most appropriate. Clinicians should consult *DSM-5*[14] for diagnostic criteria for common mental disorders, and at times it may be necessary to refer the patient for more in depth psychological assessment by a mental health professional, such as a psychologist (PhD in clinical psychology) or a licensed clinical social worker (LCSW). Ideally, the physician would then collaborate with the mental health provider in determining the best course of treatment and monitoring a patient's progress.

PSYCHOLOGICAL INTERVENTIONS FOR WEIGHT LOSS

Behavioral Weight Loss

Behavioral weight loss programs are the most widely studied and disseminated psychological treatments for obesity,[39] and BWL is the only treatment listed by Division 12 (the Society of Clinical Psychology) of the American Psychological Association (APA) as an evidenced-based practice (EBP) for obesity.[40] Although the specific protocols and delivery format may vary, there are several core components across the treatment,

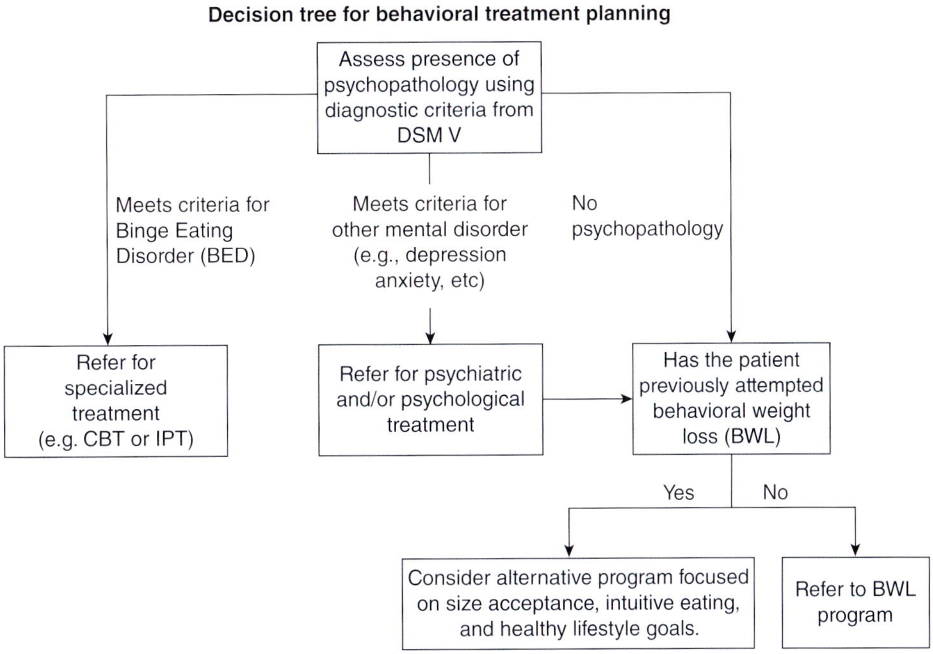

Decision tree for behavioral treatment planning

Assess presence of psychopathology using diagnostic criteria from DSM V

Meets criteria for Binge Eating Disorder (BED)

Meets criteria for other mental disorder (e.g., depression anxiety, etc)

No psychopathology

Refer for specialized treatment (e.g. CBT or IPT)

Refer for psychiatric and/or psychological treatment

Has the patient previously attempted behavioral weight loss (BWL)

Yes | No

Consider alternative program focused on size acceptance, intuitive eating, and healthy lifestyle goals.

Refer to BWL program

FIGURE 8-1. Decision tree for behavioral treatment planning.

further described in Table 8-3. The first involves use of *self-monitoring,* which involves daily logging of food intake, weight, and physical activity.[39,41,42] In addition to recording food consumption, patients are encouraged to complete a *functional analysis* of the behavior: They identify personal and environmental triggers for overeating or eating unhealthy foods.[41] Patients are then encouraged to engage in *stimulus control* techniques, by which they limit or modify these environmental stimuli.[39,41-43] Techniques for stimulus control might include removing serving dishes from the table, doing nothing else while eating, and avoiding buffet restaurants.[41] Patients are also encouraged to increase environmental stimuli that trigger the desired response, such as laying out workout clothes the night before and exercising at the same time every day or with friends.[43]

Contingency management is a behavioral technique that involves providing rewards or reinforcement once the healthy behavior is completed. It is important that individuals are able to experience that reinforcement for the *behavior* (e.g., exercising), rather than reaching a goal (e.g., a specific weight). This is because the behaviors are likely to happen more frequently, and their reinforcement will lead to further increase of healthy behaviors regardless of goal attainment, which tends to be more elusive.[43] Moreover, some healthy behaviors often have natural reinforcements, such as the "endorphin rush" following a workout, the enjoyment of a walk on a nice day, or the fun of cooking a healthy meal with one's spouse. The salience of reinforcement will differ according to personal proclivities, so providers should work with patients to develop a list of the person's most naturally rewarding healthy activities and aim

TABLE 8-3 Primary Components of Behavioral Weight Loss Treatment[a]

Component	Description	Examples
Self-monitoring	Monitoring food intake and type, physical activity, emotional state	Keeping a food journal, using a computer program or app such as My Fitness Pal or an electronic tracker such as Fitbit
Functional analysis and stimulus control	Identify triggers for overeating or other unhealthy behaviors and replace with healthier behaviors; modify environment as needed	Portion sizes too large: Use a smaller plate Eating "seconds" at dinner: Put excess food away before sitting down to eat Too tired to exercise after work: Exercise in morning Too many carbohydrates in meals: Reduce carbohydrates and increase protein consumption Overeating primarily at night when bored: Find substitute activity Overeating at a social gathering: Eat small, healthy meal beforehand
Behavioral activation	Increase activity	Gym-based exercise program, daily walking, using the stairs, parking further away, walk at lunchtime
Contingency management	Rewards for healthy behaviors (either external or "natural")	Each exercise session is rewarded with $1 put into a savings jar Eating a healthy meal gets rewarded with engaging in hobby of choice for an hour Increasing lifestyle activities that are intrinsically pleasurable and rewarding, such as visiting the farmers' market every week, taking up an active hobby such as bicycling or yoga, taking healthy cooking classes, starting a lunchtime walking group at work, etc.
Cognitive restructuring	Identify common maladaptive thoughts and replace with more adaptive ones	*Catastrophizing:* "If I don't lose 50 pounds, I'll stay miserable." *Replace with:* "Every healthy behavior I make improves my well-being." *Overgeneralization:* "I overate too much on Saturday; might as well throw in the towel." *Replace with:* "Everyone slips up once in a while; time to get back on the wagon!" *Emotional reasoning:* "I feel fat." *Replace with:* "I feel sad today, and this is distorting how I view myself." *Should statements:* "I should be able to look like that celebrity if I just try hard enough." *Replace with:* "No two people have the same body type. I'm going to try to look the best I can and accept myself as I am." *All-or-nothing thinking:* "I will eliminate all carbohydrates from my diet." *Replace with:* "It's important to have a balanced diet, including protein, healthy carbohydrates, 'good fats,' and lots of fruits and vegetables."

[a]Adapted from Anderson DA, Shapiro, JR, Lundgren JD. The behavioral treatment of obesity. *Behav Anal Today.* 2001;2(2):133–140; Jones-Cornielle LR, Stack RM, Wadden, TA. Behavioral treatment of obesity. In: Cawley J, ed. *The Oxford Handbook of the Social Science of Obesity.* Oxford, UK: Oxford University Press; 2011:771–791; Wilson GT, Brownell KD. Behavioral treatment for obesity. In: Fairburn CG, Brownell, KD, eds. *Eating Disorders and Obesity: A Comprehensive Handbook.* 2nd ed. New York: Guilford Press; 2002:524–528. https://www.myfitnesspal.com; http://www.fitbit.com.

to integrate those in the person's life as much as possible. This often dovetails with a central component of BWL, *behavioral activation,* which involves increasing exercise and physical activity.[41] Finally, BWL often includes a cognitive component, whereby patients are encouraged to identify maladaptive thoughts, such as "I'll never be able to exercise like others at the gym," and reframe them to more adaptive beliefs such as, "It's important for me to exercise some every day, no matter what it 'looks like.'"[41-43] Patients with a strong tendency to engage in cognitive distortions may benefit from further psychological counseling.

Behavioral weight loss protocols typically span 16–26 weeks,[42] and group interventions seem to yield better outcomes than individual counseling.[42] A major benefit of BWL is that people who are not mental health professionals can be trained in the interventions, making them more widely available for patients. Wadden et al. recently conducted a meta-analysis of 12 trials ($N = 3892$) of weight loss programs delivered by trained interventionists not limited to physicians, nurses, and other medical professionals working in a primary care setting.[44] They found that more frequent contact for counseling correlated with more weight loss and behavior change. The benefit of including additional counseling components to traditional BWL programs has been studied as well. For example, researchers found that adding motivational interviewing, a technique that helps patients explore and increase their level of motivation toward behavior change, increased overall weight loss and activity level.[45]

Research demonstrates that most BWL programs result in an average weight loss of 7%–15% of initial body weight immediately posttreatment.[39,41] Health benefits have been significant even with the modest amount of weight loss through BWL programs. Patients who undergo this treatment have improved hypertension, hypercholesterolemia, type 2 diabetes, and mortality[41] as well as overall psychological well-being.[39] When BWL is combined with very low calorie diets (VLCDS), more weight is lost initially, but it is quickly regained. Therefore, VLCDs are not recommended.[39,42]

While BWL programs are effective at producing weight loss in the short term, statistics on long-term maintenance of those losses are grim. At 1-year follow-up, most patients will have regained at least a third of their body weight, and longer-term follow-up data indicate that patients' weight will gradually increase until it reaches baseline.[39,42] Continued provider contact, whether face to face, over the telephone, or through electronic media, does seem to improve long-term weight maintenance.[42,46] There is also robust research support indicating that successful weight loss maintainers continue to engage in some form of regular physical activity,[42,47] so the importance of changing one's lifestyle to include frequent exercise should be stressed to patients graduating from BWL programs. Individuals who continue to self-monitor their food intake and weight daily are also more successful at maintaining long-term weight loss.[47]

Given the pervasiveness of "the maintenance problem"[46] in obesity treatment, some have called for interventions that focus less on weight loss as a goal and more on decreasing behaviors often associated with obesity, such as poor nutrition, weight cycling, and a sedentary lifestyle.[38,48] HAES includes components focused on body acceptance, replacing restricted eating with intuitive eating (e.g., eating when hungry and stopping when full), improving the nutritional quality of one's diet, integrating regular exercise, and social support.[38] Research on this program showed significant improvements in sensitization to physiological signals or hunger and satiety, improved depression and self-esteem, and lowered low-density lipoprotein (LDL) cholesterol and systolic blood pressure at posttreatment. Moreover, participants in the HAES group (vs. a diet group) had less attrition and were able to maintain all of these gains at 2-year follow-up.[38]

With the extensive research supporting the short-term success of BWL, physicians are encouraged to suggest this treatment as a "first-line" intervention, especially for patients who have never tried a structured weight loss plan and who do not engage in binge eating. Although most patients will gain weight back, 13%–22% of obese patients who participate in a weight loss program become "successful weight maintainers,"[47] so it seems worthwhile to refer "first timers" to a BWL program. For those who have tried BWL interventions and eventually returned to baseline, it may be advisable to shift focus to improving other health indicators as a goal and, if available, to refer patients to size acceptance/intuitive eating models such as HAES or a mindful eating program. Patients who have been diagnosed with BED should be referred to a specialized treatment plan to address this behavior. Various therapeutic approaches to treating BED are described in the next section.

Treatments Specific for Binge-Eating Disorder

Cognitive-Behavioral Therapy

Cognitive-behavioral therapy (CBT) is one of two psychotherapies (along with interpersonal therapy [IPT], described separately) recommended by Division 12 of the APA as an EBP for BED with "strong research support."[40] Fairburn et al. developed a manual for CBT with binge-eating patients, and this is most typically what is used in research and specialized clinical programs.[49] This 20-session protocol is divided into 3 treatment phases that may overlap with each other. Stage 1 involves setting goals for treatment, and it is stressed to the patient that the reduction and cessation of binge eating is the primary goal of treatment, rather than weight loss per se. Additional aspects of stage 1 include education about obesity and nutrition, prescribing a healthy eating schedule, and introducing regular exercise.[49]

Stage 2 focuses on restructuring problematic cognitions and beliefs, for example, that one is "addicted" to food and has "no control." Patients are instead educated about binge eating as a behavior over which they can have control and obesity as a condition over which they may have limited control. Therapists also address body image issues and attempt to reduce self-deprecating thoughts.[49] At this stage, therapists also include the behavioral technique of exposure with response prevention, by which patients are exposed to the cues that typically predicate a binge and taught behavioral techniques to refrain from engaging in the behavior. Patients may also begin daily food monitoring at this stage, and specific behavioral modifications to diet may be advised, such as eliminating high-fat desserts or making healthier food substitutions. Finally, stage 3 is focused on maintaining treatment gains and preparing for future difficulties and relapse prevention.[49]

Cognitive-behavioral therapy has been the most extensively studied treatment for BED; in general, the research has demonstrated a binge-eating abstinence rate of about 50% at posttreatment and 60% at 1-year follow-up.[50] Similar results have been found for both group and individual formats. Historically, studies have not demonstrated significant weight loss resulting from CBT or any other psychotherapy for BED.[50,51] Grilo et al. found that CBT and BWL were both equally effective in reducing binge-eating behavior, and they found no evidence that sequencing the therapies (CBT followed by BWL) yielded greater weight loss results.[51]

With regard to psychopharmacology as an adjunctive treatment, selective serotonin reuptake inhibitors (SSRIs) have been shown to be useful in decreasing binge eating, however, they have received a grade B by the National Institute for Clinical Excellence, whereas CBT is listed as a grade A treatment with the most research support.[52]

Grilo et al.[52] conducted a randomized, placebo-controlled trail with fluoxetine and CBT for BED and found that CBT plus placebo was superior to fluoxetine alone at reducing binge eating, and adding fluoxetine to CBT did not improve the treatment at posttreatment or at 12-month follow-up.

The self-help manual, *Overcoming Binge Eating*, by Fairburn is highly regarded by professionals and widely recommended to patients struggling with the disorder.[53] The use of a self-help manual is of course widely appealing, especially when the treatment of choice is not available for some patients. Therefore, Wilson et al. set out to determine whether use of the manual in conjunction with BWL (which is more widely available than specialized therapies) could be effective in treating BED.[54] Two hundred men and women who met diagnostic criteria for BED were placed into 1 of 3 treatment conditions: 20 sessions of BWL or IPT or 10 sessions of guided self-help CBT (CBTgsh) using Fairburn's manual. They found no difference between the 3 conditions on binge eating at follow-up; however, after 2 years, IPT and CBTgsh were superior to BWL in maintaining abstinence from binge eating. Because low self-esteem and high eating pathology seemed to moderate these results, the authors suggested that self-help CBT could be a "first-line treatment" for patients with BED, and those with more severe eating-related psychopathology or self-image concerns should be referred for more specialized treatments, such as IPT or full CBT.[54] Consistent with the extant research, patients who ceased binge eating entirely lost more weight than those who were unable to completely abstain, and remission from binge eating was significantly correlated with a higher number of patients who had lost and maintained the loss by 5% of their body weight at the 2-year follow up.[54]

Interpersonal Therapy

Interpersonal therapy is the only other EBT recommended for BED by Division 12 of the APA with "strong research support."[40] Like CBT, IPT is a manualized treatment protocol consisting of 12–20 sessions. Rather than focusing on maladaptive weight and eating and related cognitions, however, IPT examines an individual's interpersonal functioning, both historically and currently, to identify problems centered on unresolved grief, role transitions, interpersonal role disputes, and interpersonal deficits.[55] The approach posits that problems in these domains have an impact on one's social self-evaluation, which then leads to poor self-esteem and negative affect, which in turn triggers eating-disordered behaviors such as binge eating.[55] The therapy therefore focuses on improving one's self-esteem within a social/interpersonal context. IPT is probably the second-most-studied treatment for BED and has yielded comparable binge-eating recovery rates as CBT.[56] As with CBT, IPT has only been shown to produce some weight loss in those who are able to completely abstain from binge-eating behavior.[50]

Psychodynamic Therapy

As Tobin explained,[57] CBT tends to treat proximal triggers for binge eating, such as body image concerns, societal pressures to be thin, dieting behaviors, and negative affect. Psychodynamic therapists have historically addressed more distal influences on behavior, such as the role of childhood experiences on personality organization. Tobin advocated for approaches that integrate both psychodynamic and cognitive-behavioral techniques; he stated, "From a traditional psychodynamic perspective it is of limited use to try to directly modify the proximal triggers of binge-eating symptoms without trying to provide patients with an understanding of the more distal influences, the historical and unconscious influences on their behavior" (p. 289). He further suggested that patients with more entrenched character pathology are less likely to benefit from skills-based, symptom-reducing approaches alone and may need longer-term psychodynamic therapy to address "profound interpersonal and intrapersonal deficits" (p. 303).

Unfortunately, psychodynamic psychotherapy has not been extensively researched for BED. This reflects a larger issue in the field of psychotherapeutic research in general: Clinical researchers tend to favor manualized approaches to therapy, such as CBT, which can be more easily taught and replicated than psychodynamic approaches.[58] Although many practicing psychologists identify as psychodynamic and may achieve great success with their patients, they are often less likely in a position to do outcome research, so their evidence often remains anecdotal. Notwithstanding this, a group of Canadian researchers have developed a manualized group psychodynamic interpersonal psychotherapy (GPIP) with good initial research support.[59] In a randomized, controlled trial comparing GPIP to group CBT, they found both treatments equally effective at reducing binge eating for patients with BED. They also found the GPIP patients made positive gains with regard to their self-worth and interpersonal relationships, and they had lower symptoms of depression.[59] As with the other treatments for BED, the patients did not show any significant reductions with BMI at posttreatment.[59]

Emotion-Focused Therapy

Emotion-focused therapies (EFTs) have been gaining in popularity within the field of clinical psychology. Because binge eating has long been recognized as way to regulate affect in the absence of healthier coping skills, it follows that EFT may be beneficial in treating BED. Researchers have developed a 20-session, manualized protocol of EFT for BED; patients learn to better identify and verbally express emotions that lead to binge eating, particularly as these feelings arise within an interpersonal framework.[60] Patients who underwent a combination of dietary counseling plus a course of EFT or EFT alone had significantly reduced binge eating and weight loss at 6-month follow-up as compared to those who received dietary counseling alone.[60]

Which Patient Goes Where?

There are no established guidelines for determining which type of psychotherapy is best suited for particular subtypes of patients with BED; however, Agras[61] has suggested a *triage model*, whereby patients who seem to struggle more with maladaptive underlying beliefs about food and weight or have poor behavioral control would be referred to a CBT approach and individuals with more clear interpersonal problems would be referred to IPT. Similarly, Tobin suggested that patients who binge eat first receive a cognitive-behavioral approach to gain skills in behavior modification.[57] Those patients who continue to struggle should transition to a psychodynamic approach to allow for deeper exploration of unconscious drives and restructuring of pathological personality structures and maladaptive interpersonal patterns that also influence the behavior.

While this "buffet" ideal of psychotherapy might be conceivable in a densely populated locale where patients have access to a variety of skilled mental health practitioners, the reality in many settings is that environmental factors such as cost, payer source (i.e., insurance), and location likely dictate who is available to provide care, and the choices are often minimal. The good news is that there exists strong evidence that almost all psychotherapies have equal effectiveness as long as they are delivered by clinicians who are well trained in their treatment of choice as well as the *common factors* that occur across all therapeutic orientations.[62] This finding seems to hold true for treatment for BED as well, as Spielmans et al.'s recent meta-analysis demonstrated.[63] As long as the therapist is well trained in a particular approach for BED, compliant patients are likely to get better.

SUGGESTIONS FOR FUTURE RESEARCH

It should be clear from this review that the psychological causes for obesity are numerous, interrelated, and often idiosyncratic. In response to the great variety of factors that have been found to play a role, Friedman and Brownell suggested, "Inconsistent findings reflect an inconsistent phenomenon (i.e., the effects of being obese vary across individuals)."[64,p.293] They therefore proposed that the second and third generation of obesity research use more complex designs to better identify factors that seem to account for the vast discrepancies of psychological correlates among obese individuals. Thus, obesity research will be less concerned with "*whether* obese persons suffer psychological distress to *who* will suffer and in what *ways*."[64,p.397]

Indeed, future research should focus on the development of models for understanding the complex interplay of factors that might account for weight problems within each individual. There is also a strong need for studies using research methodology that can better determine causal pathways between the presence of psychopathology and obesity so that clinicians can tailor interventions toward prevention in either direction. Given the established intractability of obesity and the long-term "maintenance problem," any research that can offer physicians better tools to identify and address risk factors prior to significant weight gain will likely be well received and appreciated by health care consumers, providers, and public health personnel.

REFERENCES

1. Moskovich A, Hunger J, Mann T. The psychology of obesity. In: Cawley J, ed. *The Oxford Handbook of the Social Science of Obesity*. Oxford, UK: Oxford University Press; 2011:87–104.
2. Kaplan HI, Kaplan HS. The psychosomatic concept of obesity. *J Nerv Ment Dis*. 1957;125:181–201.
3. Bruch H. *Eating Disorders—Obesity, Anorexia, and the Person Within*. London: Routledge & Kegan Paul; 1973.
4. Canetti L, Bachar E, Elliot EM. Food and emotion. *Behav Process*. 2002;60:157–164.
5. Leehr EJ, Krohmer K, Schag K, Dresler T, Zipfel S, Giel KE. Emotion regulation model in binge eating disorder and obesity—a systematic review. *Neurosci Biobehav Rev*. 2015;49:125–134.
6. Schacter S. Obesity and eating. *Science*. 1968;16:751–756.
7. Stroebe W, van Koningsbruggen GM, Papies EK, Aarts H. Why most dieters fail but some succeed: a goal conflict model of eating behavior. *Psychol Rev*. 2013;120(1):110–138.
8. Nisbett RE. Hunger, obesity, and the ventromedial hypothalamus. *Psychol Rev*. 1972;79(6):433–453.
9. Herman CP, Mack D. Anxiety, restraint, and eating behavior. *J Abnorm Psychol*. 1975;84:662–672.
10. Stice E, Presnell, K, Shaw H, Rohde, P. Psychological and behavioral risk factors for obesity onset in adolescent girls: a prospective study. *J Consult Clin Psychol*. 2005;73:195–202.
11. Chapman BP, Fiscella, K, Duberstein P, Coletta M, Kawachi I. Can the influence of childhood socioeconomic status on men's and women's adult body mass be explained by adult socioeconomic status or personality? Findings from a national sample. *Health Psychol*. 2009;28(4):419–427.

12. Sutin AR, Ferrucci L, Zonderman AB, Terracciano A. Personality and obesity across the lifespan. *J Pers Soc Psychol.* 2011;101(3):579–592.

13. Marcus M. Binge eating in obesity. In: Fairburn CG, Wilson GT, eds. *Binge Eating: Nature, Assessment, and Treatment.* New York: Guilford; 1993:77–96.

14. American Psychiatric Association. *Diagnostic and Statistical Manual of Mental Disorders.* 5th ed. Washington, DC: American Psychiatric Association; 2013.

15. Yanovski SZ. Binge eating in obese persons. In: Fairburn CG, Brownell KD, eds. *Eating Disorders and Obesity: A Comprehensive Handbook.* 2nd ed. New York: Guilford Press; 2002:403–407.

16. Waller G. The Psychology of Binge Eating. In: Fairburn CG, Brownell KD, eds. Eating Disorders and Obesity: A Comprehensive Handbook, 2nd ed. New York: Guilford Press; 2002:98–102.

17. De Wit L, Luppino F, van Straten A, Penninx B, Zitman F, Cuijpers P. Depression and obesity: a meta-analysis of community-based studies. *Psychiatr Res.* 2010;178: 230–235.

18. Granberg E. Depression and obesity. In Cawley J, ed. *The Oxford Handbook of the Social Science of Obesity.* Oxford, UK: Oxford University Press; 2011:329–349.

19. Blaine B. Does depression cause obesity? A meta-analysis of longitudinal studies of depression and weight control. *J Health Psychol.* 2008;13(8):1190–1197.

20. Scott KM, McGee MA, Wells JE, Browne MA. Obesity and mental disorders in the adult general population. *J Psychosom Res.* 2008;64:97–105.

21. Mather AA, Cox BJ, Enns MW, Sareen J. Associations of obesity with psychiatric disorders and suicidal behaviors in a nationally representative sample. *J Psychosom Res.* 2009;66:277–285.

22. Lundgren JD, Rempfer MV, Lent MR, Foster GD. Perceptions of factors associated with weight management in obese adults with schizophrenia. *Psychiatr Rehabil J.* 2014;37(4):304–308.

23. Citrome L, Vreeland, B. Schizophrenia, obesity, and antipsychotic medications: what can we do? *Postgrad Med.* 2008;120(2):18–33.

24. Lundgren JD, Rempfer MV, Brown CE Goetz J, Hamera E. The prevalence of night eating syndrome and binge eating disorder among overweight and obese individuals with serious mental illness. *Psychiatry Research.* 2010;175:233–236.

25. Wardle J, Cook L. The impact of obesity on psychological well-being. *Best Pract Res Clin Endocrinol Metab.* 2005;19(3):421–440.

26. Brownell KD, Wadden TA. Etiology and treatment of obesity: understanding a serious, prevalent, and refractory disorder. *J Consult Clin Psychol.* 1992;60(4):505–517.

27. Klein D, Najman J, Kohrman AF, Munro C. Patient characteristics that elicit negative responses from family physicians. *J Fam Pract.*1982;14:881–888.

28. Price JH, Desmond SM, Krol RA, Snyder FF, O'Connell JK. Family practice physicians' beliefs, attitudes, and practices regarding obesity. *Am J Prev Med.* 1987;3:339–345.

29. Puhl R, Brownell KD. Bias, Discrimination, and Obesity. *Obesity.* 2001;9(12):788–805.

30. Kristeller JL, Hoerr RA. Physician attitudes toward man-aging obesity: differences among six specialty groups. *Prev Med.* 1997;26:542–549.

31. Adams CH, Smith NJ, Wilbur DC, Grady KE. The relationship of obesity to the frequency of pelvic examinations: do physician and patient attitudes make a difference? *Women Health.* 1993;20:45–57.

32. Olson CL, Schumaker HD, Yawn BP. Overweight women delay medical care. *Arch Fam Med,* 1994;3:888–892.

33. Fontaine KR, Faith MS, Allison DB, Cheskin LJ. Body weight and healthcare among women in the general population. *Arch Fam Med.* 1998;7:381–384.

34. Mizock L. The double stigma of obesity and serious mental illness: Promoting health and recovery. *Psychiatric Rehabilitation Journal,* 2012;35(6):466–469.

35. Volger S, Vetter ML, Dougherty M, et al. Patients' preferred terms for describing their excess weight: discussing obesity in clinical practice. *Obesity.* 2012; 20(1):147–150.

36. Brownell KD, Stunkard AJ. Goals of obesity treatment. In: Fairburn CG, Brownell KD, eds. *Eating Disorders and Obesity: A Comprehensive Handbook.* 2nd ed. New York: Guilford Press; 2002:507–511.

37. Kalarchian MA, Marcus MD. Management of the bariatric surgery patient: is there a role for the cognitive behavior therapist? *Cogn Behav Pract.* 2003;10(2):112–119.

38. Bacon L, Stern JS, Van Loan MD, Kein NL. Size acceptance and intuitive eating improve health for obese, female chronic dieters. *J Am Diet Assoc.* 2005; 105(6):929–936.

39. Wilson GT, Brownell KD. Behavioral treatment for obesity. In: Fairburn CG, Brownell, KD, eds. *Eating Disorders and Obesity: A Comprehensive Handbook.* 2nd ed. New York: Guilford Press; 2002: 524–528.

40. Loeb KL. Obesity and pediatric overweight. http://www.div12.org/psychological-treatments/ disorders/obesity-and-pediatric-overweight/. Accessed December 5, 2016.

41. Anderson DA, Shapiro JR, Lundgren JD. The behavioral treatment of obesity. *Behav Anal Today.* 2001;2(2):133–140.

42. Jones-Cornielle LR, Stack RM, Wadden TA. Behavioral treatment of obesity. In: Cawley J, ed. *The Oxford Handbook of the Social Science of Obesity.* Oxford, UK: Oxford University Press; 2011:771–791.

43. Shields AT. Examination of the obesity epidemic from a behavioral perspective. *Int J Behav Consult Ther.* 2009;5(1):142–158.

44. Wadden, Butryn, Hong, & Tsai, 2014.

45. Carels RA, Darby L, Cacciapaglia, HM, Konrad K, Coit C, Harper J, et al. Using motivational interviewing as a supplement to obesity treatment: A stepped-care approach. *Health Psychology.* 2007;26(3):369–374.

46. Perri MG. Improving maintenance in behavioral treatment. In: Fairburn CG, Brownell KD, eds. *Eating Disorders and Obesity: A Comprehensive Handbook.* 2nd ed. New York: Guilford Press; 2002:593–598.

47. Wing RR, Klem M. Characteristics of successful weight maintainers. In: Fairburn CG, Brownell KD, eds. *Eating Disorders and Obesity: A Comprehensive Handbook.* 2nd ed. New York: Guilford Press; 2002:588–592.

48. Cooper Z, Fairburn CG. A new cognitive behavioural approach to the treatment of obesity. *Behav Res Ther.* 2001;39:499–511.

49. Fairburn CG, Marcus MD, Wilson GT. Cognitive-behavioral therapy for binge eating and bulimia nervosa: a comprehensive treatment manual. In Fairburn CG, Wilson GT, eds. *Binge Eating: Nature, Assessment, and Treatment.* New York: Guilford; 1993:361–404.

50. Wilfley DE. Psychological treatment of binge eating disorder. In: Fairburn CG, Brownell KD, eds. *Eating Disorders and Obesity: A Comprehensive Handbook.* 2nd ed. New York: Guilford Press; 2002:350–353

51. Grilo CM, Masheb RM, Wilson GT, Gueorguieva R, White MA. Cognitive-behavioral therapy, behavioral weight loss, and sequential treatment for obese patients with binge-eating disorder: a randomized controlled trial. *J Consult Clin Psychol.* 2011;79(5):675–685.

52. Grilo CM, Crosby RD, Wilson GT, Masheb RM. 12-month follow-up of fluoxetine and cognitive behavioral therapy for binge eating disorder. *J Consult Clin Psychol.* 2012;80(6):108–113.

53. Fariburn CG. *Overcoming Binge Eating.* New York: Guilford; 1995.

54. Wilson GT, Wilfley DE, Agras WS, Bryson SW. Psychological treatments of binge eating disorder. *Arch Gen Psychiatry.* 2010;67(1):94–101.

55. Rieger E, Van Buren DJ, Bishop M, Tanofsky-Kraff M, Welch R, Wilfley DE. An eating disorder specific model of interpersonal psychotherapy (IPT-ED): causal pathways and treatment implications. *Clin Psychol Rev.* 2010;30:400–410.

56. Wilfley DE, Welch RR, Stein RI, et al. A randomized comparison of group cognitive-behavioral therapy and group interpersonal psychotherapy for the treatment of overweight individuals with binge-eating disorder. *Arch Gen Psychiatry.* 2002;59(8):713–721.

57. Tobin DL. Psychodynamic psychotherapy and binge eating. In: Fairburn CG, Wilson GT, eds. *Binge Eating: Nature, Assessment, and Treatment.* New York: Guilford; 1993:287–313.

58. Levy RA, Ablon, JS, eds. *Handbook of Evidence-Based Psychodynamic Psychotherapy: Bridging the Gap Between Science and Practice.* New York: Humana Press; 2010.

59. Tasca GA, Ritchie K, Conrad G, et al. Attachment scales predict outcome in a randomized controlled trial of two group therapies for binge eating disorder: an aptitude by treatment interaction. *Psychother Res.* 2006;16(1):106–121.

60. Compare A, Calugi S, Marchesini G, et al. Emotionally focused group therapy and dietary counseling in binge eating disorder. Effect on eating disorder psychopathology and quality of life. *Appetite.* 2013;71:361–368.

61. Agras WS. Short-term psychological treatments for binge eating. In: Fairburn CG, Wilson GT, eds. *Binge Eating: Nature, Assessment, and Treatment.* New York: Guilford; 1993:270–286.

62. Seligman MEP. The effectiveness of psychotherapy: the consumer reports study. *Am Psychol.* 1995;50(12):965–974.

63. Spielmans GI, Benish SG, Marin C, Bowman WM, Menster M, Wheeler AJ. Specificity of psychological treatments for bulimia nervosa and binge eating disoder? A meta-analysis of direct comparisons. *Clin Psychol Rev.* 2013;33:460–469.

64. Friedman MA, Brownell KD. Psychological consequences of obesity. In: Fairburn CG, Brownell KD, eds. *Eating Disorders and Obesity: A Comprehensive Handbook.* 2nd ed. New York: Guilford Press; 2002:393–397.

Bariatric Surgery

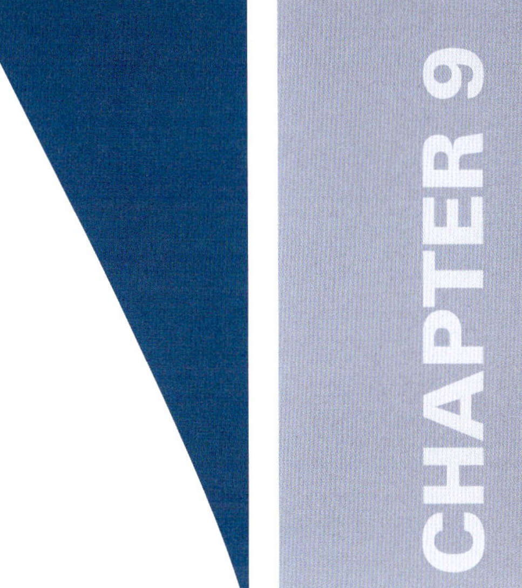

Robert N. Cooney, MD

INTRODUCTION

Obesity describes the excess accumulation of body fat and is currently endemic in the United States, afflicting over 35% of the adult population. Although the percentage of body fat (>25% in men and >32% in women) is commonly used to describe obesity, these measurements are not readily available to most clinicians. Therefore, obesity is more commonly assessed by calculating the patient's body mass index (BMI) or weight (kg) divided by their height in square meters (m^2).[1] Using these criteria, obesity is defined as having a BMI greater than 30, and clinically severe or morbid obesity is described as a having a BMI greater than 40 or a BMI greater than 35 with severe medical comorbidities.[2] Using BMI criteria, more than 50% of adult Americans are overweight or obese, and approximately 5% are morbidly obese.[3]

Although these definitions are helpful in identifying individuals who are "at risk" for obesity-related complications, neither BMI nor percentage body fat describes the regional distribution of body fat. This is important because medical consequences of obesity are related in part to the distribution of body fat. Visceral or android obesity is more common in men and associated with insulin resistance, gastroesophageal reflux, hyperlipidemia, hypertension, obstructive sleep apnea (OSA), and metabolic syndrome.[2,4,5] Gynecoid or subcutaneous obesity describes an excess accumulation of subcutaneous fat in the gluteal or buttock area and is more commonly seen in women. Degenerative joint disease, impaired mobility, dyspnea on exertion, asthma, urinary stress incontinence, and dysfunctional uterine bleeding are common medical consequences of obesity as well. Although the metabolic consequences of subcutaneous

141

adiposity are less than for visceral adiposity, complications related to wound healing and surgical site infections are more common with subcutaneous adiposity.[6–8]

INDICATIONS AND WORKUP FOR BARIATRIC SURGERY

In 1991, the National Institutes of Health published a consensus statement, entitled "Gastrointestinal Surgery for Severe Obesity."[9] In this publication, they described the generally accepted criteria for surgical weight loss or "bariatric surgery." Evaluation by a comprehensive, multidisciplinary team comprising experienced surgeons and individuals with medical, psychiatric, and nutritional expertise is recommended. The generally accepted criteria for surgical weight loss include BMI greater than 35 with severe medical comorbidities (typically type 2 diabetes or OSA) or BMI greater than 40, failure of medical weight loss, and no psychological contraindications to surgery.[9] At this time, the most commonly performed surgical procedures were vertical banded gastroplasty (VBG) and the Roux-en-Y gastric bypass (RYGB).

Although weight loss operations have changed since 1991, the process of evaluating potential candidates for bariatric surgery remains similar. Most bariatric surgery programs offer a general information session that allows potential surgical candidates a chance to learn about the different surgical procedures; the preoperative evaluation process (nutrition counseling, psychological evaluation, medical workup); and the risks and benefits of different procedures and to ask questions and the like.[10,11] One of the most controversial criteria in evaluating candidates for bariatric surgery is ascertaining whether patients have "failed medical weight loss." This problem is due in part to variable definitions of failure of medical weight loss by medical and nutrition specialists, bariatric surgeons, and third-party payers. Potential patients for bariatric surgery are commonly asked to describe previous attempts at weight loss (diet, exercise, behavior modification); duration of attempted weight loss; magnitude of weight loss; and successful maintenance of weight loss. The term *excess body weight loss* (EBWL) is commonly used to describe weight loss and is calculated using the actual and ideal body weights. Medical weight loss commonly results in 5%–10% EBWL with long-term success rates of 5% to 10%.[3,12] For a while, many insurance companies required monthly visits with a dietitian and weigh ins for 3 to 6 months with documented dietary compliance before allowing patients to be considered for surgical weight loss.[3,12] Suffice it to say, defining failure of medical weight loss remains variable in different geographic regions, by different medical specialties and different third-party payers, and among bariatric surgery programs.

It is important for patients considering surgical weight loss to understand surgery is not a "cure" for obesity; rather, it is "a tool" to help them improve their health by facilitating weight loss. For the surgery to be successful, patients need to change their eating behavior and adopt a healthier lifestyle. With that in mind, it is helpful for patients to develop some insights regarding their eating and other behaviors that contributed to their development of morbid obesity. Psychological evaluation is routinely performed by most (>80%) of bariatric surgery programs.[13] Approximately 65% to 75% of patients presenting for surgical weight loss have some type of preexisting mood disorder.

Although there is considerable variability in scope and structure, the preoperative psychological evaluation commonly includes weight history; eating behaviors;

screening and assessment of eating disorders (e.g., binge eating, nighttime eating syndrome, emotional eating, or grazing); psychosocial history; an evaluation of existing or potential mood disorder(s) and whether they are adequately controlled; and a determination of cognitive function to see if the patient understands how certain behaviors have contributed to the development of morbid obesity and whether the patient has a realistic understanding of the changes he or she will need to make for surgery to be successful. An assessment of health-related behaviors, including substance use, physical activity, expectations, and knowledge of the proposed surgery and complications is frequently performed. The most commonly identified reasons for denying surgery include substance abuse, psychotic symptoms, severe mental retardation, and patient reports of overeating to deal with stress.[14,15]

It is important to realize that even the most detailed and comprehensive psychological evaluation will not identify potentially problematic patients. The psychological evaluation is most helpful in identifying patients with "absolute contraindications" or "no contraindications for surgery" for bariatric surgical procedures. Unfortunately, when "relative contraindications" to surgery are identified, the multidisciplinary team is frequently left with a difficult decision in weighing the relative risks and benefits of surgery for the individual patient. In these situations, a physician-to-physician conversation between the surgeon, psychiatrist, and the patient's primary care physician may help to develop the best course of action to take.

Any decision to proceed with surgery requires a balanced assessment of the risks and benefits of surgery for the individual patient. While many programs have developed structured preoperative medical assessments for patients considering bariatric surgery, the individual patient's workup should be tailored based on the patient's age, functional status, underlying medical comorbidities, and previous surgical history.[11] A thorough history and physical by an experienced bariatric provider are usually the first step in the process. The need for subsequent testing and consultation is usually based on the patient's current medical diagnoses and the extent to which their "severity" and "medical control" are documented in the medical record. For example, approximately 25%–30% of patients who present for bariatric surgery have type 2 diabetes mellitus (T2DM). Many of them check their glucose levels regularly, and their hemoglobin (Hb) A_{1c} values are followed routinely and are well controlled (e.g., HbA_{1c} <7.5). It is helpful to have an assessment of T2DM control within 6 months of bariatric evaluation. This allows enough time for patients with "poorly controlled diabetes" (e.g., HBA_{1c} > 8%) to be referred back to their endocrinologist or primary medical doctor for adjustment of their medical regimen before surgery.

Many patients presenting for bariatric surgery have symptoms of OSA (e.g., snoring, daytime sleepiness, poor-quality sleep, witnessed apneic episodes, etc.), while some patients have no symptoms at all. Given the prevalence of sleep-disordered breathing in this population (>80%) and the potential risks of undiagnosed, untreated OSA in the perioperative period, we routinely refer most patients for sleep studies unless they have been previously tested or are currently being treated.[16] The need for cardiology evaluation and stress testing is decided on a case-by-case basis depending on the patient's cardiac risk factors and presence of potential cardiac symptoms. Associated medical comorbidities (e.g., chronic renal failure, fatty liver, underlying pulmonary disease, previous thromboembolic events such as deep venous thromboembolism, pulmonary embolism, or hypercoagulable state) are commonly encountered and have to be assessed in the context of the individual patient's age and other medical conditions.[10] Previous studies have identified age above 55 years, BMI above 55, male gender, and reoperative surgery as risk factors for increased morbidity and mortality in bariatric surgery patients.[17,18] Ultimately, the decision to proceed with bariatric surgery is based on a comprehensive review of the risks and benefits of surgery with the multidisciplinary team, the attending bariatric surgeon, the patient, and the patient's family. There is some evidence that surgeon and hospital volume equate with improved outcomes, and that consideration should be given for "high-risk patients" to have their bariatric surgery performed at a designated Bariatric Surgery Center of Excellence.[19]

The concept of identifying and designating Bariatric Surgery Centers of Excellence was based on the results of several studies that demonstrated decreased mortality and length of stay when bariatric surgery was performed at "high-volume hospitals" by "high-volume surgeons."[20] In an effort to decrease surgical mortality, several professional organizations (the American Society of Bariatric Surgeons and the American College of Surgeons) developed and encouraged an accreditation process for hospitals doing bariatric surgery to meet specific standards and be designated as Bariatric Surgery Centers of Excellence.

Simultaneously, the overall quality of bariatric surgery appeared to be improving. The Longitudinal Assessment of Bariatric Surgery (LABS) consortium's first study was published in 2010 and examined 30-day outcomes for 4776 patients who had bariatric surgery from 2005 to 2007 at 10 clinical sites in the United States.[21] In this study (LABS-1), the 30-day mortality for RYGB and laparoscopic adjustable gastric band (LAGB) was 0.3%, and all-cause major adverse events were 4.3%.[21] A subsequent analysis of the LABS-1 data demonstrated a reduction in risk-adjusted complications after RYGB was associated with increased surgeon volumes.[22] In contrast, analysis of gastric bypass surgery outcomes using the New York State inpatient database suggested risk-adjusted morbidity accounted for more than 80% of hospital variation compared with only 20% attributable to hospital and surgical volumes.[23]

Collectively, these data suggest bariatric surgery can be safely performed with acceptably low morbidity and mortality rates. Given the low, but potentially serious, risks of bariatric surgery, what are the long-term health benefits that patients considering bariatric surgery might expect? Several studies have examined the impact of bariatric surgery on mortality and other health parameters.[24-27] The Swedish Obesity Study (SOS) published 10-year follow-up data on 2010 bariatric surgery patients treated by gastric bypass (RYGB), VBG, or gastric banding (GB) compared with 2037 patients receiving conventional medical therapy.[27] Long-term (10-year) weight loss in the SOS was 25%, 16%, and 14%, respectively, after RYGB, VBG, and GB compared with less than 2% in the control group. The SOS also demonstrated a 29% reduction in all-cause mortality in the bariatric surgery group compared with the control group.

These results are similar to those of Adams et al., who reported a 40% reduction in mortality after gastric bypass surgery (compared with severely obese, matched controls) in a retrospective cohort study from Utah.[24] Interestingly, the study by Adams et al. demonstrated a reduction in cardiac-, diabetes-, and cancer-related mortality in the gastric bypass group, but an increase in suicide and accidental deaths relative to the control group. Consistent with these data, a retrospective, population-based study of 66,109 bariatric surgery patients examining all-cause mortality for bariatric surgery patients after 15 years confirmed these findings.[26]

The majority of these studies examined predominantly low-risk, female subjects. Of note, a retrospective Veterans Affairs (VA) system demonstrated a 24% reduction in all-cause mortality at the 10-year follow-up compared with a nonsurgical matched control group.[28] Collectively, these data suggest significant medical and long-term mortality benefits for surgical weight loss. However, additional information is needed to better understand the potential risk-benefit ratio in high-risk subsets (e.g., the predominantly male, medically complex VA population).

PERIOPERATIVE CONSIDERATIONS

Because bariatric surgery is an elective procedure, most patients expect the surgery to be performed safely with minimal or no significant risks. Despite this perception, almost by definition, morbidly obese patients having bariatric surgery procedures are at increased risk for surgical complications. Although obtaining informed consent is a standard aspect of every surgical procedure, it seems appropriate to point out that certain high-risk procedures such as bariatric surgery probably deserve additional attention to the informed consent process. Patient education about the different surgical procedures as well as the potential risks and benefits is an integral aspect of preparing patients for surgery. When asked, bariatric surgery patients routinely indicate they fully understand the risks and benefits of surgery. However, in my experience, detailed follow-up questions routinely indicate significant gaps in knowledge.

For this reason, many bariatric surgery programs routinely use preoperative true/false tests to document whether patients truly understand the actual risks of surgery as part of the informed consent process. True/false statements such as "Death is a potential complication of surgery"; "Anastomotic and staple line leaks are serious complications that may be life threatening and require additional surgery"; and "I will need to take iron and vitamin B_{12} supplements for life after surgery to prevent deficiencies" are helpful to document preoperative bariatric surgery comprehension of the potential risks related to surgery.

Many programs use clinical pathways or order sets in an effort to standardize the perioperative care of patients having bariatric surgery.[29] Clinical pathways help to minimize deviations in care by establishing routine guidelines for the care of patients having a common surgical procedure. In the case of bariatric surgery, standard operating procedures for routine laboratory testing; medications (antibiotics, pain medications, glycemic medications, antiemetics, etc.); diet; activity; physical and occupational therapy consultation; and management of OSA are established. Patients, nurses, surgery residents, and other members of the health care team are educated on the established plan of care and work together to minimize variations in care. Clinical pathways are commonly associated with fewer complications, reductions in resource utilization, and improved patient satisfaction.[29]

The perioperative management of OSA is worthy of further discussion because of its high incidence in bariatric surgery patients (>80%) and the potentially significant risks related to perioperative complications in its management. Many bariatric surgery programs, including our own, routinely screen all bariatric surgery patients for the presence of OSA. If OSA is diagnosed, we prefer to have these patients started on continuous positive airway pressure (CPAP) or bilevel positive airway pressure (BiPAP) prior to scheduling surgery. This practice is endorsed by the American Society of Anesthesiologists (ASA) practice guidelines for the perioperative management of patients with OSA, especially in patients with severe OSA.[30]

Because patients with OSA may have difficult airways, the anesthesia team should be fully prepared to deal with this potential problem. Although regional anesthesia is preferred for peripheral procedures, bariatric surgery is commonly performed under general anesthesia. Patients with OSA may demonstrate increased susceptibility to the respiratory depressant effects of inhaled anesthetics, opioids, and sedatives.[30,31] Therefore, extubation is recommended after complete reversal of neuromuscular blockade when the patient is awake and the use of upright or lateral positioning is encouraged when possible.[30,32] The data on optimal perioperative analgesia for patients with OSA is inconclusive, but support the use of regional analgesia (vs. systemic opioids) and supplemental anti-inflammatory medications to decrease systemic narcotic administration. The use of continuous opioid infusions or the administration of concurrent sedatives (e.g., benzodiazepines) is cautioned against because of the increased risks of respiratory depression.[30] Postoperatively, supplemental oxygen or CPAP should be used as needed.[33] Continuous electrocardiographic monitoring and oximetry should be strongly considered in high-risk patients after surgery.

THE OPERATING ROOM ENVIRONMENT

There are several aspects of the operating room (OR) phase of care that are worth mentioning when caring for the bariatric surgery population. Transporting and moving patients to and from the OR may require special equipment (heavy-duty wheelchairs, stretchers, etc.) to prevent patient injury. Moving bariatric surgery patients on and off the stretcher and OR table may result in patient or staff injury. Many centers use roller or specially designed bariatric transfer devices (e.g., HoverMatt, AIRPAL, etc.) to transfer patients with a high BMI on and off the OR table to prevent injuries. In addition, many facilities have special OR tables (e.g., Skytron, Maquet, etc.) to accommodate patients with a high BMI whose body weight exceeds the weight capacity of standard OR tables (normally 350 lb). Many of these tables can be "widened" in the abdominal, buttocks, or lower extremity part of the table by clamping components to the side rails. Routine perioperative procedures like obtaining intravenous access, placing epidural catheters, endotracheal intubation, blood pressure monitoring, placing urinary catheters, and so on can be more difficult than anticipated or require special equipment.

As with any surgical procedure, it is important to pay special attention to patient positioning and padding in the bariatric surgery patient. If the arms are placed on armboards, one must be careful the armboards are properly padded and not abducted or extended excessively, which can cause brachial plexus symptoms postoperatively. The patient's heels should be properly padded to avoid pressure sores during prolonged procedures, and the patient must be securely attached to the OR table. If the patient will be placed in reverse Trendelenburg position, one must be careful the OR strap(s) are also padded as patients can develop anterior femoral cutaneous nerve paresthesias or numbness if they are not. Special long instruments and heavy-duty, self-retaining retractors (e.g., Thompson Surgical Retractors) may also be required for this patient population to facilitate exposure and allow dissection and suturing in a deep operative field.

Furthermore, surgical procedures lasting more than 4–5 hours can result in rhabdomyolysis, with elevated creatine kinase and myoglobin levels. These laboratory tests should be performed in morbidly obese patients after prolonged surgical procedures, especially if urine output is poor.[34] Extubation after surgery is recommended if possible. Prolonged mechanical ventilation is associated with significant morbidity in clinically severe patients. Pressure sores in particular are a major problem (in part due to the difficulty of turning these patients in the intensive care unit), and the use of specialized bariatric air beds is recommended to minimize the risks of pressure sores if the patient requires mechanical ventilation after surgery.

BARIATRIC SURGERY PROCEDURES

A variety of surgical procedures have been performed to facilitate weight loss over the years. Some of these, including the jejunoileal bypass and VBG, are no longer performed at most centers. With that in mind, the focus here is on the most commonly performed bariatric procedures at this time, including the RYGB, the LAGB, and the laparoscopic sleeve gastrectomy (LSG).

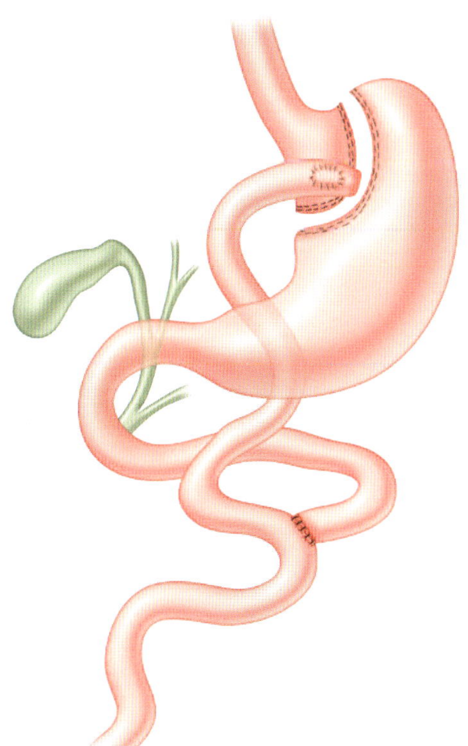

FIGURE 9-1. The Roux-en-Y gastric bypass.

The Roux-en-Y Gastric Bypass

The RYGB is among the most commonly performed and well-established bariatric surgery procedures. The RYGB procedure can be performed either open or laparoscopically with good results. With either technique, the RYGB involves several steps: creating a proximal gastric pouch (approximately 2 oz in size), constructing a Roux limb (typically 100 to 150 cm), and performing the jejunojejunostomy (between the biliopancreatic limb and Roux limb) and gastrojejunostomy (between the Roux limb and proximal gastric pouch) (see diagram in Figure 9-1). The proximal gastric pouch is fashioned by stapling perpendicular to the lesser curvature approximately 5 cm from the gastroesophageal junction, then parallel to the lesser curvature up through the angle of His. This creates a 20- to 50-mL, nondistensible, gastric pouch along the lesser curvature of the stomach. The alimentary or Roux limb is created by dividing the jejunum 40 to 50 cm distal to the ligament of Treitz and performing a side-to-side enteroenterostomy to the proximal jejunum (biliopancreatic limb) 100 to 150 cm down the Roux limb. The Roux limb is then brought behind the colon and distal stomach (retrocolic, retrogastric) or anterior to the colon and distal stomach (antecolic, antegastric), and a sutured or stapled gastrojejunostomy (approximately 12 mm) is performed. Mesenteric defects are closed, and the surgical field is drained or gastrostomy tubes are placed at the surgeon's discretion.

When laparoscopic RYGB was first described in the early 1990s, many surgeons lacked the minimally invasive technical skills to safely perform intestinal anastomoses in morbidly obese patients. Over time, with improvements in surgical technique and training, the laparoscopic RYGB became the most commonly performed bariatric surgical procedure.[22,35,36] Several studies have compared outcomes with open and laparoscopic RYGB and found the laparoscopic technique was associated with less surgical blood loss, fewer wound complications, and shorter surgical time and hospital length of stay.[37-40] Weight loss, preoperative mortality, and leak rates appear to be similar with the open and laparoscopic techniques.[40] However, anastomotic strictures, gastrointestinal hemorrhage, late small bowel obstructions, and OR costs may be somewhat higher with the laparoscopic technique.[38] Suffice it to say, the majority of patients undergoing RYGB surgery today have the surgery performed laparoscopically.

Open RYGB surgery is more commonly performed in superobese patients, in patients with multiple previous abdominal procedures, and for revisional bariatric surgical procedures. The open procedure can be performed through either a midline or a bilateral subcostal incision. Proponents of the midline approach cite muscle sparing, postoperative pain, and good upper and lower abdominal cavity exposure as advantages. Proponents of the transverse incision cite a decreased incidence of incisional hernias as a potential advantage. Ischemia and tissue loss of panniculectomy flaps has also been described in patients with bilateral subcostal incisions and should be considered in patients where subsequent panniculectomy is anticipated.

The "success rate" of the RYGB procedure is commonly mentioned as 70% and is defined as the loss and maintenance of more than 50% of EBWL. Figure 9-2 demonstrates weight loss after time following RYGB surgery. Weight loss is most rapid for 3 to 6 months after surgery; it slows for the next 6 to 12 months, and most patients reach a weight loss nadir approximately 18 months after RYGB. Mean excess weight loss after RYGB is 65% at 2 years and 68% at 3 years.[41] Long-term studies demonstrated a slight increase in weight 2–3 years after surgery (in part due to increased food tolerance, complacency, reversion to old eating habits, etc.), which reaches a plateau and seems to be maintained for many years after surgery.

The medical benefits of RYGB surgery are also significant and include remission of T2DM ($HbA_{1c} < 6.5\%$ off medications) in 67% of patients. Several studies have shown the duration of diabetes, preoperative use of insulin, and magnitude of weight loss influence the remission rate of diabetes,[42-44] so individual studies may report different rates of diabetes remission depending on the characteristics of the study population. Resolution of hypertension is seen in 38% of patients, and remission of hyperlipidemia (cholesterol < 200 mg/dL, high-density lipoproteins > 40 mg/dL, and low-density lipoproteins < 160 mg/dL) is seen in 60% of patients after RYGB.[41] Improvements in OSA, decreased risk of cancer, improvements in gastroesophageal reflux, and improved self-image are seen.[24,45,46]

Despite the medical benefits of RYGB surgery, it is considered a major surgical procedure with potential complications, and the risk-to-benefit ratio should be carefully considered before proceeding with surgery. The most common and serious complications after RYGB surgery include death (0% to 1.1%); anastomotic or staple line leaks causing sepsis (0.6% to 4.4%); gastrojejunal stricture (0.5% to 4.9%); bleeding from intestinal staple line, anastomosis, mesentery, spleen, or liver (0.6% to 3.7%);

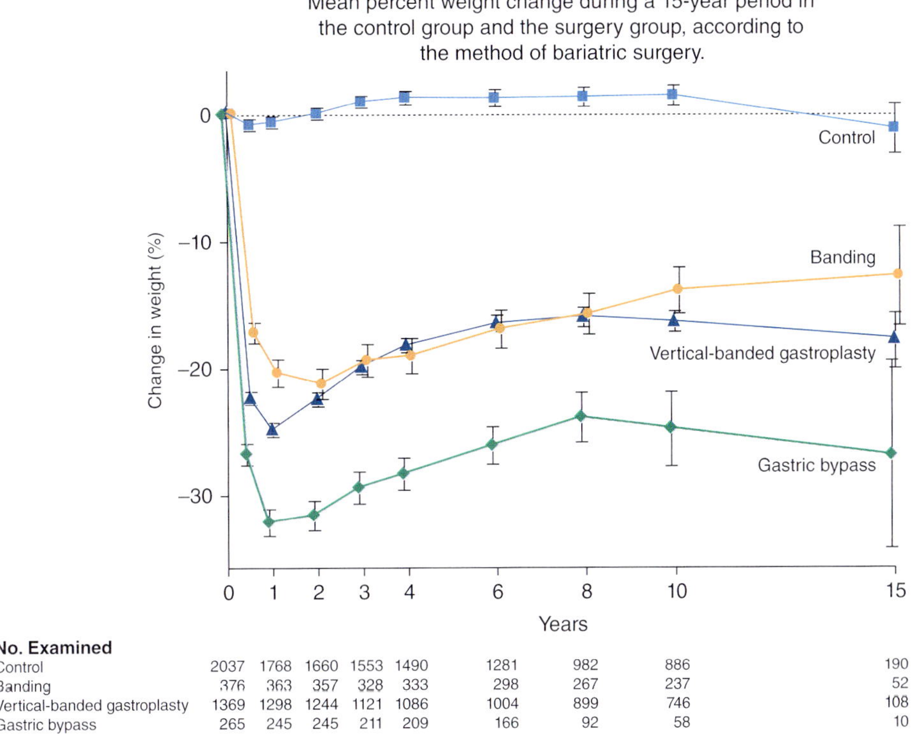

No. Examined										
Control		2037	1768	1660	1553	1490	1281	982	886	190
Banding		376	363	357	328	333	298	267	237	52
Vertical-banded gastroplasty		1369	1298	1244	1121	1086	1004	899	746	108
Gastric bypass		265	245	245	211	209	166	92	58	10

FIGURE 9-2. Weight loss after time following RYGB surgery.

and small bowel obstruction (0.4% to 5.5%).[40] The incidence of wound-related complications (e.g., seroma, surgical site infection, incisional hernia, or wound dehiscence) varies considerably depending on whether the laparoscopic technique is used.[47] Thromboembolic complications (deep venous thomboembolism or pulmonary embolism, 2%–4%), postoperative nausea and vomiting, dumping syndrome, marginal ulcers, symptomatic gallstones, micronutrient deficiencies (iron, vitamin B_{12}, and vitamin D), and protein malnutrition, although less serious, may also be seen after RYGB surgery.

Laparoscopic Adjustable Gastric Band

The LAGB is viewed as a "less-invasive and safer" bariatric procedure in which an adjustable gastric band is placed around the gastroesophageal junction to mechanically restrict food intake. Approval of the LAP-BAND system (Allergan, Inc., Irvine, CA) by the Food and Drug Administration (FDA) in 2001 resulted in a dramatic increase in the use of the LAGB as a bariatric surgical procedure. The LAGB is commonly performed using the "pars flaccida" technique. The left lateral aspect of the gastroesophageal fat pad is identified and dissected. After opening the gastrohepatic membrane and visualizing the right crus, blunt dissection is performed to develop a retrogastric tunnel toward the angle of His. Once this tunnel is established, the adjustable band is pulled through the tunnel, and the band's buckling mechanism is engaged. Next, the

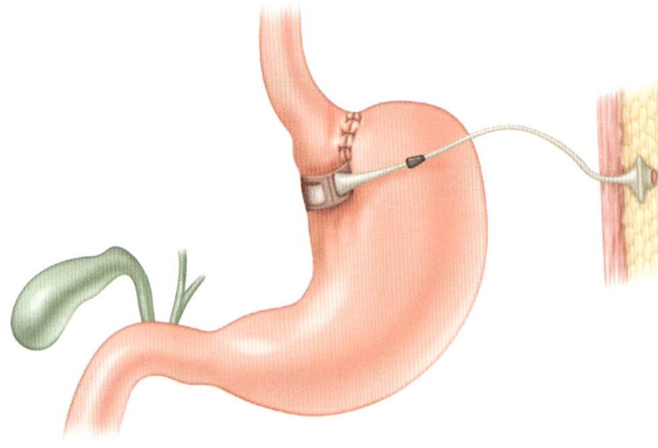

FIGURE 9-3. The laparoscopic adjustable band.

gastric fundus is plicated over the band laterally to decrease the risk of anterior slippage (Figure 9-3). Finally, the subcutaneous port is placed and fixed to the anterior abdominal wall, and the tubing is brought through the abdominal wall and attached to the port.

The "advantages" of the LAGB procedure include decreased operative mortality compared with RYGB, shorter operative time, less-complex technical procedure, the ability to adjust the magnitude of the stoma size, and the ease of "reversibility."[48] Weight loss after LAGB is more gradual over time, generally is less than with RYGB, and requires more frequent follow-up visits. The mean excess weight loss after LAGB is 42% at 2 years and 48% at 3 years.[49] The medical benefits of LAGB surgery include remission of T2DM in 28% of patients. Remission of hypertension is seen in 17% of patients, and hyperlipidemia resolves in 23% of patients after LAGB.[49]

As with any surgical procedure, there are potential complications related to LAGB placement, including mortality (0% to 0.5%), stoma obstruction (0.2% to 1.6%), band slippage (2.3% to 12.5%), band erosion (0.1% to 2.8%) and the requirement for port site revision (0.7% to 5.0%), or infection (0.4% to 1%).[48,50-52] Although the LAP-BAND experienced considerable popularity as a safe and effective alternative to the more complex RYGB procedure from approximately 2000 to 2007, more recent data suggest the requirements for frequent follow-up visits and "late complications" requiring band removal in a significant number of patients have led to decreased popularity, and the sleeve gastrectomy has emerged as an alternative, low-risk bariatric procedure.[35,36]

Laparoscopic Sleeve Gastrectomy

The sleeve gastrectomy was initially described by Almogy et al. in 1993 as a treatment for superobese male patients.[53] It was originally described as an open, longitudinal gastrectomy performed in 21 patients scheduled for duodenal switch because of unexpected intraoperative findings or hemodynamic instability.[53] The successful weight loss (45% EBWL) at 1 year and subsequent success of the LSG as part of a staged approach to the duodenal switch procedure[54] prompted the use of the LSG as a primary bariatric procedure. Over the last 10 years, the number of LSG procedures has increased dramatically, with over 18,000 cases performed in 2008 and a continued increase in subsequent years.

The LSG procedure resects the greater curvature of the stomach, creating a smaller, tubular gastric viscus, frequently using a bougie placed along the lesser curvature as a guide for resection. It is believed to be primarily a mechanically restrictive procedure but may also act by reducing ghrelin secretion and enhancing gastric emptying.[55] Several technical modifications of the LSG procedure have been described, including various bougie sizes (32F to 52F catheter), differences in distal and proximal gastric resection, suture reinforcement of the staple line, and leak testing (for review, see Reference 56).

The bougie size is felt to affect the magnitude of weight loss and intragastric pressure/leak rate. In fact, there is evidence of an inverse relationship between bougie size and leak rates, which also affect the risk of stricture and gastric emptying.[57,58] The distal gastric resection is commonly started from 2 to 7 cm proximal to the pylorus.[59] Because the blood supply near the angle of His may be decreased after resection, preserving 1–2 cm of gastric remnant in this area is recommended by many surgeons to decrease the risk of leaks. Many surgeons use suture-reinforcing materials (e.g., Peri-Strips Dry or SEAMGUARD) or biological sealants or suture between staple loads to decrease the risk of staple line leaks. Intraoperative testing with methylene blue or by endoscopic insufflation is used by many surgeons to verify intact staple lines before completing the procedure.

As mentioned, weight loss after LSG may vary depending on bougie size and other variables. The 2012 Consensus Summit on LSG in New York reported EBWL of 59% after LSG at 1 year, declining to 50% at 6 years after surgery.[60,61] Significant improvements in diabetes (33%), hypertension (58%), and hyperlipidemia (15% to 35%) are also reported after LSG.[61-63] However, "high-quality" long-term data on remission of medical complications is still somewhat "lacking" compared with RYGB and LAGB. Complications of LSG include death (0.17% to 0.49%), staple line leak (1.5% to 4.7%), bleeding (1.8% to 1.9%), and increased gastroesophageal reflux disease (0% to 30%).[58-60] It is sufficient to say that the LSG results are encouraging to date, and the number of patients undergoing LSG as a primary bariatric procedure has increased dramatically over the last several years.[35] Despite this trend, successful long-term weight loss, diabetes resolution, and improvements in gastroesophageal reflux seem better after RYGB than LSG.[61,63,64]

REPRODUCTIVE FUNCTION AND PREGNANCY AFTER BARIATRIC SURGERY

Reproductive function and pregnancy are important topics to consider because of the preponderance of women having bariatric surgery (generally 8:2, women-men) and the large number of these women who are of reproductive age.[65] Obesity is commonly associated with infertility (for review, see Reference 65). In obese women, several factors contribute to infertility. Increased adipose tissue results in the overproduction of leptin, estrogen, and testosterone.[66] Impaired leptin signaling and increased levels of estrogen appear to interfere with the hypothalamic-pituitary-ovarian (HPO) axis, resulting in dysfunctional uterine bleeding, anovulatory cycles, and reduced fertility.[66] Insulin resistance is commonly observed, with visceral adiposity resulting in increased ovarian production of testosterone and suppression of sex hormone–binding globulin (SHBG) by the liver. Collectively, these changes lead to an increase in free androgen index, hirsutism, and polycystic ovary syndrome.[65,66] Obesity also affects body image and sexual health, which have the potential to adversely affect reproductive function.[67,68] In addition, obesity is associated with multiple complications related to pregnancy, including gestational diabetes, hypertension, preeclampsia, congenital malformations, and stillbirth.[69-71]

Women who are planning to have bariatric surgery are advised to avoid pregnancy and use reliable forms of birth control for 12 to 18 months after surgery. The rapid weight loss that occurs following bariatric surgery poses increased risks for both the mother and baby.[70] Many young women undergoing bariatric surgery have been unable to get pregnant for years despite being active sexually and may not see the need for contraception. However, changes in hormonal function and fertility may occur rapidly after bariatric surgery, and the need for contraception to prevent pregnancy in the early postoperative period should be emphasized.[70] Although oral contraceptives are normally considered effective, after RYGB and other malabsorptive surgeries, oral contraceptives may not be as effective due to impaired uptake from the gastrointestinal tract. Other types of birth control, including transdermal and vaginal systems and barrier methods, should be considered. Once weight loss has stabilized, women interested in becoming pregnant should consider antepartum consultations with a dietitian, bariatric specialist, and obstetrician.[70]

Vomiting and nausea are common symptoms after bariatric surgery. These symptoms may become worse during the first trimester of pregnancy due to high levels of β-human chorionic gonadotropin (β-hCG) or decreased progesterone. The workup or intervention for severe nausea and vomiting vary with the bariatric surgical procedure. Most surgeons recommend that laparoscopic bands be fully deflated during pregnancy. If symptoms are refractory to antiemetics, upper gastrointestinal endoscopy should be performed to exclude or treat gastrojejunal stricture as a potential etiology.

Pregnancy results in increased requirements for micronutrients and vitamins.[72] Given the potential risks of micronutrient deficiency after bariatric surgical procedures, these risks are amplified during pregnancy. A comprehensive nutrition assessment should include anthropometric data (height, weight, percentage EBWL, etc.); dietary history; and blood work to assess micronutrient status (blood cell count, metabolic profile, iron profile, thiamine, folate, vitamins B_6 and B_{12}, and fat-soluble vitamins A, D, K, and zinc).[72,73] Protein intake should be approximately 1.1 g/kg of ideal body weight, and energy intake should increase from prenatal by 300 to 500 kcal/d to between 1500 and 1800 kcal/d. Current recommendations include standard prenatal vitamins with or without supplementation with daily calcium (2000 mg calcium citrate, vitamin D [50–150 μg], ferrous iron [10–65 mg], folic acid [4 mg], zinc [15 mg], and cobalamin [350–1000 μg]).[65,72] Postsurgery, BMI is commonly used to estimate desirable weight gain in this population; however, regular ultrasounds are commonly used to monitor fetal growth.[72,74]

As previously noted, obesity is associated with several adverse outcomes in pregnancy. In that regard, several studies have examined the effects of bariatric surgery on outcomes of pregnancy compared with matched controls.[69-71,75] In a recent study by Johansson et al., the risk of gestational diabetes (1.9% vs. 6.8%) and large-for-gestational-age infants (8.6% vs. 22.4%) during pregnancy were significantly decreased after bariatric surgery.[69] Although preterm birth, stillbirth, and congenital malformations were not affected by bariatric surgery, the risk of small-for-gestational-age babies (15.6% vs. 7.6%) was significantly increased.[69] These findings regarding the effects of bariatric surgery in pregnancy are similar to the results of others.[71,75]

More recently, studies by Guenard et al. suggested that surgical weight loss before pregnancy may reduce the risk of obesity and metabolic risk factors by epigenetic mechanisms involving DNA methylation.[76,77] Although these data raise potentially important questions regarding the benefits of bariatric surgery to future offspring, additional data are needed to further understand the long-term risk and benefits of maternal bariatric surgery on future offspring.[77]

REFERENCES

1. US Preventive Services Task Force. Screening for obesity in adults: recommendations and rationale. *Ann Intern Med*. 2003;139(11):930–932.
2. Haslam DW, James WP. Obesity. *Lancet*. 2005;366(9492):1197–1209.
3. Executive summary: tuidelines (2013) for the management of overweight and obesity in adults: a report of the American College of Cardiology/American Heart Association Task Force on Practice Guidelines and the Obesity Society published by the Obesity Society and American College of Cardiology/American Heart Association Task Force on Practice Guidelines. Based on a systematic review from the Obesity Expert Panel, 2013. *Obesity*. 2014;22(Suppl 2):S5–S39.
4. Vgontzas AN, Bixler EO, Chrousos GP. Metabolic disturbances in obesity versus sleep apnoea: the importance of visceral obesity and insulin resistance. *J Intern Med*. 2003;254(1):32–44.
5. Vgontzas AN, Bixler EO, Chrousos GP. Sleep apnea is a manifestation of the metabolic syndrome. *Sleep Med Rev*. 2005;9(3):211–224.
6. Lee JS, Terjimanian MN, Tishberg LM, et al. Surgical site infection and analytic morphometric assessment of body composition in patients undergoing midline laparotomy. *J Am Coll Surg*. 2011;213(2):236–244.
7. Levi B, Zhang P, Lisiecki J, et al. Use of morphometric assessment of body composition to quantify risk of surgical-site infection in patients undergoing component separation ventral hernia repair. *Plast Reconstr Surg*. 2014;133(4):559e–566e.
8. Waisbren E, Rosen H, Bader AM, Lipsitz SR, Rogers SO Jr, Eriksson E. Percent body fat and prediction of surgical site infection. *J Am Coll Surg*. 2010;210(4):381–389.
9. Hubbard VS, Hall WH. Gastrointestinal surgery for severe obesity. *Obes Surg*. 1991;1(3):257–265.
10. Ali MR, Maguire MB, Wolfe BM. Assessment of obesity-related comorbidities: a novel scheme for evaluating bariatric surgical patients. *J Am Coll Surg*. 2006;202(1):70–77.
11. Eldar S, Heneghan HM, Brethauer S, Schauer PR. A focus on surgical preoperative evaluation of the bariatric patient—the Cleveland Clinic protocol and review of the literature. *Surgeon*. 2011;9(5):273–277.
12. Appel LJ, Clark JM, Yeh HC, et al. Comparative effectiveness of weight-loss interventions in clinical practice. *N Engl J Med*. 2011;365(21):1959–1968.
13. Bauchowitz AU, Gonder-Frederick LA, Olbrisch ME, et al. Psychosocial evaluation of bariatric surgery candidates: a survey of present practices. *Psychosom Med*. 2005;67(5):825–832.
14. Wadden TA, Sarwer DB. Behavioral assessment of candidates for bariatric surgery: a patient-oriented approach. *Obesity*. 2006;14(Suppl 2):53S–62S.
15. Zimmerman M, Francione-Witt C, Chelminski I, et al. Presurgical psychiatric evaluations of candidates for bariatric surgery, part 1: reliability and reasons for and frequency of exclusion. *J Clin Psychiatry*. 2007;68(10):1557–1562.
16. Khan A, King WC, Patterson EJ, et al. Assessment of obstructive sleep apnea in adults undergoing bariatric surgery in the Longitudinal Assessment of Bariatric Surgery-2 (LABS-2) study. *J Clin Sleep Med*. 2013;9(1):21–29.
17. Gupta PK, Franck C, Miller WJ, Gupta H, Forse RA. Development and validation of a bariatric surgery morbidity risk calculator using the prospective, multicenter NSQIP dataset. *J Am Coll Surg*. 2011;212(3):301–309.
18. Maciejewski ML, Winegar DA, Farley JF, Wolfe BM, DeMaria EJ. Risk stratification of serious adverse events after gastric bypass in the Bariatric Outcomes Longitudinal Database. *Surg Obes Relat Dis*. 2012;8(6):671–677.
19. Ramanan B, Gupta PK, Gupta H, Fang X, Forse RA. Development and validation of a bariatric surgery mortality risk calculator. *J Am Coll Surg*. 2012;214(6):892–900.
20. Hollenbeak CS, Rogers AM, Barrus B, Wadiwala I, Cooney RN. Surgical volume impacts bariatric surgery mortality: a case for centers of excellence. *Surgery*. 2008;144(5):736–743.
21. Longitudinal Assessment of Bariatric Surgery Consortium, Flum DR, Belle SH, et al. Perioperative safety in the Longitudinal Assessment of Bariatric Surgery. *N Engl J Med*. 2009;361(5):445–454.
22. Smith MD, Patterson E, Wahed AS, et al. Relationship between surgeon volume and adverse outcomes after RYGB in Longitudinal Assessment of Bariatric Surgery (LABS) study. *Surg Obes Relat Dis*. 2010;6(2):118–125.
23. Dimick JB, Osborne NH, Nicholas L, Birkmeyer JD. Identifying high-quality bariatric surgery centers: hospital volume or risk-adjusted outcomes? *J Am Coll Surg*. 2009;209(6):702–706.
24. Adams TD, Gress RE, Smith SC, et al. Long-term mortality after gastric bypass surgery. *N Engl J Med*. 2007;357(8):753–761.

25. Adams TD, Pendleton RC, Strong MB, et al. Health outcomes of gastric bypass patients compared to nonsurgical, nonintervened severely obese. *Obesity.* 2010;18(1):121–130.

26. Flum DR, Dellinger EP. Impact of gastric bypass operation on survival: a population-based analysis. *J Am Coll Surg.* 2004;199(4):543–551.

27. Sjostrom L, Narbro K, Sjostrom CD, et al. Effects of bariatric surgery on mortality in Swedish obese subjects. *N Engl J Med.* 2007;357(8):741–752.

28. Arterburn DE, Olsen MK, Smith VA, et al. Association between bariatric surgery and long-term survival. *JAMA.* 2015;313(1):62–70.

29. Cooney RN, Bryant P, Haluck R, Rodgers M, Lowery M. The impact of a clinical pathway for gastric bypass surgery on resource utilization. *J Surg Res.* 2001;98(2):97–101.

30. Gross JB, Bachenberg KL, Benumof JL, et al. Practice guidelines for the perioperative management of patients with obstructive sleep apnea: a report by the American Society of Anesthesiologists Task Force on Perioperative Management of patients with obstructive sleep apnea. *Anesthesiology.* 2006;104(5): 1081–1093; quiz 1117–1088.

31. Chung SA, Yuan H, Chung F. A systemic review of obstructive sleep apnea and its implications for anesthesiologists. *Anesth Analg.* 2008;107(5):1543–1563.

32. Chung F, Liao P, Yegneswaran B, Shapiro CM, Kang W. Postoperative changes in sleep-disordered breathing and sleep architecture in patients with obstructive sleep apnea. *Anesthesiology.* 2014;120(2):287–298.

33. Liao P, Luo Q, Elsaid H, Kang W, Shapiro CM, Chung F. Perioperative auto-titrated continuous positive airway pressure treatment in surgical patients with obstructive sleep apnea: a randomized controlled trial. *Anesthesiology.* 2013;119(4):837–847.

34. Ettinger JE, de Souza CA, Santos-Filho PV, et al. Rhabdomyolysis: diagnosis and treatment in bariatric surgery. *Obes Surg.* 2007;17(4):525–532.

35. Young MT, Gebhart A, Phelan MJ, Nguyen NT. Use and outcomes of laparoscopic sleeve gastrectomy vs laparoscopic gastric bypass: analysis of the American College of Surgeons NSQIP. *J Am Coll Surg.* 2015;220(5):880–885.

36. Esteban Varela J, Nguyen NT. Laparoscopic sleeve gastrectomy leads the US utilization of bariatric surgery at academic medical centers. *Surg Obes Relat Dis.* 2015.

37. Siddiqui A, Livingston E, Huerta S. A comparison of open and laparoscopic Roux-en-Y gastric bypass surgery for morbid and super obesity: a decision-analysis model. *Am J Surg.* 2006;192(5):e1–e7.

38. Sekhar N, Torquati A, Youssef Y, Wright JK, Richards WO. A comparison of 399 open and 568 laparoscopic gastric bypasses performed during a 4-year period. *Surg Endosc.* 2007;21(4):665–668.

39. Nguyen NT, Goldman C, Rosenquist CJ, et al. Laparoscopic versus open gastric bypass: a randomized study of outcomes, quality of life, and costs. *Ann Surg.* 2001;234(3):279–289; discussion 289–291.

40. Nguyen NT, Ho HS, Palmer LS, Wolfe BM. A comparison study of laparoscopic versus open gastric bypass for morbid obesity. *J Am Coll Surg.* 2000;191(2): 149–155; discussion 155–147.

41. Puzziferri N, Austrheim-Smith IT, Wolfe BM, Wilson SE, Nguyen NT. Three-year follow-up of a prospective randomized trial comparing laparoscopic versus open gastric bypass. *Ann Surg.* 2006;243(2): 181–188.

42. Hall TC, Pellen MG, Sedman PC, Jain PK. Preoperative factors predicting remission of type 2 diabetes mellitus after Roux-en-Y gastric bypass surgery for obesity. *Obes Surg.* 2010;20(9):1245–1250.

43. Pories WJ, Swanson MS, MacDonald KG, et al. Who would have thought it? An operation proves to be the most effective therapy for adult-onset diabetes mellitus. *Ann Surg.* 1995;222(3):339–350; discussion 350–332.

44. Schauer PR, Burguera B, Ikramuddin S, et al. Effect of laparoscopic Roux-en Y gastric bypass on type 2 diabetes mellitus. *Ann Surg.* 2003;238(4):467–484; discussion 484–465.

45. Greenburg DL, Lettieri CJ, Eliasson AH. Effects of surgical weight loss on measures of obstructive sleep apnea: a meta-analysis. *Am J Med.* 2009;122(6):535–542.

46. Prachand VN, Alverdy JC. Gastroesophageal reflux disease and severe obesity: fundoplication or bariatric surgery? *World J Gastroenterol.* 2010;16(30): 3757–3761.

47. Shope TR, Cooney RN, McLeod J, Miller CA, Haluck RS. Early results after laparoscopic gastric bypass: EEA vs GIA stapled gastrojejunal anastomosis. *Obes Surg.* 2003;13(3):355–359.

48. Nguyen NT, Wilson SE. Complications of antiobesity surgery. *Nat Clin Pract Gastroenterol Hepatol.* 2007;4(3):138–147.

49. Puzziferri N, Roshek TB 3rd, Mayo HG, Gallagher R, Belle SH, Livingston EH. Long-term follow-up after bariatric surgery: a systematic review. *JAMA.* 2014;312(9):934–942.

50. Fielding GA, Ren CJ. Laparoscopic adjustable gastric band. *Surg Clin North Am.* 2005;85(1):129–140, x.

51. O'Brien PE, MacDonald L, Anderson M, Brennan L, Brown WA. Long-term outcomes after bariatric surgery: fifteen-year follow-up of adjustable gastric banding and a systematic review of the bariatric surgical literature. *Ann Surg.* 2013;257(1):87–94.

52. Brown WA, Egberts KJ, Franke-Richard D, Thodiyil P, Anderson ML, O'Brien PE. Erosions after laparoscopic adjustable gastric banding: diagnosis and management. *Ann Surg.* 2013;257(6):1047–1052.

53. Almogy G, Crookes PF, Anthone GJ. Longitudinal gastrectomy as a treatment for the high-risk super-obese patient. *Obes Surg.* 2004;14(4):492–497.

54. Gumbs AA, Gagner M, Dakin G, Pomp A. Sleeve gastrectomy for morbid obesity. *Obes Surg.* 2007;17(7):962–969.

55. Nannipieri M, Baldi S, Mari A, et al. Roux-en-Y gastric bypass and sleeve gastrectomy: mechanisms of diabetes remission and role of gut hormones. *J Clin Endocrinol Metab.* 2013;98(11):4391–4399.

56. Ferrer-Marquez M, Belda-Lozano R, Ferrer-Ayza M. Technical controversies in laparoscopic sleeve gastrectomy. *Obes Surg.* 2012;22(1):182–187.

57. Nedelcu M, Manos T, Cotirlet A, Noel P, Gagner M. Outcome of leaks after sleeve gastrectomy based on a new algorithm adressing leak size and gastric stenosis. *Obes Surg.* 2015;25(3):559–563.

58. Abou Rached A, Basile M, El Masri H. Gastric leaks post sleeve gastrectomy: review of its prevention and management. *World J Gastroenterol.* 2014;20(38):13904–13910.

59. Obeidat F, Shanti H, Mismar A, Albsoul N, Al-Qudah M. The magnitude of antral resection in laparoscopic sleeve gastrectomy and its relationship to excess weight loss. *Obes Surg.* 2015.

60. Gagner M, Deitel M, Erickson AL, Crosby RD. Survey on laparoscopic sleeve gastrectomy (LSG) at the Fourth International Consensus Summit on Sleeve Gastrectomy. *Obes Surg.* 2013;23(12):2013–2017.

61. Shabbir A, Dargan D. The success of sleeve gastrectomy in the management of metabolic syndrome and obesity. *J Biomed Res.* 2015;29(2):93–97.

62. Ruiz-Tovar J, Martinez R, Bonete JM, et al. Long-term weight and metabolic effects of laparoscopic sleeve gastrectomy calibrated with a 50F bougie. *Obes Surg.* 2015.

63. Schauer PR, Bhatt DL, Kirwan JP, et al. Bariatric surgery versus intensive medical therapy for diabetes—3-year outcomes. *N Engl J Med.* 2014;370(21):2002–2013.

64. Torgersen Z, Osmolak A, Forse RA. Sleeve gastrectomy and Roux En Y gastric bypass: current state of metabolic surgery. *Curr Opin Endocrinol Diabetes Obes.* 2014;21(5):352–357.

65. Brewer CJ, Balen AH. The adverse effects of obesity on conception and implantation. *Reproduction.* 2010;140(3):347–364.

66. Sharma A, Bahadursingh S, Ramsewak S, Teelucksingh S. Medical and surgical interventions to improve outcomes in obese women planning for pregnancy. *Best Pract Res Clin Obstet Gynaecol.* 2015;29(4):565–576.

67. Sarwer DB, Spitzer JC, Wadden TA, et al. Changes in sexual functioning and sex hormone levels in women following bariatric surgery. *JAMA Surg.* 2014;149(1):26–33.

68. Legro RS, Dodson WC, Gnatuk CL, et al. Effects of gastric bypass surgery on female reproductive function. *J Clin Endocrinol Metab.* 2012;97(12):4540–4548.

69. Johansson K, Cnattingius S, Naslund I, et al. Outcomes of pregnancy after bariatric surgery. *N Engl J Med.* 2015;372(9):814–824.

70. Magdaleno R Jr, Pereira BG, Chaim EA, Turato ER. Pregnancy after bariatric surgery: a current view of maternal, obstetrical and perinatal challenges. *Arch Gynecol Obstet.* 2012;285(3):559–566.

71. Roos N, Neovius M, Cnattingius S, et al. Perinatal outcomes after bariatric surgery: nationwide population based matched cohort study. *BMJ.* 2013;347:f6460.

72. Kaska L, Kobiela J, Abacjew-Chmylko A, et al. Nutrition and pregnancy after bariatric surgery. *ISRN Obes.* 2013;2013:492060.

73. Procter SB, Campbell CG. Position of the Academy of Nutrition and Dietetics: nutrition and lifestyle for a healthy pregnancy outcome. *J Acad Nutr Diet.* 2014;114(7):1099–1103.

74. Devlieger R, Guelinckx I, Jans G, Voets W, Vanholsbeke C, Vansant G. Micronutrient levels and supplement intake in pregnancy after bariatric surgery: a prospective cohort study. *PloS One.* 2014;9(12):e114192.

75. Uzoma A, Keriakos R. Pregnancy management following bariatric surgery. *J Obstet Gynaecol.* 2013;33(2):109–114.

76. Guenard F, Deshaies Y, Cianflone K, Kral JG, Marceau P, Vohl MC. Differential methylation in glucoregulatory genes of offspring born before vs. after maternal gastrointestinal bypass surgery. *Proc Natl Acad Sci U S A.* 2013;110(28):11439–11444.

77. Patti ME. Reducing maternal weight improves offspring metabolism and alters (or modulates) methylation. *Proc Natl Acad Sci U S A.* 2013;110(32):12859–12860.

CHAPTER 10

Obesity and Breast Development and Function

Jayne R. Charlamb, MD, FACP, IBCLC

OBESITY AND BREAST DEVELOPMENT

During preadolescent childhood, the growth of the mammary gland is isometric, keeping pace with the general growth of the child's body.[1] At *thelarche*, the onset of secondary breast development occurring at puberty, the female mammary gland undergoes significant further development of its previously primitive ductal and lobular structures. It is the deposition of adipose tissue within the mammary gland, however, that accounts for the majority of the increase in breast size associated with puberty.[2] Body mass index (BMI) has been found to relate to both the timing of thelarche and the composition of the adult female breast.

Childhood Obesity and Thelarchal Age

Age at thelarche is known to vary by race and ethnicity. A recent prospective study of a cohort of more than 1200 girls in the United States reported the median onset of thelarche (Tanner stage 2) to be 8.8 years for African American girls, 9.3 years for Hispanic girls, and 9.7 years for both white non-Hispanic and Asian girls participating in the study.[3] Excess childhood weight has also long been associated with earlier breast development, independent of race and ethnicity.[4] Some studies have relied on visual inspection as a means to assess breast development, raising the potential for excess fatty tissue deposition among obese girls to be confused with true glandular tissue, thus confounding results. However, more recent studies have made use of palpation by trained examiners to determine the onset of glandular breast development, and these studies have likewise demonstrated correlation between higher BMI and younger age at thelarche. The Breast Cancer and the Environment Research Centers (BCERC) study found a significant correlation between higher BMI and onset of breast development with girls in all BMI categories above the 50th percentile progressively more likely to have reached thelarche than those below the 50th percentile, adjusting for race and ethnicity. The authors reported that while race accounted for 4.4% of the variance in thelarchal age, BMI was the strongest predictor of earlier age at thelarche of all covariates included in their statistical model, accounting for 14.2% of the variance.[3]

There is growing evidence of a decline in age at female puberty, specifically in the age at thelarche, over the past several decades.[5,6] The concurrent trend of increasing prevalence of childhood obesity in Western populations further suggests a relationship between childhood BMI and pubertal breast development. Childhood obesity may have a direct causal impact on the timing of pubertal development through, for example, obesity's influence on endogenous hormonal levels. Studies in animal models have demonstrated causal links between feeding and pubertal development and support the possibility of a direct causal relationship between increasing obesity and earlier age at thelarche.[7] However, other potential mechanisms for the association between childhood BMI and timing of, and trends in, pubertal development have been proposed. One possible such mechanism is population exposure to environmental "endocrine-disrupting chemicals" that have the potential to independently affect both obesity and pubertal timing.[5] Certainly, further research exploring the underlying relationship between etiology of and sequelae of trends in prevalence of childhood obesity and the timing of female pubertal development is warranted.

Obesity and Breast Size and Composition

Adolescent BMI has been found to relate breast size and composition. Dual-energy x-ray absorptiometry scanning demonstrates that higher BMI correlates with greater breast area, greater breast volume, and lower breast density among adolescent girls.[8] Analysis of data from the Nurses' Health Study suggested that childhood body fatness is inversely associated with mammographic density in adulthood as well.[9] The relationship between adolescent BMI and adult breast density is of particular interest given the well-documented association between breast density and risk of breast malignancy.[10]

The percentage of fat composition within the human female breast varies greatly. One study examining fresh mastectomy specimens found fat composition ranged from 7% to 56% by volume. There was no significant correlation between BMI and percentage of fat in the breast, although the sample size was small.[11] Other studies using magnetic resonance imaging (MRI) assessment, however, have documented a positive correlation between BMI and both overall breast volume and amount of breast adipose tissue within the breast of adult women.[12,13] As discussed in the section on obesity's impact on successful breastfeeding, this additional adipose tissue may play a role in an altered breast function among obese and overweight women.

Structure and Role of Adipose Tissue Within the Breast

Many texts and figures have portrayed a distinct anatomical separation between the glandular epithelial tissue and the fatty tissues of the mature female breast. However, contemporary histological examination of fresh, fixed normal mastectomy specimens reveals that while subcutaneous fat is indeed present over the surface of the body of the breast and can be separated from the underlying breast parenchyma, there is a great deal of fat intermixed within the breast glandular parenchyma.[14] In addition, sonographic examination of the breasts of lactating women has demonstrated significant and variable fat within the glandular tissue of the breast, with only minimal subcutaneous fat noted within a 30-mm radius of the base of the nipple. Figure 10-1

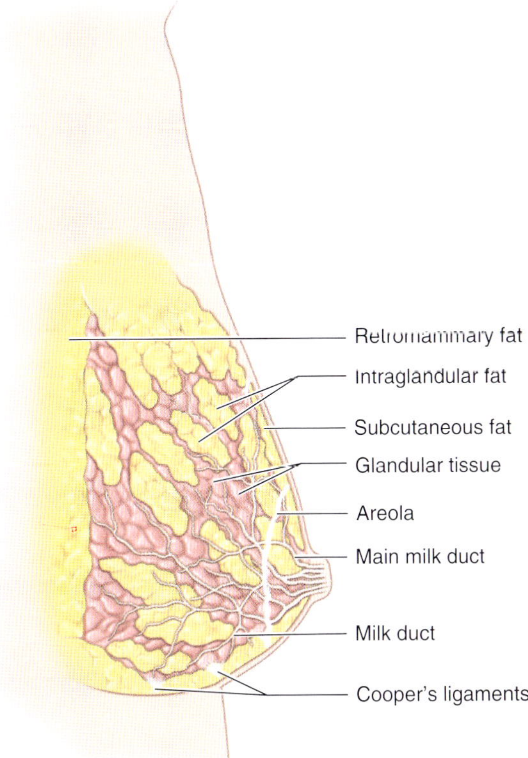

FIGURE 10-1. Drawing based on ultrasound observations. Note the presence of significant intraglandular fat. (Redrawn from Ramsay DT, Kent JC, Hartmann RA, Hartmann PE. Anatomy of the lactating human breast redefined with ultrasound imaging. *J Anat*. 2005;206(6):525–534.)

portrays the currently understood distribution of fat in the human breast, including notable amounts of fat intermixed within the glandular parenchyma.[15]

Fat within the human breast is often thought of as an inert structural component, and discussions of breast development and function typically focus on mammary epithelial tissues rather than on the mammary fat pad in which they reside. However, there is a growing recognition of the active role that mammary adipocytes seemingly play in the regulation of mammary epithelial development and function. Breast adipose tissue is thought to serve not only as a local source of lipids for the mammary epithelium, but also as a reservoir and source of paracrine and endocrine molecules affecting both breast growth and its function during lactation.[16] Although inconsistent, some evidence suggests that breast volume and the degree of breast adiposity may reflect the degree of metabolical fat elsewhere in a woman's body and may potentially serve as a marker for risk of metabolic disease.[12,13]

OBESITY AND BREAST FUNCTION: LACTATION

Lactation: The Normal Function of the Breast

Considerable attention in the medical literature is given to the breast in the context of its potential for malignant disease. However, there is a growing and important focus on issues related to the physiologic function of the breast organ: lactation. While the success of the breastfeeding relationship has the potential to significantly affect the health of all mothers and infants, it may be of special importance to obese and overweight mothers and their families.

The Importance of Breastfeeding for Infants

Exclusive breastfeeding has been well established as the normative and preferred method for the feeding of human infants. The American College of Obstetricians and Gynecologists (ACOG),[17] the American Academy of Pediatrics (AAP),[18] the American Academy of Family Physicians,[19] and the World Health Organization (WHO)[20] all recommend exclusive breastfeeding for the first half of the first year of life, followed by continued breastfeeding with complementary feedings for longer periods, ranging from at least 1 year of age to at least 2 years of age. The use of artificial breast milk substitutes (formulas) at any time, the introduction of complementary foods before approximately 6 months of age, and the discontinuation of breastfeeding before 1 to 2 years of age are all considered suboptimal breastfeeding practices. The association between lack of breastfeeding or suboptimal breastfeeding and excess morbidity and mortality in children is well documented, even in populations in the industrialized world possessing substantial economic and health care resources. Infants not breastfed or breastfed for suboptimal durations are at higher risk for otitis media, respiratory tract infection, gastrointestinal tract infections, necrotizing enterocolitis, sudden infant death syndrome (SIDS), inflammatory bowel disease, type 1 diabetes, childhood leukemias, and obesity.[18,21]

Breastfeeding as Childhood Obesity Prevention

It has been long established that breastfed infants exhibit different growth and weight-gaining patterns than their formula-fed peers, with breastfed infants overall leaner at 12 months of age.[22] A more recent literature asserts a possible relationship between breastfeeding during infancy and a child's weight beyond the breastfeeding period.

Based on evidence of an association between suboptimal breastfeeding and risk of later obesity, in a 2010 statement the US Breastfeeding Committee recommended breastfeeding as a primary prevention strategy to reduce overweight and obesity and to promote the maintenance of a healthy weight throughout the life span.[23]

Multiple plausible mechanisms for a causal relationship between breastfeeding in infancy and a lowered risk of later obesity have been purported. Among these are the exposure to components of breast milk during infancy providing determination of long-term metabolism and appetite signaling ("programming") and the infant-driven process of receiving nutrition at the breast itself leading to the development of later optimal self-regulation of energy intake.[24,25] Given that the data evidencing a relationship between breastfeeding and lowered risk of later obesity are nearly entirely observational in nature, however, it is important to carefully control for confounding variables and methodological bias when seeking to delineate the nature of this relationship. A recent extensive and careful systematic review of the literature continued to find a modest reduction in the prevalence of overweight or obesity in children exposed to longer durations of breastfeeding,[26] and a recent large meta-analysis suggested that breastfeeding may be a significant protective factor against obesity in children.[27] However, questions related to methodological and data-confounding issues persist, and the evidence related to a significant causal relationship between breastfeeding and decreased risk of obesity remains somewhat conflicting and controversial.

The Importance of Breastfeeding for Mothers

Lactation is the physiologically normal postpartum state for the human mother. Lack of breastfeeding and suboptimal breastfeeding duration and intensity are associated with excess maternal morbidity. Mothers who do not breastfeed in the immediate postpartum period have increased postpartum blood loss and a slower involution of the uterus.[18] Inverse relationships between lactation and later risks of breast malignancy, ovarian malignancy, depression, hypertension, diabetes, hyperlipedemia, and cardiovascular disease have also been documented.[18,21] The majority of evidence of these relationships arises from observational studies, however, and is therefore subject to concerns regarding methodological bias and confounding variables.

Breastfeeding in Relation to Maternal Weight and Metabolic Disease

Pregnancy is associated with numerous metabolic changes, including insulin resistance, visceral fat accumulation, and elevation in lipid and triglyceride levels. Accumulating evidence demonstrates an inverse relationship between lactation and the risk of subsequent maternal metabolic disease; therefore, breastfeeding may be of special importance for the obese mother. Stuebe and Rick-Edwards proposed the concept of lactation providing a physiologically normal and important "resetting" of the maternal metabolism after pregnancy, leading to a more rapid and more complete return to baseline metabolism.[28]

The literature relating to the effect of lactation on maternal postpartum weight loss and return to prepregnancy weight is inconclusive. Inherent confounding variables such as physical activity, dietary intake, and gestational weight gain are difficult to control. A recent systematic review found insufficient evidence to suggest a direct association between breastfeeding and postpartum weight change, although a subset of the reviewed studies the authors determined to have "higher methodologic quality" did demonstrate a positive association.[29] A recent study investigating the association between adherence to 2005 AAP recommendations for exclusive and total breastfeeding duration and maternal weight 6 years postpartum found a significant association between complete adherence to these recommendations and maternal weight among women who were obese before pregnancy compared to those who had not breastfed. No such relationship was noted among normal-weight and nonobese overweight women.[30]

Growing evidence suggests breastfeeding may play a role in postpartum maternal metabolism and related morbidities regardless of any effect it has on maternal postpartum weight specifically. Analysis of data from the Women's Health Initiative supported an inverse relationship between lactation duration and subsequent development of hyperlipidemia, hypertension, and cardiovascular disease in postmenopausal women.[31] In addition, breastfeeding has been associated with a reduced risk of subsequent development of type 2 diabetes mellitus in mothers both with and without a history of gestational diabetes mellitus (GDM), and mothers with GDM who breastfeed have improved lipid and glucose metabolic profiles for at least the first 3 months postpartum.[18,32]

Studies using computerized tomography to assess the amount of the highly metabolically active visceral fat that typically accumulates during pregnancy demonstrated an association between breastfeeding and lowered abdominal adiposity, even years after pregnancy and lactation. Controlling for known risk factors for cardiovascular disease, including BMI, premenopausal mothers who had not lactated had significantly more visceral adiposity than mothers who had lactated, while mothers who had lactated for 3 or more months after each birth had no more visceral fat than women who had never been pregnant.[33]

As with other literature related to the effects of breastfeeding, however, the observational nature of the vast majority of the studies demonstrating a relationship between breastfeeding and maternal morbidity limits the ability to assign causality. While it is plausible that suboptimal breastfeeding has a causal role in increased maternal metabolic morbidity via a failure of a physiologically normal return to baseline metabolism in the postpartum period and beyond, the relationship may also be explained by confounding variables not adequately controlled for via statistical methodologies. Alternatively, the relationship between breastfeeding success and maternal metabolism may indeed be causal, but in the opposite direction; as discussed in the following material, an inherent altered baseline metabolic state may interfere with lactation success. Thus, a woman's unsuccessful breastfeeding may be the result of the same underlying physiologic abnormalities that lead to eventual metabolically associated morbidities, rather than being a cause of these morbidities itself. Future research should attempt to further define the likely complex nature of these relationships.

The Impact of Maternal Obesity on Successful Breastfeeding

Multiple systematic reviews of the literature demonstrated an overall inverse association between maternal BMI and breastfeeding initiation and duration.[34,35] Most recently, Turcksin and colleagues reviewed prospective studies evaluating the relationship between prepregnancy maternal obesity and lactation; these authors used more stringent inclusion criteria than those used in previous reviews. They found that, overall, even when adjusting for potentially confounding factors, maternal obesity was associated with reduced intention to breastfeed, reduced initiation of breastfeeding, shortened duration of breastfeeding, less-adequate milk supply, and delayed onset of copious milk supply (*lactogenesis II*).[36] Although this and other reviews have focused on the relationship between prepregnancy BMI and breastfeeding, other evidence indicated that excessive weight gain during pregnancy may be associated with suboptimal breastfeeding regardless of prepregnancy weight status.[37]

The relationship between higher maternal BMI and decreased lactation initiation and success may not be a factor in all populations. In the United States, black women have both the lowest breastfeeding initiation and continuation rates and the highest rates of obesity compared to their white and Hispanic counterparts.[38,39] However, as detailed in the reviews previously mentioned, some of the associations between higher BMI and negative breastfeeding outcomes were noted among white or Hispanic women, but not among African American women. It is noteworthy that despite the diverse international locations of the reviewed studies, most included a majority of women of white European origin as subjects. Certainly, further research is warranted to explore and understand the seemingly complex relationships between race, obesity, and breastfeeding.

Etiology of the Impact of Maternal Obesity on Breastfeeding

Maternal obesity may have a negative impact on breastfeeding success through a number of mechanisms, and the relationship is likely complex and multifactorial. Successful lactation necessitates multiple steps, including (1) the appropriate structural development of the mammary gland during childhood and puberty, (2) further differentiation of the mammary epithelial cells under the influence of a complex of reproductive and metabolic hormones during pregnancy, (3) the initiation of copious milk secretion (lactogenesis II) triggered by a rapid decline in progesterone in the setting of prolactin and an appropriate hormonal milieu after delivery, and (4) frequent breast stimulation triggering milk synthesis and milk ejection via the release of prolactin and oxytocin, respectively, along with frequent and continued milk removal from the breast.[40,41] In addition to the hormones noted, cortisol, insulin, growth hormone, and the thyroid hormones are involved in establishing and maintaining lactation.[40–42]

Delayed onset of lactogenesis II, defined as onset of copious milk production after 72 hours after delivery of the placenta, is associated with and predictive of decreased breastfeeding success, including lowered rates of exclusive and any breastfeeding at 1 month postpartum,[43] and is often cited as a proxy for decreased lactation success. However, disruption at any step of the process outlined can have a negative impact on eventual successful lactation. Possible anatomic, physiologic, and psychosocial etiologies of the suboptimal breastfeeding success observed in obese and overweight women are discussed next and diagramed in Figure 10-2.

ANATOMIC DIFFERENCES—Anatomic differences in women with higher BMIs may play a direct role in decreased breastfeeding success. Some have noted that large-breasted women may have flattish nipples, possibly related to an excess of periareolar adipose tissue.[44,45] This, in combination with larger breasts and an overall altered upper body anatomy, may create mechanical challenges in positioning and latching a nursing infant or pumping with standard-size pump flanges. Such difficulties could

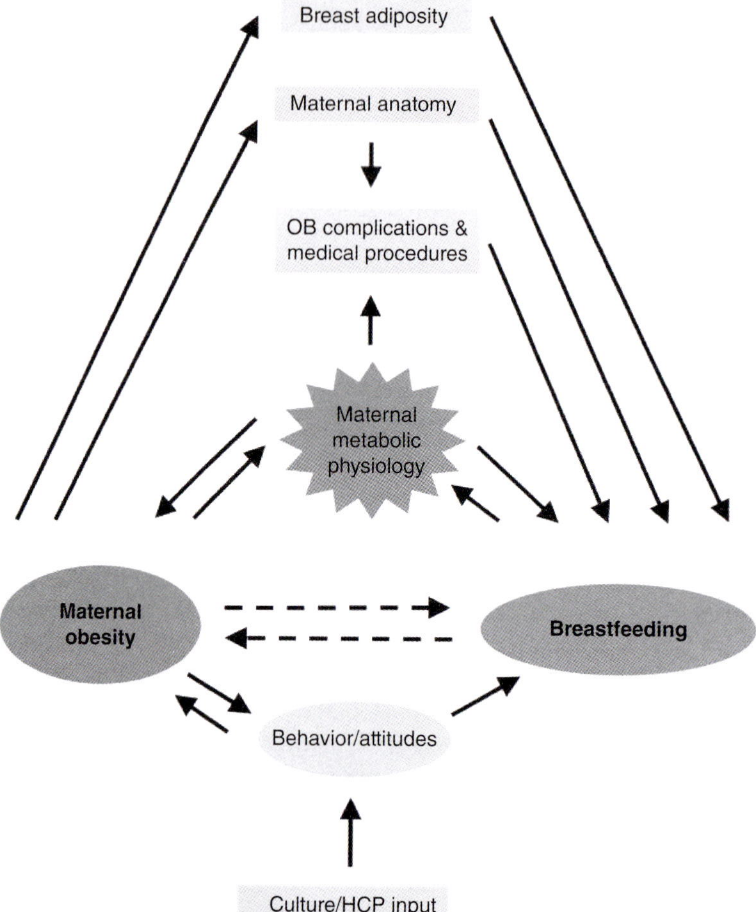

FIGURE 10-2. The complex relationships between maternal obesity and breastfeeding. Maternal obesity can affect breastfeeding success through its impact on breast composition, maternal anatomy, maternal physiology, and maternal behavior and attitudes. Abnormalities in maternal physiology and maternal anatomy can have an impact on breastfeeding success directly or through effects on obstetrical complications. Both cultural influence and input from the health care provider play a role in obesity and in breastfeeding success. Breastfeeding has a beneficial effect on maternal physiology and may possibly decrease maternal obesity. HCP, health care provider.

lead to suboptimal frequency and extent of milk transfer and significantly interfere with lactation success, especially in the early days and weeks of breastfeeding when frequent, effective feedings are essential to the development and maintenance of an optimal milk supply. In addition, mothers who have undergone breast reduction surgery in the past to alleviate the physical and emotional sequelae of their large breasts have decreased lactation performance, likely due to the anatomical disruption of fibroglandular tissue and ductal structures.[46]

BREAST ADIPOSITY—The increased breast adiposity noted among obese and overweight women[12,13] may exert a negative effect on lactation through nonmechanical means. As noted in the section on obesity and breast development and structure, breast adipose tissue is thought to serve not only as a local source of lipids for the mammary epithelium but also as a reservoir and source of paracrine and endocrine molecules affecting both breast growth and its function during lactation.[16] The extra adipose tissue found within the breasts of obese women may thereby play a role in the altered lactation function seen among obese and overweight women.

MATERNAL SYSTEMIC PHYSIOLOGY AND COMORBID CONDITIONS—Underlying maternal systemic physiologic abnormalities that occur in association with, as a cause of, or as a result of maternal obesity may have a negative impact on breastfeeding success. A growing body of literature shows evidence of a relationship between abnormalities in glucose metabolism and suboptimal lactation physiology.[35,47] Polycystic ovary syndrome (PCOS), metabolic syndrome, and thyroid disease have all been associated with decreased breastfeeding success.[42,48–50]

Some research has attempted to identify specific alterations in the endocrinologic physiology of obese women to explain decreased breastfeeding success. Controlling for confounding variables such as mode of delivery, early interaction with the infant and use of analgesia have often proven difficult.[51] One study found overweight and obese women had similar progesterone levels but a blunted prolactin response to infant suckling in the first week postpartum compared to their normal-weight peers.[52] A study of mothers with PCOS found the degree of metabolic derangement to be inversely associated with breastfeeding and breast size increment during pregnancy. However, neither androgen level nor randomized treatment with metformin was related to breastfeeding.[49] As underlying physiologic abnormalities can be lifelong, their impact on breastfeeding success may occur through affecting breast structure during development, through affecting physiologic function during the lactation process itself, or both. Further research is necessary to elucidate the nature of the relationship between abnormal maternal physiology and breastfeeding success.

ASSOCIATED OBSTETRICAL COMPLICATIONS—While it is plausible that underlying maternal systemic physiologic abnormalities among obese women themselves directly interfere with normal breast development or lactational physiology, they, along with an obese maternal anatomy, may also indirectly have a negative impact on breastfeeding success through increasing the risk of obstetrical complications and intrapartum medical procedures that hinder the establishment of lactation. For example, obese women are at increased risk of cesarean delivery and the use of exogenous oxytocin (see Chapter 21), and both of these factors have been independently associated with delayed lactogenesis II.[43,50]

Obstetrical complications and the hospital routines designed to manage them can lead to physical separation of the mother and infant during the early postpartum period, limiting the opportunity for the ideal frequency of feedings and breast stimulation associated with the development and maintenance of an optimal milk supply. Mothers undergoing cesarean delivery, for example, are not always able to initiate breastfeeding promptly. Likewise, infants of diabetic mothers are prone to macrosomia and hypoglycemia and may receive special observation requiring separation from their mothers, leading to decreased opportunity for early time at the breast.

PSYCHOSOCIAL AND BEHAVIORAL FACTORS—Although evidence for a biologic relationship between obesity and suboptimal lactation success is strong, psychosocial and behavioral factors likely play a significant role as well. Overweight and obese women have been shown to exhibit psychosocial characteristics that have been independently associated with poor breastfeeding outcomes. One recent study noted that, compared to their normal or underweight peers, overweight and obese women were less confident about reaching breastfeeding goals, reported fewer close friends or relatives who had breastfed, and experienced less-positive social influence from others to breastfeed.[53]

Issues related to negative body image may explain some of the decreased breastfeeding rates observed among obese and overweight women. Large breasts may make it difficult to breastfeed modestly or discretely in public. In addition, a woman who has negative feelings about her body at baseline may not feel confident that her breasts will be able to function properly. One recent study found higher body image concerns were associated with lower intended and actual breastfeeding durations regardless of BMI.[54] As obese and overweight women do not universally have concerns about body image, these findings might help to explain why the inverse relationship between BMI and breastfeeding has been found in some, but not all, populations.

Maternal behavior in the early postpartum period may play a role in the decreased breastfeeding success observed among women with elevated BMIs. For example, obese women have been noted to be less likely to put their infants to breast shortly after birth.[55] Breast milk expression behaviors have also been shown to differ by BMI in the early postpartum period, with obese women more likely to try milk expression but less likely to express milk successfully.[56] Given that early frequent breast stimulation is involved in the upregulation of the lactation process, the decreased breastfeeding success seen among obese mothers may be a result of behavioral, rather than purely physiologic, differences between obese and nonobese women.

Regardless of a mother's baseline psychosocial characteristics, interactions with health care providers in the prenatal, intrapartum, and postpartum time periods may have a substantial impact on her breastfeeding intent and success. Information and support from health care providers could serve to bolster a mother's confidence, allowing her to successfully nourish her infant at the breast. Alternatively, a health care provider's well-intentioned focus on identification of obesity as a risk factor for breastfeeding failure could also potentially undermine a mother's confidence, leading to a "self-fulfilling prophecy" of breastfeeding failure. Further research should attempt to explore the influence various psychosocial issues have on breastfeeding success, especially the role, positive or negative, that health care provider attitudes and interactions play in the initiation and continuation of breastfeeding.

Clinical Management of Obese and Overweight Breastfeeding Mothers

As detailed in the previous sections, although breastfeeding may be especially important for obese mothers and their infants, numerous factors put this population at risk for suboptimal lactation. The clinical picture of the obese obstetric patient may in effect present a "perfect storm" of breastfeeding challenges, including anatomical, physiologic, iatrogenic, and psychosocial factors. Although some of these challenges may be neither correctable nor avoidable, clinical care and support can serve to mitigate the negative effect they have on the lactation process, thereby maximizing the potential for breastfeeding initiation and continuation.

TABLE 10-1   WHO/UNICEF Baby-Friendly Hospital Initiative Ten Steps to Successful Breastfeeding[a]

1. Have a written breastfeeding policy that is routinely communicated to all health care staff.
2. Train all health care staff in the skills necessary to implement this policy.
3. Inform all pregnant women about the benefits and management of breastfeeding.
4. Help mothers initiate breastfeeding within a half-hour of birth.[b]
5. Show mothers how to breastfeed and how to maintain lactation, even if they are separated from their infants.
6. Give infants no food or drink other than breast milk unless medically indicated.
7. Practice rooming-in; that is, allow mothers and infants to remain together 24 hours a day.
8. Encourage breastfeeding on demand.
9. Give no artificial teats or pacifiers (also called dummies or soothers) to breastfeeding infants.
10. Foster the establishment of breastfeeding support groups and refer mothers to them on discharge from the hospital or clinic.

[a]Reprinted from WHO/UNICEF, *Protecting, Promoting and Supporting Breastfeeding: The Special Role of Maternity Services.* A joint WHO/UNICEF statement published by the World Health Organization, Geneva, Switzerland, 1989, p. iv.
[b]Baby-Friendly USA, Inc., the accrediting body for the Baby-Friendly Hospital Initiative in the United States, endorses initiation of breastfeeding within 1 hour (rather than a half-hour) after birth.[78]

It is well established that hospital policies and routines greatly influence breastfeeding outcomes.[57] The Baby-Friendly Hospital Initiative (BFHI), launched by WHO and the United Nations Children's Fund (UNICEF) in 1991 and updated in 2009, is designed to increase breastfeeding rates worldwide and is based on 10 steps hospitals can implement to protect, promote, and support breastfeeding[57] (see Table 10-1). These 10 steps, as well as many of the other clinical recommendations discussed in the following material, are evidence-based best practices for all nursing mothers but may well be especially important for obese and overweight women whose anatomy, physiology, and psychosocial perspectives can serve to challenge the successful initiation and continuation of lactation.

Unfortunately, there is a paucity of published research evaluating the effectiveness of breastfeeding support specifically in obese and overweight women. Results of published trials have been mixed. Although earlier studies were unable to demonstrate improvement with "low-intensity" interventions, one randomized trial found that targeting overweight and obese women with peer counseling before, during, and after delivery in a Baby-Friendly hospital setting was associated with increased rates of any breastfeeding and breastfeeding intensity at 2 weeks postpartum and decreased rates of infant hospitalization in the first 6 months after birth, but no impact was found on exclusive breastfeeding practices.[58] A more recent study reported that perceived physician support for breastfeeding, defined as a mother's report that her physician or her infant's pediatrician favored exclusive breastfeeding, was associated with significantly increased breastfeeding initiation and duration among both obese women and nonobese women. Physician support for breastfeeding was also associated with increased breastfeeding knowledge among obese women, but not among their nonobese peers.[59] Further research is warranted to establish how to optimize lactation success among obese and overweight mothers specifically. Table 10-2 provides clinical management information to optimize breastfeeding in the obese obstetric patient.

Prenatal Care

Prenatal discussion about the benefits of breastfeeding for both mother and baby is recommended for all pregnant women.[60] ACOG described the advice and

<table>
<tr><td>TABLE 10-2</td><td>Clinical Management to Optimize Breastfeeding in the Obese Obstetric Patient[a]</td></tr>
</table>

1. Prenatal Care
- Discuss the importance of breastfeeding and the risks of not breastfeeding for obese mothers and their infants.
- Provide education and monitoring of appropriate pregnancy weight gain and nutrition.
- Identify any physical abnormalities of breasts and nipples and any history of breast surgery.
- Identify and optimize management of underlying medical conditions, including impaired glucose metabolism, hypertension, anemia, and thyroid disease.
- Refer to prenatal breastfeeding classes and consider formal lactation consult referral.

2. Labor and Delivery and Early Postpartum Care (also see Table 11-1, WHO/UNICEF Baby-Friendly Hospital Initiative Ten Steps to Successful Breastfeeding)
- Keep the birth process as physiologically normal as possible.
- Welcome and encourage the presence of a support person for the laboring mother.
- Place the newborn in skin-to-skin contact with the mother as soon as possible after delivery.
- Avoid separation of the mother and infant throughout the hospital stay.
- Provide early and frequent assessment by a lactation consultant or other skilled health care provider.
- Encourage frequent breastfeeding, between 10 and 12 times a day, until lactogenesis II has occurred and the infant is gaining weight.

3. Discharge and Beyond
- Arrange early follow-up with the infant's health care provider.
- Refer to breastfeeding peer support organizations.
- Consider referral for outpatient lactation consultation.
- Ensure the mother has access to proper size pump flanges if she will be pumping.
- Optimize management of underlying maternal medical conditions and ensure medications are compatible with breastfeeding.
- Advise patient regarding healthy postpartum nutrition, exercise, and weight loss strategies.

[a]See text for details.

encouragement of the obstetrician-gynecologist as "critical" in a woman's decision to breastfeed.[17] Given the likely added importance of breastfeeding for obese and overweight mothers and their infants, and given the multiple challenges to successful breastfeeding these mothers face, prenatal education and discussions about infant feeding choices may be especially important for this population.

The specific language used to discuss the relative risks of breastfeeding and artificial formula feeding may have an impact on a mother's feeding decision. It may be more effective to discuss the "risks of formula feeding" than to tout the "benefits of breastfeeding," as the former language implicitly establishes breastfeeding as the normative method of nourishing a human infant.[61,62] The practitioner might find it helpful to discuss the particular importance breastfeeding has for an obese mother and her infant. Open-ended questions, such as "What are your thoughts about breastfeeding?" may allow the practitioner to identify psychosocial barriers and knowledge deficits.

Attending breastfeeding support groups and formal breastfeeding classes may be helpful for any pregnant mother planning to breastfeed. It may be prudent to educate the obese pregnant mother in particular about the impact her BMI can have on positioning during breastfeeding, the timing of lactogenesis, and her overall breastfeeding success. Prenatal referral to a lactation consultant should be considered for an obese mother to optimize breastfeeding management. However, care should be taken to avoid undermining a mother's confidence and "preordaining" breastfeeding difficulties.

As weight gain during pregnancy can have an impact on breastfeeding success,[37] obstetrical patient education related to nutrition and appropriate weight gain should begin early and continue throughout the prenatal period. In addition, assessment should be undertaken to identify any medical or physical conditions that may affect a mother's ability to breastfeed.[60] History of breast surgery or any physical abnormalities of the nipples or breast tissue should be noted. Identification and optimization of impaired glucose metabolism, hypertension, anemia, and thyroid disease may be particularly important in obese and overweight mothers.

Labor and Delivery Care

Peripartum interventions have the potential for a negative impact on breastfeeding, and efforts should be made to keep the birth process as physiologically normal as possible while maximizing the health of both infant and mother. Obese mothers are at a higher risk of exogenous oxytocin augmentation and surgical birth (see Chapter 20), both of which have been independently associated with delayed lactogenesis II.[43,50] The effect of intrapartum analgesia on breastfeeding success is unclear, although there is some evidence that epidural analgesia and intramuscular opioids are associated with decreased breastfeeding initiation.[63] The continuous presence of a support individual throughout labor and delivery may be helpful in maximizing breastfeeding outcomes. The presence of a doula has been associated with increased breastfeeding initiation and duration and has also been associated with reduced risk of other factors associated with early cessation of breastfeeding, including the use of analgesic medication and the need for surgical intervention.[60]

Early Postpartum Care

Skin-to-skin contact as soon as possible in the immediate postpartum period is recommended for all healthy newborns and may be especially important for obese and overweight breastfeeding mothers and their infants.[60] Skin-to-skin positioning allows early, frequent breastfeeding, which may negate the obesity-related blunting of the prolactin response seen in obese women and promote overall upregulation of the lactogenesis process.[51,52] In addition, skin-to-skin contact between mother and infant immediately after birth, and continuing as much as possible thereafter, is helpful in maintaining normal infant body temperature and reducing infant energy expenditures, thereby promoting maintenance of normal infant blood glucose.[64] This may be particularly important for a macrosomic infant, who is at higher risk of hypoglycemia.[51]

As with all mothers, separation of the obese or overweight mother from her newborn should be avoided whenever possible. Mother-baby rooming-in on a 24-hour basis allows opportunity for bonding and for optimal breastfeeding initiation.[60] While a breastfeeding frequency of 8 to 12 times a day is typically recommended to nursing mothers, the obese mother should be encouraged to breastfeed on the more frequent side, between 10 and 12 times a day, until lactogenesis II has occurred and the infant has been determined to be gaining weight.[45]

Positioning and Latching

Women with higher BMIs may find breastfeeding positioning and latching challenging. Early assessment by a lactation consultant or other skilled health care provider to assess and assist with the adequacy of latch is important to ensure development of the milk supply and adequate milk transfer to the infant. As obese mothers are at risk for

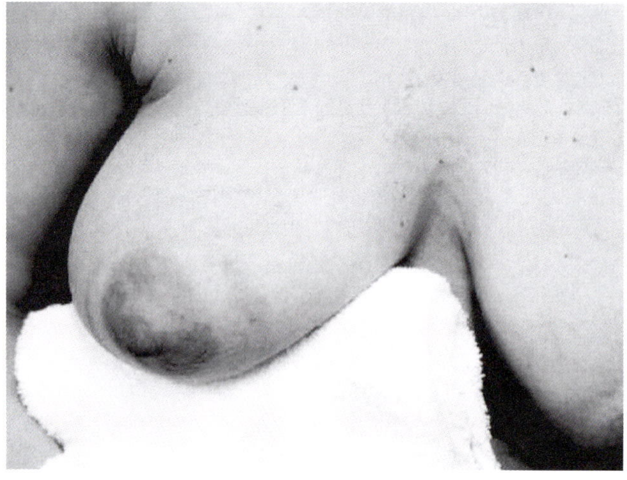

FIGURE 10-3. A rolled-up towel or small blanket under the breast can assist with stabilization of the breast during feeding.

delayed lactogenesis II, careful monitoring of breastfeeding progress and infant weights is warranted.

Obese or overweight women may require larger beds or wider chairs to obtain a comfortable nursing position.[51] Care should be taken to avoid letting a heavy breast rest on the infant's chest, and a rolled-up towel or small blanket under the breast can assist with stabilization of the breast during feeding[45] (see Figure 10-3). Due to larger breasts with short arms relative to body mass, many obese mothers find a "football hold" comfortable (see Figure 10-4). The baby's head and upper body can be supported by a pillow or by the mother's hand and arm on the same side as the nursing breast, while her opposite hand is free to support her breast.

Some obese mothers find a "laid-back" or "biologic nursing" position to be comfortable.[65] In this position, the mother is semireclined with her torso and arms well supported and the baby is placed on its stomach, securely positioned against the mother's body. Some obese mothers have large breasts with flattish nipples, possibly related to excess periareolar tissue.[44] It can be helpful for a mother to use her hand to shape a large breast into a "sandwich" to help the baby latch[66] (see Figure 10–5).

The use of a thin, flexible silicone nipple shield is sometimes recommended as a means to improve latch in mothers with flat nipples or other latching difficulties during the early postpartum period. However, published evidence supporting the safety and efficacy of the use of nipple shields to assist with latch is limited, and there is some concern regarding an associated decreased milk supply, poor infant weight gain, and shortened breastfeeding duration.[67] As the use of nipple shields has not been studied in obese lactating mothers specifically, nipple shields should be used with extra caution in this population known to be at extra risk for breastfeeding difficulties.

Discharge and Beyond

All breastfed infants should have a visit with a heath care provider at 3 to 5 days of life, or within 48 to 72 hours of discharge, to evaluate the establishment of breastfeeding as well as the infant's well-being.[60] Earlier follow-up may be considered for the breastfeeding infants of obese mothers given

FIGURE 10-4. Some obese mothers find a "football hold" comfortable. The baby's head and upper body can be supported by a pillow or by the mother's hand and arm on the same side as the nursing breast, while her opposite hand is free to support her breast. (Used with permission from Dr. Jayne Charlamb.)

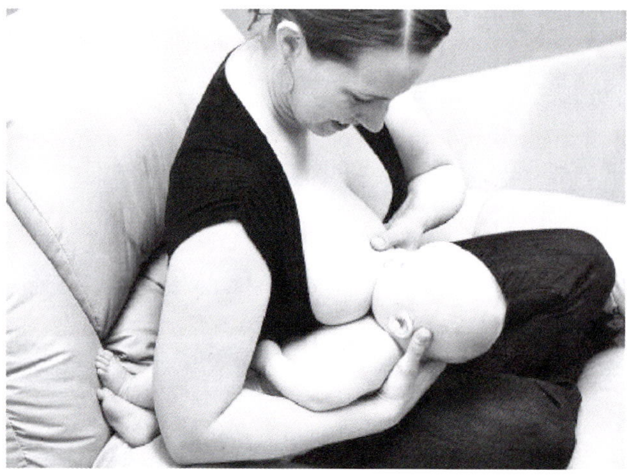

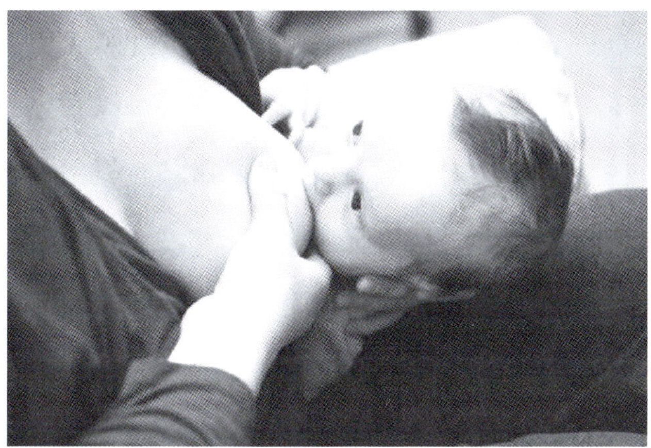

FIGURE 10-5. A mother can use her hand to shape a large breast into a "sandwich" to help her baby latch. (Used with permission from Dr. Jayne Charlamb.)

the documented risks of delayed lactogenesis and early breastfeeding cessation in this population. Referral to peer support organizations has proven helpful in promoting breastfeeding success and should be offered to all breastfeeding mothers.[60,68] Examples include La Leche League International (http://www.llli.org) and groups affiliated with hospital or governmental organizations.

Given the risk of intertrigo, obese women should be cautioned to clean and dry breast and breast skinfolds regularly. Tight bras and restrictive clothing have been associated with the development of mastitis.[45] Obese women should be cautioned to seek and wear properly fitted garments. Extra-large and custom size nursing bras can be found online and at some specialty stores. If the use of a breast pump is necessary to increase or maintain milk production, it is important to ensure that the pump flanges are of large enough size to properly fit the obese mother's breasts. Standard size flanges may be too small for some obese mothers and could both make pumping less effective and cause damage to breast and nipple tissue.[45,51] With properly fitting flanges, the nipple should be able to move freely within the flange tunnel, and pumping should be pain free.

As obese breastfeeding mothers may have chronic underlying medical conditions such as diabetes and hypertension, questions regarding the safety of maternal medication use during lactation often arise during the postpartum time period. Although only a small proportion of medications are truly contraindicated in breastfeeding mothers or are associated with adverse effects on their infants, many mothers are inappropriately advised to discontinue breastfeeding or to avoid taking essential medications.[69] Decisions regarding the selection of medications for use in the breastfeeding mother and about whether she can nurse while taking a particular medication should take into account any potential risks to the infant and to the milk supply, as well as the risks (to both infant and mother) of not breastfeeding. When there is a concern about the compatibility of a particular medication with breastfeeding, a safer medication option can often be identified. A good source of information about the safety of maternal medications during breastfeeding is the US National Library of Medicine's LactMed. Peer reviewed, and updated monthly, it is available online (http://toxnet.nlm.nih.gov).

Special Situations

BARIATRIC SURGERY AND BREASTFEEDING—The prevalence of bariatric surgery is increasing worldwide, with an estimation in 2011 of more than 340,000 procedures performed.[70] In the United States, approximately half of all bariatric surgical procedures are performed on women of childbearing age.[71] Encountering an obstetrical or lactating patient with a history of bariatric surgery is therefore not uncommon.

There is extremely limited information in the literature regarding the impact of bariatric surgery on subsequent lactation, and specific effects on supply or composition of breast milk are unknown. Any effect likely depends on the type of surgical procedure performed and on the nutritional status of the mother before and during pregnancy. Certainly, as discussed in detail previously, a mother's obesity itself, along with associated underlying medical or physiologic conditions, may also have a negative impact on lactation. Therefore, although there are concerns about nutritional deficiencies (see the discussion that follows), if bariatric surgery serves to improve a mother's BMI and her underlying physiology, it may overall have a positive impact on breastfeeding success. Further research is warranted to better establish the specific effects bariatric surgery may have on lactation.

Pregnant women who have undergone bariatric surgery are at increased risk of deficiencies in iron, vitamin B_{12}, folate, vitamin D, and calcium, and expert opinion recommends monitoring for nutritional deficiencies and for the need for vitamin supplementation during pregnancy.[72] Given the increased nutritional demands associated with lactation, post–bariatric surgery nutritional monitoring and dietary supplementation may be even more important in breastfeeding mothers. There have been case reports of failure to thrive and B_{12} deficiencies in breastfeeding infants of mothers with a history of bariatric surgery,[73] although it is difficult to determine what role inadequate exposure to nutrients during the prenatal time period played in these cases. Frequent and close monitoring for appropriate growth and development, along with consideration of laboratory monitoring of vitamin B_{12}, vitamin D, folate, calcium, and iron levels, is recommended for breastfeeding infants of mothers with a history of bariatric surgery.[73]

In addition to nutritional counseling, referral to a lactation consultant should be considered prenatally and in the immediate postpartum period to optimize breastfeeding management. A mother who has lost significant weight through bariatric surgery may face challenges in positioning and latching due to breast ptosis (sagging of the breast tissue due to loss of adipose tissue and reduction in volume).[73] As with any breastfeeding woman, skin-to-skin contact and frequent, effective latch with milk transfer during the early postpartum period are helpful in the upregulation of milk synthesis and for the development of an optimal milk supply.

REDUCTION MAMMOPLASTY AND BREASTFEEDING—Obese mothers may previously have undergone reduction mammoplasty (breast reduction) or mastopexy (breast lift). Success of breastfeeding after these procedures is variable and likely relates to the specific type of procedure performed.[45] A mother with a history of breast surgery should be referred to an experienced lactation consultant during the prenatal time period. Close postpartum monitoring and support are important to optimize milk production, monitor the infant's growth, and determine the need for infant supplementation. Women who are considering reduction mammoplasty or other surgical breast procedures should be fully informed prior to the procedure about the risks of potential decreased future lactation success.

INTENTIONAL MATERNAL WEIGHT LOSS DURING BREASTFEEDING—The medical literature and guidelines related to the safety and efficacy of intentional weight loss during lactation are limited. A 2002 review of the literature noted that moderate exercise without specific calorie reduction did not seem to promote weight loss in lactating women during the postpartum period; however, neither acute nor regular exercise was found to have adverse effects on mothers' ability to successfully breastfeed their infants.[74] A more recent systematic review assessing the benefits and harms of postpartum behavioral weight management interventions reported that the limited available evidence suggests that combined nutrition and exercise interventions can achieve weight loss during the postpartum period, but that the results from exercise-only or nutrition-only interventions are inconclusive or insufficient to determine efficacy. The authors found no evidence for an increase in adverse maternal or infant outcomes with behavioral weight management interventions.[75]

The Institute of Medicine's Subcommittee on Nutrition During Lactation published guidelines in 1991 stating that in lactating mothers who are significantly overweight, a weight loss of up to 1 to 2 kg per month should not affect milk volume, although weight gain and feeding pattern in the infant should be monitored. The report recommended against dieting in the immediate postpartum period, weight loss of more than 2 kg per month after the first postpartum month, intake of less than 1500 kcal/d, liquid diets, and weight loss medications.[76] The ACOG Committee Opinion, last reaffirmed in 2009, noted that moderate weight reduction while nursing is safe and does not compromise neonatal weight gain.[77] Future research is warranted to provide updated and more specific guidelines for lactating mothers regarding the efficacy and safety of various weight loss strategies.

FUTURE DIRECTIONS FOR RESEARCH

The relationship between obesity and breastfeeding is complex and likely multidirectional. Myriad factors affect a woman's risk of obesity and her decision and ability to initiate and continue breastfeeding. It can be difficult, if not impossible, to design and carry out randomized controlled trials exploring the relationship between these factors, and we therefore must often rely on observational studies that have limited ability to definitively determine causality. Future research should seek to clarify both the role obesity plays in the development and function of the female breast and the impact breastfeeding has on obesity and other aspects of maternal and child health.

Topics warranting further investigation were noted throughout this chapter. Specifically, further research is needed to explore the relationship between childhood obesity and both the timing of puberty and the composition of the adult female breast and to determine the role mammary adipose tissue plays in the regulation of breast development and function. In addition, future research should attempt to further elucidate the nature of the complex relationship between abnormal maternal physiology and breastfeeding success, as well as to better define the impact lack of lactation has on a mother's risk of future malignant, cardiovascular, and metabolic disease.

Most important, future research should aim to establish methods by which to optimize lactation success among obese and overweight mothers. Investigations should seek to determine the influence that various psychosocial, physiologic, and anatomic factors have on breastfeeding initiation and continuation. Whenever possible, randomized controlled trials should be designed to identify the impact specific practices and interventions during the prenatal, intrapartum, and postpartum time periods have on breastfeeding outcomes among obese and overweight women, thus moving toward establishing best practices for the support of breastfeeding in this population. Finally, given the growing numbers of obese and overweight women of childbearing age, and given the importance of supporting this population both to breastfeed and to pursue a healthy weight status, future research should seek to provide evidence to update and expand guidelines regarding the safety and efficacy of intentional maternal weight loss strategies during lactation and to determine the effects prepregnancy bariatric surgery may have on later lactation success.

REFERENCES

1. Russo J, Russo IH. Development of the human breast. *Maturitas*. 2004;49:2–15.
2. Hassiotou F, Geddes D. Anatomy of the human mammary gland: current status of knowledge. *Clin Anat*. 2013;26(1):29–48.
3. Biro FM, Greenspan LC, Galvez MP, et al. Onset of breast development in a longitudinal cohort. *Pediatrics*. 2013;132(6):1019–1027.
4. Rosenfield RL, Lipton RB, Drum ML. Thelarche, pubarche, and menarche attainment in children with normal and elevated body mass index. *Pediatrics*. 2009;123(1):84–88.
5. Biro FM, Greenspan LC, Galvez MP. Mini-review: puberty in girls of the 21st century. *J Pediatr Adolesc Gynecol*. 2012;25:289–294.
6. Herman-Giddens M. The enigmatic pursuit of puberty in girls. *Pediatrics*. 2013;132(6):1125–1126.
7. Soliman A, De Sanctis V, Elalaily R. Nutrition and pubertal development. *Indian J Endocrinol Metab*. 2014;18:S39–S47.
8. Novotny R, Daida Y, Morimoto Y, Shepherd J, Maskarinec G. Puberty, body fat, and breast density in girls of several ethnic groups. *Am J Hum Biol*. 2011;23(3):359–365.
9. Samimi G, Colditz GA, Baer HJ, Tamimi RM. Measures of energy balance and mammographic density in the nurses' health study. *Breast Cancer Res Treat*. 2008;109(1):113–122.
10. Wang AT, Vachon CM, Brandt KR, Ghosh K. Breast density and breast cancer risk: a practical review. *Mayo Clin Proc*. 2014;89(4):548–557.
11. Vandeweyer E, Hertens D. Quantification of glands and fat in breast tissue: an experimental determination. *Ann Anat*. 2002;184:181–184.
12. Janiszewski PM, Saunders TJ, Ross R. Breast volume is an independent predictor of visceral and ectopic fat in premenopausal women. *Obesity (Silver Spring)*. 2010;18(6):1183–1187.
13. Schautz B, Later W, Heller M, Müller MJ, Bosy-Westphal A. Associations between breast adipose tissue, body fat distribution and cardiometabolic risk in women: cross-sectional data and weight-loss intervention. *Eur J Clin Nutr*. 2011;65(7):784–790.
14. Nickell WB, Skelton J. Breast fat and fallacies: more than 100 years of anatomical fantasy. *J Hum Lact*. 2005;21(2):126–130.
15. Ramsay DT, Kent JC, Hartmann RA, Hartmann PE. Anatomy of the lactating human breast redefined with ultrasound imaging. *J Anat*. 2005;206(6):525–534.
16. Hovey RC, Aimo L. Diverse and active roles for adipocytes during mammary gland growth and function. *J Mammary Gland Biol Neoplasia*. 2010;15(3):279–290.
17. ACOG Committee Opinion: number 361, February 2007. Breastfeeding: maternal and infant aspects. *Obstet Gynecol*. 2007;109(2):479–480.
18. Breastfeeding and the use of human milk. *Pediatrics*. 2012;129(3):e827–e841.
19. Hauk L. AAFP releases position paper on breastfeeding. *Am Fam Physician*. 2015;91(1):56–57.
20. World Health Organization Fifty-Fifth World Health Assembly. Infant and young child nutrition global strategy on infant and young child feeding: report by the secretariat. http://apps.who.int/gb/archive/pdf_files/WHA55/ea5515.pdf?ua=1. Published April 16, 2002. Accessed March 15, 2015.
21. Ip S, Chung M, Raman G, Trikalinos TA, Lau J. A summary of the agency for healthcare research and quality's evidence report on breastfeeding in developed countries. *Breastfeed Med*. 2009;4(Suppl 1):S17–S30.
22. Dewey KG. Growth characteristics of breast-fed compared to formula-fed infants. *Biol Neonate*. 1998;74(2):94–105.
23. US Breastfeeding Committee. *Statement on Breastfeeding as a Critical Strategy for Obesity Prevention*. Washington, DC: US Breastfeeding Committee; 2010.
24. Gillman MW. Commentary: breastfeeding and obesity—the 2011 scorecard. *Int J Epidemiol*. 2011;40(3):681–684.
25. Oddy WH. Infant feeding and obesity risk in the child. *Breastfeed Rev*. 2012;20(2):7–12.
26. Horta B, Vicoria C. *Long-Term Effects of Breastfeeding: A Systematic Review*. Geneva, Switzerland: World Health Organization; 2013.
27. Yan J, Liu L, Zhu Y, Huang G, Wang PP. The association between breastfeeding and childhood obesity: a meta-analysis. *BMC Public Health*. 2014;14:1267–1267.
28. Stuebe AM, Rich-Edwards J. The reset hypothesis: lactation and maternal metabolism. *Am J Perinatol*. 2009;26(1):81–88.
29. Neville CE, McKinley MC, Holmes VA, Spence D, Woodside JV. The relationship between breastfeeding and postpartum weight change-a systematic

review and critical evaluation. *Int J Obes (Lond).* 2014;38(4):577–590.

30. Sharma AJ, Dee DL, Harden SM. Adherence to breast-feeding guidelines and maternal weight 6 years after delivery. *Pediatrics.* 2014;134(Suppl 1):S42–S49.

31. Schwarz EB, Ray RM, Stuebe AM, et al. Duration of lactation and risk factors for maternal cardiovascular disease. *Obstet Gynecol.* 2009;113(5):974–982.

32. Much D, Beyerlein A, Roß bauer M, Hummel S, Ziegler A. Review: beneficial effects of breastfeeding in women with gestational diabetes mellitus. *Mol Metab.* 2014;3:284–292.

33. Schwarz E, Bimla. Infant feeding in America: enough to break a mother's heart? *Breastfeed Med.* 2013;8:454–457.

34. Amir LH, Donath S. A systematic review of maternal obesity and breastfeeding intention, initiation and duration. *BMC Pregnancy Childbirth.* 2007;7:9–9.

35. Wojcicki JM. Maternal prepregnancy body mass index and initiation and duration of breastfeeding: a review of the literature. *J Womens Health (Larchmt).* 2011;20(3):341–347.

36. Turcksin R, Bel S, Galjaard S, Devlieger R. Maternal obesity and breastfeeding intention, initiation, intensity and duration: a systematic review. *Matern Child Nutr.* 2014;10(2):166–183.

37. Hilson JA, Rasmussen KM, Kjolhede CL. Excessive weight gain during pregnancy is associated with earlier termination of breast-feeding among white women. *J Nutr.* 2006;136(1):140–146.

38. Ogden CL, Carroll MD, Kit BK, Flegal KM. Prevalence of childhood and adult obesity in the United States, 2011–2012. *JAMA.* 2014;311(8):806–814.

39. Centers for Disease Control and Prevention (CDC). Progress in increasing breastfeedign and reducing racial/ethnic differences—United States, 2000–2008 births. *MMWR Morb Mortal Wkly Rep.* 2013;62(05):77–80.

40. Pang WW, Hartmann PE. Initiation of human lactation: secretory differentiation and secretory activation. *J Mammary Gland Biol Neoplasia.* 2007;12(4):211–221.

41. Stuebe AM. Enabling women to achieve their breast-feeding goals. *Obstet Gynecol.* 2014;123(3):643–652.

42. Speller E, Brodribb W, McGuire E. Breastfeeding and thyroid disease: a literature review. *Breastfeed Rev.* 2012;20(2):41–47.

43. Brownell E, Howard CR, Lawrence RA, Dozier AM. Original article: delayed onset lactogenesis II predicts the cessation of any or exclusive breastfeeding. *J Pediatr.* 2012;161:608–614.

44. McGuire E. Breastfeeding and high maternal body mass index. *Breastfeed Rev.* 2013;21(3):7–14.

45. Walker M. *Breastfeeding Management for the Clinician: Using the Evidence.* 3rd ed. Burlington, MA: Jones & Bartlett Learning; 2014.

46. Cruz NI, Korchin L. Lactational performance after breast reduction with different pedicles. *Plast Reconstr Surg.* 2007;120(1):35–40.

47. Nommsen-Rivers L, Dolan LM, Huang B. Timing of stage II lactogenesis is predicted by antenatal metabolic health in a cohort of primiparas. *Breastfeeding Med.* 2012;7(1):43–49.

48. Ram KT, Bobby P, Hailpern SM, et al. Research: duration of lactation is associated with lower prevalence of the metabolic syndrome in midlife—SWAN, the Study of Women's Health Across the Nation. *Obstet Gynecol.* 2008;198:268.e1–268.e6.

49. Vanky E, Nordskar JJ, Leithe H, Hjorth-Hansen A, Martinussen M, Carlsen SM. Breast size increment during pregnancy and breastfeeding in mothers with polycystic ovary syndrome: a follow-up study of a randomised controlled trial on metformin versus placebo. *BJOG.* 2012;119(11):1403–1409.

50. Hurst NM. Feature: recognizing and treating delayed or failed lactogenesis II. *J Midwifery Womens Health.* 2007;52:588–594.

51. Jevitt C, Hernandez I, Groër M. Lactation complicated by overweight and obesity: supporting the mother and newborn. *J Midwifery Womens Health.* 2007;52(6):606–613.

52. Rasmussen KMK, Chris L. Prepregnant overweight and obesity diminish the prolactin response to suckling in the first week postpartum. *Pediatrics.* 2004;113(5):e465–e471.

53. Hauff LE, Leonard SA, Rasmussen KM. Associations of maternal obesity and psychosocial factors with breastfeeding intention, initiation, and duration. *Am J Clin Nutr.* 2014;99(3):524–534.

54. Brown A, Rance J, Warren L. Body image concerns during pregnancy are associated with a shorter breast feeding duration. *Midwifery.* 2015;31:80–89.

55. Kugyelka JG, Rasmussen KM, Frongillo EA. Maternal obesity is negatively associated with breastfeeding success among hispanic but not black women. *J Nutr.* 2004;134(7):1746–1753.

56. Leonard SA, Labiner-Wolfe J, Geraghty SR, Rasmussen KM. Associations between high prepregnancy body mass index, breast-milk expression, and breast-milk production and feeding. *Am J Clin Nutr.* 2011;93(3):556–563.

57. World Health Organization. *Baby-Friendly Hospital Initiative: Revised, Updated and Expanded for Integrated Care.* Geneva, Switzerland: World Health Organization; 2009.

58. Chapman DJ, Morel K, Bermúdez-Millán A, Young S, Damio G, Pérez-Escamilla R. Breastfeeding education and support trial for overweight and obese women: a randomized trial. *Pediatrics.* 2013;131(1):e162–e170.

59. Jarlenski M, McManus J, Diener-West M, Schwarz EB, Yeung E, Bennett WL. Original article: association

between support from a health professional and breastfeeding knowledge and practices among obese women: evidence from the infant practices study II. *Womens Health Issues.* 2014;24:641-648.

60. Holmes AV, McLeod AY, Bunik M. ABM clinical protocol #5: peripartum breastfeeding management for the healthy mother and infant at term, revision 2013. *Breastfeed Med.* 2013;8(6):469-473.

61. Stuebe A. The risks of not breastfeeding for mothers and infants. *Rev Obstet Gynecol.* 2009;2(4):222-231.

62. Wiessinger D. Watch your language! *J Hum Lact.* 1996;12(1):1-4.

63. Jordan S, Emery S, Watkins A, Evans JD, Storey M, Morgan G. Associations of drugs routinely given in labour with breastfeeding at 48 hours: analysis of the cardiff births survey. *BJOG.* 2009;116(12):1622-1629.

64. Wight N, Marinelli KA. ABM clinical protocol #1: guidelines for blood glucose monitoring and treatment of hypoglycemia in term and late-preterm neonates, revised 2014. *Breastfeed Med.* 2014;9(4):173-179.

65. Colson S. Biological Nurturing: the laid-back breastfeeding revolution. *Midwifery Today.* 2012(101):9-66.

66. Wilson-Clay B, Hoover K. *The Breastfeeding Atlas.* 5th ed. Manchaca, TX: LactNews Press; 2013.

67. McKechnie A, Chevalier, Eglash A. Nipple shields: a review of the literature. *Breastfeed Med.* 2010;5:309-314.

68. Protecting, promoting and supporting breastfeeding: the special role of maternity services. A joint WHO/UNICEF statement. *Int J Gynaecol Obstet.* 1990;31(Suppl 1):171-183.

69. Sachs HC. The transfer of drugs and therapeutics into human breast milk: an update on selected topics. *Pediatrics.* 2013;132(3):e796-e809.

70. Buchwald H, Oien DM. Metabolic/bariatric surgery worldwide 2011. *Obes Surg.* 2013;23(4):427-436.

71. Willis K, Lieberman N, Sheiner E. 13: Pregnancy and neonatal outcome after bariatric surgery. *Best Pract Res Clin Obstet Gynaecol.* 2015;29(1):133-144.

72. ACOG Committee Opinion no. 549: Obesity in pregnancy. *Obstet Gynecol.* 2013;121(1):213-217.

73. Lamb M. Weight-loss surgery and breastfeeding. *Clin Lact.* 2011;2(3):17-21.

74. Larson-Meyer D. Effect of postpartum exercise on mothers and their offspring: a review of the literature. *Obes Res.* 2002;10(8):841-853.

75. Berger AA, Peragallo-Urrutia R, Nicholson WK. Systematic review of the effect of individual and combined nutrition and exercise interventions on weight, adiposity and metabolic outcomes after delivery: evidence for developing behavioral guidelines for postpartum weight control. *BMC Pregnancy Childbirth.* 2014;14:319-319.

76. Institute of Medicine (US) Subcommittee on Nutrition During Lactation, Committee on Nutrition Status During Pregnancy and Lactation, Food and Nutrition Board. *Nutrition During Lactation.* Washington, DC: National Academy Press; 1991.

77. ACOG Committee Opinion number 267, January 2002. Exercise during pregnancy and the postpartum period. *Obstet Gynecol.* 2002;99(1):171-173.

78. Baby-Friendly USA. The ten steps to successful breastfeeding. https://www.babyfriendlyusa.org/about-us/baby-friendly-hospital-initiative/the-ten-steps. Accessed August 27, 2015.

Kara C. Kort, MD

Scott P. Albert, MD

Ravi Adhikary, MD

Obesity and Benign and Malignant Disease of the Breast

CHAPTER 11

INTRODUCTION

While the epidemic of obesity in this country has well-known detrimental effects on the cardiovascular system and increased problems with arthritis and diabetes, its effect on the female breast has only more recently been realized. This chapter reviews the effects that obesity has on benign breast problems, breast imaging, and breast cancer management. A better understanding of the overall negative impact that obesity has especially on cancer prognosis, recurrence, and treatment will allow the practicing gynecologist to have a more frank discussion about the importance of maintaining a healthy body mass index (BMI).

BENIGN DISEASE

Skin Diseases

A variety of common skin conditions manifest on the breast, in the inframammary folds, and in the axilla and are exacerbated by obesity. Obesity results in numerous changes to skin, including increased sweat gland function, changes in microcirculation, and additional shearing forces in dependent areas.[1]

Intertrigo, erythematous skin plaques that develop in the inframammary skinfolds, is due to increased friction and moisture that leads to skin damage. Yeast, most commonly *Candida albicans*, often exists in these regions and requires treatment with topical antifungal powders. Some patients may require oral fluconazole for resistant cases.[2]

Other skin infections commonly seen in the obese patient include folliculitis, cellulitis, and even necrotizing soft tissue infections. The breast can be a site of these infections, especially in areas where increased skin friction leads to skin damage and susceptibility to infection. A recent study by Eggerstedt et al. examined all types and locations of necrotizing soft tissue infections; obesity and diabetes were commonly found. The mortality rate for superobese (BMI > 50) patients was 50% in this small study.[3] It is important to closely monitor and evaluate breast infections in the obese population because these patients might be more vulnerable to more significant complications, especially when diabetes accompanies obesity.

Hidradenitis suppurativa is a disease that affects the apocrine glands and can be found in areas like the axilla, inframammary region, groin, and perineum. The disease is multifactorial and difficult to manage, but manifests as chronic abscesses and subcutaneous fistula tracts, which frequently drain and become infected.[1] The disease seems to be more frequently seen in the obese population. Medical management includes topical and oral antibiotics, but these treatments often have limited efficacy. The most effective treatment is surgical excision of the affected tissue and either primary skin closure or sometimes skin grafting with widespread disease.

Breast Parenchyma and Stroma

The breast parenchyma refers to all the functional breast tissue, including the glands and breast ducts, while the stroma is essentially the support structure to the breast, such as Cooper's ligaments and the surrounding fatty tissue. A number of benign conditions affect the breast tissues; most are not associated with any increased risk for breast cancer. Some commonly seen benign breast diseases are discussed next, but there is limited published evidence that any of these "in-breast" conditions occur more often in the obese population, but instead are common in all patients.

Fat necrosis is a benign condition that occurs after breast trauma and is caused by inflammation of the adipose tissue. It can often feel like a dense mass and needs to be differentiated from cancer by imaging; occasionally, a biopsy is required. Epidermal inclusion cysts, "sebaceous cysts," can be seen in the breast and are usually superficial, well-circumscribed lesions that are easily palpable. The cyst can become infected, and definitive treatment is excision of the cyst, including the cyst wall, to reduce the likelihood of recurrence. Breast cysts are common and can be easily distinguished from solid masses by breast ultrasound. Cysts are fluid filled and can be simple; when septations or irregular walls are present, cysts are considered complex and may require a core needle biopsy for diagnosis.[4] Lipomas are benign, well-circumscribed, fatty tumors. On examination, these lesions feel soft and mobile and are not always easily seen on imaging. If there is uncertainty about the diagnosis, biopsy or surgical excision can be performed. Fibroadenomas are generally benign, well-circumscribed masses commonly seen in younger women (15–35 years old). These masses can grow slowly. Treatment includes observation for small lesions (<2 cm) and follow-up imaging to ensure stability or surgical excision for large or symptomatic lesions. A phyllode tumor is the more aggressive variant that cannot always be distinguished from a fibroadenoma until removed surgically. Therefore, a rapidly growing fibroadenoma should be removed because this may represent a phyllode tumor.

The Breast Mass After Weight Reduction Surgery

Bariatric surgery is one of the most common surgical procedures performed. On average, after gastric bypass surgery, patients lose about 60% of their body weight; for many patients, that can be greater than 100 pounds. With the marked reduction in breast adipose tissue, the fibroglandular portions of the breast become more obvious, and as a result the breast often feels more "lumpy" or dense and nodular. It is not uncommon for patients with new marked weight loss either to self-detect a new mass or to have a new mass detected on clinical breast exam. This frequently prompts immediate referral to a breast surgeon and diagnostic imaging with mammography or ultrasound. While imaging may note a change in the general appearance or density pattern, these new palpable masses are not true imaging abnormalities. These new masses should not necessarily be ignored. Clinicians should be aware of the possibility of a new breast mass in the patient with recent massive weight loss and treat the patient accordingly.

BREAST IMAGING

Obesity and Screening

Screening mammography has clearly demonstrated a decrease in the risk of death from breast carcinoma.[5] It has previously been suggested that obesity is associated with decreased compliance with routine screening mammography.[6] The current national recommendations for screening mammography[7] include mammography at least every 1–2 years beginning at about age 40. Obesity is associated with increased risk of postmenopausal breast cancer,[8] as well as an independent prognostic factor for developing distant metastasis and dying.[9] There are two questions to consider: (1) Is obesity perhaps associated with decreased compliance with routine recommended screening standards? (2) Is obesity associated with decreased sensitivity of mammography as a screening tool for breast cancer? Future research is needed to investigate these possible concerns. Both issues are discussed in the following sections.

Compliance With Screening Mammography

In one of the largest population-based analyses performed, Bertz et al. examined specifically the association between BMI and compliance with routine recommended mammographic screening; the study used data from the 2004 Behavioral Risk Factor Surveillance System (BRFSS). Using weighted analysis of over 130,000 women aged 40 and over, the proportion of women who underwent screening mammography in the previous 2 years was stratified by BMI. Interestingly, these authors found that, after adjusting for numerous factors, including age, race, smoking status, general health perception, level of education, and income level, women who were underweight (BMI < 18.5) had lower odds of complying with regular screening mammography. Overweight and obese women (class I [BMI 30 to < 35] and II [BMI 35 to < 40]) showed significantly higher association with appropriate screening mammography utilization. Obese women in class III (BMI ≥ 40) trended toward underutilization, although the findings were not statistically significant.[9] This study suggests that lack of compliance with screening recommendations does not explain the increased incidence of breast cancer in the obese population because there were no significant differences among the obese groups.

Mammography

Yearly screening mammography is recommended for average-risk women starting at the age of 40, while women who are at a higher risk may benefit from mammographic screening at a younger age. Screening may continue until the patient would be unable to act on abnormal screening results due to age or comorbid conditions or when life expectancy is less than 5–7 years.[10]

Some barriers to screening that obese women may feel include disrespectful behavior, unwanted advice to lose weight, embarrassment about being weighed, negative attitudes of providers, as well as ill-fitting gowns and small equipment.[11] Mammographic facilities may attempt to make obese women more comfortable by having sensitive personnel who are able to offer proper assistance. Waiting room chairs that are appropriate for women of all sizes as well as changing rooms and bathrooms with ample space may make the imaging experience more favorable and likely will increase compliance with screening.

In general, overweight women have less-dense breast tissue than normal-weight women on mammography, as well as larger breasts, which in turn leads to greater compression thickness.[12,13] While less-dense breasts may decrease the masking effects of dense fibroglandular tissue and improve interpretation, the increased compression thickness of the breast in obese women leads to image quality degradation when technical factors such as geometric unsharpness and contrast are measured. Subtle or small lesions may be obscured, which may be a contributing factor to the observation that tumors found in obese women tend to be larger than those found in normal-weight women.[13,14]

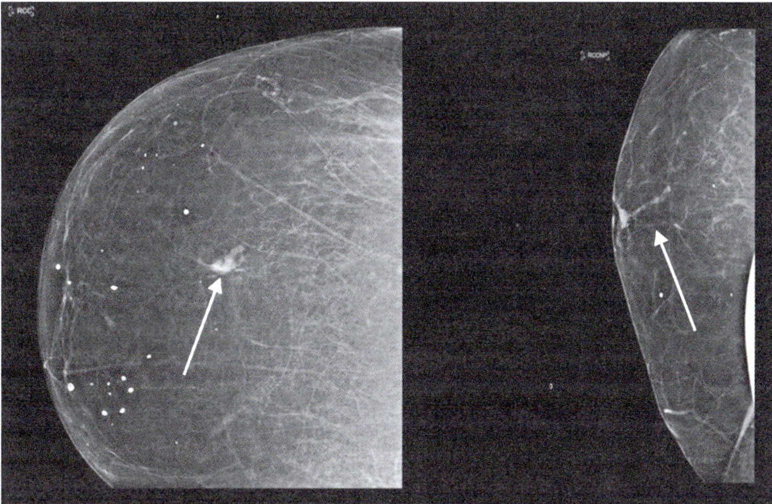

FIGURE 11-1. Multiple views are required to get the dilated duct and nipple into view on these craniocaudal mammographic images.

With larger breasts, positioning the patient for quality mammography may be challenging, and multiple additional mammograms may be required, which makes proper hanging and reading of the images difficult. Obese women with large breasts may require multiple images in a tile or mosaic fashion to image the whole breast, especially in older units, which may have smaller detectors. Multiple mammograms in the craniocaudal position may be required to obtain images with both the nipple in profile and to image the posterior breast. Multiple mammograms in the mediolateral oblique position may be required to ensure that adequate compression is achieved both posteriorly and anteriorly (see Figure 11-1). Obese patients may have smaller breasts that wrap around laterally, which may require an additional exaggerated craniocaudal view to image lateral tissue. Imaging the inframammary fold may be difficult in an obese patient with large abdominal girth. In addition, breast folds may obscure portions of the breast in obese women with large breasts.[15] The increased number of mammograms required to adequately image the entire breast as well as the increased breast thickness may result in increased radiation exposure in obese women.[13]

Evaluation of mammographic interpretation indicates obese women have higher rates of recall for additional views on screening mammogram when compared to normal-weight women, with increased rates of false-positive examinations.[12,16] Overweight women were found to have increased rates of cancer detection, with tumors that were generally larger and at a more advanced stage.[16]

Digital breast tomosynthesis is a relatively new technology utilizing multiple low-dose acquisitions in an arc to create a cross-sectional image. Initial studies have demonstrated a decrease in recall rates, which is in part due to the ability to resolve summation artifact on cross-sectional images, as well as an increase in cancer detection due to an ability to negate some of the masking effect of dense fibroglandular tissue.[17]

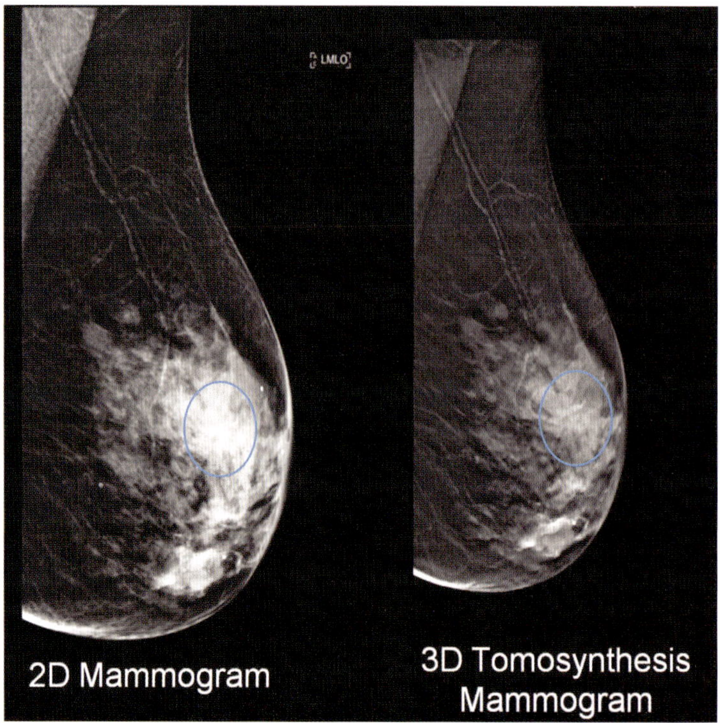

FIGURE 11-2. Comparison of traditional 2-dimensional (2-D) mammography with 3-dimensional (3-D) tomosynthesis mammography. A 3-D view shows a spiculated mass (circles).

Presumably, some of the same factors that affect obese women with standard mammography will have an impact on tomosynthesis, but further research is required (see Figure 11-2).

When a biopsy is required for calcifications or a lesion seen only on mammography, a stereotactic biopsy is recommended. Performing a stereotactic biopsy on obese patients may be challenging because of positioning, as many facilities use prone tables. Obese patients may have difficulty lying prone and staying still for the time required for a biopsy due to neck and back pain or difficulty breathing. In patients with a large abdomen, pulling the patient in far enough to access the posterior breast may be a challenge. Many prone tables also have a weight limit of 300 pounds.[15] If a site that performs upright stereotactic biopsy cannot be found for patients ineligible for prone biopsy, the patient may need to undergo a needle-localized surgical biopsy for suspicious lesions.

Ultrasound

Ultrasound of the breast may be performed for further characterization of lesions seen on mammography or on magnetic resonance imaging (MRI), in addition to evaluation of palpable masses. Screening ultrasound of the breast may also be used as an adjunct to mammography in women who are at high risk but unable to undergo MRI screening or in women with dense breasts.[10,18] Ultrasound screening in patients with dense breasts has been shown to have a relatively low positive-predictive value, indicating a high number of additional tests performed for every additional cancer found that would not have been visible on mammogram, and the best use of screening ultrasound may require more research.[18]

Quality breast ultrasound begins with high-frequency transducer, typically a linear 12-MHz transducer. A linear 17-MHz transducer may be useful to evaluate small breasts that are less than 3 cm in thickness or to evaluate superficial masses.[18] Deep lesions in a large breast may be difficult to visualize with high-frequency transducers, and a deep cyst may appear to be solid due to decreased resolution.[15] Technologists who are experienced in breast ultrasound and careful correlation of the ultrasound findings with mammographic or MRI findings are also key to a quality examination.

In obese patients who may have larger, less-dense breasts, finding smaller masses that correlate to mammographic lesions may be difficult when the breast is quite mobile. Masses may be less difficult to visualize on ultrasound in less-dense breasts, as more echogenic fibroglandular tissue offers contrast to a hypoechoic or isoechoic mass.[15]

Ultrasound-guided biopsy is generally the preferred method of biopsy in most patients, as the patient is more comfortable in a supine position and real-time imaging of the biopsy device passing through the mass allows for fewer samples to be taken with a high level of confidence that quality samples were obtained. To keep the biopsy device parallel to the chest wall and minimize the risk of pneumothorax, a remote entry site may be required in obese women with large breasts and a deep lesion.[15]

Magnetic Resonance Imaging

Magnetic resonance imaging breast screening may be used in select patients with a greater than 20% lifetime risk of breast cancer by family history, those who are *BRCA* mutation carriers, and those with a history of chest irradiation, as well as for screening of the contralateral breast in a patient with newly diagnosed breast cancer.[10] MRI may also be used as a problem-solving modality for evaluation of disease not fully assessed by mammogram and ultrasound.

Obese patients may be unable to obtain an MRI with table weight limits that range from 350 to 420 pounds, although newer tables accommodating patients weighing up to 550 pounds are available at some sites. Even though a patient may fall within the weight limit, they may be unable to obtain an MRI because of limitations on the gantry size, which has traditionally been 60 cm in diameter. Some units may offer up to a 70-cm diameter gantry size. The effective gantry size is diminished when a recommended dedicated breast coil is used.[15]

Nuclear Medicine

The use of radiopharmaceuticals with breast-specific gamma imaging (BSGI) or positron emission mammography (PEM) may be an adjunctive imaging modality in select patients,[19,20] without some of the size limitations that MRI may impose. BSGI and PEM do use significantly higher levels of radiation than other modalities,[21] and their availability is limited.

BREAST CANCER AND OBESITY

It is well known that obesity increases the risk of developing breast cancer, in particular estrogen receptor–positive disease, in postmenopausal women.[22,23] Interestingly, for reasons that are unclear, obesity seems to be protective in premenopausal women, with this subgroup of patients developing less breast cancer.[24] While the reasons for this increase in breast cancer among obese women is not completely understood, there are three plausible theories. These relate to elevated estrogen levels, elevated insulin and insulin-like growth factor (IGF) levels, and the chronic inflammatory state associated with obesity.

Physiologic Theories

Elevated Estrogen

In the absence of ovarian function in the postmenopausal woman, estrogen production occurs peripherally as circulating and androgen precursors (androstenedione) are enzymatically converted. The key enzyme for this process is aromatase. Aromatase is found largely in peripheral adipose tissue as well as adipose within the breast and breast tumors.[25] Increased adipose associated with obesity leads to increased aromatase and ultimately increased circulating biologically active estradiol.[22,23,26] Tumor necrosis factor alpha (TBF-α) and interleukin 6 (IL-6) are secreted by adipocytes to increase aromatase production. These cytokines can work in an autocrine or paracrine fashion and thus also increase the local production of estrogen in the breast.[27]

Elevated estrogen levels seem to correlate with differences in breast cancer risk, with the highest levels associated with increasing risk. Several very large reviews have shown this to be the case,[28,29] with some noting a nearly double risk in those with the highest estrogen levels.

Conversely, evidence has shown that increased exercise and physical activity may result in the lowering of serum estrone levels.[30] This helps perhaps explain the relationship between exercise and improved outcome among cancer survivors and for the practicing clinician helps reinforce recommendations for a healthy active lifestyle to our breast cancer patients for good reason.

Insulin

Obesity is a known risk factor for type 2 diabetes mellitus and as such elevated insulin levels. This chronic state of hyperinsulinemia associated with obesity leads to an associated increase in IGF. Both insulin and IGF are known to have anabolic activity and contribute to the growth and regulation of both normal mammary tissue and breast cancer. Higher levels of insulin and C-peptide have been associated with not only poor cancer outcomes in general,[31] but also, even in nondiabetic women with the highest insulin levels (compared to the lowest), with a doubled risk of breast cancer recurrence and tripled risk of death. This effect was persisted even after tumor and treatment were taken into account.[32] This finding has been coupled with the potential use of the diabetic agent metformin, which reduces glucose levels and associated hyperinsulinemia. There now is a large body of research evidence showing the potential benefit of this drug given its mechanism of action, and clinical studies showed it appears to improve outcomes in at least certain subsets of patients with breast cancer. There is ongoing research for its role not only in the adjuvant treatment setting but also in prevention.

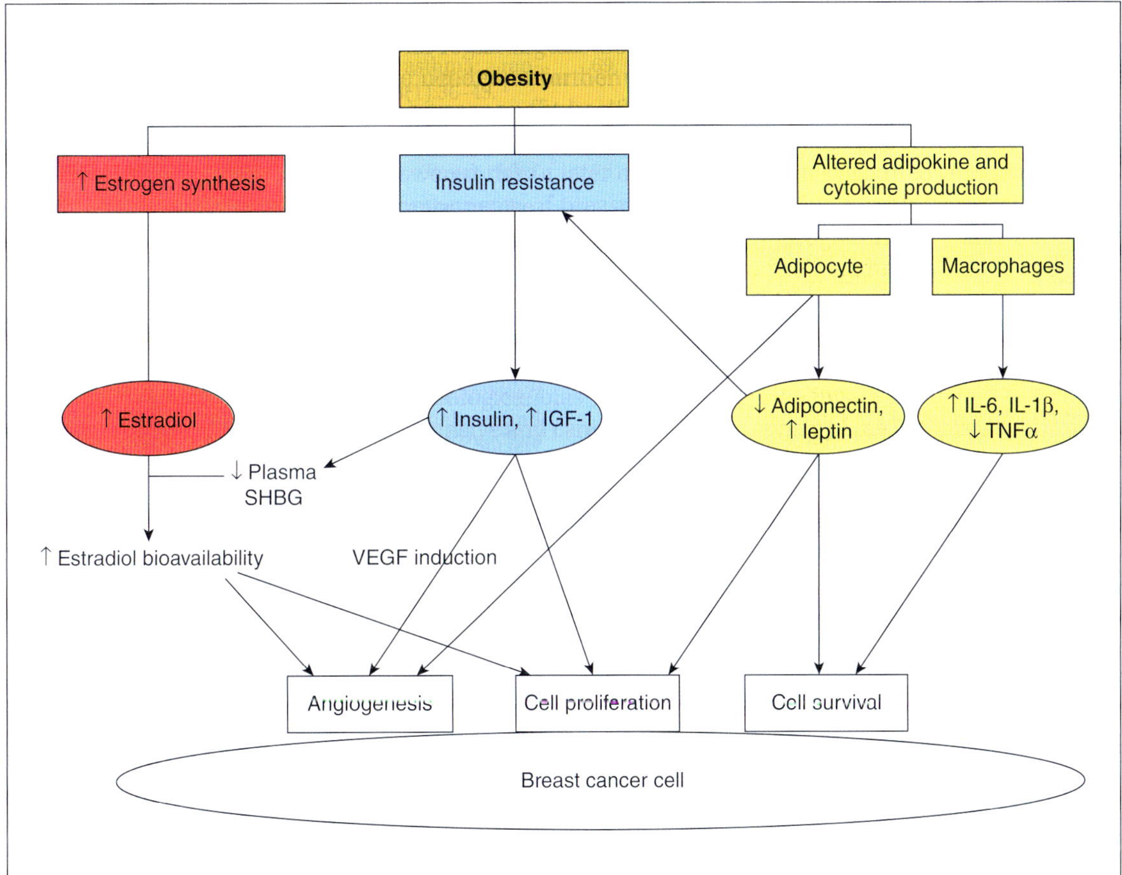

FIGURE 11-3. Schematic demonstrating the relationship and cross interaction of the three theories linking obesity to breast cancer development. VEGF, vascular endothelial growth factor.

Chronic Inflammation

The theory that chronic inflammation leads to carcinogenesis is not new. Colorectal carcinoma and inflammatory bowel disease and malignancies of lung, bladder, esophagus, and liver have all been associated with inflammation and infection.[33] Recently, it was shown that inflammatory processes exist in and around breast tumors and that within the breast of the obese woman there clearly appears to be cellular changes showing the relationship between obesity, breast inflammation, and tumorigenesis.[34] The release of inflammatory cytokines by adipocytes and activation of macrophages are key interactions for this theory (see Figure 11-3).

The theories linking obesity to breast cancer are many and, as noted, are somewhat interrelated. While a healthy lifestyle and a normal BMI are the ultimate goals for every patient, knowing the possible biologic mechanisms whereby obesity increases breast cancer risk allows future developments to target these causes.

Obesity and Breast Cancer Subtypes

Obesity is associated with not only increased risk of breast cancer but also a worse prognosis. Elevated BMI appears to be most closely associated with hormone receptor–positive tumors. Interestingly, a large meta-analysis specifically looking at obesity and breast cancer prognosis sought to determine if menopausal status or receptor subtype influenced outcome. This study was unable to show a difference between obesity, hormone receptor status, menopausal status, and breast cancer–specific outcomes. This analysis looked not only at overall survival but also at breast cancer–specific survival. Given the noted strong association between obesity and elevated estrogen levels, these findings suggest a more complex association between obesity and breast cancer prognosis, and pathways such as the insulin or IGF pathway or perhaps the inflammatory pathway may play a more significant role in breast cancer outcomes than those related to sex hormones. Future trials examining obesity and breast cancer should include both hormone receptor–positive and hormone receptor–negative tumors as well as pre- and postmenopausal women.[35]

Obesity and Triple-Negative Breast Carcinoma

While most of the reporting on the increased risk of breast carcinoma with obesity speaks to the preponderance of receptor–positive disease and the theoretical explanation regarding why, an increase in receptor-negative disease (triple negative) has been studied as well. An association between obesity and the more aggressive triple-negative breast carcinoma has been more controversial, with some groups noting elevated BMI to be a risk for the development of triple-negative breast carcinoma[36,37] and other groups unable to show this association.[38,39] In a recent systematic review and meta-analysis, Pierobon and Frankfeld showed that obese women do appear to be at increased risk for the development of triple-negative breast cancer, approximately 20% greater, than nonobese women.[40] They also noted that menopausal status may be a contributing factor, with premenopausal women at greater risk.

BREAST CANCER PROGNOSIS AND OUTCOME

As noted, there seems to be no disagreement, at least for postmenopausal women, that obesity is a risk factor for the development of breast cancer. Unfortunately, recurrence, prognosis, and survival also appear to be negatively affected by elevated BMI.[41–43] The mechanisms previously described—elevated estrogen levels, hyperinsulinemia, and chronic inflammation—contribute to recurrence and prognosis.

Several studies have shown that the obese woman tends to present with larger, more advanced tumors. In addition, studies have shown these patients present with higher-grade tumors and more nodes that are positive at surgery.[9,43]

Not surprisingly, because of the more advanced presentation, obese women appear more likely to develop distant metastasis and ultimately die of their breast cancer.[9] Not only has increasing BMI been shown to increase the risk of dying of breast cancer,[41] but also the associated worse overall and breast cancer–specific survival are noted in both pre- and postmenopausal breast cancer regardless of when BMI is ascertained.[44] Chan and colleagues looked at different time intervals from diagnosis (from before to >12 months after) and found increased risk regardless of when BMI was elevated[44] (see Figure 11-4).

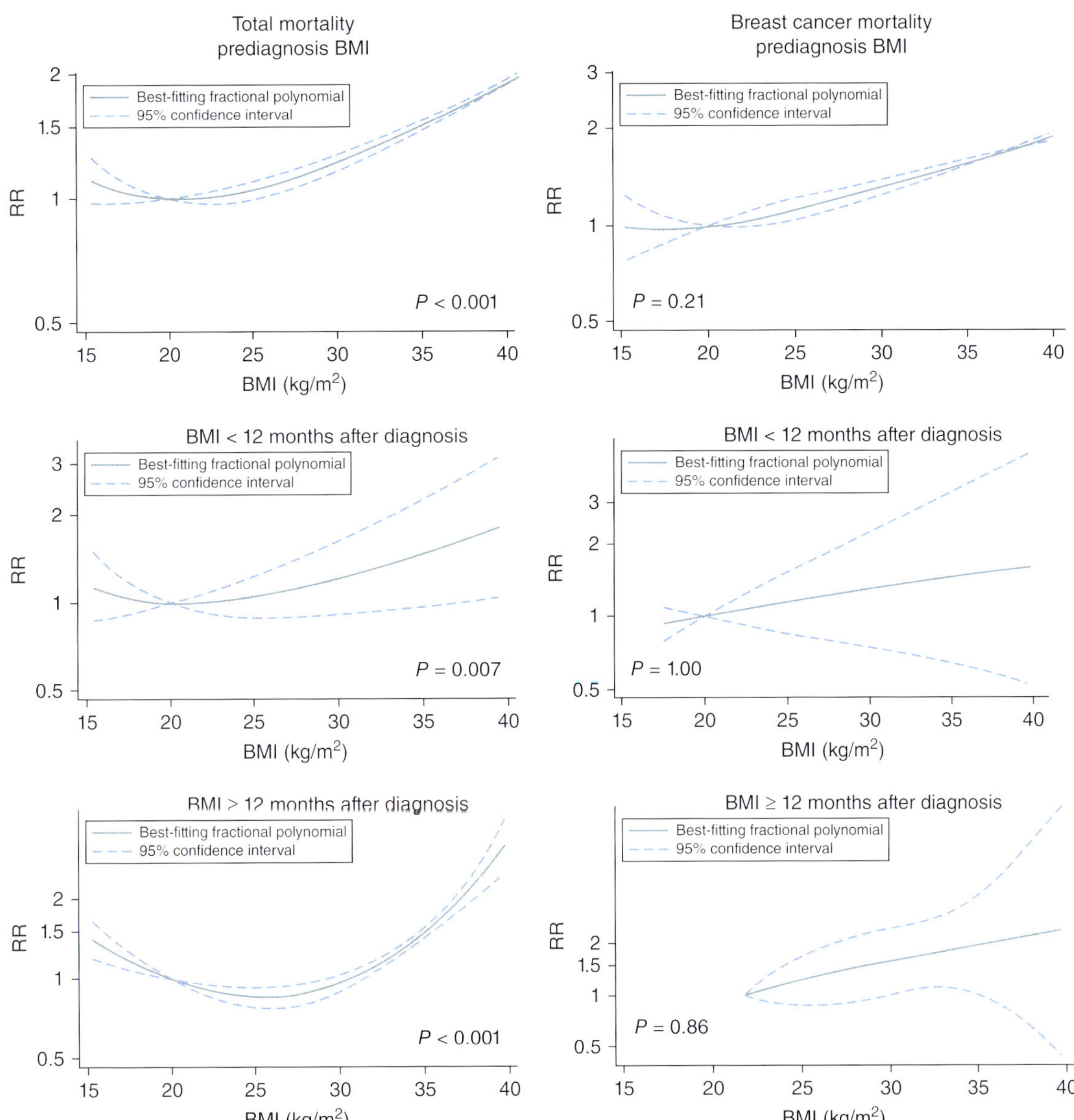

FIGURE 11-4. Total and breast cancer mortality dose-response curves as they relate to BMI. (Reprinted with permission from Chan DS, Vieira AR, Aune D, et al. Body mass index and survival in women with breast cancer—systematic literature review and meta-analysis of 82 follow-up studies. *Ann Oncol.* 2014;25(10):1901–1914.)

Gynecologists often serve as the primary providers of routine breast care and mammographic screening; obese patients should be counseled that their increased weight increases their risk of not only developing breast cancer but also dying from it or other causes once diagnosed. As breast cancer is the most common malignancy among women and obesity rates are only climbing, this will continue to be an important issue for obese patients and their primary care providers.

The Impact of Obesity on Breast Cancer Treatment

Adjuvant Chemotherapy

The worse prognosis of the obese woman with breast carcinoma has a multifactorial etiology. There appear to be direct and indirect biologic changes with regard to estrogen, insulin, and the role of inflammation. In addition, there is evidence that the obese patient, with a larger body surface area (BSA), is often underdosed with chemotherapy (given based on BSA) compared to a normal-weight patient. This may be due to fear of the underlying comorbidities that often accompany this group; it may also alter their cancer survival outcome. Griggs and colleagues specifically evaluated the impact of socioeconomic status and BMI on the quality and dosing of chemotherapy. They found BMI was associated with reduced administration of chemotherapy on both univariate and multivariate analysis.[45]

In contrast, a review of centers in the National Comprehensive Cancer Network (NCCN) over 10 years, looking at whether obesity affected the receipt of adjuvant chemotherapy, found this was not the case. This review included women with operable stages I through III breast cancer. These same authors, in a retrospective cohort study of nearly 10,000 women treated with systemic doxorubicin and cyclophosphamide over a 10-year period, reviewed the quality of chemotherapy administered. Specifically, they looked at first-dose reductions according to patient weight. They noted a progressive reduction in dosing as weight increased. This was a community-based review, looking at just over 900 practices; the authors pointed out that there was significant variation among different practices, with some groups never reducing dosing in the overweight or obese and other groups doing it routinely.

Breast cancer treatment in the obese woman poses multiple challenges to the clinician. This is a group of women by and large at greater risk of developing the disease and, once diagnosed, more likely to have advanced disease and a higher likelihood of recurrence. This is a group more likely to need and benefit from adjuvant systemic chemotherapy, but yet their obesity can affect their ability to receive the appropriate dosing to provide the benefit of this needed therapy.

Hormonal Therapy

Hormonal therapy as adjuvant treatment for receptor–positive breast carcinoma has been a standard of care for many years. Tamoxifen, a selective estrogen receptor modulator (SERM) remains the gold standard for premenopausal women, with aromatase inhibitors now serving as first-line therapy for postmenopausal women with receptor-positive disease. These effective agents have been proven to decrease the risk of recurrence of estrogen receptor–positive breast cancer and are routinely recommended to those patients without contraindication (i.e., history of deep vein thrombosis or pulmonary embolism).

Aromatase inhibitors function by a completely different mechanism than SERMs. These agents inhibit aromatase, the enzyme known to convert peripheral androstenedione to estrogen in the postmenopausal woman. With ovarian function cessation, this serves as the main source of estrogen in the postmenopausal woman.

As described previously, the obese woman is known to have increased estradiol levels as adipose is known to be a major source of aromatase . Aromatase inhibitors were recommended as first-line therapy in postmenopausal receptor–positive women in 2003 after showing improved outcomes over tamoxifen. Sestak and colleagues reviewed the original comparison trial and hypothesized, given the known increased estradiol levels in the obese postmenopausal woman, that perhaps anastrozole would be more effective in these obese patients. Comparing the impact of BMI on recurrence, this group evaluated the benefit of tamoxifen versus anastrozole according to BMI.

Unfortunately, the results again confirmed not only the increased incidence of recurrences and poorer outcome among the obese but also that the known efficacy of anastrozole over tamoxifen is greater in thin women. More specifically, anastrozole was significantly less effective in postmenopausal women with a BMI greater than 30 kg/m^2.

These authors noted that perhaps standard dosing of anastrozole (1 mg/d) is not sufficient to inhibit the increased production of estrogen in patients with increased BMI.[46] It may be that the "one-size-fits-all" dosing does not apply to those with elevated BMI and categorized as obese.

Unlike anastrozole, tamoxifen, which had always been the gold standard of hormonal therapy, has been shown not to lose efficacy in the face of obesity. Using the cohort of women from the original 1982 NSABP* B-14 Trial, Dignam et al. specifically looked at breast cancer recurrence, contralateral breast tumors, other new primary cancers, and mortality in relation to BMI. These authors found that the hazard of breast cancer recurrence was the same among obese women as compared with underweight and normal-weight woman. They also interestingly found that contralateral breast cancer was higher in obese women than in the underweight and normal-weight women, as was the risk of other primary cancers. Also, not surprisingly, obese woman had a greater all-cause mortality rate compared with normal-weight women. At least in this review, breast cancer mortality was not statistically significantly increased for obese women. Tamoxifen appears to reduce breast cancer recurrence and mortality regardless of BMI.[47]

Radiotherapy

Breast-conserving surgery for cancer revolutionized the management of breast carcinoma, allowing women the option of preserving their breasts when appropriate. Numerous trials have shown equal long-term prognosis and survival with lumpectomy and radiation when compared to mastectomy. Barring certain exceptions, radiotherapy is considered the standard of care when breast conservation is utilized for surgical management. Radiotherapy in obese breast cancer patients results in more complications, difficulties with administration, and not necessarily the improved quality of life expected with breast preservation.

With the administration of radiotherapy, the concern is always for the development of local skin toxicities. After, or even during, treatment, most women develop some element of radiation dermatitis, with or without significant moist desquamation. In the most severe case, there can be actual ulceration of the skin.[48] It has also been found that many of these initial acute skin toxicities seem to correlate with the development of some of the more long-term sequelae of radiation (chronic telangiectasia), a poor cosmetic outcome, and ultimately an adverse impact on the woman's quality of life.[48,49] Elevated BMI and bra cup size larger than D appear to be associated with greater risk of significant skin complications, such as moist desquamation. In

---

*NSABP refers to the National Surgical Adjuvant Breast and Bowel Project, it is a clinical trials cooperative group supported by the National Cancer Institute.

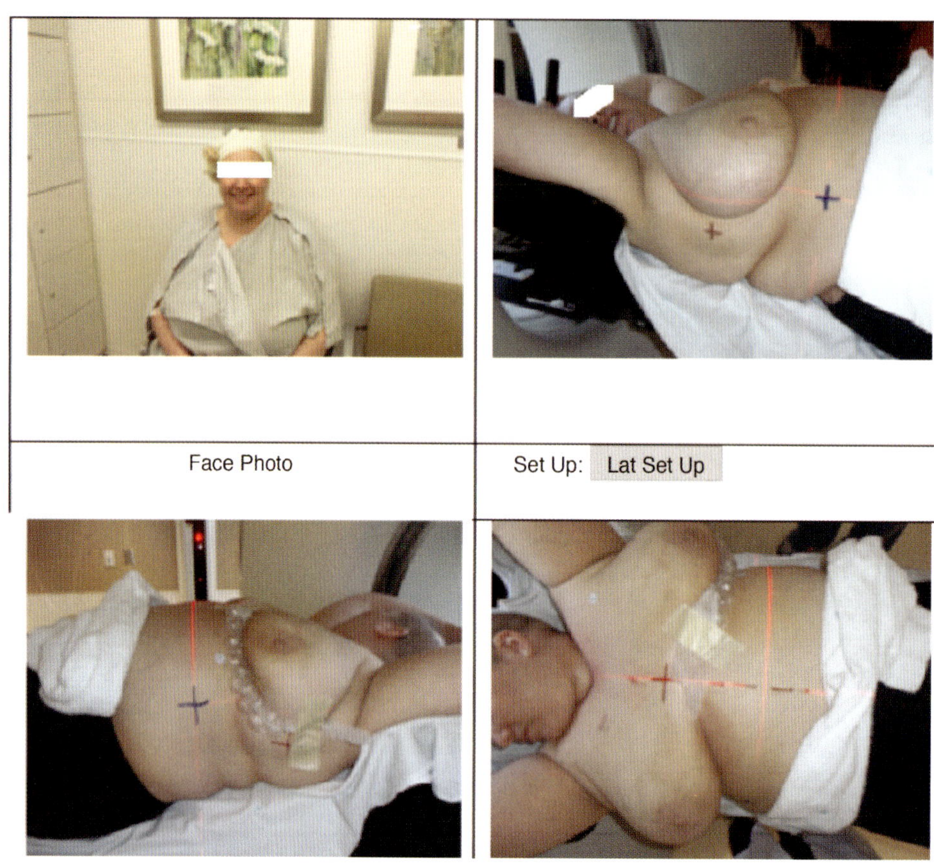

Face Photo	Set Up: Lat Set Up

FIGURE 11-5. Figure demonstrates the challenges of positioning the obese, large-breasted patient to avoid the bolus effect of redundant skinfolds. Breast is "propped" up to avoid this effect.

general, large-breasted and obese women present a challenge to the radiation oncologist in developing a treatment plan. Some of the technical challenges associated with the obese patient or very large-breasted woman include poor setup reproducibility due to size, avoiding heterogeneity of radiation dosing, and trying to limit excessive skinfolds in positioning[50] (see Figure 11-5). Administration techniques shown to be beneficial in this population to limit toxicities include hypofractionated dosing (over normofractionated) and prone positioning of the patient. Hypofractionated radiation therapy is the administration of a larger daily dose over a shorter overall course (i.e., 3 weeks vs. 6 weeks). Hypofractionated dosing administration in the obese and very large-breasted woman has been shown to result in very acceptable complication rates, with focal moist desquamation occurring in less than 10% in 1 review.[50] Prone positioning, as opposed to standard supine positioning, has been shown to greatly help overcome the technical difficulties described previously with the obese or very large-breasted patient. Prone positioning has been shown to result in improved cosmetic outcomes in this group routinely shown to be at risk for increased skin toxicity, fibrosis, poor cosmesis, and more long-term complications.[51] These techniques are not offered by all radiation oncologists. If possible, a facility that offers a full complement of techniques may be of significant benefit to this population of patients.

OBESITY AND SURGERY OF THE BREAST

Surgical Complications

Breast surgery is certainly one of the main treatment modalities of breast cancer, with almost every patient undergoing surgical therapy. Chen and colleagues specifically examined the complication rates of obese patients presenting for elective breast procedures. Using Blue Cross/Blue Shield insurance plans, these authors looked at claims filed from an identified cohort of obese patients and a control group of nonobese women over a 4-year period. A comparison was made between the proportions of patients in each group who experienced a surgical complication. Obesity was associated with an almost 12-fold increased risk of a postoperative complication (18.3% of obese patients having a claim for complication compared to 2.2% in nonobese controls). One might argue the rate was likely higher as this review reported only the cases noted as documented on claims.

The concern for increased risk of surgical postoperative complications should be addressed preoperatively with the patient, and attempts should be made perioperatively and postoperatively to address and treat expeditiously any issues that arise.[52]

Seroma Formation

The development of postoperative seroma is a relatively common complication of breast cancer surgery, with seroma occurring in the breast, axilla, and mastectomy flaps. The precise cause of seroma development is not clear. In a review by Gonzalez et al. looking at numerous variables that could be contributing to seroma formation, none was found, including patient weight.[53] Other reviews, however, looking at risk factors for the development of seroma have found obesity to be an independent risk factor for postoperative seroma.[54,55]

Axillary Nodal Evaluation and Lymphedema

It has been well and widely documented, assuming the patient is an appropriate candidate, that breast-conserving therapy with lumpectomy, sentinel node evaluation, and radiation therapy provide equally as effective outcome and survival compared to mastectomy.[56] Sentinel node biopsy is now standard of care and provides reliable and accurate staging of the affected axilla with less mortality compared to full axillary dissection when appropriate. Nonetheless, false-negative results or failure to even localize the sentinel node do still occur. Obesity has been found to be one of the factors significantly associated with failed localization of the sentinel node.[57] As such, in surgical consultation these patients should be counseled that this may occur and prepared for full axillary node dissection, which may need to be performed but not initially planned. Certainly, full axillary dissection increases the risk of arm lymphedema when compared to less-invasive sentinel node evaluation. In addition, obesity has been shown to be an independent risk factor for lymphedema associated with axillary procedures. McLaughlin and colleagues looked at the prevalence of lymphedema in patients with breast cancer 5 years out from either sentinel node biopsy or axillary dissection. Although this study showed, not surprisingly, that sentinel node biopsy resulted in a significantly lower incidence of lymphedema when compared to full axillary dissection, it still remained a risk (5% sentinel node biopsy vs. 16% axillary lymph node dissection), with greater body weight and higher BMI significant risk factors.[58]

Infection

The American College of Surgeons' (ACS') classification of wounds categorizes breast surgery as a class 1 or clean procedure. These types of cases are associated with a less than 2% risk of wound infection. As such, it is hard to justify routine use of antibiotic prophylaxis in clean cases, and there is no general recommendation for antibiotic prophylaxis in soft tissue or cutaneous procedures such as for the breast.

Despite the very low incidence of infection in clean-type cases, there have been at least some older studies showing a benefit of the use of perioperative antibiotics in reducing surgical infection with breast surgery,[59,60] in particular axillary node dissection.[60] Obesity is a known factor for increased risk of infection.

While breast surgery is classified as a clean procedure carrying a very low risk of infection, preoperative antibiotic use should at least be considered in obese patients undergoing breast-conserving therapy for early-stage breast cancer and is recommended routinely for obese women undergoing mastectomy with reconstructive surgery.

Mastectomy Challenges in the Obese

Breast Reconstruction

In the last many years, there has been what many see as a swing of the pendulum, with an almost-epidemic increase in performance of bilateral mastectomies despite the proven equivalence in survival when compared to breast-conserving surgery. While there are many theories on the reason for this apparent epidemic of mastectomies, one reason is the option and ability for immediate reconstruction. However, like any surgical procedure, obesity makes breast reconstruction more difficult, more challenging to obtain a good cosmetic outcome, and offers more complications.

In a large recent analysis using the ACS National Surgical Quality Improvement Program (NSQIP) database, Fischer and colleagues reviewed information on nearly 16,000 patients specifically looking at the impact of obesity in surgical breast reconstruction. These authors looked at both medical and surgical complications and stratified according to BMI using the World Health Organization obesity criteria. Patients were divided as nonobese (BMI = 20–29.9 kg/m^2), class I (BMI = 30–34.9 kg/m^2), class II (BMI = 35–39.9 kg/m^2), and class III (BMI $\geq$ 40 kg/m^2).

Nearly one-third of all patients were obese. This is not surprising and is in keeping with national statistics. As shown in the following material, complications were clearly greater in the obese. Progressively higher BMIs were associated with higher rates of complications. Morbidly obese patients experienced a wound complication rate of over 10.4%. Progressive increases in obesity were clearly associated with progressively increasing rates of complications. Significant increases were noted for wound complications, medical complications, major surgical complications, graft or flap loss, and return to the operating room. These authors noted that 1 of perhaps the most important findings was the markedly higher rate of major surgical complications in class III obese patients compared to nonobese patients (14.9% vs. 7.1%, $p < .0001$) A more-than-double rate, as well as an over 5% higher risk of returning to the operating room within 30 days, was seen when comparing these 2 groups. Previous

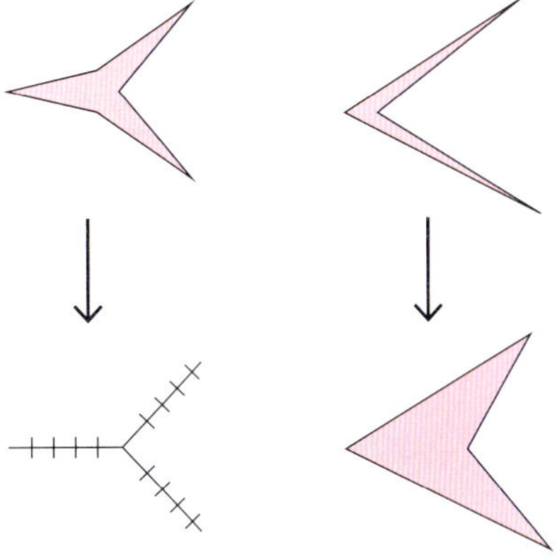

FIGURE 11-6. Y-plasty. Diagram demonstrates the final pattern of the incisional scar when the redundant breast skin out laterally by the axilla is pulled into the more medial aspect of the closure. The remaining dog-ears are trimmed and the Y pattern closed.

studies have suggested that obese women achieve greater long-term reconstructive success with autologous tissue flaps over implant-based reconstruction. Certainly, given the overall body habitus of the very obese patient, this makes sense. However, given the findings in Fischer et al.'s review and the greater magnitude of flap surgery versus implant reconstruction, one wonders if the increased medical and surgical risk is worth it.

There are many reconstructive surgeons currently refusing to take on these obese breast cancer patients for consideration of reconstruction. Although many might argue that this is ethically not appropriate, reviewing these published rates of complication it is understandable. Reconstructive complications and failure, in addition to causing great emotional distress, can often lead to marked delays in adjuvant therapies, which can affect survival. The obese, particularly morbidly obese, patient desiring breast reconstruction needs to be strongly and honestly counseled regarding her markedly increased risk of serious and potentially life-altering complications. These are difficult conversations at a fragile time for women who already struggle with body image but the conversations must take place.

Mastectomy Without Reconstruction

The obese woman with breast cancer desiring or requiring mastectomy presents a challenge not only to the plastic surgeon but also often to the general or breast surgeon when reconstruction is not chosen. The obese large-breasted woman will often have a large amount of redundant lateral soft tissue that tends to result in a large "dog-ear" of excess skin. Women will often complain of this area protruding from under the arm or as hard to fit comfortably within a bra prosthesis.

While there is no good way to avoid this issue completely, for many cases, one technique that can give more conformity to the lateral chest wall is the creation of a Y-plasty with the redundant lateral skin. In this case, the lateral-most point of the incision is pulled and tacked as medial as it comes comfortably to bring the excess skin to the chest wall. This maneuver will then create a triangular dog-ear both above and below. These are trimmed, leaving the 2 arms of the Y to be sutured. The final mastectomy scar incision will be a Y with the top arms out laterally (see Figure 11-6). The cosmetic result for the obese patient is much improved.

CONCLUSION

Because obesity in this country is estimated to be on the rise, the impact it has on breast disease and cancer warrants further research. Obesity has detrimental effects on breast cancer development, recurrence, and survival. Future studies need to be done to clarify the impact that perhaps exercise and weight loss can have to possibly improve outcomes in obese patients with cancer. In addition, our better understanding of the molecular pathways linking obesity to cancer allow for potentially significant therapeutic advances. The promising results seen with diabetic agents such as metformin suggest further targeting of the insulin pathway may be beneficial in this population. Similarly, a better understanding of the complex inflammatory mediators associated with obesity and cancer provide yet another targeted therapy. As tumor genotyping is becoming the future of medical oncology, further research can be done to look at the specific subtypes of breast cancer seen in the higher estrogen environment of the obese patient. While limiting obesity should be one of our first goals, these potential therapeutic advances may help improve the outcome in this high-risk population.

SUMMARY

Obesity is clearly an epidemic in our current society. While its effect on the cardiovascular system has been well documented for decades, its impact on benign and malignant disease of the breast is becoming increasingly clear. As obstetricians and gynecologists are often the providers overseeing breast health and screening, these findings are important.

When patients are counseled regarding good health practices and risk reduction, being overweight can be considered a risk for not only minor skin and soft tissue issues but also breast cancer with an associated poorer outcome. Counseling women about weight can be difficult, but as noted in this chapter, it can have a significant impact on their life.

REFERENCES

1. Yosipovitch G, DeVore A, Dawn A. Obesity and the skin: skin physiology and skin manifestations of obesity. *J Am Acad Dermatol.* 2007;56(6):901–916.
2. Nozickova M, Koudelkova V, Kulikova Z, Malina L, Urbanowski S, Silny W. A comparison of the efficacy of oral fluconazole, 150 mg/week versus 50 mg/day, in the treatment of tinea corporis, tinea cruris, tinea pedis, and cutaneous candidosis. *Int J Dermatol.* 1998;37(9):703–705.
3. Eggerstedt M, Gamelli RL, Mosier MJ. The care of necrotizing soft-tissue infections: patterns of definitive intervention at a large referral center. *J Burn Care Res.* 2015;36(1):105–110.
4. Guray M, Sahin AA. Benign breast diseases: classification, diagnosis, and management. *Oncologist.* 2006;11(5):435–449.
5. Nyström L, Andersson I, Bjurstam N, Frisell J, Nordenskjöld B, Rutqvist LE. Long-term effects of mammography screening: updated overview of the swedish randomised trials. *Lancet.* 2002;359(9310):909–919.
6. Ferrante JM, Chen P, Crabtree BF, Wartenberg D. Cancer screening in women: body mass index and adherence to physician recommendations. *Am J Prev Med.* 2007;32(6):525–531.
7. Smith RA, Cokkinides V, Eyre HJ. American Cancer Society guidelines for the early detection of cancer, 2006. *CA Cancer J Clin.* 2006;56(1):11–25.
8. Rose DP, Vona-Davis L. Interaction between menopausal status and obesity in affecting breast cancer risk. *Maturitas.* 2010;66(1):33–38.
9. Berz D, Sikov W, Colvin G, Weitzen S. "Weighing in" on screening mammography. *Breast Cancer Res Treat.* 2009;114(3):569–574.
10. Lee CH, Dershaw DD, Kopans D, et al. Breast cancer screening with imaging: recommendations from the Society of Breast Imaging and the ACR on the use of mammography, breast MRI, breast ultrasound, and other technologies for the detection of clinically occult breast cancer. *J Am Coll Radiol.* 2010;7(1):18–27.
11. Amy NK, Aalborg A, Lyons P, Keranen L. Barriers to routine gynecological cancer screening for white and African-American obese women. *Int J Obes.* 2006;30(1):147–155.
12. Elmore JG, Carney PA, Abraham LA, et al. The association between obesity and screening mammography accuracy. *Arch Intern Med.* 2004;164(10):1140–1147.
13. Guest AR, Helvie MA, Chan H, Hadjiiski LM, Bailey JE, Roubidoux MA. Adverse effects of increased body weight on quantitative measures of mammographic image quality. *Am J Roentgenol.* 2000;175(3):805–810.
14. Hunt KA, Sickles EA. Effect of obesity on screening mammography: outcomes analysis of 88,346 consecutive examinations. *Am J Roentgenol.* 2000;174(5):1251–1255.
15. Destounis S, Newell M, Pinsky R. Breast imaging and intervention in the overweight and obese patient. *Am J Roentgenol.* 2011;196(2):296–302.
16. Hunt KA, Sickles EA. Effect of obesity on screening mammography: outcomes analysis of 88,346

consecutive examinations. *Am J Roentgenol.* 2000; 174(5):1251–1255.

17. Skaane P, Bandos AI, Gullien R, et al. Comparison of digital mammography alone and digital mammography plus tomosynthesis in a population-based screening program. *Radiology.* 2013;267(1):47–56.

18. Hooley RJ, Greenberg KL, Stackhouse RM, Geisel JL, Butler RS, Philpotts LE. Screening US in patients with mammographically dense breasts: initial experience with connecticut public act 09-41. *Radiology.* 2012;265(1):59–69.

19. Sun Y, Wei W, Yang H, Liu J. Clinical usefulness of breast-specific gamma imaging as an adjunct modality to mammography for diagnosis of breast cancer: a systemic review and meta-analysis. *Eur J Nucl Med Mol Imaging.* 2013;40(3):450–463.

20. Schilling K, Narayanan D, Kalinyak JE, et al. Positron emission mammography in breast cancer presurgical planning: comparisons with magnetic resonance imaging. *Eur J Nucl Med Mol imaging.* 2011;38(1):23–36.

21. Hendrick RE. Radiation doses and cancer risks from breast imaging studies 1. *Radiology.* 2010;257(1):246–253.

22. Cleary MP, Grossmann ME. Obesity and breast cancer: the estrogen connection. *Endocrinology.* 2009;150(6):2537–2542.

23. van Kruijsdijk RC, van der Wall E, Visseren FL. Obesity and cancer: the role of dysfunctional adipose tissue. *Cancer Epidemiol Biomarkers Prev.* 2009;18(10):2569–2578.

24. Ursin G, Longnecker MP, Haile RW, Greenland S. A meta-analysis of body mass index and risk of premenopausal breast cancer. *Epidemiology.* 1995:137–141.

25. Miller W. Aromatase and the breast: regulation and clinical aspects. *Maturitas.* 2006;54(4):335–341.

26. Kaaks R, Rinaldi S, Key TJ, et al. Postmenopausal serum androgens, oestrogens and breast cancer risk: The European prospective investigation into cancer and nutrition. *Endocr Relat Cancer.* 2005;12(4):1071–1082.

27. Purohit A, Newman SP, Reed MJ. The role of cytokines in regulating estrogen synthesis: implications for the etiology of breast cancer. *Breast Cancer Res.* 2002;4(2):65–69.

28. Missmer SA, Eliassen AH, Barbieri RL, Hankinson SE. Endogenous estrogen, androgen, and progesterone concentrations and breast cancer risk among postmenopausal women. *J Natl Cancer Inst.* 2004;96(24):1856–1865.

29. Thomas HV, Reeves GK, Key TJ. Endogenous estrogen and postmenopausal breast cancer: a quantitative review. *Cancer Causes Control.* 1997;8(6):922–928.

30. McTiernan A, Wu L, Chen C, et al. Relation of BMI and physical activity to sex hormones in postmenopausal women. *Obesity.* 2006;14(9):1662–1677.

31. Duggan C, Irwin ML, Xiao L, et al. Associations of insulin resistance and adiponectin with mortality in women with breast cancer. *J Clin Oncol.* 2011;29(1):32–39.

32. Goodwin PJ, Ennis M, Pritchard KI, et al. Fasting insulin and outcome in early-stage breast cancer: results of a prospective cohort study. *J Clin Oncol.* 2002;20(1):42–51.

33. Iyengar NM, Hudis CA, Dannenberg AJ. Obesity and inflammation: new insights into breast cancer development and progression. *Am Soc Clin Oncol Educ Book.* 2013:46–51.

34. Morris PG, Hudis CA, Giri D, et al. Inflammation and increased aromatase expression occur in the breast tissue of obese women with breast cancer. *Cancer Prev Res.* 2011;4(7):1021–1029.

35. Niraula S, Ocana A, Ennis M, Goodwin PJ. Body size and breast cancer prognosis in relation to hormone receptor and menopausal status: a meta-analysis. *Breast Cancer Res Treat.* 2012;134(2):769–781.

36. Millikan RC, Newman B, Tse C, et al. Epidemiology of basal-like breast cancer. *Breast Cancer Res Treat.* 2008;109(1):123–139.

37. Trivers KF, Lund MJ, Porter PL, et al. The epidemiology of triple-negative breast cancer, including race. *Cancer Causes Control.* 2009;20(7):1071–1082.

38. Phipps AI, Malone KE, Porter PL, Daling JR, Li CI. Body size and risk of luminal, HER2-overexpressing, and triple-negative breast cancer in postmenopausal women. *Cancer Epidemiol Biomarkers Prev.* 2008;17(8):2078–2086.

39. Kwan ML, Kushi LH, Weltzien E, et al. Epidemiology of breast cancer subtypes in two prospective cohort studies of breast cancer survivors. *Breast Cancer Res.* 2009;11(3):R31.

40. Pierobon M, Frankenfeld CL. Obesity as a risk factor for triple-negative breast cancers: a systematic review and meta-analysis. *Breast Cancer Res Treat.* 2013;137(1):307–314.

41. Calle EE, Kaaks R. Overweight, obesity and cancer: epidemiological evidence and proposed mechanisms. *Nat Rev Cancer.* 2004;4(8):579–591.

42. Whiteman MK, Hillis SD, Curtis KM, McDonald JA, Wingo PA, Marchbanks PA. Body mass and mortality after breast cancer diagnosis. *Cancer Epidemiol Biomarkers Prev.* 2005;14(8):2009–2014.

43. Majed B, Moreau T, Senouci K, Salmon RJ, Fourquet A, Asselain B. Is obesity an independent prognosis factor in woman breast cancer? *Breast Cancer Res Treat.* 2008;111(2):329–342.

44. Chan DS, Vieira AR, Aune D, et al. Body mass index and survival in women with breast cancer—systematic literature review and meta-analysis of 82 follow-up studies. *Ann Oncol.* 2014;25(10):1901–1914.

45. Griggs JJ, Sorbero ME, Lyman GH. Undertreatment of obese women receiving breast cancer chemotherapy. *Arch Intern Med*. 2005;165(11):1267–1273.

46. Sestak I, Distler W, Forbes JF, Dowsett M, Howell A, Cuzick J. Effect of body mass index on recurrences in tamoxifen and anastrozole treated women: an exploratory analysis from the ATAC trial. *J Clin Oncol*. 2010;28(21):3411–3415.

47. Dignam JJ, Wieand K, Johnson KA, Fisher B, Xu L, Mamounas EP. Obesity, tamoxifen use, and outcomes in women with estrogen receptor-positive early-stage breast cancer. *J Natl Cancer Inst*. 2003;95(19):1467–1476.

48. Feight D, Baney T, Bruce S, McQuestion M. Putting evidence into practice. *Clin J Oncol Nurs*. 2011;15(5):481–492.

49. Lilla C, Ambrosone CB, Kropp S, et al. Predictive factors for late normal tissue complications following radiotherapy for breast cancer. *Breast Cancer Res Treat*. 2007;106(1):143–150.

50. Dorn PL, Corbin KS, Al-Hallaq H, Hasan Y, Chmura SJ. Feasibility and acute toxicity of hypofractionated radiation in large-breasted patients. *Int J Radiat Oncol Biol Phys*. 2012;83(1):79–83.

51. Bergom C, Kelly T, Morrow N, et al. Prone whole-breast irradiation using three-dimensional conformal radiotherapy in women undergoing breast conservation for early disease yields high rates of excellent to good cosmetic outcomes in patients with large and/or pendulous breasts. *Int J Radiat Oncol Biol Phys*. 2012;83(3):821–828.

52. Chen CL, Shore AD, Johns R, Clark JM, Manahan M, Makary MA. The impact of obesity on breast surgery complications. *Plast Reconstr Surg*. 2011;128(5):395e–402e.

53. Gonzalez EA, Saltzstein EC, Riedner CS, Nelson BK. Seroma formation following breast cancer surgery. *Breast J*. 2003;9(5):385–388.

54. Tomita K, Yano K, Masuoka T, Matsuda K, Takada A, Hosokawa K. Postoperative seroma formation in breast reconstruction with latissimus dorsi flaps: a retrospective study of 174 consecutive cases. *Ann Plast Surg*. 2007;59(2):149–151.

55. Kim J, Stevenson TR. Abdominoplasty, liposuction of the flanks, and obesity: analyzing risk factors for seroma formation. *Plast Reconstr Surg*. 2006;117(3):773–779.

56. Fisher B, Jeong J, Anderson S, Bryant J, Fisher ER, Wolmark N. Twenty-five-year follow-up of a randomized trial comparing radical mastectomy, total mastectomy, and total mastectomy followed by irradiation. *N Engl J Med*. 2002;347(8):567–575.

57. Goyal A, Newcombe RG, Chhabra A, Mansel RE. Factors affecting failed localisation and false-negative rates of sentinel node biopsy in breast cancer—results of the ALMANAC validation phase. *Breast Cancer Res Treat*. 2006;99(2):203–208.

58. McLaughlin SA, Wright MJ, Morris KT, et al. Prevalence of lymphedema in women with breast cancer 5 years after sentinel lymph node biopsy or axillary dissection: objective measurements. *J Clin Oncol*. 2008;26(32):5213–5219.

59. Platt R, Zucker JR, Zaleznik DF, et al. Prophylaxis against wound infection following herniorrhaphy or breast surgery. *J Infect Dis*. 1992;166(3):556–560.

60. Coit DG, Rogatko A, Brennan MF. Prognostic factors in patients with melanoma metastatic to axillary or inguinal lymph nodes. A multivariate analysis. *Ann Surg*. 1991;214(5):627–636.

Cancer in Women

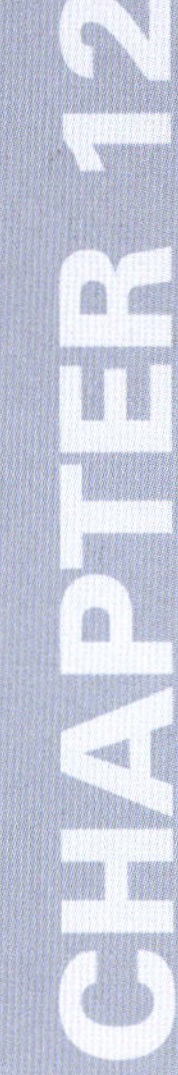

CHAPTER 12

Shaveta Malik, MD

Vanessa M. Barnabei, MD, PhD

INTRODUCTION

Cancer is the second-leading cause of death in the United States. The lifetime probability of a women being diagnosed with an invasive cancer is 38%.[1] Up to 20% of all cancers might be caused by excessive weight (overweight or obesity).[2] The burden of obesity on society continues to rise and warrants closer attention by clinicians for both cancer prevention and improved outcomes after diagnosis. The general focus of this chapter is the association of obesity with nongynecologic cancer in women. The mechanisms by which body weight influences the development of cancer are discussed. Particular emphasis is placed on the impact of increased body weight on prognosis, survival, and risk of recurrence. In addition, prevention and management strategies are discussed to aid clinicians in counseling patients regarding obesity-related cancers.

PREVALENCE AND EPIDEMIOLOGY

Surveillance, Epidemiology, and End Results (SEER) data estimates as of 2007 suggest that there will be 50,000 new cases of cancer yearly in women (7%) that are attributable to obesity.[2] More than one-third of US adults are obese (approximately 78.6 million), another third are overweight,[3] and the prevalence is increasing. The percentage of cancer cases attributable to obesity varies widely for different cancer types but is as high as 40% for some cancers, particularly adenocarcinomas of the endometrium and esophagus. A projection of the future health and economic burden of obesity in 2030 estimated that continuation of existing trends in obesity will lead to about 500,000 additional cases of cancer in the United States by 2030 (Table 12–1).[4]

A systematic review and meta-analysis were performed in 2008 to assess the strength of associations between body mass index (BMI; defined as weight in

TABLE 12-1 Estimated Cases of US Cancers Preventable per Year by Diet, Activity, and Weight Management

Cancer Type	New Cases	Percentage Prevented	Number of Cases Prevented
Breast, female	232,670	33	76,781
Prostate (advanced)	16,310	11	1,794
Gallbladder	10,650	21	2,237
Endometrial	52,630	59	31,052
Esophageal	18,170	63	11,447
Colorectal	136,830	50	68,415
Ovarian	21,980	5	1,099
Pancreatic	46,420	19	8,820
Mouth, pharyngeal, and laryngeal	38,960	63	24,545
Kidney	63,920	24	15,341
Liver	33,190	15	4,979
Stomach	22,220	47	10,443
Lung	224,210	36	80,716
Total preventable			**337,667**

kilograms divided by height in square meters) and different sites of cancer and to investigate differences in these associations between sex and ethnic groups.[5] In women, strong associations were noted between a 5-kg/m² increase in BMI and endometrial (relative risk [RR] 1.59, confidence interval [CI] 1.5–1.68), gallbladder (RR 1.59, CI 1.02–2.47), and renal (RR 1.34, CI 1.25–1.43) cancers and esophageal adenocarcinoma (RR 1.51, CI 1.31–1.74). A weaker positive association (RR < 1.20) was observed between increased BMI and postmenopausal (PMP) breast, pancreatic, thyroid, and colon cancers in women and for leukemia, multiple myeloma, and non-Hodgkin lymphoma in both sexes.

Although the relationship between obesity and cancer in women is well established, the biologic mechanisms underlying this relationship are just beginning to be elucidated. "Obesity-related cancer" is now an official designation used by the American Cancer Society and the National Cancer Institute. The list of obesity-related cancers is long and growing, with lung cancers a prominent exception to the obesity association. It is now estimated that 20% of cancer deaths are attributable to obesity-related oncogenesis. In the case of breast cancer, it was thought for many years that excess estrogen produced by adipose tissue was the major contributor to this increased risk. This was a gross oversimplification of the etiology of breast cancer, and now that we understand more about adipose tissue as an endocrine organ in and of itself, it is becoming apparent that estrogen excess may be an indirect, rather than direct, oncogenic mechanism. The metabolic abnormalities associated with excess adipose tissue and the location of that adipose tissue, and not diet or adiposity itself in most cases, are direct contributors to oncogenesis in many tissues. These metabolic abnormalities occur at both the local and systemic levels, and the variable effect of each may affect tissue-specific susceptibility to carcinogenesis.

PATHOPHYSIOLOGY

There are several pathways by which obesity contributes to excess cancer risk; these are interrelated and synergistic, including localized inflammatory changes and cytokine release, hyperinsulinemia, high leptin levels, and epigenetic changes. These are discussed in further detail in the following material.

One of the primary processes that occurs in adipose tissue of obese individuals is enlargement of adipocytes. When adipocytes reach a critical size, their blood supply is diminished, leading to localized tissue hypoxia. This tissue hypoxia and resultant tissue necrosis set off a cascade of reactions, including release of free fatty acids (FFAs) due to lipolysis, macrophage infiltration, and release of cytokines and adipokines, most importantly tumor necrosis factor alpha (TNF-α) and interleukin 6 (IL-6). Histologically, this inflammatory response can be identified as crown-like structures, or CLS-B, which are inflammatory foci that consist of a necrotic adipocyte and its surrounding macrophages. The release of inflammatory factors by these adipocytes contributes to both cancer initiation and promotion by increasing cell migration and cell invasion. The progression of these changes is shown schematically in Figure 12-1.[6]

Obesity leads to insulin resistance and the resultant increase in serum insulin causes elevations in insulinlike growth factor 1 (IGF-1) and leptin levels and, in the case of mild insulin resistance, increased adiponectin. Hyperinsulinemia causes activation of several pathways, such as via *IRS*, *ERK*, and *MYC*, which increase cellular

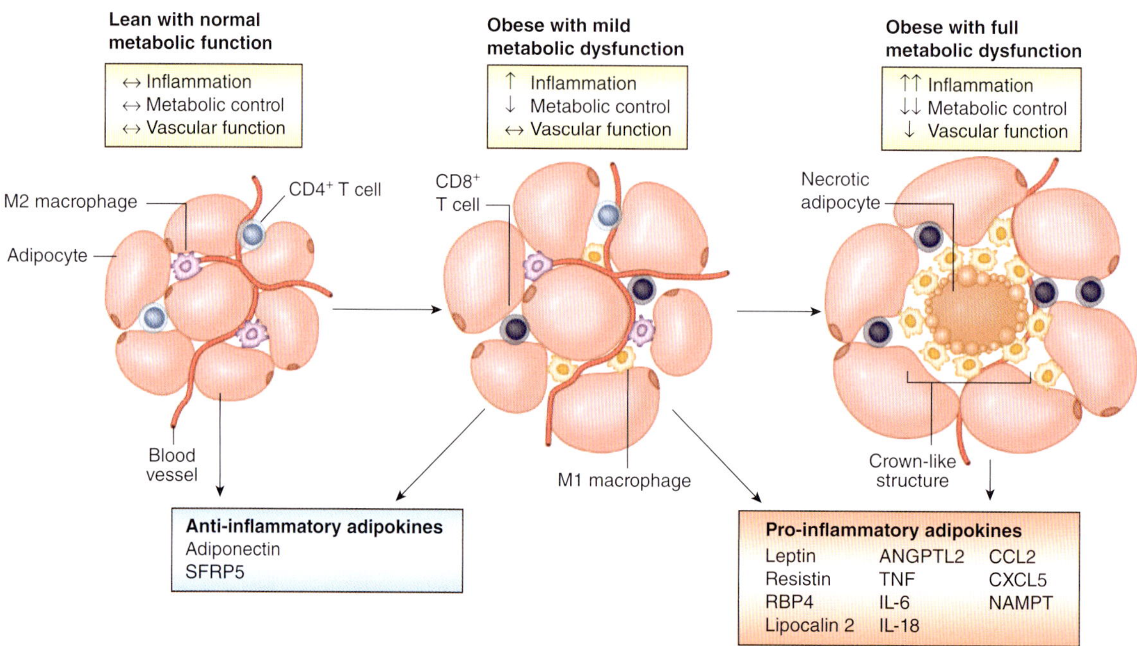

FIGURE 12-1. Relationship between obesity, metabolic function, and inflammatory changes at the level of the adipocyte. SFRPF5: secreted frizzle-related protein 5; RBP4: retinol binding protein 4; ANGPTL2: angiopoietin-like protein 2; CCL2: chemokine ligand 2; CXCL5: CXC chemokine ligand 5; NAMPT: nicotinamide phosphoribosyltransferase; IL-6: Interleukin 6. (From Ouchi N, Parker JL, Lugus JJ, Walsh K. Adipokines in inflammation and metabolic disease. *Nature Rev Immunol.* 2011;11:85–97.)

mitogenicity and cell growth and are pro-angiogenic and antiapoptotic. As insulin resistance worsens, the process shifts even further to a pro-inflammatory state.

Leptin is an important modulator of immune function through cytokine production, angiogenesis, and mitogenesis. TNF-α, which is produced by infiltrating macrophages in response to chronic inflammation in adipose tissue, leads to increases in leptin secretion, as do insulin, estrogen, and glucocorticoids. Excess TNF-α stimulates the nuclear factor kappa beta (NF-κβ) signaling pathway, which promotes cell migration and cell invasion, both pro-metastatic functions. The secretion of adiponectin, which serves to balance the effects of leptin, is decreased in the presence of these inflammatory factors. Adiponectin blocks induction of vascular endothelial growth factor (VEGF) through its suppression of TNF-α. This effect inhibits migration of vascular endothelial cells and promotes apoptosis.

As insulin resistance worsens, the ratio of adiponectin to leptin changes in favor of pro-inflammatory metabolism and the loss of the protective benefits of adiponectin. In the case of breast cancer, adiponectin levels correlate with improved survival. With unfavorable levels of adiponectin, a positive-feedback loop is created in adipose tissue that favors progression of the cycle of inflammation, cytokine release, and leptin release, leading to a pro-tumorigenic environment.[7]

Through its activation of kinases, such as Jak (Janus kinase)/STAT (signal transducer and activator of transcription), mitogen-activated protein kinase (MAPK), PI3/AKT, and others, leptin influences cell proliferation and survival. In addition,

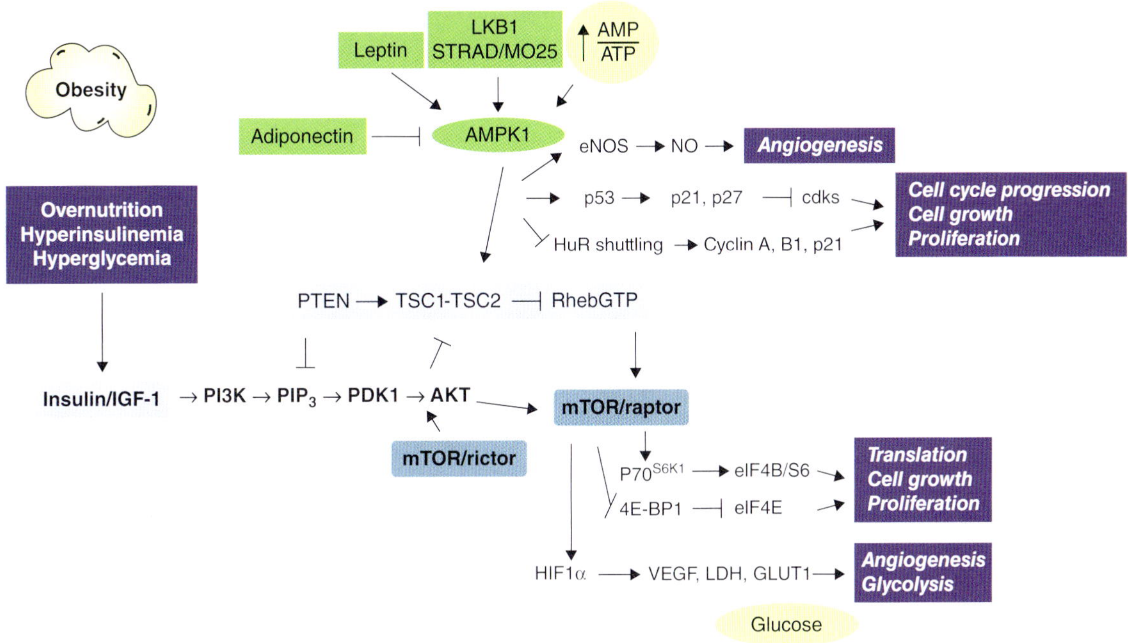

FIGURE 12-2. Interaction of insulin and leptin on cellular growth factors. LKB1: serine threonine kinase; AMPK: activated protein kinase; TOR: threonine kinase; NO: nitric oxide; eNOS: endothelial nitric oxide synthase; PTEN: phosphatase and tensin homolog; STRAD/MO25: Ste20 related adaptor protein; mTOR: mammalian target of rapamycin; RAPTOR: regulatory associated protein of mTOR; RICTOR: rapamycin-insensitive mammalian target of rapamycin; RHEB: Ras homolog enriched in brain; Ras: rat sarcoma; PIP3: phosphatidylinositol 3,4,5 triphosphate; GTP: guanosine 5-triphosphate; ATP: adenosine triphosphate; AMP: adenosine monophosphate; TSC1: tuberous sclerosus protein 1; TSC2: tuberous sclerosus protein 2; GLUT1: human glucose transporter; eIF4E: eukaryotic translation initiation factor 4E; eIF4B: eukaryotic translation initiation factor 4B; 4E-BP1: 4E binding protein 1; AKT: protein kinase B; PI3: phosphoinositide 3-kinase; LDH: lactate dehydrogenase cdks: cyclin-dependent kinases; PDK1: phosphoinositide-dependent kinase 1; PI3: phosphoinositide 3 kinase; AKT: protein kinase B. (Redrawn from Sundaram S, Johnson AJ, Makowski L. Obesity, metabolism and the microenvironment: links to cancer. *J Carcinogen.* 2013;12:19.)

leptin has been shown to stimulate all steps in the angiogenesis cascade.[8] Once a tumor is initiated, this feedback loop also promotes tumor progression by amplifying these factors in the tumor microenvironment (enhanced production of VEGF, NF-κβ, and others that promote angiogenesis, mitogenesis, and vascular permeability). A diagrammatic summary of these factors is shown in Figure 12-2.[9]

Other factors that may affect the risk of certain cancers include alterations in the microbiome, which may be particularly important in colorectal cancer, and epigenetic changes that promote the development of cancer. We expect that these changes and their effects will be elucidated in the next few years.

BREAST CANCER

Epidemiology

The risk of a obese PMP woman developing breast cancer is elevated by 20%–30% over her normal-weight peers. Current estimates suggest that up to 17% of breast cancer cases are preventable by maintenance of a normal weight. This risk seems to be related specifically to women with high central and upper body obesity, characterized by an elevated waist-to-hip ratio (WHR). Women in the lowest quartile for WHR have a decreased risk of developing breast cancer. Weight gain in adult life increases breast cancer risk, while sustainable weight loss after menopause can lead to decreased risk. These associations were particularly strong for weight gain of greater than 25 kg (RR 1.45).[10]

Breast is a fat-rich organ, and large islands of adipose tissue surround the stroma of the epithelial ducts and lobules. This proximity of biologically active adipose tissue with breast epithelium promotes crosstalk between these tissues that affects the initiation and progression of breast neoplasia. There are also data that confirm an elevated risk of breast cancer in PMP women with insulin resistance and type 2 diabetes mellitus (T2DM), independent of BMI. Emerging evidence suggests that hyperinsulinemia is a major contributor to this risk, and many, if not most, women have high insulin levels 10–15 years prior to the diagnosis of T2DM. Insulin is mitogenic and antiapoptotic, and the risk of breast cancer rises proportionally with insulin levels, independently of estradiol levels.

Pathophysiology

The pathways presented likely occur in all tissues that are at higher risk for obesity-related cancer. In the breast, these pathways also contribute to elevated bioavailable estradiol, which further contributes to increased cancer risk, especially in PMP women (Figure 12-3).[9] Adipokines, leptin, and insulin induce aromatase expression in the mesenchymal cells surrounding the adipocytes, thereby further increasing the local estrogen concentration in the breast adipose tissue by upregulating the conversion of androstenedione to estrone and testosterone to estradiol. These changes are conducive to the development of cancer that is estrogen receptor (ER) positive. An association of aromatase levels and local breast inflammation, as measured by the

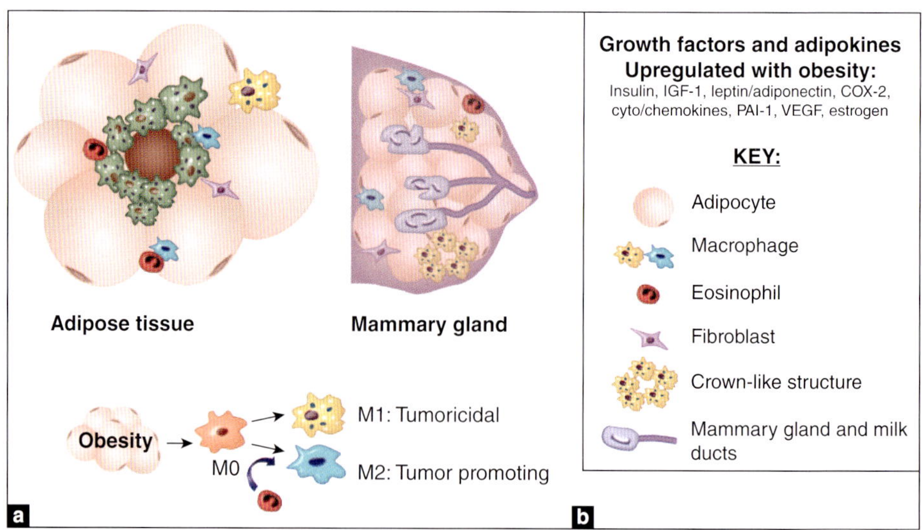

FIGURE 12-3. Obesity-related upregulation of growth factors and adipokines in mammary tissue. COX-2: cyclooxygenase 2; PAI-1: plasmingen activator inhibitor 1. (Redrawn from Sundaram S, Johnson AJ, Makowski L. Obesity, metabolism and the microenvironment: links to cancer. *J Carcinogen.* 2013;12:19.)

number of CLS-B, has been shown.[11] Estrogen promotes further cell proliferation, leading to increased expression of inflammatory mediators, thus establishing a positive-feedback loop in the breast microenvironment. This has implications for treatment and resistance to treatment in some women.

Macrophage infiltration in the microenvironment of ductal carcinoma in situ is associated with breast cancers that are high grade, ER negative (ER⁻) and progesterone receptor (PR) negative (PR⁻). The association of breast cancer and obesity in premenopausal women is less clear. Some studies supported an increased risk in obese premenopausal women, while others refuted it. A study from the National Surgical Adjuvant Breast and Bowel Project (NASBP) Cancer Prevention Trial showed that, in women over 35 years of age with a baseline elevated risk (Gail score > 1.66), the effect of overweight and obesity was additive compared to women with normal BMI.[12]

Animal models supported this association. In one study, premenopausal rats with diet-induced obesity had a 26% excess rate of mammary tumors compared to dietary-resistant rats with a higher proportion of ER⁻ tumors, a higher tumor burden, and a reduction in cancer latency.[13] There was also an adverse impact of weight gain on circulating levels of several of the factors discussed previously, including leptin, adiponectin-leptin ratio, insulin, and IGF-1.

Premenopausal women are at higher risk to develop triple-negative breast cancers [ER, PR, and human epidermal growth factor receptor 2 (*HER2/neu*)]. Paradoxically, obesity does seem to be a risk factor for triple-negative breast cancer in premenopausal women. The initial insult may be similar to that in obese PMP women with inflammatory changes and cytokine release. However, the epithelial cells in premenopausal women may undergo transition to mesenchymal cells caused in part by the leptin-induced increase in *Wnt* expression. Gene expression in these mesenchymal cells favors cell proliferation and invasion and may give rise to the triple-negative phenotype seen in premenopausal women. The details of these pathways and mechanisms remain to be elucidated.

Tumor Progression and Treatment Response

Along with being a risk factor for the development of breast cancer, obesity is a prognostic factor in stage at diagnosis and outcome. And, for most cancers in which obesity is a risk factor, the mortality risk mirrors that for incidence. In the Million Women Study, women with BMI greater than 30 had a 50% higher mortality than women with a normal BMI.[14] A similar association was found in the California Breast Cancer Survivorship Consortium.[15] In addition, breast tumors in obese women are more likely to be of higher histologic grade and more advanced stage than in women with normal BMI.

Leptin levels are significantly higher in PMP women with more advanced ER⁺ tumors, and leptin (along with BMI) is an independent predictor of stage in these women.[16] Leptin has been shown to activate ER transcription independent of estradiol, suggesting that leptin is involved in stimulation of growth of ER⁺ breast tumors through both autocrine and paracrine actions, the latter manifested as induction of aromatase in stromal cells of the breast tissue, as well as by influencing the secretion of other modulators of cell growth regulation. High leptin levels may contribute to tumor response to treatment by competing with antiestrogens at the ER and may cause antiestrogen resistance in some patients. Overexpression of leptin in breast cancer tissue may be a major factor in poor treatment response in some women because it promotes a positive-feedback loop for expression of factors essential for continued tumor promotion.

Leptin does not correlate with breast cancer stage in premenopausal women.

Risk Reduction Strategies

Maintenance of a healthy weight should be a primary disease prevention strategy as weight is one of the few modifiable cancer risk factors. Weight loss as a breast cancer prevention strategy in the United States should be promoted on a public health level; up to 17% of breast cancer cases could be prevented by weight loss, as confirmed by studies that have demonstrated a protective effect of weight loss in PMP women.[10] Unfortunately, data suggest that the incidence of obesity in the United States and worldwide continues to climb. Many women are not aware of the association between obesity and breast cancer, even women who have high awareness of other health consequences of obesity, such as hypertension and diabetes. This knowledge deficit was particularly high among black and Hispanic women, with close to 50% of these women in 1 study unaware of this association.[17]

There are multiple medical strategies under study for breast cancer treatment and possible prevention, which take advantage of anti-inflammatory and antiestrogenic properties. One strategy is the use of nonsteroidal anti-inflammatory medications (NSAIDs), such as cyclooxygenase 2 (COX-2) inhibitors. Epidemiological studies indicated that anti-inflammatory drugs reduce the risk of both ER^+ and ER^- breast cancer. CLS-Bs have been shown to produce excess amounts of COX-2-derived prostaglandin E_2, which is known to stimulate aromatase expression and estradiol production in preadipocytes. In vitro studies have shown that obesity-associated serum factors induce aromatase expression by way of induction of macrophage COX-2 expression.[18] This also led to increased ER-α activity in breast cancer cell lines. One retrospective study showed a better survival rate and longer disease-free survival in predominantly overweight and obese breast cancer patients who were taking COX-2 inhibitors than those who were not.

Another avenue that may be exploited in the fight to prevent breast cancer is the use of oral hypoglycemic agents such as metformin. Epidemiologic studies have shown an association between metformin use and decreased incidence of breast and other cancers. Metformin has been shown to induce downregulation of *ErbB2* (*HER2/ neu* equivalent in humans) expression in a mouse model.[19] *HER2/neu* is a membrane glycoprotein that is overexpressed in about 20%–30% of breast cancers and that has been correlated with poorer prognosis. Overexpression of *HER2/neu* may be associated with breakdown in the normal cell control mechanisms that would promote cell proliferation and a more aggressive tumor phenotype. Metformin may also decrease local and circulating insulin levels.

A third class of drugs, statins (used to treat hyperlipidemia), has shown potential as chemopreventive agents and has been shown to inhibit cell proliferation and induce apoptosis in in vitro models.[20] However, epidemiologic and prospective studies have revealed disappointing results. In the Women's Health Initiative (WHI), only small, nonsignificant reductions in breast cancer incidence were seen in users of a hydrophilic statin, and a small, statistically significant reduction was seen in users of a hydrophobic.[21]

Antiestrogens, such as the selective ER modulators (SERMs) tamoxifen and raloxifene, decrease the incidence of ER⁺ breast cancer in both premenopausal and PMP women by approximately 40%. The US Preventive Services Task Force (USPSTF) recommends increased use of these SERMs for primary prevention of ER⁺ breast cancer in women at high risk (5-year Gail model score > 1.67).[22] Exemestane, an aromatase inhibitor, has been shown to decrease the incidence of ER⁺ breast cancer in high-risk PMP women by approximately 70%[23] and is recommended as a primary prevention strategy by the American Society of Clinical Oncology.[24]

It is now apparent that the concept of obesity-induced overproduction of both systemic and local estrogen as the driving force for increased breast cancer risk in PMP women was a gross oversimplification. The pathways described that increase the likelihood of cancer development in obese individuals are operating in most tissues, but the enhancement of aromatase activity and estrogen production in the breast tissue add to its vulnerability to cancer initiation and progression. Future prevention strategies will likely use a multiprong approach aimed at minimizing the effects of hyperinsulinemia and excess leptin on inflammatory processes and estrogen production in the breast microenvironment.

COLORECTAL CANCER

Epidemiology

Colorectal carcinoma (CRC) is the third-leading cause of cancer-related mortality in the United States. The estimated number of new cases in US women in 2015 was 63,670, and the estimated number of deaths was 23,170. Risk factors for CRC include smoking, alcohol use, T2DM, personal history of colorectal polyps, inflammatory bowel disease (IBD), family history of colorectal cancer or adenomatous polyps, and certain familial cancer syndromes and lifestyle-related factors. Lifestyle risk factors, including diet rich in red and processed meats, physical inactivity, obesity, diabetes, and hyperinsulinemia, play a pivotal role in the etiology of the disease and account for approximately 70% of all cases. A mounting body of evidence suggests that insulin resistance and resulting hyperinsulinemia may be responsible for many of the associations of nutritional factors with CRC risk and for the high incidence of CRC in Westernized countries. A recent meta-analysis including 70,000 cases of CRC showed that individuals with a BMI of 30 or greater had a 20% greater risk of developing CRC compared with normal-weight individuals (BMI < 25 kg/m²).[25]

Obesity has emerged as a leading environmental risk factor in development of CRC, although the association of BMI with colon cancer is more evident in men (RR 1.41, CI 1.30–1.54) than in women (RR 1.08, CI 0.98–1.18). In general, abdominal obesity, measured by waist circumference (WC) and WHR, has shown the strongest association with risk of CRC compared to BMI. In the European Prospective Investigation Into Cancer and Nutrition (EPIC) study, the higher WHR was associated with an increased risk of colon cancer for women (RR 1.52) as well as for men (RR 1.51).[26]

Pathophysiology

The exact mechanism of the effect of obesity on colonic carcinogenesis is unknown. However, recent data suggest that adipocytokines could be the link between obesity and several gastrointestinal cancers. Adiponectin acts in an anticarcinogenic fashion, while leptin has more pro-tumorigenic properties. Visceral obesity is correlated with decreased adiponectin levels and increased leptin levels, which then promote carcinogenesis by the mechanisms discussed previously. In animal models, adiponectin knockout mice developed more colonic tumors when challenged with a carcinogen.[27] Also, when fed a high-fat diet, these mice developed larger tumors compared to mice fed a low-fat diet.[28]

In addition, in individuals with T2DM and metabolic syndrome, conditions characterized by long-standing insulin resistance, there are alterations in the metabolism of endogenous hormones, including insulin, IGFs, IGF-binding proteins, and sex steroids, conferring a higher risk of colon cancer. Both insulin and IGF-1 promote cell proliferation and inhibit apoptosis in colon cancer cells. Evidence also indicates that high circulating levels of C-peptide and elevated 2-hour glucose levels are associated with a greater risk of CRC or colonic adenoma.[29] It remains unclear whether this is due to direct effects of insulin on tumor growth or to closely related hormonal changes, such as an increase in bioavailable IGF-1. The understanding of the exact pathways still remains to be elucidated, but overall, the chronic inflammatory state caused by obesity combined with lifestyle factors such as poor dietary intake and limited physical activity over the life course of an individual all seem to support the development of colorectal cancer.

Tumor Progression and Treatment Response

The 5-year survival rate for 2004–2010 was 65% in the United States according to SEER data. Overall survival is highly dependent on disease stage at diagnosis, with the estimated 5-year survival rates ranging from 90% for patients with stage I disease to 13% for patients with stage IV disease. Obesity is also associated with increased rates of death and disease relapse compared to patients of normal weight. A study of survivors of stage II and stage III cancer following adjuvant chemotherapy showed that obesity was significantly associated with an increased number of metastatic regional lymph nodes compared with normal-weight patients, thus conferring an adverse prognosis. Obese patients were also more likely to have distal versus proximal colon cancers, and distal tumors have been shown to have a worse prognosis. Obese patients had higher rates of cancer recurrence, and mortality that was most evident overall for class 2 and 3 obesity (BMI ≥ 35).[30]

Risk Reduction Strategies

High BMI, visceral adiposity, and physical inactivity are consistent risk factors for colon adenoma and cancer. These factors are the major modifiable determinants of insulin resistance and hyperinsulinemia and of metabolic syndrome. Thus, an important risk reduction strategy is to increase physical activity and maintain a healthy weight. A review reported that the average reduction in risk of CRC was 40%–50% among physically active group individuals compared with the least active, independent of diet, BMI, and other potential confounders.[31] Furthermore, avoiding red and processed meat can help decrease the risk of CRC. PMP hormone therapy (HT) has also been associated with reduced risk of colon cancer, as noted in the WHI study.[32] There is some evidence that extensive use of metformin may be associated with a reduction in colon cancer risk and cancer-related mortality.

Early screening and detection/removal of polyps is an effective preventive strategy because most of the cancers arise from adenomatous polyps. Because obesity-related disorders such as T2DM and nonalcoholic fatty liver disease confer an increased risk for adenomatous polyps and CRC, more aggressive screening strategies in these individuals may be warranted. These strategies can include a recommendation to perform colonoscopy at the time of diagnosis of these disorders and have screening intervals that do not exceed 5 years in patients with T2DM.

ESOPHAGEAL CANCER

Epidemiology

Esophageal cancer is the eighth-most-common cancer worldwide and the sixth-most-common cause of cancer death. According to the American Cancer Society, the estimated number of new cases in US women in 2015 was 3450 with an estimated number of deaths of 2970. The incidence of cancer varies by gender, with a male-to-female ratio of 4:1. The lifetime risk of esophageal cancer in the United States is about 1 in 435 in women. Identified risk factors include advanced age, male gender, gastroesophageal reflux disease (GERD), Barrett's esophagus, smoking, alcohol, obesity, achalasia, Plummer-Vinson syndrome, and human papillomavirus (HPV) infection. Squamous cell type occurs in the middle of the esophagus and is the most prevalent worldwide. Adenocarcinoma occurs in the lower part of the esophagus and is the most common esophageal cancer in the United States. Its incidence has increased by 5-fold in Western countries over the last 3 decades. The reason for this dramatic increase has been linked to the rise in obesity in the United States. After endometrial cancer, it is the second-most-common cancer robustly associated with increased BMI. In data from the WHI, of 23 women with esophageal adenocarcinoma, 21 (91.3%) were in the top half of the distribution of the studied cohort with regard to WHR, WC, and BMI.[33] The prospective NIH-AARP (National Institutes of Health–AARP) Diet and Health Study found esophageal adenocarcinoma risk was highest for those with BMI above 35 kg.[34,35]

Pathophysiology

Identified risk factors for esophageal adenocarcinoma include gastroesophageal reflux disease, Barrett's esophagus, obesity, alcohol, and tobacco use. Obesity, in particular central adiposity, increases the risk for development of adenocarcinoma by two different mechanisms: reflux dependent and reflux independent.[36] Obesity promotes GERD through disruption of the gastroesophageal junction anatomy and physiology, which can lead to erosive esophagitis. Over time, squamous cells undergo metaplasia to columnar cells, resulting in Barrett's esophagus. The rate of malignant change of Barrett's esophagus to esophageal adenocarcinoma is between 0.2% and 10% per year.

In addition to this reflux-dependent mechanism, central adiposity independent of BMI has also been associated with development of esophageal disease through a reflux-independent mechanism. Thus, patients with metabolic syndrome are at higher risk. Metabolically active visceral adipose tissue releases pro-inflammatory cytokines, which may contribute to development of metaplasia and neoplasia through the pathways discussed previously. Increasing levels of adipokines are positively associated with risk of Barrett's esophagus among patients with GERD and among smokers. The exact mechanism is still unknown, but the higher concentration of adipokines possibly contributes to aberrant healing of esophageal injury caused by GERD, leading to Barrett's esophagus.[37] Obese individuals also have increased levels of epidermal growth factor, fibroblast growth factors, and transforming growth factors, all of which initiate processes that lead to esophageal metaplasia. It is also hypothesized that obesity alters the esophageal microbiome, which may further promote development of esophageal adenocarcinoma. Future studies are needed to fully elucidate the mechanisms involved.

Male propensity of esophageal cancer is likely secondary to the differences in fat storage between the two genders. Male adiposity is a measure of visceral fat compared to female adiposity being a measure of subcutaneous fat. Visceral fat has been linked specifically to the development of esophageal adenocarcinoma, as suggested by a study that utilized computed tomographic (CT) scan measurement of visceral fat versus subcutaneous fat. Patients with excess visceral fat were more prone to development of esophageal adenocarcinoma.

Tumor Progression and Treatment Response

Regardless of the histology, esophageal cancer is associated with poor prognosis. Only about 1 in 5 patients survive 5 years or more beyond the date of diagnosis. The estimated 5-year survival rate in the United States is only 18%. Secondary to the poor survival of patients with esophageal carcinoma, there is a greater need for emphasis on prevention and early detection. If the cancer is localized at time of detection, 5-year survival is up to 40%.

Risk Reduction Strategies

Primary prevention involves lifestyle changes, such as smoking cessation, avoidance of alcohol, diet rich in fruits and vegetables, maintenance of an active lifestyle to prevent obesity and central adiposity, and treatment of GERD with proton pump inhibitors. Secondary prevention involves chemopreventive agents and increased surveillance in patients with Barrett's esophagus, leading to earlier diagnosis and intervention. Some studies have found a decreased risk of esophageal adenocarcinoma in patients with Barrett's esophagus who take NSAIDs or statins, but these drugs are not advised as chemopreventive agents secondary to their side-effect profile.

PANCREATIC CANCER

Epidemiology

Pancreatic adenocarcinoma is the fourth-leading cause of cancer death. The estimated number of new cases in US women in 2015 was 25,400, and the estimated number of deaths was nearly as high, 20,330. Nonmodifiable risk factors include age, male gender, African American race, family history, genetic syndromes, long-standing T2DM, chronic pancreatitis, and liver cirrhosis. Modifiable risk factors include smoking, alcohol, overweight, and obesity. It has been estimated that the population-attributable percentage of obesity-associated pancreatic cancer is 26.9% for the US population.[37]

Pathophysiology

Obesity has been considered a risk factor for pancreatic diseases, including pancreatitis and pancreatic cancer. Severe acute pancreatitis is significantly more frequent in obese individuals. Numerous studies have investigated the role of overweight and obesity as a risk factor for pancreatic cancer. Although no definite mechanism is yet established, hyperinsulinemia and insulin resistance have been hypothesized as contributing factors. Obesity and physical inactivity increase insulin resistance. In a state of hyperinsulinemia, increased circulating levels of IGF-1 induce proliferation of islet cells and inhibit apoptosis, thus contributing to tumorigenesis. These mechanisms have been examined in hamster models, in which insulin resistance appears to play a key role; in these models, correction of insulin resistance prevented tumor development. The role of oxidative stress initiated by hyperglycemia also deserves further attention.[38]

A case-control study of 841 patients with pancreatic adenocarcinoma and 754 healthy individuals concluded that individuals who were overweight from the ages of 14 to 39 years or obese from the ages of 20 to 49 years had an increased risk of pancreatic cancer, independent of diabetes status.[39]

Tumor Progression and Treatment Response

Pancreatic cancer is a fatal malignancy and has one of the lowest survival rates of any cancer. The 5-year survival rate for 2004–2010 was around 7% in the United States according to SEER data. Radical surgery is the only treatment with curative intent that affects survival. Overweight or obesity not only increase the risk of developing pancreatic cancer but also are associated with decreased age of onset and with poor survival in patients with pancreatic cancer. Obesity at an older age or shortly before the cancer diagnosis was associated with a reduced overall survival time regardless of disease stage and tumor resection status.[39]

The survival rate has improved slightly in recent years secondary to increased use of resection, improved surgical techniques, and increased use of adjuvant chemotherapy. In general, the high mortality is due to advanced disease stage at the time of diagnosis and the limited effectiveness of systemic therapies. Only a small percentage of patients, about 15%–20%, have a resectable tumor. Recurrence and death from disease occur in the vast majority of patients.

Risk Reduction Strategies

Smoking and obesity are two major risk factors. Smoking is responsible for 20%–30% of pancreatic cancers and obesity for another 25%. Thus, major risk reduction strategies include smoking cessation; staying at a healthy weight by diet and exercise, including a diet rich in fruits and vegetables; as well as avoidance of processed meat and red meat.

GALLBLADDER CANCER

Epidemiology

The estimated number of new cases of gallbladder cancer (GBC) in US women in 2015 was 6150, and the estimated number of deaths was 2080. The main risk factors for gallbladder cancer are age greater than 65, female gender, gallstones, gallbladder polyps, porcelain gallbladder, primary sclerosing cholangitis, abnormalities of the bile duct, endogenous and exogenous estrogens, overweight, and obesity. Most of the aforementioned risk factors are related in some way to chronic inflammation, leading to scarring and irritation of the gallbladder mucosa. The higher incidence of gallbladder disease and cancer in women can partly be explained by the effect of endogenous and exogenous estrogen on the biliary tract, including long duration of use of oral contraceptive pills and PMP HT.

Pathophysiology

Obesity increases risk of gallbladder diseases and GBC. The EPIC study involved a mean follow-up of 8.6 years, in which 86 cases of GBC were diagnosed. A case-control study using a subset of patients in the EPIC study found an association of general and abdominal obesity with risk of GBC.[40] The mechanism is not well established, but there are several plausible explanations. Obesity-related metabolic disorders such as insulin resistance and hyperinsulinemia promote hepatic cholesterol secretion, leading to supersaturation of cholesterol in bile, thus promoting gallstone formation. Obese individuals are also likely to have large gallbladder volume, leading to slower evacuation of the gallbladder and mucosal abnormalities, both of which are associated with gallstone formation. In addition, obesity-induced chronic inflammation caused by inflammatory products and oxidative stress may contribute to biliary tissue damage and predispose to malignant transformation of gallbladder epithelial cells.

In a meta-analysis of prospective studies, the relative risk of biliary cancer increased by 1.11 for each increment of 5 kg/m^2 increase in BMI.[41] Several studies have demonstrated that, as BMI increases, the relative risk of GBC increases. A Norwegian study with 1715 cases of GBC showed that the RR of GBC in women with BMI 35–39.9 was 2.56, and in women with BMI of 40 or greater, the RR for GBC was 2.77.[42] Another case-control study, with 627 patients with biliary tract cancer, showed that adults with a BMI of 25 or greater had a 1.6-fold higher RR of GBC than normal subjects.[43]

Tumor Progression and Treatment Response

Biliary tract cancer is a highly lethal neoplasm and is associated with a poor prognosis because of late diagnosis and few effective treatment options. Lack of good screening tests, lack of symptoms at an early stage, and inability to palpate any abnormalities during a routine physical exam are some of the factors that contribute to advanced-stage cancer at the time of diagnosis. Only 20% are diagnosed at an early stage. Survival rate at stage I is 50%, while stage IV survival is 2%–4%. Overall 5-year survival rate is less than 20%.

Risk Reduction Strategies

Control of obesity through measures such as lifestyle modification, healthy diet, and regular exercise may prove useful in the prevention of GBC. Prophylactic cholecystectomy for patients with a long-standing history of gallstones or patients with porcelain gallbladder should be considered.

KIDNEY CANCER

Epidemiology

The incidence of kidney cancer is increasing worldwide. In the United States, 61,560 new cases of kidney cancer were expected to be diagnosed in 2015, of which 23,050 would be in women with a death rate of 5000. Improvement in diagnostic modalities has definitely played a role but does not account for the increased incidence entirely. Renal cell carcinoma (RCC) is the major type of kidney cancer and accounts for 80%–90% of all cases. The etiology of RCC is still largely undefined, although potential risk factors have been recognized, including tobacco smoking, obesity, genetic and hereditary risk factors like Von Hippel-Lindau disease, exposure to certain substances like cadmium and trichloroethylene, hypertension, and a family history of kidney cancer. Several studies worldwide have demonstrated the influence of BMI on renal carcinogenesis.

In the Million Women Study,[14] which recruited 1.2 million women who were followed for the development of cancer and cancer mortality, a significant correlation was found between kidney cancer and increased BMI. RCC was the third-highest cancer most robustly associated with increased BMI, following endometrial and esophageal adenocarcinoma. In the EPIC trial involving 348,550 individuals, women with a weight or BMI in the top quintile had a 2-fold increased risk of RCC after adjusting for smoking and other risk factors.[44] Among women, all measures of obesity, including BMI, body weight, and waist and hip circumference, were related to an increased risk of RCC. Clear cell cancer is the histologic subtype most strongly associated with obesity. The risk for the development of RCC has been directly correlated with increased weight in a dose-response manner, with an estimated increase of 34% for women for every 5 kg/m^2 increase in BMI.

Pathophysiology

The exact mechanism of obesity-related development of RCC is unclear, but several mechanisms have been proposed. Obese patients have higher levels of adipose tissue, which lead to increased levels of insulin and IGF-1, known to have cancer-promoting effects. Upregulation of leptin and downregulation of adiponectin play a major role in RCC pathogenesis.[45] In addition, obese patients tend to have other comorbidities, such as hypertension and diabetes, which are known risk factors for RCC. Other mechanisms include increased estrogen levels and decreased immune function in patients with metabolic syndrome and or obesity.

Tumor Progression and Treatment Response

The 5-year survival rate varies based on the stage of diagnosis, with a survival rate of 92% for local disease but only 12% for distant disease. Unfortunately, approximately one-fourth of patients have metastatic disease at time of diagnosis.

Risk Reduction Strategies

In many cases, the cause of kidney cancer is not known. Heritable conditions that raise the risk of RCC are not modifiable. The most important risk reduction strategies include smoking cessation and maintenance of a healthy weight. Avoiding workplace exposure to harmful substances may also help reduce risk.

THYROID CANCER

Epidemiology

Thyroid cancer is the most common endocrine-related malignancy and accounts for approximately 9% of solid-organ malignancies in women. The incidence of thyroid cancer is estimated to be 2–3.8/100,000 women. The estimated number of new cases in US women in 2015 was 49,350, and the estimated number of deaths was 1070. The main risk factors for thyroid cancer are age, female gender, iodine deficiency, exposure to ionizing radiation, a history of benign thyroid disease like goiter, thyroid nodules, Hashimoto thyroiditis, and a family history of thyroid cancer. Thyroid cancer occurs 3 times more often in women than in men.

Recently, chronic inflammatory conditions such as obesity have been shown to be an independent risk factor for the development of thyroid cancer. Since 1980, the incidence of thyroid cancer in the United States has nearly tripled,[46] concurrent with the doubling of obesity. This increase in incidence of thyroid cancer is partly due to not only increased diagnostic scrutiny but also secondary to an increase in differentiated thyroid carcinomas, and more specifically, papillary thyroid carcinomas.[47] This suggests that an increasing exposure to risk factors may be contributing to this noticeable surge.

Results from case-control studies,[48] as well as prospective studies,[49] have suggested a moderate positive association between BMI and thyroid cancer risk, notably in women. A meta-analysis of relevant published cohort studies done in 2012 demonstrated a statistically significant association between BMI and thyroid cancer risk for males (overweight, $p = .007$; obesity, $p < .001$; excess body weight, $p < .001$) and females (obesity, $p = .002$; excess body weight, $p < .001$). The strength of the association increases with increasing BMI.[50]

Pathophysiology

The mechanism by which obesity effects development of thyroid cancer is largely unknown. There is a complex interplay of five important factors (thyroid hormones; adipokines; inflammation; insulin resistance; and sex hormones, mainly estrogen) in individuals with excess weight (Figure 12-4).[51] Insulin resistance (IR) may be a central mediator of risk. Expanding adipose tissue leads to IR, an abnormal cytokine profile, and inflammation, which creates a vicious cycle and may contribute to the pathogenesis of thyroid cancer, a theme that is repeated throughout this chapter. The exact understanding of the mechanism by which they interfere with thyroid hormones is still poor, but these factors not only lead to onset of thyroid tumor but also affect progression and aggressiveness of such tumors.[51] Estrogen is a potent growth factor for both benign and malignant thyroid cells and plays a role in the regulation of angiogenesis and metastasis, thus contributing to the difference in clinical evolution of thyroid cancer between genders.

Tumor Progression and Treatment Response

Thyroid cancer has one of the highest survival rates of any cancer in women. The 5-year survival rate for 2004–2010 was around 98% in the United States. Obesity not only is associated with an increased risk of thyroid cancer but also could exert an influence on tumor presentation. A 5-kg/m^2 increase in BMI was associated with papillary thyroid cancers larger than 1 cm, microscopic extrathyroidal invasion, and advanced tumor/node metastases.[52] The high survival rate is secondary to availability of excellent treatment modalities involving any combination of surgery, radioactive iodine, radiation, and chemotherapy.

Risk Reduction Strategies

Most people with thyroid cancer have no known risk factors; thus, prevention is challenging. In the United States, most people get enough iodine in their diet secondary to iodination of salt and other foods. Limiting childhood radiation exposure and increased surveillance of patients with family history will help with prevention and early detection. An increased awareness and a better understanding of the pathogenic mechanisms linking obesity and insulin resistance with thyroid cancer would enable

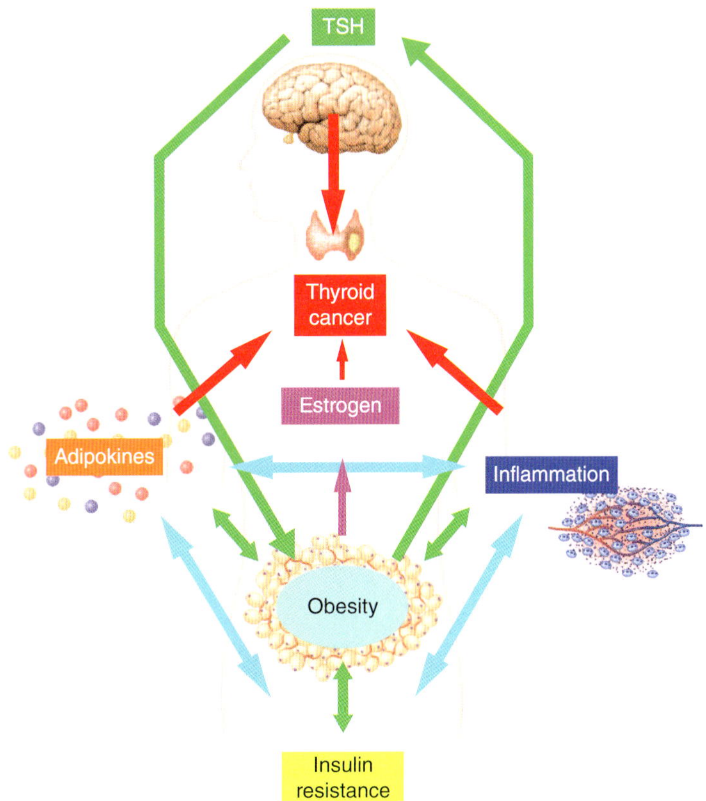

FIGURE 12-4. Factors contributing to obesity-related thyroid cancer. (From Marcello MA, Cunha LL, Batista FA, Ward LS. Obesity and thyroid cancer. *Endocr Relat Cancer*. 2014;21:255–271.)

the clinician to use a guided approach combining various modalities in the prevention and treatment of thyroid cancer. It is crucial to identify the at-risk population and perform early screening to help decrease morbidity, mortality, and recurrence risks. Risk-based ultrasound screening has been proposed in the obese population and was found to be cost effective in a subgroup of obese patients with 1 or more of the 4 identifiable risk factors for thyroid cancer: family history of thyroid cancer, radiation exposure, Hashimoto thyroiditis, and elevated thyroid-stimulating hormone (TSH). A combination of lifestyle changes and pharmacological methods can further aid in prevention of thyroid cancer and its risk of recurrence. Risk-based ultrasound screening in overweight/obese at-risk patients can aid in early detection of thyroid cancer.

SUMMARY

Cancer Mortality

Increasingly, evidence suggests that being overweight or obese raises the risk of cancer recurrence and may lower the chances of survival for many cancers. Thus, both during and after cancer treatment, people should try to become and to stay at a healthy weight whenever possible.

Risk Reduction Strategies

The American Cancer Society recommends maintaining a healthy weight throughout life, best achieved by primary prevention of overweight through a balance of food intake with energy expenditure by physical activity. However, faced with our current prevalence of obesity in the United States, prevention strategies that go beyond lifestyle modification will be needed. Pharmacologic and surgical modification of risk is already possible for some cancers, such as breast cancer, and evidence suggests that these may affect the risk of many other obesity-related cancers.

Diet

Overweight patients are encouraged to decrease portion sizes, limit between-meal snacking, and limit drinks containing high calories, fat, and added sugars. Diet modifications should also include replacement of fried foods and high-sugar/high-carbohydrate foods with vegetables and fruits, whole grains, beans, and lower-calorie beverages. Even if an ideal weight is not reached, studies have shown that modest weight loss still has health benefits.

Exercise

Adults should get at least 150 minutes of moderate-intensity or 75 minutes of vigorous-intensity activity each week (or a combination of these). Increased physical activity is important in promoting weight loss and in keeping weight off. Limiting sedentary behavior is recommended. If every adult reduced his or her BMI by 1%, which would be equivalent to a weight loss of roughly 1 kg (or 2.2 lb) for an adult of average weight, this would prevent the increase in the number of cancer cases and actually result in the avoidance of about 100,000 new cases of cancer over the next several years.

Future Research

Future research is crucial in many different facets of obesity-related cancer, including pathophysiology, prevention strategies, and, last, treatment modalities. A better understanding of the complex mechanisms, such as the roles of leptin, hyperinsulinemia, and various adipocytokines, on obesity-related cancers will be helpful. In addition, therapies directed at patient-specific adipocytokine and genetic profiles should be considered. The role of medications such as NSAIDs, statins, and antiestrogens in the prevention of cancer deserves continued attention. Effect of interventions such as bariatric surgery on reduction of cancer risk should further be elucidated to aid in counseling women about effective risk reduction strategies. This will help improve patient and clinician knowledge of the role of obesity in relation to cancer risk and motivate individuals to maintain a healthy lifestyle.

REFERENCES

1. Siegel RL, Miller KD, Jemal A. Cancer statistics, 2015. *CA Cancer J Clin.* 2015;65(1):5–29.
2. Wolin KY, Carson K, Colditz GA. Obesity and cancer. *Oncologist.* 2010;15:556–565.
3. Ogden CL, Carroll MD, Kit BK, Flegal KM. Prevalence of childhood and adult obesity in the United States, 2011–2012. *JAMA.* 2014;311(8):806–814.
4. American Cancer Society, Inc. *Surveillance Research 2015.*
5. Renehan AG, Tyson M, Egger M, Heller RF, Zwahlen M. Body-mass index and incidence of cancer: a systematic review and meta-analysis of prospective observational studies. *Lancet.* 2008;371(9612):569–578.
6. Ouchi N, Parker JL, Lugus JJ, Walsh K. Adipokines in inflammation and metabolic disease. *Nature Rev Immunol.* 2011;11:85–97.
7. Rose DP, Vona-Davis L. Biochemical and molecular mechanisms for the association between obesity,

chronic inflammation, and breast cancer. *BioFactors*. 2013;40:1–12.

8. Park J, Schere PE. Leptin and cancer: from cancer stem cells to metastasis. *Endocr Relat Cancer*. 2011;18:C25–C29.

9. Sundaram S, Johnson AJ, Makowski L. Obesity, metabolism and the microenvironment: links to cancer. *J Carcinogen*. 2013;12:19.

10. Eliassen AH, Colditz GA, Rosner B, et al. Adult weight change and risk of postmenopausal breast cancer. *JAMA*. 2006;296:193–201.

11. Morris PG, Hudis CA, Morrow M, et al. Inflammation and increased aromatase expression occur in the breast tissue of obese women with breast cancer. *Cancer Prev Res*. 2011;4(7):1021–9.

12. Cecchini RS, Costantino JP, Cauley JA, et al. Body mass index and the risk of developing invasive breast cancer among high-risk women in NASPB P-1 and STAR breast cancer prevention trials. *Cancer Prev Res*. 2012;5:583–592.

13. Matthews SB, Zhu Z, Jiang W, et al. Excess weight gain accelerates 1-mtethyl-1-nitrosourea-induced mammary carcinogenesis in a rat model of premenopausal breast cancer. *Cancer Prev Res*. 2014;7:310–318.

14. Reeves GK, Pirie K, Beral V, et al. Cancer incidence and mortality in relation to body mass index in the Million Women Study; cohort study. *BMJ*. 2007;335(7630):1134–1144.

15. Kwan ML, John EM, Caan BJ, et al. Obesity and mortality after breast cancer by race/ethnicity: the California Breast Cancer Survivorship Consortium. *Am J Epidemiol*. 2014;179:95–111.

16. Maccio A, Mededdu C, Gramignano G, et al. Corrleation of body mass index and leptin with tumor size and stage of disease in hormone-dependent postmenopausal breast cancer: preliminary results and therapeutic implications. *J Mol Med*. 2010;88:677–686.

17. Winston GJ, Caeser-Phillips E, Peterson JC, et al. Knowledge of the health consequences of obesity among overweight/obese black and Hispanic adults. *Patient Educ Counsel*. 2014;94:123–127.

18. Bowers LW, Maximo IXF, Brenner AJ, et al. NSAID use reduces breast cancer recurrence in overweight and obese women: role of prostaglandin-aromatase interactions. *Cancer Res*. 2014;74:4446–4457.

19. Zhu P, Davis M, Blackwelder AJ, et al. Metformin selectively targets tumor-initiating cells in *ErbB-2*-overexpressing breast cancer models. *Cancer Prev Res*. 2013;7:199–210.

20. Seeger H, Wallwiener D, Mueck AO. Statins can inhibit proliferation of human breast cancer cells in vitro. *Exp Clin Endocrinol Diabetes*. 2003;111:47–48.

21. Cauley JA, McTiernan A, Rodabough RJ, et al. Statin use and breast cancer: prospective results from the Women's Health Initiative. *J Natl Cancer Inst*. 2006;98:700–707.

22. Nelson HD, Smith ME, Griffin JC, Fu R. Use of medications to reduce risk for primary breast cancer: a systematic review for the US Preventive Services Task Force. *Ann Int Med*. 2013;158:604–614.

23. Goss PE, Ingle JN, Martinez A, et al. Exemestane for breast cancer prevention in postmenopausal women. *N Engl J Med*. 2011;364:2381–2391.

24. Visavanthan K, Hurley P, Bantug E, et al. Use of pharmacologic interventions for breast cancer risk reduction: American Society of Clinical Oncology clinical practice guideline. *J Clin Oncol*. 2013;31:2942–2962.

25. Moghaddam A, Woodward M, Huxley R. Obesity and risk of colorectal cancer: a meta-analysis of 31 studies with 70,000 events. *Cancer Epidemiol Biomarkers Prev*. 2007;16(12):2533–2547.

26. Pischon T, Lahmann PH, Boeing H, et al. Body size and risk of colon and rectal cancer in the European Prospective Investigation into Cancer and Nutrition (EPIC). *J Natl Cancer Inst*. 2006;98:920–931.

27. Saxena A, Baliga MS, Ponemone V, et al. Mucus and adiponectin deficiency: role in chronic inflammation-induced colon cancer. *Int J Colorectal Dis*. 2013;28:1267–1279.

28. Moon HS, Liu X, Nagel JM, et al. Salutary effects of adiponectin on colon cancer: in vivo and in vitro studies in mice. *Gut*. 2013;62:561–570.

29. Wei E, Ma J, Pollak M, et al. A prospective study of C-peptide, insulin like growth factor-1, insulin-like growth factor binding protein-1, and the risk of colorectal cancer in women. *Cancer Epidemiol Biomarkers Prev*. 2005;14(4):850–855.

30. Sinicrope FA, Foster NR, Sargent DJ, O'Connell MJ, Rankin C. Obesity is an independent prognostic variable in colon cancer survivors. *Clin Cancer Res*. 2010;16(6):1884–1893.

31. Friedenrich CM. Physical activity and cancer prevention: from observational to interventional research. *Cancer Epidemiol Biomarkers Prev*. 2001;10:287–301.

32. Rossouw JE, Anderson GL, Prentice RL, et al. Risks and benefits of estrogen plus progestin in healthy postmenopausal women: principal results from the Women's Health Initiative randomized controlled trial. *JAMA*. 2002;288(3):321–333.

33. Bodelon C, Anderson GL, Rossing MA, Chlebowski RT, Ochs-Balcom HM, Vaughan TL. Hormonal factors and risks of esophageal squamous cell carcinoma and adenocarcinoma in postmenopausal women. *Cancer Prev Res*. 2011;4(6):840–850.

34. O'Doherty MG, Freedman ND, Hollenbeck AR et al. A prospective cohort study of obesity and risk of oesophageal and gastric adenocarcinoma in the NIH-AARP Diet and Health Study. *Gut*. 2012;61(9):1261–1268.

35. Singh S, Sharma AN, Murad MH, et al. Central adiposity is associated with increased risk of esophageal inflammation, metaplasia, and adenocarcinoma: a systematic review and meta-analysis. *Clin Gastroenterol Hepatol.* 2013;11:1399–1412.

36. Alemán JO, Eusebi LH, Ricciardiello L, Patidar K, Sanyal AJ, Holt PR. Mechanisms of obesity-induced gastrointestinal neoplasia. *Gastroenterology.* 2014;146(2):357–373.

37. Calle EE, Kaaks R. Overweight, obesity and cancer: epidemiological evidence and proposed mechanism. *Nat Rev Cancer.* 2004;4(8):579–591.

38. Giovannucci E, Michaud D. The role of obesity and related metabolic disturbances in cancers of the colon, prostate and pancreas. *Gastroenterology.* 2007;132:2208–2225.

39. Li D, Morris J, Liu J, et al. Body mass index and risk, age of onset, and survival in patients with pancreatic cancer. *JAMA.* 2009;301(24):2553–2562.

40. Schlesinger S, Aleksandrova K, Pischon T, et al. Abdominal obesity, weight gain during adulthood and risk of liver and biliary tract cancer in a European cohort. *Int J Cancer.* 2013;132:645–657.

41. Park M, Song DY, Je Y, Lee JE. Body mass index and biliary tract disease: a systematic review and meta-analysis of prospective studies. *Prev Med.* 2014;65:13–22.

42. Engeland A, Tretli S, Austad G, et al. Height and body mass index in relation to colorectal and gallbladder cancer in two million Norwegian men and women. *Cancer Causes Control.* 2005;16:987–996.

43. Hsing AW, Sakoda LC, Rashid A, et al. Body size and the risk of biliary tract cancer: a population-based study in China. *Br J Cancer.* 2008;99:811–815.

44. Pischon T, Lahmann PH, Boeing H, et al. Body size and risk of renal cell carcinoma in the European Prospective Investigation Into Cancer and Nutrition (EPIC). *Int J Cancer.* 2006;118:728–738.

45. Altekruse SF, Kosary CL, Krapcho M, et al., eds. *SEER Cancer Statistics Review, 1975–2007.* Bethesda, MD: National Cancer Institute. http://seer.cancer.gov/csr/1975_2007. Based on November 2009 SEER data submission; posted to the SEER website 2010.

46. Drabkin HA, Gemmill RM. Obesity, cholesterol and clear-cell renal cell carcinoma. *Adv Cancer Res.* 2010;107:39–56.

47. Pellegriti G, Frasca F, Regalbuto C, Squatrito S, Vigneri R. Worldwide increasing incidence of thyroid cancer: update on epidemiology and risk factors. *J Cancer Epidemiol.* 2013;2013:965212.

48. Clero E, Leux C, Brindel P, et al. Pooled analysis of two case-control studies in New Caledonia and French Polynesia of body mass index and differentiated thyroid cancer: the importance of body surface area. *Thyroid.* 2010;20(11):1285–1293.

49. Kitahara CM, Platz EA, Freeman LE, et al. Obesity and thyroid cancer risk among US men and women: a pooled analysis of five prospective studies. *Cancer Epidemiol Biomarkers Prev.* 2011;20(3):464–472.

50. Zhao ZG, Guo XG, Ba CX, et al. Overweight, obesity and thyroid cancer risk, a meta-analysis of cohort studies. *J Int Med Res.* 2012;40(6):2041–2050.

51. Marcello MA, Cunha LL, Batista FA, Ward LS. Obesity and thyroid cancer. *Endocr Relat Cancer.* 2014;21:255–271.

52. Kim HJ, Kim NK, Choi JH, et al. Associations between body mass index and clinico-pathological characteristics of papillary thyroid cancer. *Clin Endocrinol.* 2013;78(1):134–140.

CHAPTER 13

Critical Care

David Landsberg, MD, FACP, FCCP

INTRODUCTION

The "obesity paradox," as it is termed, may at first glance seem counterintuitive, but on reflection by the experienced intensive care unit (ICU) clinician, it quickly is found to be consistent with clinical observation. The obesity paradox refers to a literature body that supports decreased mortality in obese ICU patients when compared to nonobese patients of otherwise-matched demography and complexity of illness. While the morbidly obese patient may need more complex care and may be more apt to suffer certain complications, the obese patient has also been shown to be more likely to survive. More simply, it has been shown that despite the increased morbidity associated with obese ICU patients, there is also an association of decreased mortality.

It is the goal of this chapter to highlight these potential areas of increased morbidity as well as areas where usual management schema will need to be adjusted to these patients' unique physiology. Wherever possible, I draw attention to any available data specific to the obese female population, although the overwhelming bulk of available literature on this topic is not gender specific (Figure 13-1).

SEPSIS

Infections and Antimicrobials

Obesity has been recognized as a risk factor for both morbidity and mortality in patients infected with H1N1 influenza. The Centers for Disease Control and Prevention (CDC) considers morbid obesity a high-risk condition for 2009 H1N1-related

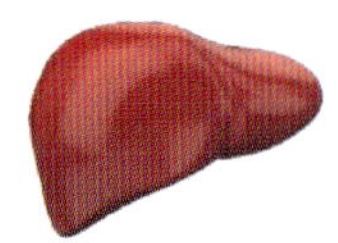
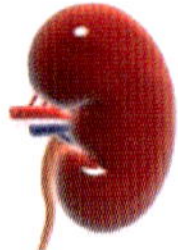
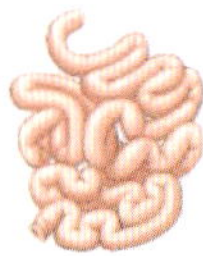
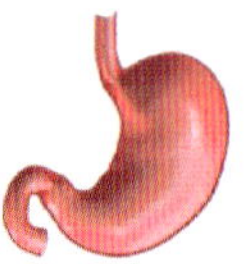

Reduced hepatic metabolism due to steatosis; variable effect on cytochrome P-450	Increased glomerular filtration rate; obesity-associated kidney failure	Increased lipophilic intestinal absorption	Delayed gastric emptying decreasing absorption

FIGURE 13-1. Physiological effects of obesity.

hospitalization and possibly death.[1] A study of 534 patients in California with H1N1 in 2009 found that, at a body mass index (BMI) of 40, the odds ratio (OR) of death was 2.8; for those patients with BMI greater than 45, the OR for death increased a further 50% to 4.2.[1] During the same year, a study of 1520 patients in the United Kingdom also identified obesity as an independent risk factor for H1N1-associated morbidity greater than that associated with delayed admission, pneumonia, and the need for supplemental oxygen.[2] There is also evidence that vaccination may be less effective in obese patients, with the rate of titer decay having been shown to be significantly more rapid in this population.[3]

Bacterial pneumonia as both a primary and a secondary infection has inconsistently been associated with obesity, but even in the studies that favored obesity as a risk factor for pneumonia, the paradox of increased survival generally remained present.[4-6] The development of community-acquired *Clostridium difficile* infection was associated with obesity in a 2013 Boston study.[7] A 2008 randomized controlled trial found a higher rate of infection associated with femoral catheters placed in obese as compared to nonobese patients, while a 2009 study of over 2000 ICU patients found severe obesity to be a risk factor for catheter-related (OR 2.2) and other bloodstream infections (OR 3.2).[8,9] It is not known whether the biology of obesity is responsible for the aforementioned associations or if habitus itself is the progenitor of these complications.

I have long used whole-body chlorhexidine bathing for the morbidly obese population in the ICU. Anecdotally, we have had great success with this strategy, with the underlying assumption that increased skin surface and areas of intertrigo predispose to colonization and substantial bioburdens. In more recent years, there is evidence to suggest this practice be adopted to prevent central line–associated blood stream infections (CLABSIs) for all patients.[10,11] If the strategy is, in fact, effective, then one could postulate that patients with greater body surface area (BSA) should stand to enjoy the benefit from the intervention.

We know that obesity can, itself, predispose to infection.[12-14] We also know that the treatment of infection may be complicated by morbid obesity when one endeavors to adequately dose antibiotics, especially in the setting of life-threatening infection. Antimicrobials are often dosed by ideal or actual body weight, but this becomes problematic when the distribution volume of some antibiotics will so vastly exceed that predicted by any body weight dosing schema. This runs the risk of clinically important underdosing of antibiotics not only affecting the index patient but also contributing to resistance through pathogen exposure to subtherapeutic inhibitory concentrations.

There are data for piperacillin-tazobactam in patients with BMIs over 40 (study group mean BMI of 57) that showed that the dosing regimen of 4.5 g every 6 hours was adequate for minimum inhibitory concentration (MIC) attainment for likely pathogens in this population.[15] Interestingly, the study found that the half-life of the drug was approximately 3-fold historical controls of normal BMI, which actually increased the area under the curve for time above MIC. This decreased clearance coupled with dosing at the highest end of the recommended range resulted in adequate dosing of piperacillin-tazobactam and is a theme seen with β-lactams in general.[15]

In a study of 48 critically ill patients on vancomycin, it was found that standard pharmacokinetic modeling was more likely to be inaccurate in obese patients.[16] A 2014 literature review found that obesity was a significant confounder for accuracy of aminoglycoside dosing but, most troublingly, also found that the inaccuracy resulted in both subtherapeutic and supratherapeutic dosing.[17] A study of carbapenem dosing was published in 2013 that concluded that the use of extended infusions could minimize the effects of patient weight and large volumes of distribution on achievement of adequate MICs.[18] There are also data to implicate that almost 3-fold dosing can be required for lipophilic antibiotics (fluoroquinolones, macrolides, glycylcyclines, and lincosamides) in the obese population due to the enhanced adipose volume of distribution.[19,20] In obese patients on continuous renal replacement therapy, there are recommendations to dose ciprofloxacin as high as 800 mg every 12 hours.[21]

While there is a paucity of literature, overall general guidelines to aid the practitioner should be based on the pharmacokinetic data referenced above. Of note, a 2010 study found no correlation between increasing body weight and in vivo volume of distribution for the metabolite of oseltamivir with the plasma concentration exceeding the needed threshold many fold throughout the dosing interval.[22]

Renal Failure

Renal failure has been observed to occur disproportionately in the obese critically ill patient. A study of 751 patients with acute respiratory distress syndrome (ARDS) found that the OR of acute kidney injury (AKI) increased by 1.2 for every 5 kg/m^2 increase in BMI. The same study also found that the OR for mortality was 0.81 for every 5 kg/m^2 increase in BMI.[23] Among 562 critically ill Canadian patients with H1N1, the OR for obesity as an independent predictor of AKI was 2.94, and the OR was 2.25 for renal replacement therapy.[24] Among 400 trauma patients, obesity was found to confer an OR of 4.72 for AKI.[25] The apparent propensity for renal failure in the obese patient may be biology, or it may be related to a tendency to underresuscitate in this population due to barriers in perception of what defines an adequate volume of crystalloid in an obese patient.

Hemodynamic Support

The first and most important reality to digest is that the volume of fluid that will be required to adequately resuscitate a morbidly obese patient may be in the tens of liters. The Surviving Sepsis Campaign recommends 30 kg/m^2 of initial bolus resuscitation to adequately challenge a patient in septic shock.[26] Some quick math yields some extraordinary numbers. These volumes, while they may seem extreme, are appropriate and suited to the extreme sizes to which they are ascribed. To use less in the face of ongoing hypoperfusion in respect of arbitrary norms of resuscitation would be inappropriate and an injustice to these patients. It should also be understood that the prevalence of obstructive sleep apnea (OSA) and obesity hypoventilation syndrome (OHS) in the population of patients with BMIs exceeding 40 is as high as 70% and 30%, respectively, in some studies.[27–29]

This becomes important in a discussion of hemodynamic support when one realizes the prevalence of pulmonary hypertension and subsequent right heart failure this will engender. In practice, I assume embarrassed right heart function in the presence of morbid obesity and venous stasis of the lower extremities until echocardiography refutes that assessment. The presence of right heart dysfunction will generally magnify the usual fluid requirements in resuscitation of a vasodilatory shock.

The use of bedside ultrasonography often yields a technically limited evaluation in these patients due to their habitus further complicating their management by confounding, while not completely incapacitating, this tool that has become so common in the practice of critical care. If a pulmonary artery catheter is in place, some guidance can be gleaned from a 2006 study of 700 consecutive patients taken for angiography who had clean coronaries and a cardiac output (CO) measurement during the angiography. BMI was found to positively correlate with CO and stroke volume (SV). Each 1 kg/m^2 increase in BMI was found to give a 0.08 L/min increase in CO and 1.35 mL increase in SV.[30]

Given the increased risk for AKI in this population, hemodynamic support and adequacy of resuscitation volume should be followed vigilantly by whatever means one chooses. There are no conclusive data to support one over another.

On the note of measurement, I would challenge the dogma of the superiority of invasive monitoring. There are no high-quality data in the literature to support improved outcomes with invasive versus noninvasive approaches of monitoring in critical care.[31,32] That said, upper arm girth may be a practical limitation to reliable blood pressure measurement; certainly, in absence of any other means to measure blood pressure, an arterial line will give you not only a reading but also a gold standard reading. Alternatively, there are relatively new products available designed to take forearm blood pressure measurements. At least one of these devices is clinically validated specifically for measuring blood pressure in the forearm of obese patients. (Critikon Radial-Cuf by GE Healthcare). Beyond these pitfalls, the principles of hemodynamic monitoring and resuscitation remain the same.

RESPIRATORY FAILURE

The primary pitfalls in the respiratory management of the obese patient relate to the weight of the chest wall, especially while supine, and its effect on the airway as well as mechanics of respiration. Obese patients are more prone to hypoxia than leaner individuals as a result of reductions in multiple pulmonary function parameters. They include forced vital capacity (FVC), forced expiratory volume in 1 second (FEV$_1$), expiratory reserve volume (ERV), functional residual capacity (FRC), and maximum voluntary ventilation (MVV).[33] Pregnancy also results in substantial reductions in ERV and FRC.[34] It is not known whether the usual increase in tidal volume of 30%–40% in pregnancy is attenuated in the obese patient by lower baseline ERV and FRC.

Pulmonary complications of obesity include OSA and OHS and some have suggested asthma, although others have argued it is more a subjective dyspnea than true reactive airway disease.[35-37] This chapter also addresses the life-threatening pulmonary complications specific to pregnancy and where their diagnosis and management may be complicated by obesity.

Noninvasive Ventilation

The prevalence of OSA and OHS in this population is substantial, as mentioned previously, and should be anticipated when caring for the obese patient irrespective of initial indications for admission. This can include interventions such as screening with simple questions all the way to subspecialist consultation. Obese patients who are expected to receive sedatives or analgesics during their stay are at especially high risk for respiratory complications as any tendency for hypoventilation will be magnified by these drugs. These patients should be considered for more careful monitoring through means such as remote oximetry and capnography as well as tighter nursing ratios.

I recommend, in those patients for whom a surgical procedure is elective who screen positive for the possibility of OSA, that there be consideration given for deferment of elective surgery. Where surgery should not be deferred, patients should be considered for empiric monitoring and subspecialist consultation for the provision of empiric noninvasive positive pressure ventilation (NIPPV) in the postoperative setting. Certainly, for those patients who already carry the diagnosis of OSA or OHS, any outpatient management strategies already instituted should be carried over meticulously to the inpatient setting. In the patient who reports noncompliance with their prescribed continuous positive airway pressure (CPAP) or bilevel positive airway pressure (BiPAP) at home, it will be important to ensure compliance while hospitalized as their native dependence will only be magnified by the indications for and process of hospitalization. Further, I advocate for the aggressive use of NIPPV in this population for both chronic and acute indications.

The complexity of invasive airway instrumentation and invasive ventilation in these patients increases the potential for associated complications.[38-41] Therefore, if presented with an acute clinical scenario that is judged likely to improve in the coming hours to the point that the need for positive-pressure ventilation is expected to wane, it is reasonable to consider NIPPV for sedate patients who are judged to adequately protect their airway. These patients must be managed in an ICU setting where the ongoing level of sedation and response to therapy can be vigilantly monitored. Avoiding an intubation or reintubation in this population is of great benefit to the patient if it can be done safely.

Airway

In the upper airway, glottic visualization may be complicated by excess fatty tissue in the mouth and pharynx as well as by difficulty in placing the patient in the optimal position. The literature would suggest the "ramped" position to be superior to sniffing in this population.[42] Ramped positioning requires the placement of towels, blankets, or pillows to elevate the head, neck, and upper back until the external auditory meatus and the sternal notch are on the same horizontal plane. This position has been shown to improve visualization during direct laryngoscopy.[42] It is important to recognize that proper patient positioning prior to any elective attempts at airway instrumentation in the obese patient carries an extra imperative.

Movement of the obese patient, compared to leaner patients, after sedation will be more difficult and potentially impossible. As always, a clear plan for difficult airway should be in place, with the proper equipment and personnel at bedside prior to any elective airway attempts. A difficult airway plan must be in place for all facilities, with extra attention to the bariatric airway in those facilities that specialize in the care of these patients.

While avoiding a review of all available airway adjuncts that are not necessarily unique to the bariatric airway, it merits specific mention that the laryngeal mask airway (LMA) may be an invaluable tool in temporizing airway control in the obese population when visualization proves elusive and bag valve mask ventilation is inadequate. Specifically, the intubating LMA has been shown to have 96.5% and 100% intubation success via blind and fiber-optic approaches.[43] The intubating LMA has the advantage of temporizing the airway while providing a very high success rate conduit through which to pass an endotracheal tube.

In the lower airway, tracheomalacia has been increasingly recognized as a source for respiratory failure. Obesity has been implicated in multiple studies as a contributing factor to this disease.[44,45] Stenting of proximal large airways is occasionally performed with varying success in the literature, but in my experience with little durable effect. The most durable treatment for the obese patient with tracheomalacia in my view is tracheostomy as a bridge to weight loss. Anecdotally, I have had great success with this approach in the limited number of patients who durably lose weight. The finite treatment for tracheomalacia associated with obesity is to provide positive pressure to stent the airways open.

Pulmonary Parenchyma

The reader is well acquainted with the gravid patient's risk for pneumonia and viral pneumonia in particular, with some studies implicating a 5-fold increased risk for the latter.[46] Maravi-Poma and colleagues described that 20% of reproductive age female ICU admissions during the 2009 H1N1 outbreak in Spain were pregnant.[46] The outcomes for influenza in the morbidly obese are discussed elsewhere in this chapter and are an exception to the obesity paradox wherein obesity in the setting of H1N1 clearly confers increased mortality.[47–49] It is not known whether this added hazard is conferred for other strains.

The gravid patient is at increased risk for aspiration from a host of pregnancy-associated factors, including the gravid uterus, delayed gastric emptying, lower gastric pH, and progesterone-mediated lower esophageal sphincter relaxation.[49] This risk would seem to only be magnified in the presence of obesity, where the increased risk for hypercapnia and sedation may now coexist with pregnancy. Lee and colleagues in 2014 looked at over 5500 patients with lung injury and found, perhaps counterintuitively, that neither obesity nor gastroesophageal reflux disease (GERD) were associated with aspiration.[50]

It has been shown, however, that obesity and GERD are associated with tracheomalacia.[45] In those patients who require mechanical ventilation, there are available outcomes data. Overall, the mortality data are favorable, with ORs for mortality consistently ranging from 1.0 to 0.75 when compared to nonobese cohorts.[51–53] Some studies link obesity with increased incidence of ARDS, but even the bulk of those studies fail to demonstrate excess mortality.[39,50]

Both pregnancy and obesity are risk factors for venous thromboembolic (VTE) disease.[54–56] The prevention and management of VTE are not generally different in this population than others beyond the choice of anticoagulant with respect to fetal harm and dosing with respect to obesity as discussed previously in this chapter.

Amniotic fluid embolism (AFE) remains a rare complication with high associated mortality with clear associations to placental abnormalities and induction of labor.[57] A review of the literature does not reveal a clear association between obesity and risk for AFE; however, there is a clear association between obesity and risk for failed trial of labor and cesarean delivery.[58,59] The statistics of a rare disease presenting in a special population may limit the recognition of the same without interrogation of an extremely large cohort, but the suggestion by association of known risk factors for each is an association of which to be aware as it may inform differential diagnosis in the acute setting. The management of AFE remains supportive.

The mortality associated with both VTE and AFE has improved significantly with the advent of modern critical care. The ultimate expression of this evolution can be seen in the growing availability of extracorporeal membrane oxygenation (ECMO) for adults.[60,61] Previously universally fatal cases of pulmonary embolism (PE) and AFE can now be supported with high rates of survival, but it should be understood that obesity can be seen to limit the use of ECMO. Historically, obesity has been seen as a limiting factor to the use of ECMO for a host of technical reasons, including cannulation and provision of adequate CO, but there is a growing literature base of successful use of ECMO in this population.[60,62] I would advocate for its use in a peripartum patient of almost any size. In addition, rescue therapy with emergent pulmonary thromboendarterectomy in obese patients reported by Fernandes found no increase in complications or difference in mortality in a review of 476 consecutive operations over a 3.5-year period.[63]

SURGICAL PATIENTS

Preoperative Evaluation

Preoperative evaluation not only centers on the same risks discussed in the respiratory section but also integrates the cardiovascular and endocrine risks so strongly associated with obesity. Many of the comorbid conditions of obesity are also significant risk factors for coronary disease, and there is a strong association between congestive heart failure and obesity as well as the better-known association of diabetes and obesity.[64,65] Whether these diseases are present and whether they are adequately controlled will significantly affect the patient's risk for surgery and general anesthesia.[66] The balance of the preoperative evaluation should focus on anticipation of the postoperative complications and limiting their impact, as discussed previously.

Surgical Outcomes

Ten years ago, much of the trauma literature reflected increased mortality among obese patients, but in the last 10 years there have been many articles suggesting protective effects of obesity, perhaps owing to better management of ICU complications to which this population is predisposed. This strong trend toward concordance with the obesity paradox reflects the general tone of the more modern literature base.

On balance, there are 2 recent articles implicating substantial associated excess mortality risk in the obese population. One in particular, reported by Weinlein and colleagues,[67] found an OR of mortality in morbidly obese patients with femoral shaft fractures to be an excruciatingly high 46.77. Much of this was likely due to an observed OR of 35 for the development of ARDS in this study. The second article found an OR of mortality at a comparatively paltry 1.5, but the statistical analysis was robust; having looked at the national trauma databank for 4 years, they were able to compare 16,000 morbidly obese trauma patients to 16,000 nonobese.[68] We may need a little more time to divine the truth, but even in the articles that are at odds on mortality, there is a consistent trend of longer hospitalizations, more complications, more ICU days, and more ventilator days.[69,70]

The incidence of prolonged mechanical ventilation increases the incidence of tracheostomy and its own set of increased complications in this population.[71] Regarding tracheostomy, El Solh and Jaafar reviewed 89 surgical tracheostomies performed in morbidly obese patients and compared them to nonobese and ascribed a hazard ratio of 4.4 for complications to the morbidly obese cohort.[72] In contrast, McCaque et al. reported no increase in complications among obese patients who underwent percutaneous dilatational tracheostomy at the bedside when analyzing 426 patients over a 6-year period.[73] In a review of 102 obese patients who underwent tracheostomy, Byrd et al. reported the most common outcome, 49% of patients, to be tracheostomy dependence.[74] These are important factors for the practitioner to understand to both effectively anticipate complications and accurately inform families about expectations when a decision point is reached for tracheostomy.

As outlined previously, obese patients are at increased risk for AKI; this holds true among surgical patients as well. A hazard ratio of 2.39 for AKI after cardiopulmonary bypass in the morbidly obese has been reported as has an increased incidence of rhabdomyolysis among 96 obese patients compared to 102 nonobese admitted to a single trauma center over a 2-year period.[75,76]

Hemorrhagic Shock and Coagulopathy

The risk of hemorrhage is ever present in the gravid patient and only increases as the pregnancy progresses. The reader is familiar with the progressive increases in plasma volume in pregnancy, and this volume is only magnified by the presence of obesity. While the principles of management of hemorrhage and associated coagulopathy, whether hemorrhagic or consumptive, are not different in the obese patient, it must be emphasized that the volumes of blood products necessary to restore circulating intravascular volume and correct coagulopathy will be proportionally increased as the size of the patient increases. Using fresh frozen plasma (FFP) as an example, the standard dosage of FFP is 10–20 mL/kg of body weight.[77,78] An actively bleeding patient in hemorrhagic shock may easily require the higher dose, if not more.[79] Quick math yields a dose of 4 L of FFP for a 200-kg patient. In the case of consumptive coagulopathy complicated by coexistent hemorrhage, one can easily deplete a large hospital's storage rapidly. Many hospitals today have massive transfusion protocols designed to free up and anticipate resource usage from the blood bank. In the setting of morbid obesity, it would be good practice to make the blood bank aware of the special circumstances and the anticipated need for volumes that may be substantially outside the norm.

CONCLUSION

In sum, the preponderance of the literature supports an inverse relation between BMI and mortality in the setting of critical illness. It is important for the practitioner to be aware that despite the acute magnitude of illness in the obese population from either medical or surgical causes, there is the expectation of excess morbidity but with the compensation of excess survival in the end. The obese patient presents a set of unique management challenges. It is in the recognition and anticipation of these challenges that excess morbidity and mortality may be minimized. We have seen that this is a durable cohort of patients who, despite longer stays and higher complexity, are anything but frail.

REFERENCES

1. Louie JK, Acosta M, Winter K, et al. Factors associated with death or hospitalization due to pandemic 2009 influenza A(H1N1) infection in California. *JAMA*. 2009;302(17):1896–1902. doi:10.1001/jama.2009.1583.

2. Myles PR, Semple MG, Lim WS, et al. Predictors of clinical outcome in a national hospitalised cohort across both waves of the influenza A/H1N1 pandemic 2009–2010 in the UK. *Thorax*. 2012;67(8):709–717. doi:10.1136/thoraxjnl-2011-200266.

3. Sheridan PA, Paich HA, Handy J, et al. Obesity is associated with impaired immune response to influenza vaccination in humans. *Int J Obes (Lond)*. 2012;36(8):1072–1077. doi:10.1038/ijo.2011.208.

4. Kahlon S, Eurich DT, Padwal RS, et al. Obesity and outcomes in patients hospitalized with pneumonia. *Clin Microbiol Infect*. 2013;19(8):709–716. doi:10.1111/j.1469-0691.2012.04003.x.

5. Singanayagam A, Singanayagam A, Chalmers JD. Obesity is associated with improved survival in community-acquired pneumonia. *Eur Respir J*. 2013;42(1):180–187. doi:10.1183/09031936.00115312.

6. Corrales-Medina VF, Valayam J, Serpa JA, Rueda AM, Musher DM. The obesity paradox in community-acquired bacterial pneumonia. *Int J Infect Dis*. 2011;15(1):e54–e57. doi:10.1016/j.ijid.2010.09.011.

7. Leung J, Burke B, Ford D, et al. Possible association between obesity and *Clostridium difficile* infection. *Emerg Infect Dis*. 2013;19(11):1791–1798. doi:10.3201/eid1911.130618.

8. Parienti J-J, Thirion M, Mégarbane B, et al. Femoral versus jugular venous catheterization and risk of nosocomial events in adults requiring acute renal replacement therapy: a randomized controlled trial. *JAMA*. 2008;299(20):2413–2422. doi:10.1001/jama.299.20.2413.

9. Dossett LA, Dageforde LA, Swenson BR, et al. Obesity and site-specific nosocomial infection risk in the intensive care unit. *Surg Infect (Larchmt)*. 2009;10(2):137–142. doi:http://dx.doi.org/10.1089/sur.2008.028.

10. Miller SE, Maragakis LL. Central line-associated bloodstream infection prevention. *Curr Opin Infect Dis*. 2012;25(4):412–422. doi:10.1097/QCO.0b013e328355e4da.

11. Latif A, Halim MS, Pronovost PJ. Eliminating Infections In the ICU: CLABSI. *Curr Infect Dis Rep*. 2015;17(7):491. doi:10.1007/s11908-015-0491-8.

12. Falagas ME, Kompoti M. Obesity and infection. *Lancet Infect Dis*. 2006;6(7):438–446. doi:10.1016/S1473-3099(06)70523-0.

13. Huttunen R, Syrjänen J. Obesity and the risk and outcome of infection. *Int J Obes*. 2012 May:333–340. doi:10.1038/ijo.2012.62.

14. Kanneganti T-D, Dixit VD. Immunological complications of obesity. *Nat Immunol*. 2012;13(8):707–712. doi:10.1038/ni.2343.

15. Sturm AW, Allen N, Rafferty KD, et al. Pharmacokinetic analysis of piperacillin administered with tazobactam in critically ill, morbidly obese surgical patients. *Pharmacotherapy*. 2014;34(1):28–35. doi:10.1002/phar.1324.

16. Aubron C, Corallo CE, Nunn MO, Dooley MJ, Cheng AC. Evaluation of the accuracy of a pharmacokinetic dosing program in predicting serum vancomycin concentrations in critically ill patients. *Ann Pharmacother*. 2011;45(10):1193–1198. doi:10.1345/aph.1Q195.

17. Velissaris D, Karamouzos V, Marangos M, Pierrakos C, Karanikolas M. Pharmacokinetic changes and dosing modification of aminoglycosides in critically ill obese patients: a literature review. *J Clin Med Res*. 2014;6(4):227–233. doi:10.14740/jocmr1858w.

18. Roberts JA, Lipman J. Optimal doripenem dosing simulations in critically ill nosocomial pneumonia patients with obesity, augmented renal

clearance, and decreased bacterial susceptibility. *Crit Care Med.* 2013;41(2):489–495. doi:10.1097/CCM.0b013e31826ab4c4.

19. Erstad BL. Dosing of medications in morbidly obese patients in the intensive care unit setting. *Intensive Care Med.* 2004;30(1):18–32. doi:10.1007/s00134-003-2059-6.

20. Hanley MJ, Abernethy DR, Greenblatt DJ. Effect of obesity on the pharmacokinetics of drugs in humans. *Clin Pharmacokinet.* 2010;49(2):71–87. doi:10.2165/11318100-000000000-00000.

21. Utrup TR, Mueller EW, Healy DP, Callcut RA, Peterson JD, Hurford WE. High-dose ciprofloxacin for serious gram-negative infection in an obese, critically ill patient receiving continuous venovenous hemodiafiltration. *Ann Pharmacother.* 2010;44(10):1660–1664. doi:10.1345/aph.1P234.

22. Ariano RE, Sitar DS, Zelenitsky SA, et al. Enteric absorption and pharmacokinetics of oseltamivir in critically ill patients with pandemic (H1N1) influenza. *CMAJ.* 2010;182(4):357–363. doi:10.1503/cmaj.092127.

23. Soto GJ, Frank AJ, Christiani DC, Gong MN. Body mass index and acute kidney injury in the acute respiratory distress syndrome. *Crit Care Med.* 2012;40(9):2601–2608. doi:10.1097/CCM.0b013e3182591ed9.

24. Bagshaw SM, Sood MM, Long J, Fowler RA, Adhikari NK, Canadian Critical Care Trials Group HNC. Acute kidney injury among critically ill patients with pandemic H1N1 influenza A in Canada: cohort study. *BMC Nephrol.* 2013;14:123. doi:10.1186/1471-2369-14-123.

25. Shashaty MGS, Meyer NJ, Localio AR, et al. African American race, obesity, and blood product transfusion are risk factors for acute kidney injury in critically ill trauma patients. *J Crit Care.* 2012;27(5):496–504. doi:10.1016/j.jcrc.2012.02.002.

26. Dellinger RP, Levy MM, Rhodes A, et al. Surviving sepsis campaign: international guidelines for management of severe sepsis and septic shock: 2012. *Crit Care Med.* 2013;41(2):580–637. doi:10.1097/CCM.0b013e31827e83af.

27. Lee W, Nagubadi S, Kryger MH, Mokhlesi B. Epidemiology of obstructive sleep apnea: a population-based perspective. *Expert Rev Respir Med.* 2008;2(3):349–364. doi:10.1586/17476348.2.3.349.

28. Lopez PP, Stefan B, Schulman CI, et al. Prevalence of sleep apnea in morbidly obese patients who presented for weight loss surgery evaluation: more evidence for routine screening for obstructive sleep apnea before weight loss surgery. *Am Surg.* 2008;74(9):834–838. PMID:18807673.

29. Sareli AE, Cantor CR, Williams NN, et al. Obstructive sleep apnea in patients undergoing bariatric surgery—a tertiary center experience. *Obes Surg.* 2011;21(3):316–327. doi:10.1007/s11695-009-9928-1.

30. Stelfox HT, Ahmed SB, Ribeiro RA, Gettings EM, Pomerantsev E, Schmidt U. Hemodynamic monitoring in obese patients: the impact of body mass index on cardiac output and stroke volume. *Crit Care Med.* 2006;34(4):1243–1246. doi:10.1097/01.CCM.0000208358.27005.F4.

31. Arora S, Singh PM, Goudra BG, Sinha AC. Changing trends of hemodynamic monitoring in ICU—from invasive to non-invasive methods: are we there yet? *Int J Crit Illn Inj Sci.* 2014;4(2):168–177. doi:10.4103/2229-5151.134185.

32. Ramsingh D, Alexander B, Cannesson M. Clinical review: does it matter which hemodynamic monitoring system is used? *Crit Care.* 2013;17(2):208. doi:10.1186/cc11814.

33. Biring MS, Lewis MI, Liu JT, Mohsenifar Z. Pulmonary physiologic changes of morbid obesity. *Am J Med Sci.* 1999;318(5):293–297. PMID:10555090.

34. Bobrowski RA. Pulmonary physiology in pregnancy. *Clin Obstet Gynecol.* 2010;53(2):285–300. doi:10.1097/GRF.0b013e3181e04776.

35. Ali Z, Ulrik CS. Obesity and asthma: a coincidence or a causal relationship? A systematic review. *Respir Med.* 2013;107(9):1287–1300. doi:10.1016/j.rmed.2013.03.019.

36. Beuther DA, Sutherland ER. Overweight, obesity, and incident asthma: a meta-analysis of prospective epidemiologic studies. *Am J Respir Crit Care Med.* 2007;175(7):661–666. doi:10.1164/rccm.200611-1717OC.

37. Farah CS, Salome CM. Asthma and obesity: a known association but unknown mechanism. *Respirology.* 2012;17(3):412–421. doi:10.1111/j.1440-1843.2011.02080.x.

38. Frat J-P, Gissot V, Ragot S, et al. Impact of obesity in mechanically ventilated patients: a prospective study. *Intensive Care Med.* 2008;34(11):1991–1998. doi:10.1007/s00134-008-1245-y.

39. Gong MN, Bajwa EK, Thompson BT, Christiani DC. Body mass index is associated with the development of acute respiratory distress syndrome. *Thorax.* 2010;65(1):44–50. doi:10.1136/thx.2009.117572.

40. Griesdale DEG, Bosma TL, Kurth T, Isac G, Chittock DR. Complications of endotracheal intubation in the critically ill. *Intensive Care Med.* 2008;34:1835–1842. doi:10.1007/s00134-008-1205-6.

41. Weig T, Schubert MI, Gruener N, et al. Abdominal obesity and prolonged prone positioning increase risk of developing sclerosing cholangitis in critically ill patients with influenza A-associated ARDS. *Eur J Med Res.* 2012;17(1):30. doi:10.1186/2047-783X-17-30.

42. Collins JS, Lemmens HJM, Brodsky JB, Brock-Utne JG, Levitan RM. Laryngoscopy and morbid obesity: a comparison of the "sniff" and "ramped" positions. *Obes Surg.* 2004;14(9):1171–1175. doi:10.1381/0960892042386869.

43. Ferson DZ, Rosenblatt WH, Johansen MJ, Osborn I, Ovassapian A. Use of the intubating LMA-Fastrach in 254 patients with difficult-to-manage airways. *Anesthesiology.* 2001;95(5):1175–1181. doi:10.1097/00000542-200111000-00022.

44. Kandaswamy C, Balasubramanian V. Review of adult tracheomalacia and its relationship with chronic obstructive pulmonary disease. *Curr Opin Pulm Med.* 2009;15(2):113–119. doi:10.1097/MCP.0b013e328321832d.

45. Kandaswamy C, Bird G, Gill N, Math E, Vempilly JJ. Severe tracheomalacia in the ICU: identification of diagnostic criteria and risk factor analysis from a case control study. *Respir Care.* 2013;58(2):340–347. doi:10.4187/respcare.01866.

46. Maravi-Poma E, Martin-Loeches I, Regidor E, Laplaza C, Cambra K. Severe 2009 H1N1 influenza in pregnant women in Spain. *Crit Care Med.* 2011;39(5):945–951.

47. Louie JK, Acosta M, Samuel MC, et al. A novel risk factor for a novel virus: obesity and 2009 pandemic influenza A (H1N1). *Clin Infect Dis.* 2011;52(3):301–312. doi:10.1093/cid/ciq152.

48. Morgan OW, Bramley A, Fowlkes A, et al. Morbid obesity as a risk factor for hospitalization and death due to 2009 pandemic influenza A(H1N1) disease. *PLoS One.* 2010;5(3):e9694. doi:10.1371/journal.pone.0009694.

49. Hill Malfertheiner S, Malfertheiner M V, Kropf S, Costa S-D, Malfertheiner P. A prospective longitudinal cohort study: evolution of GERD symptoms during the course of pregnancy. *BMC Gastroenterol.* 2012;12(1):131. doi:10.1186/1471-230X-12-131.

50. Lee A, Festic E, Park PK, et al. Characteristics and outcomes of patients hospitalized following pulmonary aspiration. *Chest.* 2014;146(4):899–907. doi:10.1378/chest.13-3028.

51. Kumar G, Majumdar T, Jacobs ER, et al. Outcomes of morbidly obese patients receiving invasive mechanical ventilation: a nationwide analysis. *Chest.* 2013;144(1):48–54. doi:10.1378/chest.12-2310.

52. Lee CK, Tefera E, Colice G. The effect of obesity on outcomes in mechanically ventilated patients in a medical intensive care unit. *Respiration.* 2014;87(3):219–226. doi:10.1159/000357317.

53. O'Brien JM, Philips GS, Ali NA, Aberegg SK, Marsh CB, Lemeshow S. The association between body mass index, processes of care, and outcomes from mechanical ventilation: a prospective cohort study. *Crit Care Med.* 2012;40(5):1456–1463. doi:10.1097/CCM.0b013e31823e9a80.

54. Battinelli EM, Bauer KA. Thrombophilias in pregnancy. *Hematol Oncol Clin North Am.* 2011;25(2):323–333. doi:10.1016/j.hoc.2011.02.003.

55. McLintock C, Brighton T, Chunilal S, et al. Recommendations for the diagnosis and treatment of deep venous thrombosis and pulmonary embolism in pregnancy and the postpartum period. *Aust N Z J Obstet Gynaecol.* 2012;52(1):14–22. doi:10.1111/j.1479-828X.2011.01361.x.

56. Fontaine G V, Vigil E, Wohlt PD, et al. Venous thromboembolism in critically ill medical patients receiving chemoprophylaxis: a focus on obesity and other risk factors. *Clin Appl Thromb Hemost.* 2016;22(3):265–273. doi:10.1177/1076029615604048.

57. Conde-Agudelo A, Romero R. Amniotic fluid embolism: an evidence-based review. *Am J Obstet Gynecol.* 2009;201(5):445.e1-e445.e13. doi:10.1016/j.ajog.2009.04.052.

58. Barau G, Robillard PY, Hulsey TC, et al. Linear association between maternal pre-pregnancy body mass index and risk of caesarean section in term deliveries. *BJOG.* 2006;113(January 2001):1173–1177. doi:10.1111/j.1471-0528.2006.01038.x.

59. Poobalan AS, Aucott LS, Gurung T, Smith WCS, Bhattacharya S. Obesity as an independent risk factor for elective and emergency caesarean delivery in nulliparous women—systematic review and meta-analysis of cohort studies. *Obes Rev.* 2009;10(1):28–35. doi:10.1111/j.1467-789X.2008.00537.x.

60. Brodie D, Bacchetta M. Extracorporeal membrane oxygenation for ARDS in adults. *N Engl J Med.* 2011;365(20):1905–1914. doi:10.1056/NEJMct1103720.

61. Pellegrino V, Hockings LE, Davies A. Veno-arterial extracorporeal membrane oxygenation for adult cardiovascular failure. *Curr Opin Crit Care.* 2014;20(5):484–492. doi:10.1097/MCC.0000000000000141.

62. Makdisi G, Wang I W. Extra corporeal membrane oxygenation (ECMO) review of a lifesaving technology. *J Thorac Dis.* 2015;7(7):E166–E176. doi:10.3978/j.issn.2072-1439.2015.07.17.

63. Fernandes TM, Auger WR, Fedullo PF, et al. Baseline body mass index does not significantly affect outcomes after pulmonary thromboendarterectomy. *Ann Thorac Surg.* 2014;98(5):1776–1781. doi:10.1016/j.athoracsur.2014.06.045.

64. Bahrami H, Bluemke DA, Kronmal R, et al. Novel metabolic risk factors for incident heart failure and their relationship with obesity. The MESA (Multi-Ethnic Study of Atherosclerosis) study. *J Am Coll Cardiol.* 2008;51(18):1775–1783. doi:10.1016/j.jacc.2007.12.048.

65. Mokdad AH, Bowman BA, Ford ES, Vinicor F, Marks JS, Koplan JP. The continuing epidemics of obesity and diabetes in the United States. *JAMA.* 2001;286(10):1195–1200. doi:10.1001/jama.286.10.1195.

66. Sankar A, Johnson SR, Beattie WS, Tait G, Wijeysundera DN. Reliability of the American Society of Anesthesiologists physical status scale in clinical practice. *Br J Anaesth.* 2014;113(3):424–432. doi:10.1093/bja/aeu100.

67. Weinlein JC, Deaderick S, Murphy RF. Morbid obesity increases the risk for systemic complications in patients with femoral shaft fractures. *J Orthop Trauma*. 2015;29(3):e91–e95. doi:10.1097/BOT.0000000000000167.

68. Ditillo M, Pandit V, Rhee P, et al. Morbid obesity predisposes trauma patients to worse outcomes: a National Trauma Data Bank analysis. *J Trauma Acute Care Surg*. 2014;76(1):176–179. doi:10.1097/TA.0b013e3182ab0d7c.

69. Bochicchio GV, Joshi M, Bochicchio K, Nehman S, Tracy JK, Scalea TM. Impact of obesity in the critically ill trauma patient: a prospective study. *J Am Coll Surg*. 2006;203(4):533–538. doi:10.1016/j.jamcollsurg.2006.07.001.

70. Brown CVR, Neville AL, Rhee P, Salim A, Velmahos GC, Demetriades D. The impact of obesity on the outcomes of 1,153 critically injured blunt trauma patients. *J Trauma*. 2005;59(November):1048–1051; discussion 1051. doi:10.1097/01.ta.0000189047.65630.c5.

71. Cheung NH, Napolitano LM. Tracheostomy: epidemiology, indications, timing, technique, and outcomes. *Respir Care*. 2014;59(6):895–915; discussion 916–919. doi:10.4187/respcare.02971.

72. El Solh AA, Jaafar W. A comparative study of the complications of surgical tracheostomy in morbidly obese critically ill patients. *Crit Care*. 2007;11(1):R3. doi:10.1186/cc5147.

73. McCague A, Aljanabi H, Wong DT. Safety analysis of percutaneous dilational tracheostomies with bronchoscopy in the obese patient. *Laryngoscope*. 2012;122(May):1031–1034. doi:10.1002/lary.22505.

74. Byrd JK, Ranasinghe VJ, Day KE, Wolf BJ, Lentsch EJ. Predictors of clinical outcome after tracheotomy in critically ill obese patients. *Laryngoscope*. 2014;124(5):1118–1122. doi:10.1002/lary.24347.

75. Kumar AB, Bridget Zimmerman M, Suneja M. Obesity and post-cardiopulmonary bypass-associated acute kidney injury: a single-center retrospective analysis. *J Cardiothorac Vasc Anesth*. 2014;28(3):551–556. doi:10.1053/j.jvca.2013.05.037.

76. Chan JL, Imai T, Barmparas G, et al. Rhabdomyolysis in obese trauma patients. *Am Surg*. 2014;80(10):1012–1017. PMID:25264650.

77. A. J. The development of a dosage calculation tool for fresh frozen plasma (FFP). *Transfus Med*. 2011;21:43.

78. Roback JD, Caldwell S, Carson J, et al. Evidence-based practice guidelines for plasma transfusion. *Transfusion*. 2010;50(6):1227–1239. doi:10.1111/j.1537-2995.2010.02632.x.

79. Mitra B, Mori A, Cameron PA, Fitzgerald M, Paul E, Street A. Fresh frozen plasma (FFP) use during massive blood transfusion in trauma resuscitation. *Injury*. 2010;41(1):35–39. doi:10.1016/j.injury.2009.09.029.

Pain Management in the Obese Population

Brendan McGinn, MD

PAIN MANAGEMENT
PREGNANCY
· Medication Considerations
· Musculoskeletal Pain Considerations

· Headache Considerations
· Anesthesia Considerations
GYNECOLOGY

PAIN MANAGEMENT

Chronic pain, like other medical comorbidities such as cardiovascular disease and diabetes, is more prevalent in obese patients than in the overall population. One recent study showed close to 40% of obese people suffer from chronic pain, with an increased incidence as body mass index (BMI) increases.[1] A survey of more than 1 million people showed that overweight individuals had approximately 20% more pain compared to normal weight individuals, increasing to 254% more pain in individuals with BMIs greater than 40.[2]

Acute and chronic pain that develops during pregnancy as well as chronic pain related to gynecologic disorders or within pelvic structures can be challenging to manage in the obese population. As is the case with many other comorbid conditions related to obesity, weight reduction first and foremost can at least help correct some of the metabolic and physical derangements that contribute to pain, if not provide relief of pain symptoms in and of itself.[3]

PREGNANCY

Given the high prevalence of chronic pain disorders in obese patients plus the overall increased incidence of new musculoskeletal pain in pregnancy, addressing acute or chronic pain during pregnancy can be challenging in the obese woman. Although there are numerous texts and publications discussing pain and pain management during pregnancy, the focus here is on specific aspects as they relate to the obese pregnant patient.

The interplay between increased mechanical loading, increased inflammation, and a negative psychological state mediates some of the relationships between pain

and obesity.[4] Adipose tissue itself as well as high loading pressures on bones, joints, and muscles, can cause an increase in inflammatory markers that results in pain. Depression can also cause increases in systemic inflammation as well as unhealthy lifestyle choices that can lead to further weight gain. Obesity is associated not only with depression and anxiety but also with pain catastrophizing that can amplify the pain experience and hinder the physical activity required for weight loss due to a fear of causing more pain. As these factors are already an issue in the obese patient, the extent to which they affect the obese pregnant patient, for whom further weight gain, systemic inflammation and labile psychological states are generally inevitable, can be more extreme.

Medication Considerations

In general, it is always better to exhaust all nonpharmacologic means of treatment before prescribing any new medication to the pregnant patient. As polypharmacy may already be an issue given the comorbidities associated with obesity (e.g., hypertension, diabetes, and depression), avoiding additional medications that may have adverse side effect profiles for the mother or that may cross the placenta is always best if possible.

Nonsteroidal anti-inflammatory drugs (NSAIDs) are relatively contraindicated during the third trimester of pregnancy due to their association with decreased fetal urine production, resulting in low amniotic fluid levels and constriction of the ductus arteriosus, both via inhibition of prostaglandin synthesis. This unfortunately removes one of the most effective classes of medications to treat musculoskeletal pain from a clinician's armamentarium at a stage of pregnancy when pain complaints can be most severe. Indomethacin and ibuprofen are associated with a higher incidence of ductal closure than aspirin.[5] However, aspirin has platelet-inhibiting properties along with its physiologic effects on the fetus as an NSAID. On top of an increased risk of bleeding in the parturient, aspirin at doses above 80 mg is associated with an increased risk of intracranial hemorrhage in the premature infant and should be avoided if possible.[6] NSAID use after 34 weeks' gestation has also been associated with pulmonary hypertension of the newborn.[7]

As a general rule based on the risks mentioned, it is prudent to discontinue any NSAID use at the start of the third trimester and encourage limited use during earlier stages of pregnancy. The use of low-dose aspirin in other obstetric or chronic medical conditions unrelated to musculoskeletal pain poses the least risk of any type of NSAID. However, it should probably still be avoided in the treatment of pain given the overall relative risk of bleeding from platelet dysfunction. Figure 14-1 outlines some of the pharmacokinetics and dosing recommendations for the most commonly prescribed NSAIDs. Although short-term use of NSAIDs may not pose an imminent risk to the fetus, in the absence of liver disease the clinician should consider acetaminophen first as it lacks any of the neonatal side effects of NSAIDs while providing similar analgesia for the mother.

Generally, NSAIDs are the first line of treatment for pain associated with uterine fibroids. Obesity is associated with an increased incidence of uterine fibroids, likely from increased circulating estrogen. Existing fibroids tend to increase in size during pregnancy due to even higher levels of circulating estrogen, leading to a concomitant

Drug	Half-Life (hours)	Urinary Excretion of Unchanged Drug	Recommended Anti-inflammatory Dosage
Aspirin	0.25	<2%	1200–1500 mg tid
Salicylate[1]	2–19	2%–30%	See footnote 2
Celecoxib	11	27%[3]	100–200 mg bid
Diclofenac	1.1	<1%	50–75 mg qid
Diflunisal	13	3%–9%	500 mg bid
Etodolac	6.5	<1%	200–300 mg qid
Fenoprofen	2.5	30%	600 mg qid
Flurbiprofen	3.8	<1%	300 mg tid
Ibuprofen	2	<1%	600 mg qid
Indomethacin	4–5	16%	50–70 mg tid
Ketoprofen	1.8	<1%	70 mg tid
Ketorolac	4–10	58%	10 mg qid[4]
Meloxicam	20	Data not found	7.5–15 mg qd
Nabumetone[5]	26	1%	1000–2000 mg qd[6]
Naproxen	14	<1%	375 mg bid
Oxaprozin	58	1%–4%	1200–1800 mg qd[6]
Piroxicam	57	4%–10%	20 mg qd[6]
Sulindac	8	7%	200 mg bid
Tolmetin	1	7%	400 mg qid

[1]Major anti-inflammatory metabolite of aspirin.
[2]Salicylate is usually given in the form of aspirin.
[3]Total urinary excretion including metabolites.
[4]Recommended for treatment of acute (e.g., surgical) pain only.
[5]Nabumetone is a prodrug; the half-life and urinary excretion are for its active metabolite.
[6]A single daily dose is sufficient because of the long half-life.

FIGURE 14-1. NSAIDs from Lange. Taken from Morgan and Mikhail's Clinical Anesthesiology. 5th ed.

increase in pelvic pain. However, aside from short courses (24–48 hours) before the third trimester, NSAIDs should again be avoided to address this pain syndrome during pregnancy if possible.

Because they lack the physiologic side effects of NSAIDs, opioid analgesics can be a good alternative to address acute pain exacerbations during pregnancy. They should always be utilized sparingly as chronic use can lead to maternal as well as neonatal dependence, with abrupt stoppage precipitating withdrawal-type symptoms, such as fetal tachycardia, which can be life threatening in the later stages of pregnancy.

Aside from these risks, the choice to address acute pain with opioids in the obese patient should be carefully weighed against the risks posed by the inherent sedating side effects, especially given the increased incidence of obstructive sleep apnea (OSA) in these patients. The transient hypoxic episodes that accompany this condition can result in decreased placental blood flow and over time affect fetal growth and development. Opioids can further depress the respiratory drive that forces obese patients with OSA to breathe during apneic episodes and therefore worsen the amount and duration of hypoxia.

Given the fact that there is an increased incidence of type 2 diabetes mellitus in obese women compared to the general population, any preexisting diabetic neuropathy in an obese woman can potentially be worsened by the increased insulin resistance that occurs during pregnancy itself. In a prospective multicenter study of more than 16,000 patients, a BMI of 30–39.9 was associated with an increased risk of gestational diabetes mellitus and fetal macrosomia when compared with a BMI of less than 30.[8] Patients with diabetic neuropathy are often treated with a combination of medications, which may include anticonvulsants or, more recently, antidepressants. The use of selective serotonin reuptake inhibitors or serotonin-norepinephrine reuptake inhibitors has increased overall not only in the treatment of depression but also in the management of chronic migraine headaches and as adjuvant therapy in the management of chronic pain, including painful diabetic neuropathy. With the incidence of depression and chronic pain higher in the obese population overall, one can expect the use of these medications to be increased as well.

Most anticonvulsants and antidepressants fall under Food and Drug Administration categories C and D, meaning their use needs to be critically evaluated to address the risks of teratogenicity versus therapeutic benefit. Despite these medications being profoundly beneficial in certain chronic pain conditions, it is probably best to address pain syndromes and symptoms with therapies that pose less theoretical risk to the fetus. In conditions where the medications are being used to primarily treat seizure disorders or depression, discussion concerning discontinuation is best left to a patient's treating neurologist or psychiatrist.

Musculoskeletal Pain Considerations

Musculoskeletal changes during pregnancy that can lead to chronic pain conditions include an increase in lumbar lordosis and neck flexion with decreased shoulder height, all to compensate for the gradually enlarging gravid uterus. These are all changes that occur to some extent in the obese woman depending on the amount of abdominal adiposity present prior to pregnancy. The twofold (or more) increase in force that presses down on joints and muscles in the obese woman can be amplified many times during pregnancy in this context.[9]

Although the hormone relaxin is known to contribute to myometrial relaxation and pubic diastasis (which can itself be a source of pain), increased levels do not correlate with laxity in other joints. However, joint pain and laxity are associated with increased levels of estradiol and progesterone.[10]

Obesity is not a purported risk factor for pubic diastasis in pregnancy. However, fetal macrosomia *is* a risk factor, which itself is associated with obesity.[11] Weight bearing alone can exacerbate pain from pubic diastasis in the postpartum period, and although the pelvis usually returns to normal in 4–12 weeks, the inactivity that it promotes can further contribute to weight gain in the obese postpartum patient.

Obesity itself has been shown to be an independent risk factor for osteoarthritis of the knee.[12] The joint laxity that occurs during pregnancy can affect the ligaments of the knee, which, already under stress from chronic loading pressures, experiences larger loading pressures as pregnancy progresses at the same time joint support decreases. Any underlying arthritis will inevitably worsen in this context.

The increased risk of osteoporosis due to elevated circulating estrogen levels in the obese woman can contribute to chronic hip and knee pain that can worsen during pregnancy. More worrisome is the risk of developing osteonecrosis of the hip as glucocorticoid levels and loading pressures further increase during pregnancy.[13] Although this is rare, the risk is greater in the obese pregnant patient and can manifest as a progressive worsening of hip pain radiating to the groin that may be associated with dislocation or fracture of the femoral head.

Back pain manifests almost 50% of the time at some point during pregnancy.[14] Low back pain already has a higher incidence in the obese population due to the increase in axial loading pressures.[15] This is exacerbated in pregnancy, especially in the low back, due to the weight of the gravid uterus causing not only increased axial loading but also increased lumbar lordosis with associated painful facet arthropathy.

The increases in axial loading pressure and joint laxity can manifest along the lumbar spine's anterior and posterior longitudinal ligaments, with the resulting instability leading to further paraspinous muscle strain and spasm that can already be present in the obese patient.

Pain in the sacroiliac (SI) joint can be caused by increased axial loading pressures as well and can often be misinterpreted as posterior pelvic pain emanating from internal visceral structures. Higher levels of estrogen circulating in the obese patient prior to pregnancy may already contribute to a widening of the SI joint, predisposing these patients to painful SI joint arthropathy as pregnancy progresses.

Although the prevalence of lumbar disk disease is not increased during pregnancy compared to nonpregnant women, it *is* increased in obese women versus women with normal BMIs. Radiculopathy is rarely due to nerve root compression. In fact, the incidence of a "slipped disk" or herniated nucleus pulposus during pregnancy that may lead to lumbar nerve root impingement is only around 1 in 10,000.[16] The radicular symptoms in the lower extremities that are often associated with low back pain in pregnancy may be due to mass effect on the lumbar and sacral plexuses by the gravid uterus.[17]

Conservative therapies for low back pain in the pregnant patient are the same as those for the general population. The American College of Obstetricians and Gynecologists recommends exercise in pregnancy to maintain proper posture to address low back pain.[18] As preexisting pain is often already a major barrier to increasing physical activity in obese women, exercise in pregnancy becomes even more of a challenge. Other conservative modalities include heat, massage, and acupuncture.

Generators of musculoskeletal pain in the obese pregnant patient can often be injected with local anesthetic with or without a long-acting formulation of corticosteroid if standard medical management with short courses of anti-inflammatory medications is ineffective. Types include epidural, intra-articular, and intramuscular injections, with peripheral nerve blocks employed to temporarily relieve severe acute pain exacerbations. Short courses of low-potency opioids such as hydrocodone may be indicated for severe exacerbations as well, often as a bridge to an injection. Many patients opt for injections initially to avoid any systemic medication while pregnant.

Meralgia paresthetica (MP) and carpal tunnel syndrome (CTS) have an increased incidence in obesity.[19] These often-painful mononeuropathies can also manifest during pregnancy. In MP, the expanding abdominal wall along with generalized edema impinge on the lateral femoral cutaneous nerve beneath the iliacus fascia as it courses under the inguinal ligament. In CTS, like MP, the increase in overall total body fluid can cause impingement on the median nerve as it courses beneath the flexor retinaculum in the wrist. Neuropathies such as these also have an increased incidence in diabetic patients, emphasizing the need to aggressively treat chronic diabetes and address new-onset gestational diabetes to prevent worsening painful neuropathic symptoms in the obese pregnant patient.

Abdominal pain during pregnancy can be due to multiple causes, the most concerning of which is miscarriage and the sequelae that can follow. This should be high on the clinician's list of differentials in the obese woman of childbearing age as obesity is linked to an increased risk of spontaneous abortion. It also may sometimes be difficult to recognize the existence of a pregnancy in this patient population until later in pregnancy, especially in the context of any preexisting menstrual irregularities, as the expanding gravid uterus does not readily show externally due to the overlying abdominal adiposity.

Causes of focal abdominal wall pain already associated with obesity that may be exacerbated by the gravid uterus and expanding abdominal wall include anterior cutaneous nerve entrapment (ACNE) in the foramen of the rectus muscle aponeurosis. In addition, any added stretch imposed on the abdominal wall muscles may cause a dehiscence or rupture of the epigastric veins within the rectus sheath, leading to a painful localized hematoma.[20] Figure 14-2 shows the innervation of the anterior abdominal wall, with each dermatome consisting of both an anterior and a lateral cutaneous nerve branch. The course of these nerves before they pierce the subcutaneous tissue of the abdominal wall is between the transversus abdominis and internal oblique muscles. The rectus sheath, where painful hematomas can develop, is formed by the aponeuroses of the transversus abdominis and the external and internal oblique muscles (Figure 14-3).

Although rest and heat may suffice as treatment for either condition, ACNE can be treated with a low-volume injection of local anesthetic with or without steroid at the point of maximal tenderness near the abdominal midline.

Headache Considerations

Chronic migraine headaches occur more commonly in patients who are obese, female, and of reproductive age.[21] This triple hit is somewhat attenuated during pregnancy; many women report an improvement in migraine frequency and severity. This may be due to a sustained elevation in estradiol levels during pregnancy, which is essentially the opposite of the sudden drop in estrogen that occurs during menses when there is an increased occurrence of migraines.

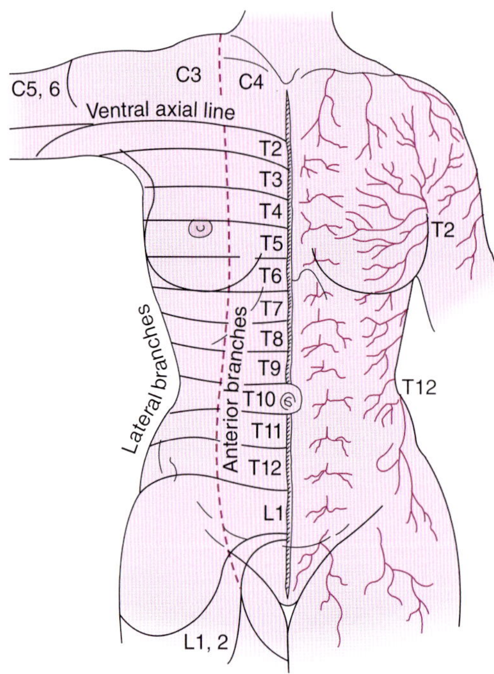

FIGURE 14-2. Abdominal cutaneous nerve distributions.

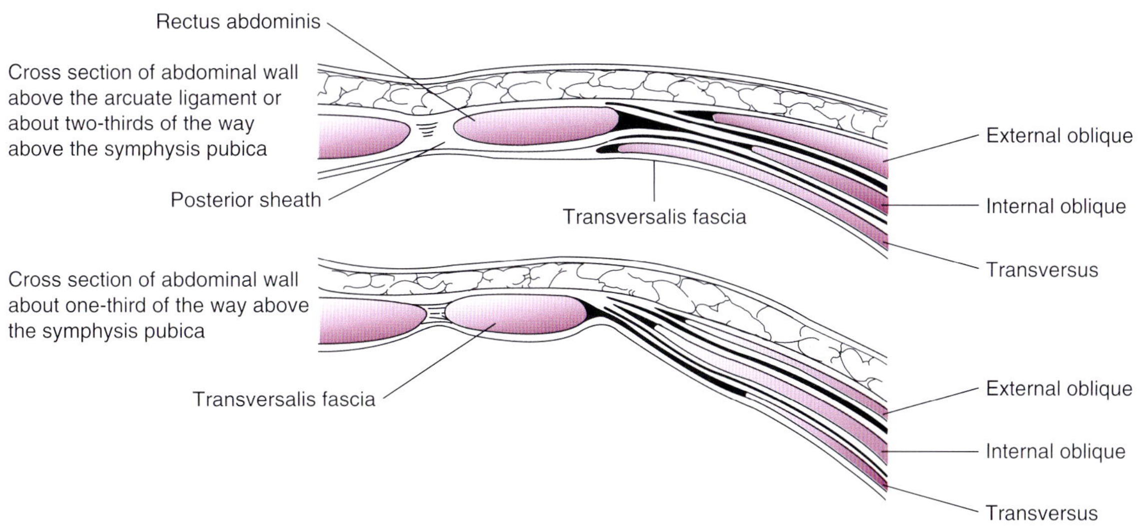

FIGURE 14-3. Abdominal cross section.

With the decreased frequency and severity of migraine headaches that can occur in pregnancy, new-onset headaches during pregnancy need to have a thorough workup to rule out other critical conditions, such as preeclampsia, cerebral venous thrombosis, and pseudotumor cerebri, all of which also have a higher incidence in the obese patient.

Obese women who are at higher risk of coming into pregnancy with a history of chronic migraines will similarly have a higher incidence of taking triptans and ergot alkaloids, both contraindicated in pregnancy, for abortive therapy. If nonpharmacologic therapy such as relaxation techniques or biofeedback is ineffective, a pharmacologic approach employing acetaminophen and caffeine is indicated. If this is not effective, a short course of NSAIDs prior to the third trimester can be given a trial, as can opioid analgesics.

Anesthesia Considerations

During the labor process itself, epidural anesthesia has a much higher incidence of initial failure and accidental dural puncture in the obese versus normal parturient.[22] Although dural punctures may occur more often in obese women, a postdural puncture headache (PDPH) does not occur more often in obese women versus women of normal BMI. Risk factors for developing PDPH include female gender, pregnancy, and young age. If hydration, caffeine, and acetaminophen are ineffective, the standard of care for persistent PDPH is an epidural blood patch (EBP). Given that a difficult epidural placement was likely the reason for the initial dural puncture in the parturient, the placement of an EBP will no doubt be difficult as well. In extremely obese women or in the presence of spine pathology, fluoroscopy or other interventional radiologic imaging may be required to place an EBP.

Because epidural and spinal anesthesia may be technically difficult to provide to the obese parturient and because the rate of cesarean section is significantly higher in this population, general anesthesia is often required to safely deliver the neonate. Given the comorbidities and altered airway anatomy associated with obese patients that can make tracheal intubation difficult, general anesthesia in the obese parturient can be especially tenuous, with the potential for hemodynamic instability and hypoxia that can affect both the mother and the fetus. Pain management in labor and delivery is discussed in further detail in Chapter 25, Obesity in Pregnancy and Anesthesia.

GYNECOLOGY

The etiology of pelvic pain is a challenge for the clinician to diagnose, let alone treat. There are many causes of pelvic pain, with some taking on a more complex presentation in the obese patient. Although numerous texts and publications discuss the causes of and treatments for pelvic pain, the focus here is on a few specific aspects as they relate to the obese patient.

One small cross-sectional study involving 91 women showed an increased risk of pelvic pain associated with obesity.[23] However, a systematic review looking at 15 studies showed no association between pelvic pain in the context of dysmenorrhea and obesity.[24] In another large cohort of premenopausal women using data collected from the Nurses' Health Study II, there was evidence of a decreased incidence of laparoscopically confirmed endometriosis in childhood and early adulthood as BMI increased.[25] Taken together, it is unclear what, if any correlation exists between obesity and pelvic pain. Regardless, there are some conditions and comorbidities associated with obesity that do relate to pelvic pain.

Both obesity and type 2 diabetes are associated with polycystic ovarian syndrome (PCOS), with up to 80% of women in the United States with PCOS reported to be overweight or obese.[26] Due to the hyperandrogenism that accompanies PCOS, adiposity is usually distributed in the abdomen, contributing to the so-called apple shape, unlike in the buttocks and hips in "pear-shaped" obesity that is usually associated with women (Figure 14-4). The location of this abdominal weight can directly cause other painful symptoms. Low back muscle strain and degenerative disk disease are more likely to manifest with the accentuation of lumbar lordosis that occurs to compensate for the abdominal fat pulling the body forward. Pain in PCOS can also arise from the visceral stretch of the polycystic ovaries themselves.

Because PCOS is also strongly associated with type 2 diabetes, diabetic neuropathy can predispose obese patients with

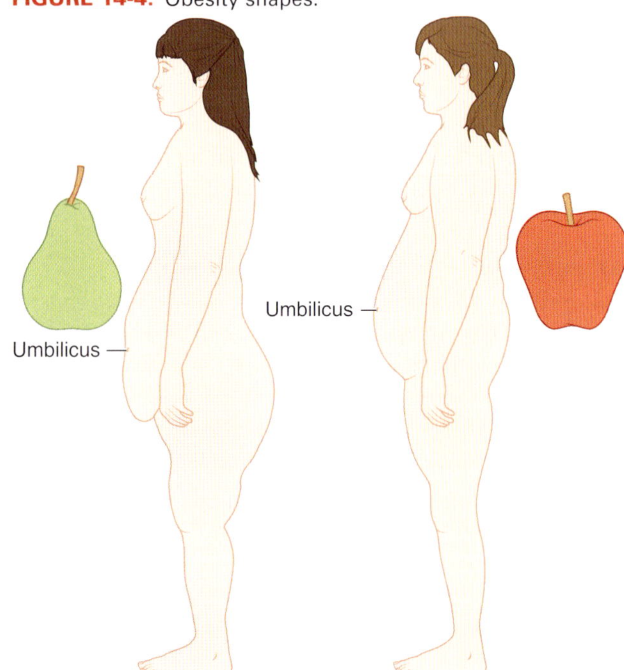

FIGURE 14-4. Obesity shapes.

PCOS to neuropathic pain within various other pelvic structures and along the distal extremities.

Neuropathy is likely responsible for the majority of pelvic pain for which an organic cause cannot be easily detected with physical findings or laboratory testing. Often, a peripheral neuropathy of the obturator, pudendal, or genitofemoral nerves can be both diagnosed and treated with the injection of local anesthetic around the nerve at its course proximal to the area of pain. Pudendal neuropathy, which is most often due to anatomical nerve compression between the sacrospinous and sacrotuberous ligaments, has been shown to respond to neural blockade. Injections spaced out in month-long intervals can reduce symptoms, but this has been shown in only small, uncontrolled studies.[27] The excessive weight from gluteal adiposity that is consistently distributed over the ischial tuberosity when sitting in most obese women puts them at higher risk for developing pudendal neuralgia. In the event that neural blockade is ineffective or if the clinician chooses to be more conservative initially, neuropathic medications such as the anticonvulsant gabapentin or the tricyclic antidepressant amitriptyline can be used as first line.

Pain can arise from muscles that line the pelvic cavity, including the internal and external obturators, levator ani, and even the iliopsoas. Strain and muscle spasms can be triggered by increased loading pressures on the pelvis in the obese patient. These muscles can be injected, anti-inflammatory medications can be given a trial, and a physical therapist can recommend strengthening exercises to prevent worsening of myofascial pain. However, nothing can substitute for weight loss itself.

Pelvic pain can be frustrating to endure as a patient due to the often-difficult ability to treat, which is frequently due to the difficult ability to diagnose. Referrals by gynecologists to pain clinics often lead to trials of unproven medical therapies, occasional diagnostic procedures, and usually a return to the gynecologist without many answers. Depression and dysthymia as well as panic and catastrophizing disorders are linked to chronic pelvic pain. Treatment for these conditions includes psychotherapy and potentially medications, as well as biofeedback, hypnosis, and group therapy. The high incidence of depression associated with obesity is additive in these patients.

As can be seen with most pain scenarios previously discussed, weight loss is the first line of "treatment," yet this can be unrealistic in the obese pregnant patient and incredibly difficult to achieve in the patient with chronic pelvic pain with associated depression. Pain can inhibit the physical activity that, along with diet, is required for weight loss, which results in a more sedentary lifestyle, more deconditioning, and worsening of underlying chronic pain and depression in a detrimental feedback cycle. A combination of medical, interventional, physical, and psychological therapies are usually required to make any positive change in these patients. They remain some of the most difficult to treat from a pain perspective.

REFERENCES

1. Coaccioli S, Masia F, Celi G, et al. Chronic pain in the obese: a quali-quantitative observational study. *Recenti Prog Med*. 2014;105:151–154.
2. Stone AA, Broderick JE. Obesity and pain are associated in the United States. *Obesity (Silver Spring)*. 2012;20:1491–1495.
3. Guh DP, Zhang W, Faith MS, et al. The incidence of co-morbidities related to obesity and overweight: a systematic review and meta-analysis. *BMC Public Health*. 2009;9:88.
4. Vincent HK, Adams MCB, Vincent KR, et al. Musculoskeletal pain, fear avoidance behaviors, and

functional decline in obesity: potential interventions to manage pain and maintain function. *Reg Anesth Pain Med*. 2013;38(6):481–491.

5. Koren G, Florescu A, Costei AM, et al. Nonsteroidal anti-inflammatory drugs during third trimester and the risk of premature closure of the ductus arteriosus: a meta-analysis. *Ann Pharmacother*. 2006;40:824.

6. Briggs GG, Freeman RK, Yaffe SJ. *Drugs in Pregnancy and Lactation*. Baltimore, MD: Williams & Wilkins; 1990.

7. Alano MA, Ngougmna E, Ostrea EM Jr, et al. Analysis of nonsteroidal anti-inflammatory drugs in meconium and its relation to persistent pulmonary hypertension of the newborn. *Pediatrics*. 2001;107:519–523.

8. Weiss JL, Malone FD, Emig D, et al. Obesity, obstetric complications and cesarean delivery rate—a population-based screening study. FASTER Research Consortium. *Am J Obstet Gynecol*. 2004;190:1091–1097.

9. Karzel RP, Freedman MJ. Orthopedic injuries in pregnancy. In: Artal R, Wiswell RA, Drinkwater BL, eds. *Exercise in Pregnancy*. 2nd ed. Baltimore, MD: Lippencott, Williams & Wilkins; 1991.

10. Marnach ML, Ramin KD, Ramsey PS, et al. Characterization of the relationship between joint laxity and maternal hormones in pregnancy. *Obstet Gynecol*. 2003;101:331.

11. Snow RE, Neubert AG. Peripartum pubic symphysis separation: a case series and review of the literature. *Obstet Gynecol Surv*. 1997;52:438.

12. Felson DT, Anderson JJ, Naimark A, et al. Obesity and knee osteoarthritis: the Framingham Study. *Ann Intern Med*. 1988;109:18–24.

13. Hungerford DS, Lennox DW. The importance of increased interosseous pressure in the development of osteonecrosis of the femoral head: implications for treatment. *Orthop Clin North Am*. 1985;16:635–654.

14. Ostgaard HC, Andersson GBJ, Karlsson K. Prevalence of backpain in pregnancy. *Spine*. 1991;16:549–552.

15. Nilsen TIL, Holtermann A, Mork PJ. Physical exercise, body mass index, and risk of chronic pain in the low back and neck/shoulders: longitudinal data from the Nord-Trondelag health study. *Am J Epidemiol*. 2011;174(3):267–273.

16. Laban MM, Perrin JCS, Latimer FR. Pregnancy and the herniated lumbar disc. *Arch Phys Med Rehabil*. 1983;64:319–321.

17. Fast A, Shapiro D, Ducommun EJ, et al. Low back pain in pregnancy. *Spine*. 1987;12:368–371.

18. American College of Obstetricians and Gynecologists. *Planning for Pregnancy, Birth and Beyond*. New York, NY: Dutton; 1996:92–95.

19. Parisi TJ, Mandrekar J, Dyck PJ, et al. Meralgia paresthetica: relation to obesity, advanced age and diabetes mellitus. *Neurology*. 2011;77(16):1538–1542.

20. Peleg R, Gohar J, Koretz M, et al. Abdominal wall pain in pregnant women caused by thoracic lateral cutaneous nerve entrapment. *Eur J Obstet Gynecol Reprod Biol*. 1997;74:169–171.

21. Chai NC, Scher AI, Moghekar A, et al. Obesity and headache: part I—systematic review of the epidemiology of obesity and headache. *Headache*. 2014;54(2):219–234.

22. Hood DD, Dewan DM. Anesthetic and obstetric outcome in morbidly obese parturients. *Anesthesiology*. 1993;79(6):1210–1218.

23. Gurian MB, Mitidieri AM, da Silva JB, et al. Measurement of pain and anthropometric parameters in women with chronic pelvic pain. *J Eval Clin Pract*. 2015; 21(1):21–27.

24. Ju H, Jones M, Mishra G. The prevalence and risk factors of dysmenorrhea. *Epidemiol Rev*. 2014;36:104–113.

25. Vitonis AF, Baer HJ, Hankinson SE, Laufer MR, Missmer SA. A prospective study of body size during childhood and early adulthood and the incidence of endometriosis. *Hum Reprod*. 2010;25(5):1325–1334.

26. Sam S, Dunaif A. Polycystic ovary syndrome: syndrome XX? *Trends Endocrinol Metab*. 2003;14:365–370.

27. Antolak SJ Jr, Hough DM, Pawlina W, Spinner RJ. Anatomical basis of chronic pelvic pain syndrome: the ischial spine and pudendal nerve entrapment. *Med Hypotheses*. 2002;59:349–353.

CHAPTER 15

Electronic Tools

Amy R. Slutzky, PhD, MLIS

John Epling, MD, MSEdk

INTRODUCTION

The use of handheld and computer-based technology has revolutionized many aspects of the clinical practice of medicine as well as patients' experience of health care. The pace of development of this technology is extremely rapid, and busy clinicians often struggle with important questions about these innovations. How do I find and afford the best new devices and technologies? What are the best practices and rules for interacting with patients using these technologies? Are there security issues to consider? Will my patients like them or benefit from them? Despite these questions and concerns, there is evidence that clinicians and patients are adopting these technologies rapidly.[1] The adoption of electronic health records, for example, was progressing slowly until 2011, when use began doubling for hospitals and clinician offices, due largely to incentives and legislation.[2]

Patients use Internet sources for medical information, especially about nutrition and weight management, at a high rate and often do not discuss this use with their clinicians.[3,4] While increased use of computers and devices is thought to be associated with the sedentary activity that promotes obesity, both patients and clinicians are embracing the use of these methods.[5] The proliferation of smartphones, with their always-on connection to the Internet, large data storage capacity, and camera and video capabilities, gives clinicians and patients enormous potential for using computing in daily clinical practice.

Clinicians have been grappling with the management of obesity for years, and obesity complicates many aspects of care for women, such as contraception, fertility, pregnancy, mental health, cancer, and cardiovascular disease.[6,7] In addition to commonly holding negative attitudes toward obese patients, clinicians have lacked the appropriate tools and resources for referral to their patients for education, motivation, and support in achieving their weight management goals.[8-10] The advent of these electronic tools—from industry, from entrepreneurs, and as part of national guideline efforts—has opened a new realm of possibility for clinicians to educate themselves and their patients about obesity, to help motivate these patients for change, and to support them in their journey.

We begin this chapter by discussing the categories and uses of electronic tools to manage obesity. In general, we focus on the issue of obesity in women's health, but use more general sources when more specific data or recommendations were not available. Given the pace of change in this field, we do not attempt to create a list of the current or popular applications and sites but may use occasional specific examples. We discuss tools used by both patients and clinicians and make note of the theoretical basis of these technologies, where applicable. We then review the current "snapshot" of the evidence behind the use of these electronic tools to manage obesity to give the reader a sense of the empirical research behind their use. We discuss the use of electronic tools for obesity in the general population of adults and children or adolescents first, as women are well represented in these studies and there is a paucity of women-only studies. Finally, we close with some comments about the new directions in this field and "things to watch for."

Terminology is an important concern in the world of technology. We adopt the following conventions for simplicity (Figure 15-1). *Computers* refers to desktop, laptop, or notebook computers. The term *tablets* is used to refer to portable devices that are larger than phones but operate on mobile software platforms rather than full operating systems. *Smartphones* are digital, handheld telephones with mobile operating systems that can run small applications ("apps"). We distinguish smartphones from more basic *mobile phones*—admittedly a technologically outdated term—which lack the major mobile operating systems and computing capacity and are used primarily for telephone calls and text messaging. *Personal digital assistants* (PDAs) are the predecessors of smartphones; they use mobile operating systems and applications but do not have cellular or Wi-Fi connectivity. *Text messaging* here includes both SMS (simple [or short] message service) and MMS (multimedia messaging service) applications,

- Computers
    - Desktop, Laptop, or Notebook
    - Any operating system
- Tablets
    - Larger-sized mobile devices
    - Touch screens
    - Mobile operating system
    - Wi-fi and/or cellular data network connectivity
- Smartphones
    - Smaller mobile devices
    - Cellular data network +/− wifi connectivity
    - Mobile operating systems
- Mobile phones
    - Small mobile devices
    - Cellular data network only
    - Telephone and text messaging capability only
- Personal Digital Assistants (PDA)
    - Small mobile devices
    - No cellular data network access, +/− WiFi connectivity
    - Mobile operating systems
- (Mobile) Apps
    - Small-footprint software designed to run on mobile operating systems
- Text messaging
    - Over cellular data networks
        - Short/Simple Messaging Service (SMS)
        - Multimedia Messaging Service (MMS)
    - Over Wi-Fi connections
        - Internet-only Messaging Services
- Telehealth
    - The use of (usually videoconferencing) technology to conduct a health encounter
- "mHealth"
    - Health applications and devices that are focused on mobility
- "eHealth"
    - Health applications involving any computer or device

FIGURE 15-1. Terminology for electronic tools.

whether available over the telephone company networks or through Internet connections, and using open or closed messaging networks. The term *telehealth* refers to the use of (usually video teleconference) technology to conduct one-on-one or group education or treatment sessions. The newer terms *mHealth* and *eHealth* are meant to distinguish the use of electronic applications and devices in health care; the former is restricted to mobile applications and devices, the latter is more inclusive of all electronic tools in health care.

THE SPECTRUM OF ELECTRONIC TOOLS IN OBESITY MANAGEMENT

We have constructed four broad categories of electronic technology currently used or marketed for the management of obesity. First is "information management." This category includes databases of guidelines and medical knowledge (including electronic textbooks), calorie information and diet plans, and exercise information.

The second category is "social support." With the varied modes of communication available with these technologies, a variety of new social support options exists, including online support communities and enhanced methods of synchronous and asynchronous communication between the patient and the patient's doctor or office staff (e.g., nurse, care manager). The third category of use of these electronic tools is "support for behavior change." From automated reminder systems, to online communities, to tracking of food and physical activity details, these tools can facilitate monitoring and habit formation, which are key to managing obesity. Finally, there are more specific "miscellaneous uses" of technology—applications that address an entire care episode—from information, to scheduling, to postoperative instructions.

Information Management

Medical Knowledge for Clinicians

As the computing power of handheld devices and prevalence of computers have increased over the last decade, clinicians are using the data storage power of electronic tools to replace the various paper-based textbooks, quick references, and handbooks. The promise of these tools is contained in the following characteristics: comprehensiveness, authoritativeness, currency, and ease of search. Computer tools' ability to hold a large amount of data should enable quick access to comprehensive amounts of information with increasingly less regard for cost and technological limitation. Large databases of drug and clinical information can theoretically support practice by enabling better retrieval of diagnoses, pharmaceutical and other therapy options, and potential adverse effects. The use of search and cross-referencing functionality further leverages the comprehensiveness of these databases by allowing both directed inquiries about a given topic and drug interaction information or likelihood of disease given a certain combination of symptoms. This comprehensiveness can, of course, be a challenge if the information is not appropriately indexed and outlined.

Knowledge for Patients

Patients also have benefitted from this explosion of easily accessible information. Some of the most popular Internet sites and mobile apps feature dietary recommendations for weight loss as well as recommendations for physical activity (complete with video demonstrations). These sites are heavily advertised on the Internet and on mobile devices. An unfortunate downside to this information, however, has been the proliferation of misinformation: fad diets, ineffective weight loss plans, and, potentially even more harmful, availability of a relatively unregulated universe of sites offering weight loss "supplements" and "dietary aids." Patients consult these information sources frequently, often without disclosing that information to their clinicians.[3]

Electronic tools can also help extend the reach of more traditional patient education methods. Both individual and group education can be enhanced by multimedia and distance education technologies (telehealth, webinars, etc.) available through both computers and mobile devices.[11]

Social Support

Online Communities

From even the early days of the Internet, computers provided a way to seek community. From the pioneering "bulletin board services" to the enormous and varied social networking sites of today, people with similar interests and needs can gather to share information and provide social support and motivation for each other. In the realm of obesity and weight management, this has spurred the development of new weight loss sites (focusing on healthy eating, physical activity or both) as well as conversion of traditional face-to-face groups (like Weight Watchers®) to online communities. These sites at their basic, usually free, levels not only can offer community assistance from the other members, but also can offer enhanced resources (personal coaching, expert online classes, diets, etc.), often through a premium subscription service. As with other Internet sites, these groups may be moderated (with varying degrees of control), but the quality of information and advice found on these sites can vary considerably.

Engagement with online services and communities can vary considerably, with many demographic factors: age, race, or socioeconomic status. However the results of existing studies are not consistent, and there is considerable engagement among populations that are traditionally considered to have low engagement with technology.[3,12–14] Some of the existing research has targeted traditionally difficult-to-reach or underserved populations. Use of mHealth technologies has been found, for example, to be a promising method for engaging in healthy behaviors patients with serious mental illness (e.g., schizophrenia, depression, bipolar disorder) and patients with developmental or acquired disabilities.[15–17]

Enhanced Communication With Health Care

The dramatic increase in the use of electronic health records by clinicians coupled with monetary incentives to drive specific communications uses (e.g., "meaningful use" payments from government insurers), as well as an emphasis on population health, have created new opportunities for clinicians' offices to engage in multiple new communications strategies with patients. Health information messages and reminders from a clinician's office can keep patients focused on their efforts to effect healthy change in their lives. The ability to ask questions and obtain minor services online from the clinician's office can create more communication around the desired behavior change and can help keep patients on the path toward wellness. The advent of health care reform has ushered in a new focus on care management utilizing other-than-clinician health care professionals to track a group of patients carefully and ensure their ongoing engagement with the practice, compliance with medications and laboratory monitoring, and attendance at scheduled follow-ups. Each of these electronic tools extends the patients' support systems beyond the traditional family and social circle to the clinicians' office and to online communities—theoretically allowing access to a broader and more compatible and committed set of social supporters to help patients eat healthier, get more physical activity, and lose weight. These tools—often multidevice or multiplatform—can also support enhanced communications between patients and a number of different health professionals: clinicians, dieticians/nutritionists, and so on.[18,19] For patients with a more defined significant psychological basis for their obesity, such as binge-eating disorder, telehealth (usually video communication with patients at a distance) can expand the access and reach of behavioral health providers to target populations.[20,21]

Support for Behavior Change

Supporting healthy behavior change is a key component of most clinician-patient relationships, yet many clinicians feel inadequately prepared and compensated for this work. A good deal of the support for behavior change can be found simply in the social support and communication interventions described previously. Online social support and enhanced contact with clinicians' offices can help patients with goal setting, provide recommendations for reaching and maintaining goals, and support and motivate patients to enact and sustain their change. Electronic tools also provide easy-to-use automation for reminders and prompts and motivational messaging and monitoring that can help keep patients on track with their desired change.

Change Theories Addressed With Electronic Tools

Overall, behavioral change interventions for obesity, while only partially effective on their own, are an important set of tools in the clinician's management of obesity. A comprehensive behavioral approach to weight loss can lead to as much as 10% weight loss, enough to effect positive clinical outcomes,[22] and electronic tools can be important in supporting the length and frequency of engagement of this behavioral treatment and can automate some of it. Electronic tools, arising as they do from a variety of sources (companies, organizations, individual developers), have a wide array of theoretical bases for their construction. The more useful tools will use either accepted psychological theories or proven models of care in their design and application.

An important caveat to consider is that the use of these electronic tools most often does not result in behavior change on its own. The tools must be integrated into a thoughtful plan for patient engagement around the behavior change and used as facilitators for this engagement.[23] Theories of behavioral change, such as the theory of self-efficacy, health belief model, the information-processing paradigm, social learning, theory of planned action, and motivational interviewing, are incorporated into the design of many apps and devices and the designs of studies evaluating them.[24,25]

Enhancing motivation for difficult personal behavioral change is an important part of this theoretical basis for the use of electronic tools, and many of the tools allow a significant amount of personalization and customization, from generating suggestions based on personal data and setting individual health goals to virtual environments and gaming.[26] Wearable accelerometer bands engage the highly effective behavioral conditioning theory of "variable reinforcement" by rewarding the user with a "buzzing" on achievement of a step goal, usually without displaying the exact count of steps leading up to the goal. The result is users "chasing" this reward, often by engaging in simple physical activity at the end of a day to achieve the goal.[27] The impact of these tools' effect on behavior change, however, can be moderated by the user's initial expectations for their success; it remains to be seen whether clinicians can affect these expectations by actively discussing these technologies with patients.[28]

Monitoring

A host of electronic tools have been created for monitoring food and calorie intake, exercise and physical activity, and other obesity-related behaviors, such as screen time, sedentary activity, and sleep. The accuracy of these electronic tools in measuring physical activity has improved significantly over the years—with even smartphone accelerometers achieving high levels of accuracy in detecting specific differences in exercise intensity.[29,30] Further progress will be made as the requirements for manual data entry will be replaced with the increasing capability of sensors, for instance, replacing manual entry of foods in a diet log with automatic sensing of ingestion activity or with analysis of digital photographs of food consumed followed by immediate feedback.[31,32] The US Food and Drug Administration (FDA) has determined that apps that can function as a medical device or that will integrate with medical devices fall under their purview for regulation.[33] The full meaning and impact of this regulation is still evolving.

The potential for electronic tools goes beyond the single sensor to the emerging field of "wireless body-area networks" and "wireless personal-area networks"—a system of sensors simultaneously tracking different parameters to provide coordinated physiologic information to the patient and clinician to support weight loss. In the case of obesity management, a single network could simultaneously track movement, heart rate, blood pressure, weight, and calorie intake and perform continually updating calculations to provide the patient with choices for the patient to increase calorie expenditure or decrease intake. The technology for these networks is currently being refined and optimized to ensure proper operation and security.[34–36]

Reminders and Motivational Messaging

PATIENTS—The tools used for monitoring frequently also contain motivational messages and feedback based on goals set by the app or by the patient. These goals are frequently configurable: weight loss, weight maintenance, increasing exercise, decreasing unhealthy eating, increasing healthy foods, and so on.[37] Text messaging, either as a primary intervention or as an adjunct to other clinical or population health efforts, is a popular method that is assumed to be more universally available—relying only on an SMS-capable phone rather than requiring a smartphone for an app.[38–40] Apps that support a specific weight loss plan (whether diet, physical activity, or both) are used by the promoters of these plans and by patients as value-added components of a subscription service or product.[41] Interactive voice response technology can be a relatively low-technology solution that provides both monitoring and directed feedback for patients who only have access to telephones.[42]

CLINICIANS—A proven strategy for changing clinician behavior is the use of reminder systems in the patient chart. With the increased penetration and capabilities of electronic health records, along with the ubiquity of handheld devices used as clinical decision aids, these reminders can be more sophisticated, targeted, and powerful.[43] Research into the acceptability of these reminders, however, has raised concerns about reminder "fatigue" (especially due to any logistical issues with the reminders themselves), as well as questions about the source and evidence base of recommendations. Greater attention needs to be paid to the refinement of these reminder systems and to thorough education on their use.[44]

Miscellaneous Uses

A study reviewing smartphone apps related specifically to the broad application store search topic of "bariatric surgery" found a variety of apps—many in the categories discussed. A substantial number, however, were focused on bariatric surgery itself: knowledge about the procedure, online communities, postsurgery meal trackers, or gastric band volume trackers. The reviewers in this study bemoaned the lack of medical professional involvement and lack of consumer review of these apps.[45,46]

Barriers to Use

There are many potential barriers to using electronic tools to manage any health condition. The multiplicity of sources of apps and tools combined with the lack of a single, reliable source for critical consumer-oriented review results in a general knowledge gap about available, high-quality tools. Another barrier is the lack of available technology to employ electronic tools. The technology—whether it is sensor technology like wrist-worn monitoring devices or an app that requires a capable smartphone or computer—can be cost prohibitive, especially for those whose obesity is already due to difficult socioeconomic circumstances. In addition, problems with the interoperability of devices, apps, and computers can increase cost. Health or technology illiteracy and concerns about privacy of health information and personal details (age, location, etc.) are important issues that are not always well addressed. Unfortunately, the enthusiasm for the capability of this technology can often overwhelm caution about equal access and the privacy of personal data.[47]

Usability is a particular concern in technology adoption. Usability is a broad term comprising the quality of content and the ease of use of a technical device or application and is thought to play an important role in determining the adoption of technology by the end user. Several studies have looked at particular categories of technology in this field and found a variety of results. Factors affecting usability of technology in specific populations (e.g., pregnant women in the care of midwives) include an accurate appraisal of risks and benefits for specific populations as well as the accessibility and availability of the technology and influence over the content and frequency of messaging.[48,49]

EFFECTIVENESS OF ELECTRONIC TOOLS IN MANAGING OBESITY

Overview and Methods

Despite the relatively recent development of many of the tools described, a sizable existing body of literature examines the effectiveness of these tools in combating obesity. Often, the designs of these studies involve a combination of technological methods, so their evaluation and results will frequently not promote the use of a single technology in isolation, but a combination of electronic tools as well as combining these tools with more traditional aspects of care. During the 10-year period from 2005 to 2015, over 100 relevant studies were published, including several systematic reviews and at least 2 systematic reviews of reviews.[50,51] As a group, these studies suggested that electronic tools can be valuable in helping people lose weight in the short term. However, the usefulness of the findings of these studies thus far has been somewhat limited by both methodological and reporting issues.

Because they involve comprehensive review of existing research as well as methodological assessment of individual studies, systematic reviews can provide valuable, high-level evidence to guide clinical practice. More than a dozen such reviews have been published on the use of electronic tools in the treatment and management of obesity. The relatively large number of available systematic reviews, and the breadth of their coverage, improves the chance that all available evidence about these tools has been found and that there has been some assessment of the included studies. We have therefore based much of our overview of the effectiveness of existing electronic tools on the findings of current systematic reviews.

The reviews summarized here have, as expected, varied in their scope and focus. Some have used broad selection criteria—such as all "technology-based,"[52,53]

"-assisted,"[54,55] or "-supported"[56] interventions—in selecting studies to include in their reviews, while others have restricted their focus to the use of specific types of tools, such as computers,[57] mobile phones,[58,59] or smartphones.[60] Most of the studies included in these reviews have reported at least one physical measure of weight loss (e.g., change in weight, waist circumference, or body mass index [BMI]). Others have focused on change in related behaviors (e.g., physical activity, healthy eating), and a few have included measures of psychosocial variables. The majority of the studies lasted 3 to 12 months, with a few including follow-up data for longer periods. All reviews provided narrative summaries of results; 3 employed meta-analytic techniques to combine quantitative results of individual studies.[57,61,62] Regardless of the specific focus, most systematic reviews have found mixed-quality studies, with weak-to-moderate evidence of short-term benefits of electronic tools in promoting weight loss.

We elected to present evidence from the use of electronic tools without regard to gender initially because women are overrepresented in most studies of weight loss interventions, and the number of female-only studies is still small. We examine systematic review data for adults first, then children and adolescents (because the data are difficult to parse into adolescent age groups only). We then look at the findings of recent studies that have focused on the effectiveness of these tools specifically for women.

Adults—Both Sexes

Allen and colleagues[54] reviewed clinical trials of technology-assisted weight management interventions in a variety of outpatient and population-based settings. The 39 trials selected for inclusion in their review employed a variety of electronic tools, including text or e-mail messaging, online chat rooms, or self-monitoring with smartphones or other mobile devices. Duration for most trials was 3, 6, or 12 months, with only 4 of the 39 studies reporting follow-up data greater than 12 months. Of the trials, 53% reported statistically significant weight loss for intervention groups as compared with control groups, but the magnitude of the weight loss seen ranged in the low single digits for both absolute loss (in kilograms) and percentage loss.

Levine et al.,[55] also looking at technology-assisted weight loss interventions, limited their focus to interventions implemented in an ambulatory primary care setting. Sixteen studies qualified for inclusion in their review. Similar to the review by Allen et al., the duration of included studies ranged from 3 to 12 months, with only 4 lasting longer than 12 months. Twelve of the 16 studies that met the review's inclusion criteria reported greater weight loss for intervention groups than for control groups, with weight loss in intervention groups ranging from 0.08 to 5.4 kg (0.8%–5.8% of initial body weight, respectively). Of note, there were 5 studies in common between the Allen and Levine reviews.

A Cochrane systematic review by Wieland et al. focused specifically on computer-based interventions for weight loss in obese adults.[57] The reviewers included in their study only randomized controlled trials (RCTs) or quasi-RCTs, in which follow-up data were available for at least 80% of participants. Their literature search was unusually comprehensive, including searches of a federally funded biomedical research database, a registry of controlled trials, and reference lists of included studies and review articles, as well as consultation with study authors and experts in the field.

Eighteen studies were included: 14 that focused on weight loss and 4 that focused on weight maintenance. Because of the great variability in study design across the included studies, reviewers grouped individual studies according to treatment type, control condition, outcomes, and time frames and performed several separate analyses using meta-analytic (quantitative) techniques. Overall, they found that interactive computer-based interventions led to greater short-term weight loss compared to minimal or no treatment (mean differences of 1–2 kg between groups). However, computer-based interventions were found to be *less* effective than in-person interventions.

Other reviews have focused specifically on the use of mobile devices. Khokhar et al.[61] examined the effectiveness of electronic mobile devices in combating weight loss. They found only 6 RCTs that met their study's inclusion criteria: 4 trials that involved the use of mobile phones and 2 that involved the use of PDAs. Meta-analysis found a weighted mean difference in weight attributed to device use of –1.09 kg (95% confidence interval [CI] –2.12 to –0.05). However, further analysis that grouped studies by the type of device used revealed that the change was significant for studies involving mobile phones (weighted mean difference: –1.78 kg [95% CI –2.92 to –0.63]), but *not* for studies employing PDAs (weighted mean difference: –0.23 kg [95% CI –0.87 to 0.41). Moreover, the significant impact of mobile phone use was influenced heavily by a single study that used a mobile phone app, whereas the comparator studies used only text messaging.

In a systematic review of mobile phone interventions, Liu and colleagues[62] found 14 relevant RCTs (including 3 studies that were also included in the review by Khokhar et al.). Included studies lasted from 1 to 12 months. Meta-analysis found small but significant reductions in both body weight (–1.44 kg, 95% CI –2.12 to –0.76 kg) and BMI (–0.024 kg/m^2, 95% CI –0.40 to –0.08 kg/m^2).

The findings of narrative (non systematic) reviews are generally consistent with these findings. McTigue and Conroy,[63] for example, reviewed RCTs of weight loss interventions that included an online (Internet) component, limiting their discussion to those studies reporting follow-up data 12 months or longer. Ten studies were included, and reviewers found that "only about half of the studies showed a significant difference in weight loss between study arms" (p. 101). The authors noted, however, that the studies varied considerably in design, and nonsignificant results were "partially mitigated by the fact that some studies compared more than one active study arm."[63]

Children and Adolescents—Both Sexes

Several systematic reviews have focused on the effectiveness of electronic tools in the prevention and treatment of pediatric obesity; we include a summary of these here because most studies included adolescent females in their study populations. Chen and Wilkosz[52] reviewed studies of technology-based interventions for obesity prevention in adolescents. Only 6 of the 14 identified studies (4 involving web-based activities and 2 involving video games) found significant decreases in either BMI or percentage body fat. All significant effects were short term, with durations ranging from immediately after the intervention to 9 months later. The one study that recorded long-term outcomes—24 months after the intervention—reported that significant differences found at 6 months had disappeared 18 months later.[64]

A review by An et al.[65] examined web-based weight management programs for children and adolescents. Of 8 identified RCTs, 6 reported statistically significant effectiveness of their interventions (either stand-alone programs or combined interventions) on measures of BMI, weight loss, physical activity, or dietary fat intake.

A review by Smith et al. looked at 13 studies evaluating the use of different types of health information technology in preventing childhood obesity.[66] Two of the studies compared weight loss in families receiving diet and exercise counseling delivered in person or by telemedicine. Neither of these two studies showed a significant difference in weight loss between the intervention and control groups. Three studies examined the use of text messaging or telephone support for weight loss in children and adolescents. While 2 of the 3 studies found no significant effect of the messaging/telephone support, one study found larger decreases in children's BMI at 1-year follow-up, but only for families with more intensive involvement in the intervention, and this study was focused on preteen children.

A 2015 systematic review by Turner et al. examined the effectiveness of mobile and wireless technologies in preventing and treating pediatric obesity.[67] Participants in 95% of identified studies were 12–15 years of age. Forty-one articles (reporting on 32 studies) fit the review's selection criteria. However, only 7 articles (describing 3 studies) were RCTs; the others were all categorized by the authors as either pilot interventions or technology use and design studies. In all 3 RCTs, SMS messaging was used in addition to other modes of treatment (e.g., group sessions, in-person visits, website). Results indicated that the addition of SMS messaging to other treatment modes added no significant effect in terms of BMI, weight-to-height ratio, adiposity, physical activity, diet, or psychosocial outcomes.

Focusing on behavior change, Lau and colleagues[53] reviewed technology-based interventions for promoting physical activity in children and adolescents. Nine RCTs were selected for review (including 2 studies that were also included in the review by Chen and Wilcosz, described previously[52]). Only 3 of those 9 studies reported significantly greater change (i.e., more physical activity) in intervention groups versus comparison groups. One study, however, reported significantly greater change in the comparison group.

Key Features of Effective Electronic Tools

Several review articles identified one or more features that appeared to be key to the success of the technology-assisted interventions in the studies they reviewed. Two features, in particular, were repeatedly cited as critical to successful weight loss interventions:

- self-monitoring (of weight, diet, activity)[51,55,57,58,67–69] and
- feedback, preferably from a (human) counselor or clinician.[51,54,55,57,67–70]

Other features noted as important to successful technology-assisted interventions include:

- social support and encouragement from others,[58,63,67,70]
- the ability to set specific goals,[51,68,70] and
- customization and personalization of the goals and device/software settings.[58,71]

This is consistent with findings of an oft-cited review by Khaylis et al.,[72] the goal of which was the identification of those program components that were most effective in facilitating weight loss. The authors reviewed 21 relevant studies that employed either randomized controlled or experimental pretest-posttest designs. Based on the findings of these studies, they identified 5 key intervention components that seemed to correlate best with successful outcomes: self-monitoring, counselor feedback and communication, social support, a structured program, and an individually tailored program.

The findings of these reviews point to the importance of human involvement in facilitating weight loss. Several reviews noted that, regardless of delivery mode (e.g., e-mail, text, face-to-face), feedback is most effective as part of a weight loss intervention when delivered by a person, rather than as fully automated messages.[55,73,74] For example, in a review of electronic health interventions for weight management among racial and ethnic minorities, Bennett et al. noted that, with one exception, all studies (included in their review) that reported significant outcomes involved interventions that also included support from a (human) counselor.[74] In addition, the consistent results of Wieland's comprehensive meta-analysis highlight the inability of most technology-assisted interventions to achieve the results of intensive in-person treatment.[57]

In addition to these key features, An et al.[65] suggested an additional factor important to the success of pediatric weight loss programs. In their review of weight management programs for children and adolescents, they noted that several of the successful programs included in their review involved the participation of one obese parent in the intervention along with the child. Citing other research in which parent or family involvement contributed to effective weight loss interventions, they recommended that family/parental involvement be included as a key factor in future web-based weight management programs for childhood obesity.

Limitations of Existing Systematic Reviews

With few exceptions, the authors of systematic reviews in this area have attached strong qualifications to their stated conclusions, warning of numerous characteristics of the reviewed studies that threaten the validity and thus the usefulness of those conclusions. Reviewers noted small sample sizes, high attrition rates, and the use of "completer" instead of "intent-to-treat" analyses in many of the studies, all potential sources of significant bias. Several report quantifiers of "risk of bias" (i.e., validity concerns) for included studies, most finding wide variability and an overall moderate risk of bias.

Levine et al.,[55] for example, found that 10 of the 16 studies included in their review scored 6 or fewer of 9 possible points on the Delphi[75] and Cochrane Effective Practice and Organization of Care (EPOC)[76] criteria. Liu et al.[62] assessed the methodological quality of the RCTs included in their review using the Jadad scoring system[77]; they found that 12 of the 14 studies scored 3 of a possible 5 points, with one scoring higher and one scoring lower. In reviews involving pediatric populations, Chen and Wilkosz[52] found that half of the studies selected for their review (7 of 14) scored 6 or fewer of 9 possible points on an adapted version of a scale used by the Cochrane Effective Practice and Organization of Care Review Group. Smith et al.[66] assessed the methodological quality of the studies included in their review using a 10-point scoring system; quality scores ranged from 1 to 10, with a mean score of 3.7. In their review of *review* articles, Tang et al. summarized that the "overall methodological quality of included reviews was relatively poor."[51] Most of the reviews that they examined failed to assess the methodological quality of individual studies or to consider potential reporting biases, and only 7 of the 20 reviews scored highly on the Overview Quality Assessment Questionnaire (OQAQ). All of these observations raise caution in interpreting and generalizing the findings of much of the current research.

In addition to more general methodological issues, heterogeneity in both interventions and control groups among existing studies make drawing strong conclusions difficult, if not impossible. As would be expected, interventions varied across studies with regard to the specific technology used (e.g., websites, text messaging, online group meetings), making generalizations about optimal methods or platforms difficult.[54,57,58,74,78] Even more confounding, however, is the fact that some studies examined technology-assisted interventions as *stand-alone* treatments, while others studied the impact of one or more electronic tools used in *combination* with one or more standard treatment techniques (e.g., in-person counseling, group meetings).[51,53,59,67,79] Some studies also included financial compensation (incentives, payments, or fees)[78] in their intervention programs. Such study designs make it extremely difficult to distinguish which component(s) of the intervention can be credited with any measured improvements.

Comparison groups in existing studies also varied in important ways that affect interpretation of results. In some studies, control and comparison groups received no treatment at all; in others, they received "minimal" or "standard" treatments, and in still others, control groups received intensive in-person treatment.[67] (Moreover, it has been noted that standard treatment for obesity varies considerably by setting, particularly across different countries.[78]) All of these are valid "control" groups for purposes of internal validity. These differences, however, complicate the interpretation and external validity of the combined results.

The review undertaken by Wieland et al.[37] comprised an ambitious effort to overcome this wide variation in study design. In this review, the authors divided individual studies, and even individual study "arms," into groups with similar treatment type (computer-based intervention as a sole intervention vs. as a part of a combined intervention); control conditions (minimal or no intervention vs. intensive in-person intervention); outcomes measured; and time frames and then conducted separate meta-analyses combining results within these smaller groups. The authors noted that it was difficult to draw firm conclusions from these analyses because they were based on very small numbers of studies. Another methodological consequence of this approach is the problems presented by multiple comparisons. Nonetheless, this method helps to disentangle the possible impact of various treatments, and the consistency of the review's findings is noteworthy.

Finally, reviewers have discussed the difficulties posed by incomplete reporting *within* studies and inconsistent reporting *across* studies. Several noted, for example, that many research reports have failed to include adherence rates (i.e., rates of exposure to, or engagement with, the intervention).[53,57,68,74] Others noted limitations caused by failure of researchers to include results for subgroup analyses, such as race/ethnicity[74] or gender.[59] Moreover, even when information *is* reported for variables such as adherence, definitions and metrics used have often varied across studies,[54,68,74] further complicating attempts to compare or combine results across studies. Unfortunately, all of these issues preclude our ability to draw strong conclusions from the results of existing studies in this area.

Effectiveness of Electronic Tools for Weight Management in Women

Having completed the review of the broad landscape concerning the effectiveness of electronic tools in managing obesity in populations that included women and adolescent girls, we now turn to focus on studies of effectiveness targeting women in particular. Single studies for obesity in women's health particularly fall into two major categories: women with overweight or obesity (often focusing on specific target populations) and prevention of excessive weight gain in pregnant women.

Many recent studies have examined the potential of electronic tools in assisting women in combating weight gain and obesity. Several have focused on weight loss for women within specific minority groups. In 1 RCT, overweight/obese African American women participated in an intervention that included instruction, reminders, support, and exercise videos, all provided via home Internet-enabled digital video recorders, along with telephone counseling and support.[80] At 9-month follow-up, weight loss in the intervention group was not significantly different from weight loss in the control group. Another randomized controlled study examined the effectiveness of text messaging in promoting weight loss among racial and ethnic minority women.[81] Using a fully automated messaging system, participants logged behaviors related to tailored health-related goals and received feedback, reminders, and reinforcement by text messaging and e-mail. After 6 months, average weight loss in the intervention group was higher than in the control group, but the difference was not significant. Authors of both of these studies noted that low adherence rates may have limited their findings.

Other studies have targeted women who have survived cancer. In a study by McCarroll et al.,[82] overweight/obese survivors of endometrial or breast cancer used a mobile application to log daily food intake, body weight, and exercise type and duration. Participants received individualized feedback and reminders via phone, e-mail, or push notification. At the end of the 4-week study, researchers found a significant reduction in weight, with an average weight loss of 2.3 kg. In another study,[83] overweight/obese rural breast cancer survivors recorded food intake using e-mail, fax, or voice message; received feedback; and participated in weekly group telephone sessions. After 6 months, researchers observed a significant average weight loss of 12.5 kg. Unfortunately, however, the interpretation of the findings of these 2 studies is unclear because neither study included a control group.

Two systematic reviews have examined the usefulness of electronic tools specifically for weight management in women. Derbyshire and Dancey[60] reviewed the literature on the use of smartphone applications for women's health. Of the 15 RCTs selected for inclusion in their review, 10 involved smartphone applications designed to assist with weight loss. Interventions in these 10 studies included various combinations of self-monitoring/reporting of weight, diet, or exercise; information or counseling; and personalized feedback or reinforcement via text or twitter messaging, podcasts, mobile applications, or the Internet. Two of the 10 studies lasted for 12 months; durations of all others ranged from 2 to 6 months. Eight of the 10 studies reported significantly greater weight loss for groups using the smartphone applications than for control groups.

O'Brien et al.[56] reviewed the literature on technology-supported interventions for healthy pregnant women. Acknowledging the small number of RCTs on this topic, the reviewers included cross-sectional observational studies, feasibility studies, and ongoing trials, as well as RCTs in their selection criteria. They found 5 RCTs and 2 cross-sectional observational studies. The 2 observational studies (which both evaluated the same national health promotion program) both focused on program usage or appreciation, rather than effectiveness; neither recorded information on clinical or behavioral outcomes. Four of the 5 RCTs reported on studies that were ongoing at the time of the search (March 2013) and thus had incomplete data. The one remaining study, which assessed the impact of an interactive, computerized teaching and counseling tool, found no statistically significant difference between intervention and control group with regard to gestational weight gained. Some significant differences were found, however, with regard to self-reported physical activity, healthy eating behaviors, nutritional knowledge, and frequency of patient-clinician discussions about these topics.

The findings of these reviews are not notably different from the findings of reviews involving the general population. Like those reviews, discussed previously, these women-specific studies revealed some weak-to-moderate evidence of short-term effectiveness, with key success features that are very similar to those in the more general reviews. The similarity is not surprising because women are overrepresented among subjects in most studies in this field. And, like the studies included in the reviews described in the previous section, the studies included in these two reviews present methodological issues (including small sample sizes, high attrition rates, short follow-up durations, combination interventions, and varying control conditions) that make it difficult to draw strong conclusions. Thus, research results in this area demonstrate the promising potential of the role electronic tools can play in the management and treatment of obesity, but, at this point, our conclusions must remain cautious.

Public Health Impact of Electronic Tools

The state of the research in this field is overall poor. Most studies measure only immediate outcomes and fail to address true population health impact. The RE-AIM (reach, effectiveness, adoption, implementation, maintenance) framework has been adopted as a measure of the true public health impact of population health and clinical interventions.[84] A review of physical health-promoting applications categorized the existing research by their outcomes in the RE-AIM framework and found that the outcomes studied focused primarily on reach, effectiveness, and implementation and rarely on adoption and maintenance. Of course, the true evaluation of behavior change interventions hinges on these longer-term outcomes of adoption and maintenance, so the real test of many of these interventions has yet to be performed.[85]

Adverse Effects/Risks of Electronic Tools

While much research has pointed to the potential benefits of the use of electronic tools in this field, some researchers have warned of possible adverse effects, particularly regarding the widespread use of commercially available mobile apps by patients. Most concerns have focused on potential health risks for patients due to inaccurate or unreliable health information, threats to privacy and confidentiality of sensitive information, or liability risks for clinicians.

Potential Health Risks for Patients

Recent research has demonstrated that numerous commercially available weight management apps lack a clear evidence base and thus may provide incomplete, inaccurate, or out-of-date health information to users. Breton and colleagues assessed 204 weight loss apps according to their adherence to 13 evidence-based practices common to 4 governmental agencies (Centers for Disease Control and Prevention [CDC], National Institutes of Health [NIH], FDA, and US Department of Agriculture [USDA]).[86] They found that 124 (61%) of the 204 apps included only 2 or fewer of the 13 evidence-based guidelines, and only 10 of the 204 apps included 8 or more of the 13 guidelines. In another study, Gan and Allman-Farinelli assessed the quality of the content of smartphone apps related to weight loss by calculating a composite score based, in part, on measures of topic coverage, scientific accuracy, and author accountability.[87] (Calculation of their composite score also included a measure of applicability to the Australian population, which may or may not be relevant to other populations.) Based on composite scores, only 8 of the 54 reviewed apps were rated as "good"; 32 were rated as "fair" and 14 as "poor." Stevens et al. looked at the degree to which medical professionals have been involved in app development. They identified 28 apps related to weight loss surgery, including 26 apps targeting patients and 2 intended for clinician use.[45] Only 12 of the 28 apps reported input from health professionals in determining the content provided.

Similar findings have been reported for apps focusing on other health-related topics. In a review of 39 melanoma detection apps, Kassionos et al.[88] found little evidence of clinician input and no evidence that any of the apps had been checked for accuracy. Rosser and Eccleston[89] reviewed 111 smartphone apps for pain management. Of these, 86% did not report any involvement of a health care professional in app development, and the great majority of those did not report the source of the health information provided by the app. Pandey et al.[90] reviewed cancer-related apps and reported that only 43 of 77 reviewed apps included scientifically validated information. Of the 46 apps targeting the general public (vs. health care workers), only 32% were based on scientifically validated information. In a review of apps relevant to breast disease, Mobasheri et al.[91] found that only 21 (14%) of 148 apps had a documented evidence base, and only 19 (13%) of the 148 apps reported the involvement of a medical professional in the development of the app. While these studies did not specifically involve the treatment or management of obesity, they provide one indication of a lack of quality of content found in health-related mobile apps for women and suggested that many of these apps may not be appropriate for evidence-based practice in women's health.

Threats to Privacy and Confidentiality

The field of eHealth and mHealth has a dearth of studies that look at actual outcomes related to privacy, security, and liability in the use of electronic applications and devices. The studies reviewed here have looked instead at the landscape of potential threat from these applications. A German informatics group has produced 2 reviews of potential security and privacy issues. The first study performed an automated and exhaustive search of health and medical app categories in the Apple iTunes® store and the Android Play® store.[92] The privacy policies of 600 of the most frequently used applications in these stores were analyzed for their content. Only 31% of the applications had privacy policies, and of those, the average policy contained 1755 words. The reading level generally recommended for patient education materials is between 5th- and 8th-grade level,[93] but most of these policies were written at the reading level of a 16-year-old (10th or 11th grade). Some policies were written so generically that they did not even mention the specific features of the apps they covered.

A second study by this group reviewed all available mHealth apps in the same 2 app stores and analyzed them for the level of potential risk posed by the apps' stated capabilities, storage, and communication requirements. There was no detailed analysis of the code of these apps, and the authors did not actually use the apps. The authors analyzed approximately 25% of the apps found in the stores based on their assessment of significant use through reviews and ratings. They assessed the level of potential risk by categorizing apps into 12 "archetypes" or categories based on their principal function (e.g., treatment guides, fitness trackers, health records) and analyzing each archetype's potential risk in categories: the specificity of health information (as opposed to other personal information); the impact of loss of data (important data being unavailable for management decisions); change in management based on inaccurate data; disclosure of data (embarrassment, threats to employment, etc.); and value of stolen data (identity theft, employment decisions, etc.).[94] Of all apps, 96% were assessed as posing at least some security risk using this method, with risks ranging from minimal to severe. Also, 16% were found to pose high levels of privacy risk based on their categorizations as health records, health monitors, and personalized treatment reminders.

A review of current laws in the United States and Europe and proposals for eHealth and mHealth policies found a regulatory and policy environment that is wanting. The review found too few applicable laws in the European Union. The laws found in the United States were dated and too random in focus and were applicable principally to eHealth, not specifically to mHealth applications and devices. The authors recommended the following security precautions for app developers: standard electronic security measures (strong passwords, suitable encryption, etc.); patient-controlled access based on specific roles; erasure of personal health information when it is no longer needed; and some procedure for notification and compensation in the case of a security breach.

Liability Concerns for Clinicians

Many innovations in medicine bring concern about liability for clinicians. The stories of privacy concerns with routine Internet and social networking use coupled with the explosion of interest in mHealth and eHealth applications has magnified this concern. A study by McGraw et al. studied the liability concerns voiced by clinicians during a research project focused on the design of specific eHealth applications.[95] This study found the primary concerns to be timeliness and adequacy of the response to electronic patient information, the potential volume of data to be dealt with, and the accuracy of patient-reported or device-reported data for making medical decisions. The principal caveat to conclusions from this research is the lack of a definition of "standard of care" in dealing with innovative technologies, which is the standard against which liability determinations are made in health care. The authors advised that clinicians (1) review with their patients and agree on the types of data to be transferred electronically, (2) assign a specific staff member to monitor the flow of this data,

(3) devise a specific medical emergency protocol, and (4) actively review the appropriateness of each piece of the patient's electronic information for inclusion in the record.

A legally oriented review by Yang and Silverman summarized both the privacy and liability concerns with electronic tools, noting the "patchwork of legal and liability issues" in the United States. Their summary recommendations for clinicians were to demand appropriate data security from any app provider and establish clear protocols for monitoring the information from these apps and devices.[96]

Cautions

In this exciting new world of technological support for health, a few cautions are in order. The evidence base, as seen in the previous section, is largely immature and depends on studies with proxy and short-term outcomes.[97] New frameworks for evaluation of electronic tools have been suggested,[98] but this field will continue to evolve. Legal liability for information contained in or transmitted by these tools is an evolving field also. If an application transmits data or information to a medical office, systems should be set up to ensure data security, proper integration into medical records, and a protocol for identifying and handling emergent results.[95]

Adolescents, particularly females, are at risk when online in social media situations, so caution about the dangers of predatory sexual activity and bullying are important to consider when recommending technological interventions. The American College of Cardiology guideline concerning use of technology and social media to combat obesity in children suggests active engagement by clinicians by offering to act as an additional information resource for parents and children when they are engaging in social media about health issues.[99]

CONCLUSIONS

Recommendations for Use

In the tradition of Hippocrates, the first recommendation for use of the electronic tools described in this chapter must be "Do no harm." In the field of technology, this harm relates first to privacy. Do not use yourself, and advise patients not to use, unencrypted e-mail or apps that do not provide encryption when patient health information is communicated from device to device. Minimize the transfer of personal health information between devices and use established methods (such as existing electronic health record patient portals or interfaces designed specifically for the device) to exchange that information when necessary. Ensure that storage of such data is enhanced with encryption and strong passwords. Ensure that wireless networks used for clinical purposes to transmit data use the strongest available security.

Be careful about your online presence and social network activity, remaining aware that the provision of medical information can constitute medical advice and avoiding the use of any personal health information on these networks. If you choose to provide medical information online, review any provided information online carefully with legal counsel and encourage readers to discuss this information with their health care providers before using the information.[100] Advise your patients, especially teens, to exercise extreme care on social networks to avoid bullying or accidental disclosure of personal information and to disclose any harassment or bullying to parents or guardians.

Encourage the use of monitoring devices (when approved) and apps—from accelerometers to diet and weight logs—as ways to support behavior change. The accuracy of most accelerometers is good enough for the patient to use them for goal setting and behavior reinforcement.[29,30] Encourage your patients to share their information with you so you can engage in open discussions about their behavior change and can provide the necessary support and encouragement.

For online communities and apps containing weight loss information or strategies beyond diet and weight logs, advise your patients to look for more well-known and reviewed applications and to discuss the recommendations and information with you so that you can counter any misinformation and provide any necessary context for recommendations found in them. Work against the tendency for patients not to disclose the use of these technologies by asking about their use, congratulating the patient for the commitment to weight management, and encouraging the open discussion of information.

State of the Literature

The field of electronic tools for the management of obesity is still relatively new. The existing body of research reflects this with its plethora of pilot and feasibility studies and studies with small sample sizes and short-term outcomes. The outcomes seen to date, however, show some promise for the judicious use of these tools to (1) encourage conversations between the clinician and patient around weight loss and (2) support patients in their behavioral change with monitoring, goal setting, and community support.

The clinician's goal should be to try to remain abreast of the changes in this field by asking patients about any new tools they are using and looking for more definitive research on their effectiveness. The more valuable research will consist of RCTs with longer-term outcomes (preferably greater than 1 year) and will look at weight lost and maintained, as well as reduction in weight-related morbidity (or mortality), and will have a clear assessment of adverse effects.

REFERENCES

1. Ventola CL. Mobile devices and apps for health care professionals: uses and benefits. *P T.* 2014;39(5):356–364.
2. US Department of Health and Human Services. Doctors and hospitals' use of health IT more than doubles since 2012. http://www.hhs.gov/news/press/2013pres/05/20130522a.html. Published May 22, 2013. Accessed January 25, 2015.
3. Diaz JA, Griffith RA, Ng JJ, Reinert SE, Friedmann PD, Moulton AW. Patients' use of the Internet for medical information. *J Gen Intern Med.* 2002;17(3):180–185.
4. Hearn L, Miller M, Fletcher A. Online healthy lifestyle support in the perinatal period: what do women want and do they use it? *Aust J Prim Health.* 2013;19(4):313–318.
5. Gilmore LA, Duhé AF, Frost EA, Redman LM. The technology boom: a new era in obesity management. *J Diabetes Sci Technol.* 2014;8(3):596–608.
6. Kulie T, Slattengren A, Redmer J, Counts H, Eglash A, Schrager S. Obesity and women's health: an evidence-based review. *J Am Board Fam Med.* 2011;24(1):75–85.
7. Lash MM, Armstrong A. Impact of obesity on women's health. *Fertil Steril.* 2009;91(5):1712–1716.
8. Epling JW, Morley CP, Ploutz-Snyder R. Family physician attitudes in managing obesity: a cross-sectional survey study. *BMC Res Notes.* 2011;4:473. doi:10.1186/1756-0500-4-473.
9. Foster GD, Wadden TA, Makris AP, et al. Primary care physicians' attitudes about obesity and its treatment. *Obes Res.* 2003;11(10):1168–1177.
10. Fujioka K, Bakhru N. Office-based management of obesity. *Mt Sinai J Med.* 2010;77(5):466–471.
11. Chang M, Nitzke S, Brown R, Resnicow K. A community based prevention of weight gain intervention (Mothers in Motion) among young low-income

overweight and obese mothers: design and rationale. *BMC Public Health.* 2014;14:280.

12. Demment MM, Graham ML, Olson CM. How an online intervention to prevent excessive gestational weight gain is used and by whom: a randomized controlled process evaluation. *J Med Internet Res.* 2014;16(8):e194.

13. Kontos E, Blake KD, Chou WS, Prestin A. Predictors of eHealth usage: insights on the digital divide from the health information national trends survey 2012. *J Med Internet Res.* 2014;16(7):e172.

14. Walker LO, Im EO, Vaughan MW. Communication technologies and maternal interest in health-promotion information about postpartum weight and parenting practices. *J Obstet Gynecol Neonatal Nurs.* 2012;41(2):201–215.

15. Naslund JA, Aschbrenner KA, Barre LK, Bartels SJ. Feasibility of popular m-health technologies for activity tracking among individuals with serious mental illness. *Telemed e-Health.* 2015;21(3):213–216.

16. Ptomey LT, Sullivan DK, Lee J, Goetz JR, Gibson C, Donnelly JE. The use of technology for delivering a weight loss program for adolescents with intellectual and developmental disabilities. *J Acad Nutri Dietet.* 2015;115(1):112–118.

17. Lee H, Kane I, Brar J, Sereika S. Telephone-delivered physical activity intervention for individuals with serious mental illness: a feasibility study. *J Am Psychiatr Nurses Assoc.* 2014;20(6):389–397.

18. Barnett J, Harricharan M, Fletcher D, Gilchrist B, Coughlan J. myPace: an integrative health platform for supporting weight loss and maintenance behaviours. *IEEE J Biomed Health Inform.* 2015;19(1):109–116.

19. Daugherty BL, Schap TE, Ettienne-Gittens R, et al. Novel technologies for assessing dietary intake: evaluating the usability of a mobile telephone food record among adults and adolescents. *J Med Internet Res.* 2012;14(2):e58.

20. Castelnuovo G, Manzoni GM, Villa V, Cesa GL, Pietrabissa G, Molinari E. The STRATOB study: design of a randomized controlled clinical trial of cognitive behavioral therapy and brief strategic therapy with telecare in patients with obesity and binge-eating disorder referred to residential nutritional rehabilitation. *Trials.* 2011;12:114.

21. Dunn C, Whetstone LM, Kolasa KM, et al. Using synchronous distance-education technology to deliver a weight management intervention. *J Nutr Educ Behav.* 2014;46(6):602–609.

22. Butryn ML, Webb V, Wadden TA. Behavioral treatment of obesity. *Psychiatr Clin North Am.* 2011;34(4):841–859.

23. Patel MS, Asch DA, Volpp KG. Wearable devices as facilitators, not drivers, of health behavior change. *JAMA.* 2015;313(5):459–460.

24. Musgrove M. Voxiva launches US text service to aid pregnant women. *The Washington Post.* February 9, 2010: Business. http://www.washingtonpost.com/wp-dyn/content/article/2010/02/08/AR2010020803680.html. Accessed December 22, 2014.

25. US Department of Health and Human Services. *Physical Activity Evaluation Handbook.* Atlanta, GA: US Department of Health and Human Services, Centers for Disease Control and Prevention; 2002.

26. Carrino S, Caon M, Angelini L, et al. PEGASO: a personalised and motivational ICT system to empower adolescents towards healthy lifestyles. *Stud Health Technol Inform.* 2014;207:350–359.

27. Delgado M. How fit is that fitbit? *Berkeley Science Review.* December 19, 2014. http://berkeleysciencereview.com/fit-fitbit/. Accessed December 19, 2014.

28. Kim HK, Niederdeppe J, Guillory J, Graham M, Olson C, Gay G. Determinants of pregnant women's online self-regulatory activities for appropriate gestational weight gain. *Health Commun.* 2015;30(9):922–932.

29. Arif M, Bilal M, Kattan A, Ahamed SI. Better physical activity classification using smartphone acceleration sensor. *J Med Syst.* 2014;38(9):95.

30. Lee J, Kim Y, Welk GJ. Validity of consumer-based physical activity monitors. *Med Sci Sports Exerc.* 2014;46(9):1840–1848.

31. Fontana JM, Farooq M, Sazonov E. Automatic ingestion monitor: a novel wearable device for monitoring of ingestive behavior. *IEEE Trans Biomed Eng.* 2014;61(6):1772–1779.

32. Martin CK, Nicklas T, Gunturk B, Correa JB, Allen HR, Champagne C. Measuring food intake with digital photography. *J Hum Nutri Dietet.* 2014;27:72–81.

33. Kampfrath T. Food and drug administration starts treating mobile medical apps as medical devices. *Clin Chem.* 2014;60(2):428.

34. Alrajeh NA, Lloret J, Canovas A. A framework for obesity control using a wireless body sensor network. *Int J Distrib Sensor Networks.* 2014; Article ID 534760.

35. Federal Communications Commission. Amendment of the commission's rules to provide spectrum for the operation of medical body area netwoks. *Fed Regist.* Dec 22, 2014;ET Docket No. 08-59; FCC 14-124. http://www.fcc.gov/document/commission-finalizes-rules-operation-medical-body-area-networks. Accessed December 22, 2014.

36. Federal Communications Commission. Medical body area network—final rule. *Fed Regist.* 2014; 79(193):60092. http://www.gpo.gov/fdsys/pkg/FR-2014-10-06/pdf/2014-23519.pdf. Accessed December 23, 2014.

37. Appel HB, Huang B, Cole A, James R, Ai AL. Starting the conversation—a childhood obesity knowledge project using an app. *Br J Med Med Res.* 2014;4(7):1526–1538.

38. Bouhaidar CM, DeShazo JP, Puri P, Gray P, Robins JL, Salyer J. Text messaging as adjunct to community-based weight management program. *Comput Inform Nurs*. 2013;31(10):469–476.

39. Faghanipour S, Hajikazemi E, Nikpour S, Shariatpanahi SA, Hosseini AF. Mobile phone short message service (SMS) for weight management in iranian overweight and obese women: a pilot study. *Int J Telemed Appl*. 2013;2013:785654.

40. Gerber BS, Stolley MR, Thompson AL, Sharp LK, Fitzgibbon ML. Mobile phone text messaging to promote healthy behaviors and weight loss maintenance: a feasibility study. *Health Informatics J*. 2009;15(1):17–25.

41. Brindal E, Hendrie G, Freyne J, Coombe M, Berkovsky S, Noakes M. Design and pilot results of a mobile phone weight-loss application for women starting a meal replacement programme. *J Telemed Telecare*. 2013;19:166–174.

42. Steinberg DM, Levine EL, Lane I, et al. Adherence to self-monitoring via interactive voice response technology in an eHealth intervention targeting weight gain prevention among black women: randomized controlled trial. *J Med Internet Res*. 2014;16(4):e114.

43. Ayash CR, Simon SR, Marshall R, et al. Evaluating the impact of point-of-care decision support tools in improving diagnosis of obese children in primary care. *Obesity (Silver Spring)*. 2013;21(3):576–582.

44. Dryden EM, Hardin J, McDonald J, Taveras EM, Hacker K. Provider perspectives on electronic decision supports for obesity prevention. *Clin Pediatr (Phila)*. 2012;51(5):490–497.

45. Stevens DJ, Jackson JA, Howes N, Morgan J. Obesity surgery smartphone apps: a review. *Obes Surg*. 2014;24(1):32–36.

46. Connor K, Brady RRW, Tulloh B, de Beaux A. Smartphone applications (apps) for bariatric surgery. *Obes Surg*. 2013;23(10):1669–1672.

47. Bipartisan Policy Center. *Improving Quality and Reducing Costs in Health Care: Engaging Consumers Using Electronic Tools*. Washington, DC: Bipartisan Policy Center; December 2012.

48. Jeon E, Park HA, Min YH, Kim HY. Analysis of the information quality of Korean obesity-management smartphone applications. *Healthc Inform Res*. 2014;20(1):23–29.

49. Soltani H, Furness PJ, Arden MA, et al. Women's and midwives' perspectives on the design of a text messaging support for maternal obesity services: an exploratory study. *J Obes*. 2012;2012:835464. doi:10.1155/2012/835464.

50. Stephens SK, Cobiac LJ, Veerman JL. Improving diet and physical activity to reduce population prevalence of overweight and obesity: an overview of current evidence. *Prev Med*. 2014;62:167–178.

51. Tang J, Abraham C, Greaves C, Yates T. Self-directed interventions to promote weight loss: a systematic review of reviews. *J Med Internet Res*. 2014;16(2):e58:4.

52. Chen J, Wilkosz ME. Efficacy of technology-based interventions for obesity prevention in adolescents: a systematic review. *Adolesc Health Med Ther*. 2014;5:159–170.

53. Lau PW, Lau EY, Wong del P, Ransdell L. A systematic review of information and communication technology-based interventions for promoting physical activity behavior change in children and adolescents. *J Med Internet Res*. 2011;13(3):e48.

54. Allen JK, Stephens J, Patel A. Technology-assisted weight management interventions: systematic review of clinical trials. *Telemed J E Health*. 2014;20(12):1103–1120.

55. Levine DM, Savarimuthu S, Squires A, Nicholson J, Jay M. Technology-assisted weight loss interventions in primary care: a systematic review. *J Gen Intern Med*. 2015;30(1):107–117.

56. O'Brien OA, McCarthy M, Gibney ER, McAuliffe FM. Technology-supported dietary and lifestyle interventions in healthy pregnant women: a systematic review. *Eur J Clin Nutr*. 2014;68(7):760–766.

57. Wieland LS, Falzon L, Sciamanna CN, et al. Interactive computer-based interventions for weight loss or weight maintenance in overweight or obese people. *Cochrane Database Systc Rev*. 2012;8:CD007675.

58. Aguilar-Martínez A, Solé-Sedeño JM, Mancebo-Moreno G, Medina FX, Carreras-Collado R, Saigí-Rubió F. Use of mobile phones as a tool for weight loss: a systematic review. *J Telemed Telecare*. 2014;20(6):339–349.

59. Stephens J, Allen J. Mobile phone interventions to increase physical activity and reduce weight: a systematic review. *J Cardiovasc Nurs*. 2013;28(4):320–329.

60. Derbyshire E, Dancey D. Smartphone medical applications for women's health: what is the evidence-base and feedback? *Int J Telemed Appl*. 2013;2013:782074.

61. Khokhar B, Jones J, Ronksley P, Caird J, Rabi D. The effectiveness of mobile electronic devices in weight loss among overweight and obese populations: a systematic review and meta-analysis. 2013;28:S201.

62. Liu F, Kong X, Cao J, et al. Mobile phone intervention and weight loss among overweight and obese adults: a meta-analysis of randomized controlled trials. *Am J Epidemiol*. 2015;181(5):337–348. doi:kwu260 [pii].

63. McTigue KM, Conroy MB. Use of the Internet in the treatment of obesity and prevention of type 2 diabetes in primary care. *Proc Nutr Soc*. 2013;72(1):98–108.

64. Williamson DA, Walden HM, White MA, et al. Two-year Internet-based randomized controlled trial for weight loss in african-american girls. *Obesity (Silver Spring)*. 2006;14(7):1231–1243.

65. An J, Hayman LL, Park Y, Dusaj TK, Ayres CG. Web-based weight management programs for children

and adolescents: a systematic review of randomized controlled trial studies. *ANS Adv Nurs Sci.* 2009;32(3):222–240.

66. Smith AJ, Skow Á, Bodurtha J, Kinra S. Health information technology in screening and treatment of child obesity: a systematic review. *Pediatrics.* 2013;131(3):c894–e902.

67. Turner T, Spruijt-Metz D, Wen CKF, Hingle MD. Prevention and treatment of pediatric obesity using mobile and wireless technologies: a systematic review. *Pediatr Obes.* 2015;10(6):403–409.

68. Coons MJ, Demott A, Buscemi J, et al. Technology interventions to curb obesity: a systematic review of the current literature. *Curr Cardiovasc Risk Rep.* 2012;6(2):120–134.

69. Thomas JG, Bond DS. Review of innovations in digital health technology to promote weight control. *Curr Diab Rep.* 2014;14(5):485–485.

70. Bort-Roig J, Gilson N, Puig-Ribera A, Contreras R, Trost S. Measuring and influencing physical activity with smartphone technology: a systematic review. *Sports Med.* 2014;44(5):671–686.

71. Michie S, Abraham C, Whittington C, McAteer J, Gupta S. Effective techniques in healthy eating and physical activity interventions: a meta-regression. *Health Psychol.* 2009;28(6):690.

72. Khaylis A, Yiaslas T, Bergstrom J, Gore-Felton C. A review of efficacious technology-based weight-loss interventions: five key components. *Telemed J E Health.* 2010;16(9):931–938.

73. Thomas JG, Bond DS. Review of innovations in digital health technology to promote weight control. *Curr Diab Rep.* 2014;14(5):485–485.

74. Bennett GG, Steinberg DM, Stoute C, et al. Electronic health (eHealth) interventions for weight management among racial/ethnic minority adults: a systematic review. *Obes Rev.* 2014;15(suppl 4):146–158.

75. Verhagen AP, de Vet HCW, de Bie RA, et al. The delphi list. *J Clin Epidemiol.* 1998;51(12):1235–1241.

76. Cochrane Effective Practice and Organisation of Care Group. Suggested risk of bias criteria for EPOC reviews. http://epoc.cochrane.org/sites/epoc.cochrane.org/files/uploads/14%20Suggested%20risk%20of%20bias%20criteria%20for%20EPOC%20reviews%2009%2002%2015_0.pdf. Accessed March 22, 2015.

77. Jadad AR, Moore RA, Carroll D, et al. Assessing the quality of reports of randomized clinical trials: is blinding necessary? *Control Clin Trials.* 1996;17(1):1–12.

78. Bacigalupo R, Cudd P, Littlewood C, Bissell P, Hawley MS, Buckley Woods H. Interventions employing mobile technology for overweight and obesity: an early systematic review of randomized controlled trials. *Obes Rev.* 2013;14(4):279–291.

79. Hutchesson MJ, Morgan PJ, McCoy P, Collins CE. Response to: Self-directed interventions to promote weight loss: a systematic review of reviews. *J Med Internet Res.* 2014;16(7):e178. doi:10.2196/jmir.3476.

80. Gerber BS, Schiffer L, Brown AA, et al. Video telehealth for weight maintenance of African-American women. *J Telemed Telecare.* 2013;19(5):266–272. doi:10.1177/1357633X13490901.

81. Steinberg DM, Levine EL, Askew S, Foley P, Bennett GG. Daily text messaging for weight control among racial and ethnic minority women: randomized controlled pilot study. *J Med Internet Res.* 2013;15(11):e244. doi:10.2196/jmir.2844.

82. McCarroll ML, Armbruster S, Pohle-Krauza RJ, et al. Feasibility of a lifestyle intervention for overweight/obese endometrial and breast cancer survivors using an interactive mobile application. *Gynecol Oncol.* 2015;137(3):508–515.

83. Befort CA, Klemp JR, Austin HL, et al. Outcomes of a weight loss intervention among rural breast cancer survivors. *Breast Cancer Res Treat.* 2012;132(2):631–639. doi:10.1007/s10549-011-1922-3.

84. Glasgow RE, Vogt TM, Boles SM. Evaluating the public health impact of health promotion interventions: the RE-AIM framework. *Am J Public Health.* 1999;89(9):1322–1327. Accessed March 28, 2015. doi:10.2105/AJPH.89.9.1322.

85. Blackman KC, Zoellner J, Berrey LM, et al. Assessing the internal and external validity of mobile health physical activity promotion interventions: a systematic literature review using the RE-AIM framework. *J Med Internet Res.* 2013;15(10):e224.

86. Breton ER, Fuemmeler BF, Abroms LC. Weight loss—there is an app for that! But does it adhere to evidence-informed practices? *Transl Behav Med.* 2011;1(4):523–529.

87. Gan KO, Allman-Farinelli M. A scientific audit of smartphone applications for the management of obesity. *Aust N Z J Public Health.* 2011;35(3):293–294.

88. Kassianos AP, Emery JD, Murchie P, Walter FM. Smartphone applications for melanoma detection by community, patient and generalist clinician users: a review. *Br J Dermatol.* 2015;172(6):1507–1518.

89. Rosser BA, Eccleston C. Smartphone applications for pain management. *J Telemed Telecare.* 2011;17(6):308–312.

90. Pandey A, Hasan S, Dubey D, Sarangi S. Smartphone apps as a source of cancer information: changing trends in health information-seeking behavior. *J Cancer Educ.* 2013;28(1):138–142.

91. Mobasheri MH, Johnston M, King D, Leff D, Thiruchelvam P, Darzi A. Original article: smartphone breast applications—what's the evidence? *Breast.* 2014;23:683–689.

92. Sunyaev A, Dehling T, Taylor PL, Mandl KD. Availability and quality of mobile health app privacy policies. *J Am Med Inform Assoc.* 2014;0:1–4.

93. Cotugna N, Vickery CE, Carpenter-Haefele KM. Evaluation of literacy level of patient education pages in health-related journals. *J Community Health.* 2005;30(3):213–219.

94. Dehling T, Gao F, Schneider S, Sunyaev A. Exploring the far side of mobile health: information security and privacy of mobile health apps on iOS and android. *JMIR Mhealth Uhealth.* 2015;3(1):e8.

95. McGraw D, Belfort R, Pfister H, Ingargiola S. Going digital with patients: managing potential liability risks of patient-generated electronic health information. *J Particip Med.* 2013, Dec 23;5.

96. Yang YT, Silverman RD. Mobile health applications: the patchwork of legal and liability issues suggests strategies to improve oversight. *Health Aff.* 2014;33(2):222–227.

97. Fiordelli M, Diviani N, Schulz PJ. Mapping mHealth research: a decade of evolution. *J Med Internet Res.* 2013;15(5):e95.

98. Kumar S, Nilsen WJ, Abernethy A, et al. Mobile health technology evaluation. *Am J Prev Med.* 2013;45(2):228–236.

99. Li JS, Barnett TA, Goodman E, Wasserman RC, Kemper AR. Approaches to the prevention and management of childhood obesity: the role of social networks and the use of social media and related electronic technologies: a scientific statement from the American Heart Association. *Circulation.* 2013;127(2):260–267.

100. Cucina R. E4: information technology in patient care. In: Papadakis MA, McPhee SJ, Rabow MW, eds. *Current Medical Diagnosis and Treatment 2015.* New York: McGraw-Hill Education; 2015. http://accessmedicine.mhmedical.com/content.aspx?bookid=1019&Sectionid=56908841. Accessed December 22, 2014.

Obstetrics

Nutrition and Weight Gain in Pregnancy: Weight Loss Strategies/ Nutritional Management

Sherry L. Blumenthal, MD, MSEd, FACOG

INTRODUCTION

Due to the increasing prevalence of obesity, interest in nutrition has increased. Every 5 years, the US Department of Agriculture (USDA) revises the nutrition guidelines; the last publication was in 2015. The "pyramid" from 2005 has been changed to a graphic similar to the "My Plate" diagram recommended for weight control (http://www.chosemyplate.gov) and not only reflects the known requirements and "conventional" scientific wisdom for nutrients, but also, to some extent, represents a realistic and simplified recommendation based on what the American public is willing to accept and follow (Figure 16-1). The ChooseMyPlate website also contains recommendations for pregnancy. The nutrition guidelines may unfortunately reflect pressure from the food industry, according to many nutrition advocates.

The overall body of evidence examined by the 2015 Dietary Guidelines Advisory Committee (DGAC) identified that a healthy dietary pattern is higher in vegetables, fruits, whole grains, low- or nonfat dairy, seafood, legumes, and nuts; moderate in alcohol (among nonpregnant adults); lower in red and processed meats; and low in sugar-sweetened foods and drinks and refined grains.[1]

The practicing obstetrician/gynecologist has the responsibility to be well versed in nutrition. We are sometimes the only physicians women see on a regular basis. Also, women usually make the food decisions for the family, so educating them may result in benefits to men and children. It appears that once obese, an individual has a difficult time achieving a normal weight. Therefore, prevention of obesity is a crucial goal.

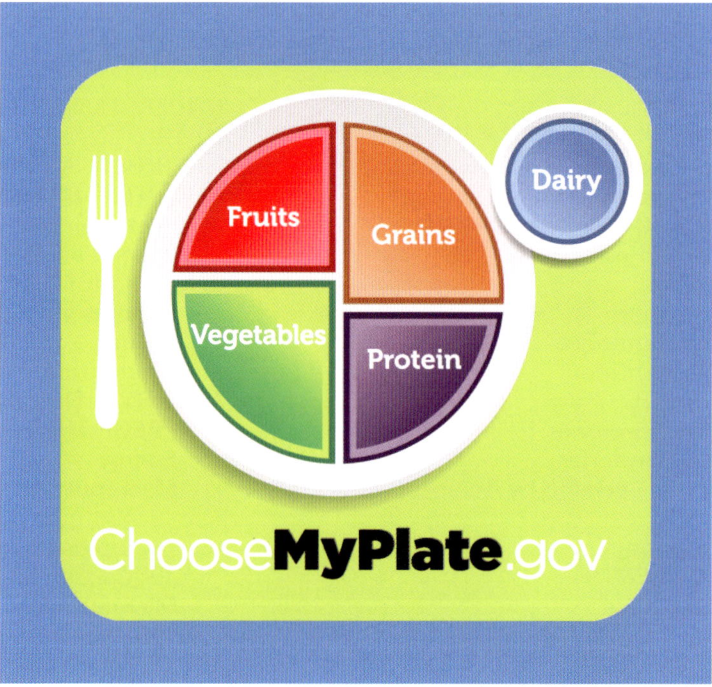

FIGURE 16-1. The USDA ChooseMyPlate representation. (From the USDA's Center for Nutrition Policy and Promotion, myplate.gov.)

Another reason that we are important in battling this disease is that obesity affects every aspect of obstetrical/gynecological practice. The increase in morbidity and mortality in pregnancy,[2] infertility issues, gynecologic cancers (with poorer survival[3]), and complications of surgery in the obese woman impels us to contribute to the prevention and treatment of obesity. The cornerstones of prevention and treatment are proper nutrition, exercise, and education of both the patient and physician.

BASIC PRINCIPLES OF NUTRITION

Energy Concepts and Metabolism

The Human "Machine"

As machines, we are obligated to obey the laws of thermodynamics. The first law of thermodynamics states that the total amount of energy in the universe remains constant; therefore, our bodies cannot independently produce energy but must obtain it by ingesting nutrients and converting the energy obtained into other forms. The second law of thermodynamics states that any energy transformation is always in the direction of increased entropy, or disorder, and cannot be recovered for later use. The goal of our metabolism is to preserve a steady state. In our bodies, we actually do not obtain equilibrium, the complete reversibility of all reactions, but a "near" state, called energy balance. The energy content of the body and its composition stay constant only at the expense of needing renewed supplies (intake of fuel) and disposal of waste products (energy dissipation). Complete equilibrium would equal death, but the steady state allows renewal by the input and output of substances as described The body takes in fuel (macronutrients) and converts the chemical energy of that fuel into other forms of energy, such as mechanical energy and heat. Energy is liberated primarily by the process of oxidation by reactions in the mitochondria of the cells. There may also be partial oxidation (anaerobic reactions, i.e., glycolysis) of fuel, which is later converted and may be completely oxidized or stored. Glycolysis proceeds without the mitochondria or oxygen. An example is glucose conversion to pyruvate or lactate.

While macronutrients are metabolized by different pathways, the common pathway converges at acetyl coenzyme A (acetyl-CoA). In the mitochondria, the Krebs cycle leads to oxidation of acetyl-CoA, production of "reducing equivalents" (e.g., nicotinamide adenine dinucleotide, NAD), CO_2, and a molecule of adenosine triphosphate (ATP).[4] The energy produced is used for bodily functions: synthesis of structures and compounds, cellular pumping mechanisms used for muscle contraction, physical activity, and the aforementioned heat production. The chemical products of this oxidation are carbon dioxide, water, and nitrogen oxides (waste). Waste or "by-products" of our metabolism are excreted by the lungs (carbon dioxide) or kidneys (water and urea). We do not excrete other metabolic products, such as amino acids, ketones, or lactate, at any significant rate.[2]

HORMONES ACTIVE IN METABOLISM

There are a number of hormones active in metabolism.[4,5] This section discusses these hormones.

Pancreatic Hormones

Insulin

Insulin is essentially an anabolic hormone. Its secretion by the islets (β cells) is regulated primarily by blood glucose concentrations. After a meal, insulin secretion is potentiated by intestinal hormones, the incretins. Incretins are peptides secreted by the gut after a carbohydrate-containing meal and include glucagon-like peptide (GLP-1) and gastric inhibitory peptide (GIP). They account for the difference in insulin response when glucose is ingested orally versus infused intravenously. Insulin acts to regulate enzymatic actions (dephosphorylation) and affects long-term regulation of gene transcription. Insulin has the effect of deposition of glycogen in liver and muscle, synthesis of protein in skeletal muscle, and storage of fat in adipose cells.

Glucagon

Glucagon, secreted by α cells, exerts its major effect on the liver. Its secretion increases when blood glucose levels fall or a meal high in protein is ingested. Stored glycogen is converted to glucose as needed.

Adrenal Hormones

Epinephrine

Epinephrine (adrenaline) release is stimulated by a fall in blood glucose concentration. Stimuli for its release are stress, anxiety, exercise, and blood loss. It is produced in the adrenal medulla and responds to hypothalamic signals. Through a chain of signals, increasing epinephrine raises glucose and esterified fatty acid levels in the bloodstream from stored glycogen and fat breakdown.

Norepinephrine is a neurotransmitter that acts on the same cell receptors as epinephrine and responds to the same stimuli. It is present at high concentrations during strenuous exercise. While its basic presence is at the sympathetic nerve terminal and is reabsorbed by it, it can leak into the circulation and act as a hormone.

Cortisol

Cortisol is highly bound to plasma proteins, such that only 5% of the cortisol circulates as free, active hormone. It regulates gene expression and is mostly catabolic. It increases fat mobilization, increases skeletal muscle dissolution, and increases gluconeogenesis in the liver. Its release is stimulated by pituitary adrenocorticotropic hormone (corticotropin, ACTH).

Pituitary Hormones

Growth hormone is mainly anabolic. It increases the synthesis of cartilage and increases bone length. Secretion is increased by a fall in plasma glucose, stimulating gluconeogenesis and fat mobilization. It also acts to stimulate production of insulin-like growth factors 1 and 2 (IGF-1 and IGF-2, respectively), mediators of the effects of growth hormone.

The pituitary gland also produces thyroid-stimulating hormone (TSH), which drives the thyroid gland, and ACTH, which increases production of cortisol.

Thyroid Hormones

The thyroid hormones thyroxine (T_4) and triiodothyronine (T_3) have longer-term effects than other hormones involved in metabolism. They are primarily catabolic, stimulating energy expenditure and influencing the breakdown of muscle protein.

Action is believed to be at the level of the mitochondria. Deficiency of these hormones decreases the metabolic rate but alone is not considered responsible for significant obesity. The third form of thyroid hormone, reverse T_3, is metabolically inactive but may be involved in energy conservation during stress or starvation, when its production increases.

Hormones Secreted by Adipose Tissue

Leptin

Leptin is a peptide hormone secreted by fat cells. The larger the adipocyte, the more leptin it produces. Leptin appears to cross the blood-brain barrier and exert its effect at the hypothalamus, decreasing appetite. The feedback mechanism that operates creates an increase in appetite when fat stored in adipocytes is low, therefore stimulating increased food intake. Of interest is that mutation in either the leptin gene or its receptor is associated with morbid obesity; however, few cases of obesity are associated with the gene mutation.

Adiponectin

Adiponectin is a peptide also secreted by fat cells. It protects against insulin resistance, usually by decreasing it. Larger adipocytes secrete less adiponectin; therefore, obese women produce less of this hormone.

There are other related hormones called "adipokines," including some inflammatory cytokines, such as tumor necrosis factor alpha (TNF-α) and interleukin 6 (IL-6).[5]

MACRONUTRIENTS

The basic essential nutrients in our diet are carbohydrates, protein, and fats (Figure 16-2). In addition, we require vitamins and minerals to catalyze metabolic processes.

Carbohydrates

Carbohydrates consist of two groups, simple and complex. Both groups supply energy for metabolism. Glucose is the simple carbohydrate to which basic nutrients are reduced for energy production. Exogenous simple carbohydrates, such as sucrose, a dimer of glucose and fructose, are rapidly absorbed and rapidly raise blood sugar. These two components have slightly different effects on stimulating insulin production but are considered to have a "high glycemic index" due to causing a rapid rise in insulin. Simple carbohydrates are consumed in large amounts by the American public; the estimate ranges from 22% to 25% of our total calorie intake.

Simple carbohydrates are also found naturally in many foods, such as milk (lactose) and fruit. An important issue is the fact that simple carbohydrates, which occur naturally in foods such as fruit, come in a "package," which often contains other vital nutrients and fiber.

Complex carbohydrates are exemplified by starches and "fiber." Starches are polysaccharides, meaning they are many

FIGURE 16-2. Understanding food labels: the current label.

Nutrition Facts

Serving Size 2/3 cup (55g)
Servings Per Container About 8

Amount Per Serving

Calories 230   Calories from Fat 40

	% Daily Value*
Total Fat 8g	**12**%
Saturated Fat 1g	**5**%
Trans Fat 0g	
Cholesterol 0mg	**0**%
Sodium 160mg	**7**%
Total Carbohydrate 37g	**12**%
Dietary Fiber 4g	**16**%
Sugars 1g	
Protein 3g	

Vitamin A	10%
Vitamin C	8%
Calcium	20%
Iron	45%

* Percent Daily Values are based on a 2,000 calorie diet. Your daily value may be higher or lower depending on your calorie needs.

	Calories:	2,000	2,500
Total Fat	Less than	65g	80g
Sat Fat	Less than	20g	25g
Cholesterol	Less than	300mg	300mg
Sodium	Less than	2,400mg	2,400mg
Total Carbohydrate		300g	375g
Dietary Fiber		25g	30g

units of glucose joined together by acetyl linkages. They are considered to have a lower glycemic index than simple sugars; they raise blood sugar more slowly because more metabolic steps are required to break down the compounds before absorption. Complex carbohydrates occur naturally in grains and vegetables as well as in refined foods.

All carbohydrates provide 4 Calories of energy per gram. A Calorie equals 1 kilocalorie of energy released per gram when a substance is ignited in a Caloric bomb.

Any excess carbohydrate ingested will be stored in 1 of 2 ways: converted to glycogen and stored in the liver or stored in adipocytes as fat. Because the brain requires about 100 g of glucose per day, which is close to the amount that can be stored in the liver, the major residual storage form is fat, triacylglycerol (TAG). TAG is hydrophobic and coalesces into small droplets for ease of storage. The efficiency of energy storage of fat is 8 times higher per gram than carbohydrate or protein.

Protein

Protein, consisting of amino acids, is the nutrient that, while also providing energy, has primarily a structural and enzymatic function. There are 9 amino acids that cannot be produced by the body and therefore must be obtained through food. These, the "essential" amino acids, are histidine, isoleucine, leucine, lysine, methionine, phenylalanine, threonine, tryptophan, and valine. All amino acids have the same basic structure, differing only in a side group. The simplest amino acid, glycine, has a hydrogen as its side group.

Animal sources of protein contain all of the essential amino acids, but many plant-based foods do not. An exception is soy. To obtain all of the essential amino acids, vegetarians need to consume a combination of foods that together will supply all of them.

The body's protein is not generally used as a fuel beyond the amount ingested daily. Each gram of protein contains 4 kcal of energy.

Fats

Fats (lipids) are composed of chains of fatty acids. They provide energy that can be used fairly rapidly or stored. In fact, any energy remaining after basic metabolic functions are performed is stored as fat. The survival value of this is obvious unless the food consumer is already "overnourished."

Included in the category of lipids are saturated/trans and unsaturated fats, the former being found in processed foods as well as naturally in most animal products.

Butyric acid is one of the fatty acids responsible for the flavor in butter. Of the approximately 40 naturally occurring fatty acids, those without carbon-carbon double bonds are classified as saturated, and those containing carbon-carbon double bonds are classified as unsaturated. Palmitic and stearic acids are the most common saturated fatty acids, and oleic and linoleic acids are the most common unsaturated fatty acids. Oleic acid is monounsaturated because it has only 1 carbon-carbon double bond. Linoleic, linolenic, and arachidonic acids are polyunsaturated because they have 2, 3, and 4 carbon-carbon double bonds, respectively. Examples of where saturated fats occur in nature are dairy, meat, and eggs.

Unsaturated fats are most commonly found in vegetable oils, nuts, and seeds. Polyunsaturated and monounsaturated fats are considered to be healthier. Saturated fats are believed to increase levels of low-density lipoprotein (LDL) cholesterol and contribute to the risk of coronary artery disease (CAD).[8]

Among the fatty acids, omega-3 and omega-6 appear to promote heart health. They are found mainly in fish, vegetable products, and nuts. They are both *cis-* isomers rather than in the *trans-* configuration. Trans fats are deleterious to heart health.[10,11]

Each gram of fat produces 9 kcal of energy, that is, has a greater "calorie density" than carbohydrate or protein. This information is valuable in counseling about eating patterns. Fats are essential, however. Many vitamins are fat soluble and therefore are not available to our bodies unless we consume some fat. As mentioned, fat is our major form of energy storage.

MICRONUTRIENTS (VITAMINS AND MINERALS)

Vitamins and minerals are naturally occurring chemicals that are vital for catalyzing metabolic reactions, incorporating into body structures, and functioning of many body systems. Some, such as vitamin D, promote absorption of other substances, such as the mineral calcium. For each vitamin, there is an official recommended daily allowance (RDA) (Table 16-1), more recently expressed as Dietary Reference Intake (DRI), a recommended minimum intake suiting the needs of most individuals. The RDA is actually that quantity per day needed to avoid "deficiency" diseases, for example, scurvy, rickets, beriberi, and pellagra. Most naturally occurring foods contain enough vitamins (in a balanced, varied diet) to meet the RDA for all vitamins except D.

Vitamin D is produced in skin cells when acted on by the ultraviolet (UV) in sunlight. Vitamin D deficiency is common in areas 45° degrees above or below the equator,[6,7] and supplementation is often recommended. Most people in general meet the RDA for vitamin D sufficiency, although there are variables such as season, time and length of day, use of sunscreen, skin pigmentation, smog, and cloud cover. Individuals with limited exposure due to being homebound, wearing robes and head coverings for religious reasons, or having occupations that limit overall sun exposure are at greater risk of insufficiency.

Women of African American ancestry show lower levels of serum vitamin D and yet have a lower risk of fracture and osteoporosis. Older adults, those with certain

TABLE 16-1 USDA Recommendations for RDAs of Vitamins and Minerals[a]

Recommended Daily Allowances for Adults (19 Years and Up)

Nutrient	*Male 19–50 Years*	*Male > 50 Years*	*Female 19–50 Years*	*Female > 50 Years*
RDA Vitamins (Per Day)				
Vitamin A: retinol	900 μg	900 μg	700 μg	700 μg
Vitamin C: ascorbic acid	90 mg	90 mg	75 mg	75 mg
Vitamin D	5* μg	10* μg	5* μg	10* μg
Vitamin E	15 mg	15 mg	15 mg	15 mg

(Continued)

TABLE 16-1 USDA Recommendations for RDAs of Vitamins and Minerals[a] (*Continued*)

Recommended Daily Allowances for Adults (19 Years and Up)

Nutrient	Male 19–50 Years	Male > 50 Years	Female 19–50 Years	Female > 50 Years
Vitamin K	120* µg	120* µg	90* µg	90* µg
Vitamin B_1: thiamin	1.2 mg	1.2 mg	1.1 mg	1.1 mg
Vitamin B_2: riboflavin	1.3 mg	1.3 mg	1.1 mg	1.1 mg
Vitamin B_3: niacin	16 mg	16 mg	14 mg	14 mg
Vitamin B_5: pantothenic acid	5* mg	5* mg	5* mg	5* mg
Vitamin B_6: pyridoxine	1.3 mg	1.7 mg	1.3 mg	1.5 mg
Vitamin B_{12}	2.4 µg	2.4 µg	2.4 µg	2.4 µg
Biotin	30* µg	30* µg	30* µg	30* µg
Choline	550* mg	550* mg	425* mg	425* mg
Folate: folic acid	400 µg	400 µg	400 µg	400 µg

Recommended Daily Allowances for Minerals

Nutrient	Male 19–50 Years	Male > 50 Years	Female 19–50 Years	Female > 50 Years
Calcium	1000* mg	1200* mg	1000* mg	1200* mg
Chromium	35* µg	30* µg	25* µg	20* µg
Copper	900 µg	900 µg	900 µg	900 µg
Fluoride	4* mg	4* mg	3* mg	3* mg
Iodine	150 µg	150 µg	150 µg	150 µg
Iron	8 mg	8 mg	18 mg	8 mg
Magnesium	400/420 mg	420 mg	310/320 mg	320 mg
Manganese	2.3* mg	2.3* mg	1.8* mg	1.8* mg
Molybdenum	45 µg	45 µg	45 µg	45 µg
Phosphorus	700 mg	700 mg	700 mg	700 mg
Selenium	55 µg	55 µg	55 µg	55 µg
Zinc	11 mg	11 mg	8 mg	8 mg
Potassium	4.7* g	4.7* g	4.7* g	4.7* g
Sodium	1.5* g	1.3* g	1.5* g	1.3* g
Chloride	2.3* g	2.0* g	2.3* g	2.0* g

[a]From the USDA.

chronic diseases affecting the kidney, and those with inflammatory bowel disease, cystic fibrosis, and celiac disease may require vitamin D supplementation.

Women who are obese may need larger dietary amounts of vitamin D to achieve serum levels equal to those women of normal weight. While the ability of the skin to synthesize the vitamin is unaffected by obesity, vitamin D is sequestered in subcutaneous fat and therefore may not be released into the circulation as well. Women who have undergone gastric bypass may become deficient due to bypass of the upper small intestine, where Vitamin D is absorbed; it is unknown whether mobilization of the vitamin from fat stores will compensate.[4]

The Food and Nutrition Board (FNB) has evaluated the relationship of vitamin D to multiple health measures and has found no cause-and-effect relationship between vitamin D and any outcome other than bone health.

There are also maximum recommendations for certain vitamins to avoid toxicity. For example, excess vitamin B_6 results in neurologic damage, and excess vitamin C results in kidney stones.

Examples of foods high in certain vitamins include leafy green vegetables (B vitamins, C, and K). Folate, a B vitamin, is added to many baked products, such as breads and cereals. Dairy products contain some vitamin D but are usually fortified to increase the amount.[4] It is unlikely for an individual to achieve toxic levels of any vitamin if ingested in a balanced diet.

Minerals are usually found in the environment as positive or negative ions in compounds such as sodium chloride (NaCl), potassium chloride (KCl), and calcium carbonate ($CaCO_3$). They are naturally incorporated into food through the soil or water. Many foods contain enough of the required minerals, but this varies by environment and the available foods in that setting. For example, iodine occurs naturally in seaweed and fish.

Deficiency in that mineral is common in inland societies where access to seafood is limited. Many types of salt (NaCl) available have added iodine to prevent deficiency because iodine is essential for thyroid gland functioning.

Foods high in certain minerals include dairy products (calcium), red meat (iron), and bananas (potassium). Calcium, for example, is incorporated into bone for structural integrity and is essential for the functioning of muscle.

UNDERSTANDING FOOD LABELS

Most commercial foods are required to have labels with nutritional information (Figure 16-3). Reading these helps in determining energy intake and nutrients contained in that food. Required are serving size, calories per serving, and amount of various nutrients, such as carbohydrates and protein, usually measured in grams.

Food labeling can be confusing to the consumer. One problem is that the sugar content of food may only reflect

FIGURE 16-3. The new Nutrition Facts label proposed by the FDA.

Nutrition Facts

8 servings per container

Serving size — 2/3 cup (55g)

Amount per 2/3 cup

Calories — 230

% DV*

12%	**Total Fat** 8g
5%	Saturated Fat 1g
	Trans Fat 0g
0%	**Cholesterol** 0mg
7%	**Sodium** 160mg
12%	**Total Carbs** 37g
14%	Dietary Fiber 4g
	Sugars 1g
	Added Sugars 0g
	Protein 3g
10%	Vitamin D 2mcg
20%	Calcium 260mg
45%	Iron 8mg
5%	Potassium 235mg

* Footnote on Daily Values (DV) and calories reference to be inserted here.

TABLE 16-2 Calculation of Daily Estimated Energy Requirements[a]

Physical Activity Coefficients for Females 19 Years and Older[b]

Sedentary	*Low Active*	*Active*	*Very Active*
1	*1.12*	*1.27*	*1.45*

Nonpregnant females 19 years and older:
354 − (6.91 × Age in years) + Physical activity coefficient × (9.36 × Weight in kilograms) + (726 × Height in meters)

Sedentary = Usual daily activities; low active = additional 30–60 minutes of moderate activity (walking); active = additional 60 minutes of moderate activity; very active = additional 120 minutes of moderate activity.
[a]From Lanham-New SA, Macdonald IA, Roche HM, eds. *Nutrition and Metabolism.* 2nd ed. Hoboken, NJ: Wiley-Blackwell; 2011.
[b]Per day.

added sugar, not naturally occurring sugar; however, the listing of ingredients in a product can be helpful. If sugar is the first ingredient on a label, this signals the consumer that the product might be one to avoid. The Food and Drug Administration (FDA) has recently required listed the added sugar as percentage of daily recommended amount.

Another important consideration is interpreting the claim that a product is "whole grain." If refined flour is the first ingredient, then the product should not be considered whole grain for the purposes of nutrition. The percentages are based on a diet containing 2000 Cal/d. This number may not be appropriate for all women, especially the obese, very active, or pregnant woman. While this information is important for the consumer, especially serving size, it needs to be individualized based on energy needs (Table 16-2). There is an equation proposed by the Institute of Medicine (IOM) to assist in calculation of energy needs for an individual. Once appropriate energy needs are calculated, serving size of a specific food will need modification to apply to that individual. Although an oversimplification, the basic principle is that to maintain body weight, energy "in" must equal energy "out." Overweight and obesity result when more energy (Calories) is ingested than expended in metabolic processes and activity.

NUTRITIONAL PROBLEMS

Over two-thirds of women in the United States are overweight or obese. This means that the most pressing nutritional issue in this country is "overnutrition." Obesity is a major cause of morbidity and mortality in general and more specifically affects pregnancy complications, both maternal and fetal; increases the risk of gynecologic cancers and survival in those afflicted; and affects fertility and urogynecologic issues.

Most dietary modifications in nonpregnant women rest primarily on decreasing caloric intake so that it is less than output. This results in weight loss. As mentioned, the formula is not quite as straightforward as this, but as a basic guideline, it is valuable. We now have information that many factors contribute to the individual's energy balance and weight. Physical activity to increase energy output is a long-known and essential part of any weight loss or weight maintenance strategy.

Body habitus, however, is also influenced by intrauterine environment, genetics and epigenetics, inflammation, bowel flora,[8] number of adipocytes and the hormones they produce, and the types of nutrients ingested. "Obesity before pregnancy is an independent risk factor for adverse pregnancy outcomes" (V), and there are suggested interventions that may limit weight gain and improve outcomes.

For example, obese pregnant women have an intrauterine environment that imprints on the fetus. Hyperglycemia is known to have effects on organ formation in the first trimester and on subsequent fetal growth in later trimesters. (This is partly due to increases in IGF.)

Fetuses that are large for gestational age (LGA) have a greater proportion of body fat than fetuses of appropriate weight. They have a greater risk of childhood obesity and metabolic syndrome. One result of this suboptimal environment is "turning on and off" certain regions of some genes by methylation or acetylation (i.e., epigenetics).

Many families have a predisposition to obesity that is independent of energy balance, and they may require less energy than others. Inflammatory markers, such as TNF-α, are higher in obese individuals, although this may be an effect rather than a cause. Weight loss decreases inflammatory markers.

Childhood obesity, with the increase in adipocytes, results in increases in aromatase, IGF, and free fatty acids and a decrease in leptin and adiponectin. While the fat content in adipocytes may decrease with weight loss, the number of adipocytes may not, making it much easier to reaccumulate fat in them.

It has been standard practice in raising livestock for food to administer antibiotics to decrease infections and stimulate more rapid weight gain. The apparent mechanism lies in a change in bowel flora. In mouse experiments, change in fecal flora results in weight gain with a similar diet.[13] In the United States, antibiotics are commonly used, sometimes inappropriately. This may be a factor contributing to obesity. More human research is needed, of course.[13]

Regardless of these factors, it remains true that decreasing intake relative to output will reduce weight. Nutritional requirements do change with age and pregnancy status.

NUTRITION IN PREGNANCY

Nutrition recommendations differ in women depending on whether they are not pregnant, anticipating or could become pregnant, or have achieved pregnancy. Recommendations also vary by trimester of pregnancy. While basic nutritional requirements (i.e., intake of essential nutrients) may not vary by BMI class, certainly recommendations for weight gain during pregnancy do vary by BMI.

The IOM has issued recommendations for weight gain in pregnancy (Table 16-3).[14] These are also the recommendations of the American Congress of Obstetricians and Gynecologists (ACOG). These consider BMI, whereas earlier recommendations, before the "obesity epidemic" was recognized, did not.

Insufficient preconception energy stores have a negative effect on ovulation, conception, and subsequent pregnancy. The same is true of excessive fat stores, that is, obesity. The latter interferes with fertility by its relative insulin insensitivity, excess of

TABLE 16-3 New IOM Recommendations for Total and Rate of Weight Gain During Pregnancy by Prepregnancy BMI[a]

	Total Weight Gain, kg (lb)	Rates of Gain in 2nd and 3rd Trimesters, in kg/wk (Range)	Rates of Gain in 2nd and 3rd Trimesters, lb/wk
Underweight (<18.5 kg/m^2)	12.5–18 (28–40)	0.51 (0.44–0.58)	1 (1–1.3)
Normal weight (19–24.9 kg/m^2)	11.5–16 (25–35)	0.42 (0.35–0.50)	1 (0.8–1)
Overweight (25–29.9 kg/m^2)	7–11.5 (15–25)	0.28 (0.23–0.33)	0.6 (0.5–0.7)
Obese (>30 kg/m^2)	5–9 (11–20)	0.22 (0.17–0.27)	0.5 (0.4–0.6)

[a]This assumes a 0.5- to 2.0-kg (1.1- to 4.4-lbs.) weight gain in the first trimester (based on Siega-Riz et al., 1994; Abrams et al., 1995; Carmichael et al., 1997).

estrogen and testosterone, and changes in leptin levels. In the first trimester, hyperglycemia acts as a teratogen, increasing the incidence of fetal anomalies.

Components of weight gain in pregnancy (Table 16-4) include products of conception (fetus, amniotic fluid, and placenta); increased maternal fat stores; and increased extracellular fluid, uterine weight, breast enlargement and development, and blood.

Whatever the maternal BMI, energy and nutrient requirements exceed those of the non-pregnant woman (Table 16-5). There are current sources that suggest that the morbidly obese woman should gain no weight during pregnancy, based on recent studies.[15]

TABLE 16-4 Weight of Components of Pregnancy at Term[a]

Component	Weight (g)
Products of conception	4850
Placenta	650
Amniotic fluid	800
Fetus	3400
Maternal fat stores	3345
Maternal tissues	4305
Extracellular fluid	1680
Uterus and breasts	1375
Blood	1250
Total	12,500

[a]From Yao R, Ananth CV, Park BY, Pereira L, Plante LA; Perinatal Research Consortium. Obesity and the risk of stillbirth: a population-based cohort study. *Am J Obstet Gynecol.* 2014;210(5):457.e1-9.

TABLE 16-5 Equations for Calculation of Energy Needs[a]

First trimester	EER = Nonpregnant EER + 0
Second trimester	EER = Nonpregnant EER + 340
Third trimester	EER = Nonpregnant EER + 452

Abbreviation: EER, estimated energy requirement in kilocalories per day.
[a]From Lanham-New SA, Macdonald IA, Roche HM, eds. *Nutrition and Metabolism.* 2nd ed. Hoboken, NJ: Wiley-Blackwell; 2011.

NUTRITION BY TRIMESTER

During implantation, in the first 2 weeks, there is a negligible increase in nutritional needs. However, physiology differs in the trimesters of pregnancy; therefore, nutrient requirements and energy requirements differ as well.

First Trimester

In the first trimester, organogenesis takes place. Early pregnancy is anabolic, during which maternal fat stores increase and nutrients are stored. There are small increases in insulin sensitivity.[5] The embryonic cells begin to differentiate into various organs (e.g., heart, liver, and kidneys), and the skeletal system begins to form. The neural tube closes in the first 4 weeks of pregnancy, a reminder that timing of sufficient nutrients is key to proper fetal development. Nourishment and energy at this stage are provided by the maternal blood supply.

Maternal energy requirements do not increase during the first trimester; however, several specific nutrients are crucial. For example, adequate folate is recommended before conception (or if women are at risk of conception). Many women are unaware that they have conceived when the neural tube is already beginning to close. For this reason, 400 µg per day are recommended for all reproductive-aged women until requirements increase after the first trimester. Many foods, as mentioned previously, are fortified with folic acid, but many sources recommend a multivitamin containing the fortification amount as a precaution.

Riboflavin (vitamin B_2) is vital for proper skeletal development. Neuromotor problems can result from inadequate pyridoxine (vitamin B_6) and manganese. Several B vitamins, niacin (B_3) and vitamin B_{12}, affect central nervous system (CNS) development.

A recent randomized controlled trial of myoinositol, a naturally occurring cyclitol found in plants and animal foods, showed that supplementation starting the first trimester in obese women lowered the incidence of gestational diabetes and macrosomia.[17]

Second and Third Trimesters

The second and third trimesters comprise what may be considered the "growth period." Late pregnancy can be considered catabolic, accompanied by decreased insulin sensitivity. There is therefore greater availability of glucose and free fatty acids for fetal growth.[5]

The first phase of this period is hyperplasia, when the number of cells rapidly increases. Folate and B_{12} are crucial to this process. In the second phase, hyperplasia is joined by hypertrophy, an increase in cell size. Adequate amino acids are required to form fetal protein and are requirement for vitamin B_6 increases. In the third phase of growth, cellular hypertrophy without significant cellular division dominates. This requires an increase in energy supply through an increase in basic essential nutrient intake.

ENERGY METABOLISM IN PREGNANCY

In pregnancy, energy expenditure may decrease due to lowered physical activity, but there does not appear to be a major change in energy metabolism to produce actual conservation. There are, however, changes in the body's use of various nutrients when there are both maternal and fetal requirements.[7]

Proteins

Amino acids appear to be conserved for fetal growth. Nitrogen is retained due to decreased excretion (decreased urea synthesis), and that retention increases in later pregnancy when the fetal demand for protein is greatest. There is no apparent maternal storage of protein for later fetal use; therefore, increased dietary protein is needed. Changes in protein metabolism are complex, and any adaptation to increase maternal intake of protein is a subject for further research.

Lipids

The concentration of serum lipids increases during pregnancy as early as the first trimester.

Micronutrients

Metabolism of nutrients changes early in pregnancy, even though the major fetal demand occurs during the growth period. In the first trimester, concentration of circulating micronutrients shows a decrease that persists throughout pregnancy. This is partly due to increased plasma volume but begins before that increase.

While the mechanism is unknown, there seems to be an increase in absorption of micronutrients during pregnancy. There is a resultant increase in the total amounts of vitamins and minerals in the bloodstream. It is important to understand the changes in "levels" in pregnancy when interpreting laboratory results.

Plasma levels of vitamin D_3 rise early in pregnancy and probably are the result of the doubling of calcium absorption in the gut. While total calcium levels fall, ionized calcium and phosphate remain constant and in the normal range. The decrease of albumin due to increasing plasma volume may be the cause of the unionized calcium decrease.

NUTRITION RECOMMENDATIONS FOR PREGNANCY

Increasing food intake can compensate for the increased energy demands of pregnancy. Well-nourished women require only modest changes in consumption, and overnourished women may actually benefit from maintaining or decreasing current intake. It appears that excess weight gain in the first trimester may cause more neonatal maternal morbidity than weight gain in the second or third trimester.[12]

Food cravings and "aversions" may influence dietary choices; however, there is no evidence that they are harmful or reflect actual physiologic needs. There are apparent changes in taste and smell due to hormonal variations that influence food preferences in pregnancy.

Universal supplement use is not recommended by nutritionists or by the IOM when a woman has a well-balanced diet. Supplementation is not evidence based and must be individualized. Interestingly, women with adequate intake (AI) of nutrients are most likely to use supplements, whereas those at greatest risk of malnutrition in pregnancy are less likely to use a supplement.[4] This may be due to lack of access to supplements in developing countries and in the United States when prenatal care is difficult to obtain. There are actually few data on the benefits and risks of supplements during pregnancy, other than to "supplement" an inadequate intake of micronutrients. Certainly, eating fish rather than supplementing with DHA (docosahexaenoic acid) to provide essential fatty acids is an option.

Energy

The required increase in energy intake is negligible in the first trimester. After that, recommendations need to be individualized based on nutritional status when entering pregnancy and level of energy expenditure (i.e., level of physical exercise). Table 16-5 takes these factors into account and can be used to advise women regarding necessary increases that are appropriate for them.

Energy requirements vary by ethnic group, BMI, and environment. It should be noted that the IOM recommendations for gestational weight gain in the obese gravida are based on the group with a BMI of 30–34.9 (class I).

Research is needed to determine causes of variances and what changes in recommendations (Table 16-6) should be made.[16]

Macronutrients

Protein

As with energy requirements, needs do not increase in the first trimester. In the second two trimesters, protein deposition is estimated to total 925 g. The requirement therefore is approximately 0.8 g of protein/kg/d, and the recommended dietary intake is 1.00 g/kg/d in pregnancy. This would equal 65 g/d in the average 65-kg (143-pound) woman.

TABLE 16-6 Recommended Daily Allowances for Pregnant/Lactating Women[a]

Nutrient	Pregnancy 14–18 Years	Pregnancy 19–50 Years	Lactation 14–18 Years	Lactation 19–50 Years
Recommended Daily Allowances for Vitamins				
Vitamin A: retinol	750 µg	770 µg	1200 µg	1300 µg
Vitamin C: ascorbic acid	80 mg	85 mg	115 mg	120 mg
Vitamin D	5* µg	5* µg	5* µg	5* µg
Vitamin E	15 mg	15 mg	19 mg	19 mg
Vitamin K	75* µg	90* µg	75* µg	90* µg

(*Continued*)

TABLE 16-6 Recommended Daily Allowances for Pregnant/Lactating Women[a] (*Continued*)

Nutrient	Pregnancy 14–18 Years	Pregnancy 19–50 Years	Lactation 14–18 Years	Lactation 19–50 Years
Recommended Daily Allowances for Vitamins				
Vitamin B_1: thiamin	1.4 mg	1.4 mg	1.4 mg	1.4 mg
Vitamin B_2: riboflavin	1.4 mg	1.4 mg	1.6 mg	1.6 mg
Vitamin B_3: niacin	18 mg	18 mg	17 mg	17 mg
Vitamin B_5: pantothenic acid	6* mg	6* mg	7* mg	7* mg
Vitamin B_6: pyridoxine	1.9 mg	1.9 mg	2.0 mg	2.0 mg
Vitamin B_{12}	2.6 µg	2.6 µg	2.8 µg	2.8 µg
Biotin	30* µg	30* µg	35* µg	35* µg
Choline	450* mg	450* mg	550* mg	550* mg
Folate: folic acid	600 µg	600 µg	500 µg	500 µg
Recommended Daily Allowances for Minerals				
Calcium	1300* mg	1000* mg	1300* mg	1000* mg
Chromium	29* µg	30* µg	44* µg	45* µg
Copper	1000 µg	1000 µg	1300 µg	1300 µg
Fluoride	3* mg	3* mg	3* mg	3* mg
Iodine	220 µg	220 µg	290 µg	290 µg
Iron	27 mg	27 mg	10 mg	9 mg
Magnesium	400 mg	350/360 mg	360 mg	310/320 mg
Manganese	2.0* mg	2.0* mg	2.6* mg	2.6* mg
Molybdenum	50 µg	50 µg	50 µg	50 µg
Phosphorus	1250 mg	700 mg	1250 mg	700 mg
Selenium	60 µg	60 µg	70 µg	70 µg
Zinc	12 mg	11 mg	13 mg	12 mg
Potassium	4.7* g	4.7* g	5.1* g	5.1* g
Sodium	1.5* g	1.5* g	1.5* g	1.5* g
Chloride	2.3* g	2.3* g	2.3* g	2.3* g

[a]From Otten JJ, Helwig JP, Meyers LD, eds. *DRI, Dietary Reference Intakes: The Essential Guide to Nutrient Requirements.* Institute of Medicine. Washington, DC: National Academies Press; 2006.

Lipids

The only recommendations for fat consumption apply to certain essential fatty acids. They are required by both the placenta and the fetus. Pregnant women need approximately 25% more of omega-6 and omega-3 fatty acids to foster membrane and brain development. DHA is the most important omega-3 fatty acid for brain development and is provided by fish. While there are concerns that certain fish may have dangerous levels of mercury, many do not (e.g., catfish, light tuna, shrimp, salmon, pollock, and catfish).

Recommendations for consumption of about 360 g (12 oz) of fish, also an excellent protein source, provide enough DHA. If that is not possible, a supplement can be used.

A recent meta-analysis about supplementation with DHA (omega-3 fatty acids) was performed, and there was no advantage in prevention of delivery at less than 37 weeks, although latency and birth weight were positively affected.[18]

The health benefits of DHA supplementation are actively under study. For long-chain fatty acids, the recommended total amount in pregnancy is 115 mg/d, with 10 g/d for linoleic acid and 1 g/d for α-linolenic acid.

Carbohydrates

There are no specific additional recommendations for carbohydrates or added fiber in pregnancy. The recommended AI of carbohydrates, however, does increase from 25 g/d for nonpregnant women to 28 g/d for those who are pregnant.

Micronutrients

Vitamins

There is a small increase in the AI for vitamin A. This fat-soluble vitamin is stored in the fetal liver, and the AI increase ensures adequate fetal reserves. High intakes during pregnancy can be toxic to the fetus as well as the mother.

Vitamin D crosses the placenta and is active in calcium metabolism. No increase in vitamin D intake is required if dairy intake is adequate. If not, or if sunlight exposure is limited, a supplement of 1000–2000 IU/d is recommended. For those who have adequate vitamin D levels, there is insufficient evidence to recommend supplementation in pregnancy beyond the amount in a prenatal vitamin, 400 IU/d, and there is no evidence for screening all pregnant women.[19,20]

Vitamins E and K, also fat soluble, are adequate at nonpregnant intakes.[21,22]

The AI for water-soluble vitamins, the B vitamins, may be increased up to 50%. These vitamins, as opposed to the fat-soluble ones, are not stored and must be replenished daily. Folate requirements are markedly increased. Folic acid, as a source of folate, is more efficient in providing adequate levels and is the form usually contained in supplements. Excess folate (over 1 g/d) can mask symptoms of B_{12} deficiency and increase the risk of neurologic damage.

Choline acts in membrane and neurotransmitter synthesis and in methylation reactions. It is also a precursor to acetylcholine. The recommendation for choline increases to 440 mg/d in pregnancy due to fetal demand. Inadequate choline intake in early pregnancy has been associated with neural tube defects (NTDs).[23]

Minerals

Minerals transferred to the fetus come from a variety of sources. Some are transferred to the fetus from maternal stores, some from increased absorption or increased maternal consumption.

A total of 30 g of calcium crosses the placenta during gestation, the major amount in the last trimester. There is a suggestion that due to increased maternal calcium absorption in pregnancy, supplemental calcium above that recommended in nonpregnant women may not be necessary.

In pregnancy, up to 400 mg of iron must be transferred to the fetus and stored in its liver. Iron is also required by the woman for additional hemoglobin formation to partly compensate for plasma expansion in pregnancy. Iron is required for formation of the placenta. Fortunately, maternal iron absorption is more efficient in pregnancy, especially in the second half. In addition, there are no menstrual losses. On the other hand, iron intake must also be sufficient to compensate for blood loss at delivery. Taking all of these factors into account, the recommendation for ingested iron is increased relative to the nonpregnant state. Iron from animal sources is better absorbed than that from plant sources; therefore, accommodations must be made for vegetarians.[24] Iodine requirements increase 60% relative to nonpregnancy so that there are adequate stores in the fetal thyroid gland.

Recommendations for zinc are to increase intake of this mineral. The same applies for its absorption as for iron. Therefore, vegetarians will need more supplementation.

Special Considerations in Pregnancy

The prepregnancy nutritional status of the woman and other individual risk factors in her health, or in genetic risks for the fetus, may require a change in nutrient recommendations.

An example is adding folic acid for prevention of NTD for high-risk woman or in the case where the woman has a previous baby with an NTD. The recommendation is a daily intake of 4 mg (400 µg).

There is some evidence that additional calcium supplementation might lower the risk of preeclampsia in high-risk women.

Woman who are deficient in certain vitamins or iron before pregnancy may need to supplement with larger amounts than usually recommended. Care should be taken to monitor levels, however, so that toxicity does not result. It would be preferable to replenish nutrients before pregnancy if possible.

Carbohydrate recommendations may need modification in women with pregestational type 2 diabetes mellitus.

Obesity is another diagnosis that needs careful consideration.[25] While the IOM recommendations for weight gain in pregnancy are lower in women with elevated BMIs, several studies showed that no weight gain for the morbidly obese woman (BMI 40+) is associated with less morbidity (e.g., diabetes, hypertension, and LGA babies) with the concomitant higher risk of birth trauma. There was an increase in small-for-gestational-age (SGA) fetuses, but it was not significantly greater than in the IOM recommendations.[16]

Also, serum measurements of fat-soluble vitamins, specifically D, may be lower in the obese than in the gravida with normal BMI. This is in part because increased maternal fat stores increase storage of vitamin D, lowering serum levels while total body levels are the same. The impact of this is unclear, and as mentioned, supplementation of vitamin D in pregnancy is controversial. Prepregnancy obesity appears to predict poor vitamin D status based on serum measurements in mothers and their neonates.[19]

Vegetarians do not need encouragement to add animal products to their diets. Those who eat dairy and eggs differ from vegans, who ingest no animal products. Vegans must take care to obtain sufficient protein, with all the essential amino acids. This can be achieved by pairing certain foods such as rice and beans or by consumption of soy products. Together, they provide all of the essential amino acids for synthesis of protein. Another good protein source is nuts. Also, as mentioned, care must be taken to ingest adequate zinc, calcium, B_{12}, and iron. Eggs and dairy provide these nutrients, but vegans need to add legumes for zinc and fortified foods or supplements for B_{12} and iron.

Women who have had bariatric surgery may have specific nutritional needs. The type of procedure may influence the risk of deficiencies, being lower with laparoscopic banding and higher with gastric bypass or biliopancreatic diversion (not commonly done at this time). Levels of nutrients may need to be measured and monitored. Those of particular concern are B_{12}, iron, folate, and calcium.[25]

SUMMARY

Obesity is a complex medical condition that causes morbidity in pregnant and non-pregnant women. Proper nutrition is essential to prevent and treat this disease. Food intake in both amount and calorie density is only part of the problem. Other issues are genetics, epigenetics, inflammation, bowel flora, exercise, and psychological make-up.

Weight gain recommendations differ in pregnancy among women who are normal weight, overweight, and obese. IOM recommendations may be too high for obese parturients.

Recommendations for energy intake and for specific nutrients change in pregnant women, influenced by trimester. There are special considerations for women with medical conditions such as Diabetes, and those who have had bariatric surgery.

FDA requirements for package labeling and revisions in the food "pyramid" may assist patients in choosing healthy options. Physician understanding of nutrition is important in counseling women as to the accepted recommendations and can allow for individualization.

REFERENCES

1. DGAC Recommendations. Scientific Report of the 2015 Dietary Guidelines Advisory Committee. Part B, *Chapter 2: Themes and Recommendations: Integrating the Evidence*. Washington, DC: Department of Health and Human Services; 2015:1–12.

2. Yao R, Ananth CV, Park BY, Pereira L, Plante LA; Perinatal Research Consortium. Obesity and the risk of stillbirth: a population-based cohort study. Presented at the 2014 SMFM Annual Meeting, New Orleans, LA, February 3–8, 2014. *Am J Obstet Gynecol*. 2014 March 24;210(5):457.e1-9.

3. Frumovitz, Jhingran A, Soliman PT, Klopp AH, Schmeler KM, Eifel PJ. Morbid obesity as an independent risk factor for disease-specific survival in cervical cancer. *Obstet Gynecol*. 2014 Dec;124(6):1098–1104.

4. Lanham New SA, Macdonald IA, Roche HM, eds. *Nutrition and Metabolism*. 2nd ed. Hoboken, NJ: Wiley-Blackwell; 2011.

5. Lain KY, Catalano PM. Metabolic changes in pregnancy. *Clin Obstet Gynecol*. 2007 Dec;50(4):938–948.

6. Steele KE, Burke AE. Clinical updates in women's health care. *Obesity*. 2013 Jan;12(1):8.

7. Siega-Riz AM, Mehta U. Nutrition. *Clinical Updates in Women's Health*. 2014 July;13(3):4.

8. Jensen MD, Ryan DH, Apovian MA, et al. 2013 AHA/ACC/TOS guideline for the management of overweight and obesity in adults: a report of the American College of Cardiology/American Heart Association Task Force on Practice Guidelines and the Obesity Society. *J Am Coll Cardiol*.

2014;63(25, pt B):2985–3023. PMID:24239920. http://www.ncbi.nlm.nih.gov/pubmed/24239920.

9. Otten JJ, Helwig JP, Meyers LD, eds. *DRI, Dietary Reference Intakes: The Essential Guide to Nutrient Requirements.* Institute of Medicine. Washington, DC, National Academies Press; 2006.

10. Hanley DA, Davison KS. Vitamin D insufficiency in North America. *J Nutr.* 2005 Feb 1;135(2):332–337.

11. Lite J. Vitamin D deficiency soars in the US. *Scientific American.* March 23, 2009.

12. Karachaliou M, Georgiou V, Roumeliotaki T, et al. Association of trimester-specific gestational weight gain with fetal growth, offspring obesity and cardiometabolic traits in early childhood. *Am J Obstet Gynecol.* 2015;212:502.e1-14.

13. Catiriona M, Cotter PD. Role of the gut microbiota in health, understanding a hidden metabolic organ. *Ther Avd Gastroenterol.* 2013;6(4):295–308.

14. Rasmussen KM, Yaktine AL, eds. *Weight Gain During Pregnancy: Reexamining the Guidelines.* Washington, DC: Committee to Reexamine IOM Pregnancy Weight Guidelines; Institute of Medicine, National Research Council.

15. AAP Committee on Fetus and Newborn and ACOG Committee on Obstetric Practice. Preconception and antepartum care. In: *Guidelines for Perinatal Care.* 7th ed. Elk Grove Village, IL: American Academy of Pediatrics; and Washington, DC: American College of Obstetricians and Gynecologists; 2012:95–168.

16. Truong YN, Yee LM, Caughey AB, et al. Weight gain in pregnancy: does the Institute of Medicine have it right? *Am J Obstet Gynecol.* 2015;212:362.e1-8.

17. D'Anna R, Di Benedetto A, Scilipoti A, et al. Myo-inositol supplementation for prevention of gestational diabetes in obese pregnant women. *Obstet Gynecol.* 2015 Aug;126(2):310-315.

18. Saccone G, Berghella V. Omega-3 supplementation to prevent recurrent preterm birth: a systematic review and metaanalysis of randomized controlled trials. *Am J Obstet Gynecol.* 213(2):135–140.

19. American College of Obstetricians and Gynecologists, Committee on Obstetric Practice. ACIG Committee Opinion No. 495: Vitamin D: screening and supplementation during pregnancy. *Obstet Gynecol.* 2011 July;118(1):197-198.

20. Institute of Medicine of the National Academies (US). *Dietary Reference Intakes for Calcium and Vitamin D.* Washington, DC: National Academies Press; 2010.

21. Institute of Medicine. *Dietary Reference Intakes for Vitamin C, Vitamin E, Selenium, and Carotenoids.* Washington, DC: National Academies Press; 2000.

22. Institute of Medicine. *Dietary Reference Intakes for Vitamin A, Vitamin K, Arsenic, Boron, Chromium, Copper, Iodine, Iron, Manganese, Molybdenum, Nickel, Silicon, Vanadium, and Zinc.* Washington, DC: National Academies Press; 2001.

23. Institute of Medicine. Dietary Reference Intakes for *Thiamine, Riboflavin, Niacin, Vitamin B_6, Folate, Vitamin B_{12},* Pantothenic Acid, Biotin and Choline. Washington, DC: National Academies Press; 1998. https://www.nap.edu/read/6015/chapter/1.

24. Institute of Medicine. *Dietary Reference Intakes for Calcium, Phosphorous, Magnesium, Vitamin D, and Fluoride.* Washington, DC: National Academies Press; 1997.

25. Burke A. Obesity. *Clinical Updates in Women's Healthcare.* 2013 Jan;12(1):49, 51–54.

CHAPTER 17

Prenatal Care and Fertility Testing

Shawky Z. A. Badawy, MD

INTRODUCTION
ETIOLOGY OF INFERTILITY IN OBESE
    PATIENTS

INFERTILITY WORKUP
CONCLUSION

INTRODUCTION

Obesity is on the rise in the United States, with an incidence of 50% of women who are obese and 30% who are overweight. Obesity affects the reproductive system and the endocrine system. Obesity leads to infertility and repeated miscarriages.[1]

Since ancient civilization, obesity has been described as a cause of infertility. Hippocrates wrote that people of such constitution cannot be prolific. Fatness and flabbiness are to blame. The womb is unable to receive the semen and they menstruate infrequently and little.[2]

Endocrinologically, obesity could be part of a disease process, such as polycystic ovarian syndrome, Cushing disease, and hypothyroidism. Therefore, in the evaluation of obese women, we have to take this into consideration and to order the proper endocrine testing so that treatment will be directed toward correcting these factors. Ovulatory dysfunction can be an important factor leading to infertility in obese women. In addition, there is an increased incidence of insulin resistance; these patients might develop a prediabetic or diabetic condition that will have a negative effect on fertility and pregnancy.[3–5]

Obesity could also affect men; the result will be a low testosterone level, which will lead to sperm abnormalities. The endocrine abnormality in men might also contribute to ejaculatory dysfunction, and this will lead to infertility.[6] Obesity in men may lead to DNA abnormalities, thus affecting the fertilization process. Also, obesity may affect the offspring, leading to obesity genetic factors.[7] Obesity leads to increased testicular heat, which negatively affects sperm motility and function.[8]

It is estimated that obesity in women will lead to 6% of primary infertility according to a recent report by the American Society of Reproductive Medicine. Reproductive endocrinologists and infertility specialists must consider proper counseling of obese women who present for infertility evaluation because that could be the main issue. If they achieve pregnancy, there will be problems related to continuation of the pregnancy or related to the fetus and its progression in pregnancy.

ETIOLOGY OF INFERTILITY IN OBESE PATIENTS

One of the major effects of obesity in women is ovulatory dysfunction. These women become oligomenorrheic or amenorrheic. This is due to extragonadal estrogen synthesis, which leads to suppression of gonadotropins and of ovarian follicle development, causing anovulation. This is a major cause of infertility in obese patients.[9]

The use of fertility medications to induce ovulation may be helpful. However, the dosage of these medications may be somewhat higher that would be used for a normal-weight patient. In addition, pregnancy in obese women will subject the patient as well as the fetus to risk factors, especially if the woman develops diabetes or hypertension. For this reason, the patient would be referred to a perinatologist for prenatal counseling to understand the problems that may be present during pregnancy. Therefore, one of the goals is to counsel the patient to join a weight reduction program to avoid all these problems. Weight loss has been shown to improve ovulation and conception.[10–12]

Obesity has also been shown to be a significant factor in male infertility. One of the major findings is abnormality in the sperm picture, with a decrease in the concentration, motility, and normal morphology. In some reports, also DNA fragmentation has been demonstrated, and this may lead to failure to achieve pregnancy or cause fetal wastage.[13,14] Furthermore, obesity in men has been associated with erectile dysfunction. This might be the result of hypogonadism and increased concentrations of inflammatory cytokines.[15] Evaluation of the male factor is essential in the study of etiology of infertility because this contributes to about 30%–40% of the causes.

Obesity due to increase in subcutaneous fat increases the activity of aromatase and therefore the conversion of androgens into estrogens. The high levels of estrogens in obese women and men has a negative feedback on the hypothalamic-pituitary gonadal access, which leads to hypogonadism and subsequently to anovulation in women and decreased spermatogenesis in men. In addition, testosterone level in men decreases, causing some problems related to sperm function and erectile dysfunction in men.

Obesity is associated with an increase in insulin levels due to insulin resistance. This leads to a decrease in steroid hormone-binding globulin synthesis by the liver. The end result is the increase in free sex steroid levels, which leads to their metabolic clearance. As a result, there will be an increase in androgen synthesis that contributes to ovulatory dysfunction, irregular cycles, and infertility. Another factor in obesity is the increase in the messenger protein leptin, which in high concentrations leads to an inhibitory effect on the hypothalamic-pituitary axis. The end result is ovulatory dysfunction and infertility. The same phenomenon will affect testicular function and spermatogenesis, resulting in infertility.[16–18]

INFERTILITY WORKUP

Because of the factors mentioned, the workup of the infertile couple who have obesity as a problem in the male, female, or both needs special consideration to address all the problems and manage them properly (see Table 17-1). The female obese patient with anovulatory dysfunction requires endocrine studies in the form of thyroid studies and examination of prolactin level, total testosterone level, and cortisol and dehydroepiandrostene sulfate levels. Serum follicle-stimulating hormone (FSH) level is also recommended to evaluate ovarian reserve.[19,20] Metabolic studies in the form of liver enzymes, fasting blood sugar, and hemoglobin A_{1C} are also needed to help manage these patients.

For the standard evaluation to check for uterine and tubal disease, a hysterosalpingogram should be performed to complete the workup.[21] The hysterosalpingogram is usually performed in the proliferative phase of the menstrual cycle. The patients are scheduled within the week following the end of the menstrual cycle. The endometrium will be thin, and there is no bleeding and no interference with the flow of the dye. As such, it will not lead to any false-positive or false-negative effect. The patient is usually placed in the dorsal lithotomy position, and the speculum is placed in the vagina. The cervix and vagina are cleaned using antiseptic lotion. A thin intrauterine catheter with a balloon is introduced into the cervical canal into the lower segment of the uterine cavity. The balloon is inflated with 1–2 mL of air. In other situations, a cannula with a plastic tip is used to deliver the dye through the cervix into the uterine cavity. The fluoroscopy is activated, and the radiopaque dye will be injected slowly; it will be seen on the monitor traveling into the uterine cavity and into the fallopian tubes to outline these structures. Any pathology in the uterine cavity will show a filling defect. In addition, any obstruction in the fallopian tubes will be seen clearly and help in future management of these situations. The patients are instructed to take a dose of antiprostaglandins about 1 hour before the procedure to alleviate any discomfort as a result of the injection of the dye.

The dye used for hysterosalpingogram is made up of organic iodine compound. Its mode of action is to block x-rays directed toward the organ to be visualized, thus allowing the treating physician to identify pathology in the uterus such as congenital anomalies or tumors inside the cavity. It also identifies the pathology related to the

TABLE 17-1 Infertility Workup in Obese Patients

Endocrine studies
- T_4, TSH
- Prolactin
- Testosterone
- Dehydroepiandrostene sulfate
- Cortisol

Metabolic studies
- Fasting blood sugar
- Hemoglobulin A_{1c}

Hysterosalpingogram
Semen analysis

blockage in the fallopian tubes. After the test is completed, the dye in the uterine cavity will drain in the vagina. The dye in the tubes and peritoneal cavity will be absorbed and eliminated in the urine.

The results of the hysterosalpingogram will reveal any uterine anomaly as a result of failure of fusion of the paramesonephric ducts with conditions such as septate uterus, bicornuate uterus or didelphic uterus. The tubal disease that is diagnosed by hysterosalpingogram could be in the form of distal obstruction as hydrosalpinx. It could also be in the form of proximal tubal obstruction as a result of spasm, endometriosis, or salpingitis isthmica nodosa.[22,23] In cases of proximal tubal obstruction, it is suggested that transcervical tubal catheterization be performed to see if this is a spasm or fibrosis and if it could be recanalized without resorting to major surgery.[24]

Another aspect of evaluation of female infertility is to check for ovulation. This is usually accomplished by one of two methods. The first method is recording of the basal body temperature daily during the cycle. This is usually done in the morning before the patient gets out of bed. This is to ensure that this is a basal body temperature. You find that if the patient is ovulatory, around ovulation time the basal body temperature will rise about 0.5°F–1°F, and that temperature measurement will remain as it is and will continue if pregnancy occurs. If there is no pregnancy, the temperature will decrease prior to the menstrual flow. However, this method is not usually accurate when compared to endocrine studies.[25] In obese women with anovulatory cycles, expect a monophasic temperature chart. Further studies, such as endometrial biopsy or serum progesterone level, will confirm the diagnosis.

The midluteal serum progesterone level is a quick method for diagnosing ovulation. If the level is 3 ng/mL or above, it indicates that the patient definitely ovulated.[26] However, this test does not reflect on endometrial changes or presence of chronic infection.

Ovulation may also be diagnosed by performing a midluteal endometrial biopsy. The sample will be sent to the pathologist for evaluation of the progesterone effect. This is related to changes of the endometrial glands to reflect the secretory changes, starting as subnuclear, then supranuclear. In addition, stroma cells enlarge with increased vascularity. The pathologist reports on these changes in the form of dating of the endometrium according to the established criteria put forward by Noyes et al. The endometrial biopsy can also show if there is any chronic inflammatory pathology in the endometrium that prevents pregnancy.[27] Chronic inflammatory changes may be due to tuberculosis, bilharziasis, or chronic nonspecific bacterial disease.

For the male partner, we recommend endocrine studies for FSH, testosterone, thyroid hormones, and prolactin level. A semen analysis must be done in an andrology laboratory that is well staffed with highly specialized andrologists to look at the count, motility, and morphology according to the World Health Organization (WHO) criteria; in addition, the lab must check for DNA fragmentation. WHO criteria were introduced in 1980 and are revised every few years. The last revision was in 2010. These are followed by all andrology laboratories in their reporting. The normal criteria accordingly include the following:

- Volume 1.5 mL
- Sperm count 15 million/mL
- Total sperm count 39 million/mL

- Total motility 40%
- Progressive motility 32%
- Sperm viability 58%
- Sperm morphology over 4%
- Leukocytes less than 1/mL

These WHO criteria are different from the previous ones but should be followed by andrology laboratories at the present time.[28] Furthermore, metabolic studies are performed to rule out diabetes and insulin resistance.

It is clear that the evaluation of the obese infertile patient is different from evaluation of patients with normal weight because of the added endocrinopathies and metabolic abnormalities related to weight increase.

An extensive workup will assist the infertility specialist in counseling these patients and helping them to try to achieve weight loss before embarking on fertility treatment.

CONCLUSION

Obesity is a serious health hazard for men and women. It leads to development of metabolic diseases such as diabetes and hypertension. In addition, it is a significant factor in the etiology of infertility. The major cause of infertility is ovulatory dysfunction in women and defective spermatogenesis in men.

One of the areas of research to help understand the disease process and its effect on ovulation and steroidogenesis is the relationship between leptins and obesity. Another area of research is related to methods, both medical and surgical, to be adopted for weight loss. Further studies are needed in these areas. Certainly, weight loss in obese women has been shown to correct the metabolic syndrome and to improve fertility potential; it should be encouraged in all patients with a body mass index greater than 30.

REFERENCES

1. Pasquali R, Patton L, Gambineri A. Obesity and infertility. *Curr Endocrin Diabets Obes*. 2007;14(6): 482–487.
2. Brower CJ, Balen AH. The adverse effect of conception and implantation. *Reproduction*. 2010;140:347–364.
3. Pasquali R, Gambineri A. Metabolic effect of obesity on reproduction. *Reprod Biomed Online*. 2006;12(15): 542–551.
4. Wike S, Murdoch A. Obesity and female fertility: a primary care perspective. *J Fam Plan Reprod Health Care*. 2009;35(3):181–185.
5. Pasquali R, Pelusi C, Genghini S, et al. Obesity and reproductive disorders in women. *Hum Reprod Update*. 2003;9(4):359–372.
6. Hammoud AO, Meikle W, Oliviera Reis L, et al. Obesity and male infertility. *Semin Reprod Med*. 2012;30(6): 486–495.
7. Palmer NO, Bakos HW, Fullston T, et al. Impact of obesity on male fertility, sperm function and molecular composition. *Spermatogenesis*. 2012;2(4):253–263.
8. Robinson D, Rock J, Menkin MF. Control of human spermatogenesis by induced changes of intrasacrotal temperature. *JAMA*. 1968;204:290–297.
9. Green BB, Weiss NS, Daling JR. Risk of ovulatory infertility in relation to body weight. *Fertil Steril*. 1988; 50: 721–726.
10. Huber-Buchholz MM, Carey DG, Norman RJ. Restoration of reproductive potential by lifestyle modification in obese polycystic ovary syndrome: role of insulin sensitivity and luteinizing hormone. *J Clin Endocrinol Metab*. 1999;84:1470–1474.
11. Crosignani PG, Colombo M, Vegetti W, et al. Overweight and obese anovulatory patients with polycystic ovaries: parallel improvements in anthropometric indices, ovarian physiology and fertility rate induced by diet. *Hum Reprod*. 2003;18:1928–1932.
12. Clark AM, Thornley B, Tomlinson L, et al. Weight loss in obese infertile women results in improvement in reproductive outcome for all forms of fertility treatment. *Hum Reprod*. 1998;13:1502–1505.

13. Bakos HW, Thompson JG, Feil D, et al. Sperm DNA damage is associated with reproductive technology pregnancy. *Int J Androl.* 2008;31:518–526.

14. Brahem S, Mehdi M, Landolsi H, et al. Semen parameters and sperm DNA fragmentation as causes of recurrent pregnancy loss. *Urology.* 2011;78:792–796.

15. Giugliano F, Esposito K, DiPalo C, et al: Erectile dysfunction associates with endothelial dysfunction and raised pro-inflammatory cytokine levels in obese men. *J Endocrinol Invest.* 2004;27(7):665–669.

16. Agarwal SK, Voegel K, Weitsman SR, et al. Leptin anatoagonizes the insulin like growth factor-1 augmentation of steroidogenesis in granulose and the Ca cells of the human oveary. *J Clin Endocrinol Metab.* 1998;84:1072–1076.

17. Farooq R, Lutfullah S, Ahmed M. Serum leptin levels in obese infertility men and women. *Pak J Pharm Sci.* 2014;27(1):67–71.

18. Farooq R, Lutfullah S, Ishaq H. Relation of serum leptin with sex hormones of obese infertile men and women. *J Appl Pharm Sci.* 2013;3(1):60–65.

19. Abdalla H, Thum MY: An elevated basal FSH reflects a quantitative rather than a qualitative decline of the ovarian reserve. *Hum Reprod.* 2004;19:893.

20. Practice Committee of the American Society for Reproductive Medicine. Testing and interpreting measures of ovarian reserve: a committee opinion. *Fertil Steril.* 2012;98:1407.

21. Lim CP, Hasafa Z, Bhattacharya S, et al. Should a hysterosalpingogram be a first-line investigation to diagnose female tubal subfertility in the modern subfertility workup? *Hum Reprod.* 2011;26:967.

22. Swart P, Mol BW, van der Veen F, et al. The accuracy of hysterosalpingography in the diagnosis of tubal pathology: a meta-analysis. *Fertil Steril.* 1995;64:486.

23. Papaioannou S, Bourdrez P, Varma R, et al. Tubal evaluation in the investigation of subfertility: a structured comparison of tests. *BJOG.* 2004;111:1313.

24. Thurmond AS. Fallopian tube catheterization. *Semin Intervent Radiol.* 2008;25(4):425–431.

25. Bauman JE. Basal body temperature: unreliable method for anovulation detection. *Fertil Steril.* 1981;36(6):729–733.

26. Wathen NC, Perry L, Lilford RJ, et al. Interpretation of single progesterone measurement in diagnosis of anovulation and defective luteal phase: observations on analysis of the normal range. *Br Med J (Clin Res Ed).* 1984;288:7.

27. Noyes RW, Hertig AT, Rock J. Dating the endometrial biopsy. *Fertil Steril.* 1950;1:3–25.

28. Cooper TG, Noonan E, von Eckardstein S, Auger J, Baker HW, Behre HM, Haugen TB, Kruger T, Wang C, Mbizvo MT, Vogelsong KM. World Health Organization reference values for human semen characteristics. *Hum Reprod Update.* 2010 May-Jun;16(3): 231-45.

CHAPTER 18

Preconceptual Counseling and Prenatal Diagnosis

Jeffrey R. Johnson, MD

Vanessa Barnabei, MD, PhD

OVERVIEW

The prevalence of obesity has increased substantially over the past 10 years and affects more than one-third of the population in the United States. The rates of extreme obesity (body mass index [BMI] > 40) have had the fastest rate of increase, now affecting up to 8% of the population. All levels of obesity affect more persons in the southern United States than in other regions, and non-Hispanic black women are disproportionately represented compared to other ethnicities, with 50% affected. Mexican American women follow closely at 45%, and 33% of non-Hispanic Caucasian women are obese.

Obesity presents many challenges prior to pregnancy, and weight loss prior to conception has many proven benefits. Preconception counseling is of benefit in these patients. There are risks to pregnancy at the time of conception, as well as during the first trimester, and counseling about these risks prior to pregnancy would allow the patient the opportunity to make lifestyle changes that would benefit her and improve obstetrical outcome. There are several limitations during pregnancy in regard to prenatal diagnosis, and accurate determination of certain risks to the fetus may be more difficult to ascertain than in the nonobese population. The risks of certain prenatal diagnostic procedures are increased, and the limitations of prenatal imaging by ultrasound for diagnosis of certain types of fetal abnormalities worsen. This chapter focuses on preconception counseling as well as the difficulties of prenatal testing in this group of patients. Difficulties later in pregnancy are covered elsewhere in this book.

PRECONCEPTION COUNSELING

Obesity is defined by BMI level, and normal weight is defined as a BMI of 18.5–24.9. The Institute of Medicine (IOM) recently published pregnancy weight gain guidelines based on prepregnancy BMI.[1] The recommendations are independent of age, parity, smoking history, race, and ethnic background. The IOM guidelines define overweight as a BMI of 25–29.9, and obesity as a BMI greater than 30. IOM does not differentiate between the higher classes of obesity, which are separated into class I (BMI 30–34.9), class II (BMI 35–39.9), and class III (BMI > 40). The risks during pregnancy are affected by extreme obesity and increase with increasing degree of obesity.

Preconception counseling is important for all women, but especially for obese women, particularly as they reach class II or class III obesity. The risk of gestational diabetes, for example, increases from an odds ratio of 2.6 (confidence interval [CI] 1.2–3.9) for women who are class I to (CI 1.5–5.9) for women with class III (OR = 4). The risk of preeclampsia increases from 1.6 (class I) to 3.7 (class III) (CI 0.90–2.2 and 1.85–4.4, respectively), and fetal macrosomia increases from an odds ratio of 1.7 (class I) to 2.9 (class III) (CI 1.3–2.6 and 1.8–3.8, respectively). The risk of Cesarean section ranges from 20.7% for women with a BMI of 29.9 or less to 33.8% for women with a BMI of 30–34.9 and 47.4% for women with a BMI of 40.[2] There is also an increased risk of spontaneous abortion in obese women, in both those who conceive spontaneously and those undergoing fertility treatments.

Encouraging weight loss in these women may substantially reduce their risk of obstetric complications. All studies that have compared pregnancy outcomes for obese women to those for patients who underwent an active weight loss program prior to conception showed a significantly decreased rate of obstetric complications in those who lost at least 10% of their prepregnancy weight or decreased their class of obesity by 1 level. There does not appear to be any threshold below which there is a higher chance of better outcomes, but it appears that in the obesity class III set of patients, even a modest weight loss of 5% shows a decrease in the rate of development of gestational diabetes, premature delivery, and hypertensive complications.[3]

As with any nonpregnant obese individual, a baseline electrocardiogram (ECG) and echocardiogram are suggested when a women presents for preconception or prenatal care. This is particularly true in the first trimester of pregnancy, as these patients may have underlying cardiomyopathy from prolonged obesity and may have hypertension. The higher-class obese patients may exhibit a "Pickwickian"-type syndrome and be chronically short of breath, be polycythemic, and have hypertrophic cardiomyopathy. In addition, if a patient requires more than 2 pillows to sleep at night or there is evidence of excessive snoring or sleep apnea, a sleep study should be undertaken to determine if there are any issues with chronic airway obstruction. These obstructive airway issues will worsen during the course of pregnancy with the gravid uterus and physiologic airway changes, and many of these patients will benefit from a continuous positive airway pressure (CPAP) machine for sleep.

Counseling of these women is also important to inform them of potential fetal risks. The risks of stillbirth[4] and certain congenital defects, such as neural tube defects

(NTDs), are increased, and 1 study of 2900 obese women suggested a lower rate of prematurity.[5] Other studies[4,6] have suggested higher rates of premature delivery in obese women compared to normal-weight women. Many of these preterm deliveries are iatrogenic due to pregnancy complications caused by obesity, such as preeclampsia, hypertension, and gestational diabetes. A Swedish study[4] showed that if women with a BMI greater than 25 optimized their BMI prior to pregnancy, there was a 13% reduction in risk of stillbirth. A meta-analysis of 9 observational studies showed that women who were overweight or obese before pregnancy were at greater risk of stillbirth. The odds ratio for overweight women was 1.47 (CI 1.08–1.94) and for obese women was 2.07 (CI 1.59–2.74). As women are more likely to remain obese at the time of conception and during pregnancy, it is unclear if weight loss during pregnancy confers the same benefit.

Obese women are more likely to give birth to an infant with certain congenital anomalies; the most frequent are NTDs. The risk of an NTD is double that compared to normal-weight women,[6] and this association persists after controlling for diabetes as a potential confounding factor. Folic acid administration in doses higher than the usual recommended 400 μg daily has not been studied in women without diabetes, and whether this would confer any reduction in risk of NTDs in obese women is not known.

Other congenital defects are noted with increased frequency in obese women, and in decreasing order are congenital cardiac defects; orofacial defects, including cleft lip, cleft lip and palate, but not cleft palate alone; and limb abnormalities.[7] The mechanism for the development of these types of defects and how they relate to obesity are not known.

An important factor in preconception counseling is to inform patients of potential lifelong implications in their offspring related to maternal obesity. The relationship between maternal obesity and diabetes in later life in both mothers and offspring is already well established.[8] The exact cause of this relationship is not completely understood, and there may be multiple factors involved in the development of this relationship. There is certainly a strong genetic component, and a family history of type 1 and type 2 diabetes will significantly increase the rates of diabetes in progeny within these families. However, there also appears to be mechanisms, such as epigenetic modification of the fetal genome, that increase the rates of diabetes even in those without a family history of diabetes.

A 2012 study[9] reported higher rates of impaired glucose tolerance of offspring in 21% of Caucasian women with gestational diabetes and 11% in Caucasian women with type 1 diabetes. These studies have shown impaired glucose tolerance that persists through at least 16 years of age, and other studies have found this association much later in life.[10] There is a correlation with fetal hyperinsulinemia that leads to pancreatic overgrowth; excessive fat formation, leading to chronic inflammation; and development of metabolic syndrome. These correlations vary in degree of risk but are seen in age- and sex-matched controls across many populations and ethnicities. This risk remains unchanged after adjustment for demographic variables, socioeconomic status, and maternal prepregnancy BMI among populations studied.

The pathophysiology of the association between stillbirth and obesity is not entirely certain, but there may be several mechanisms involved. These include placental dysfunction, placental inflammation, impaired glucose tolerance and fetal insulin resistance, and hyperlipidemia. In many animal models, there are mechanisms that are known as programming effects. These are mechanisms by which an exposure to an outside agent or condition will activate certain genes within the genome, such that development of disease may occur. For example, the genes that control low-density lipoprotein (LDL) metabolism become activated.[8] This may occur in utero, and offspring show cholesterol streaks within large vessels such as the aorta, renal arteries, and mesenteric arteries. These high-density LDL molecules are strong producers of vascular atherosclerotic plaques, and even though most will recede in newborns and children, there is increasing evidence[8] that in utero, these genes confer a lifelong risk for the development of atherosclerotic disease.

Placental dysfunction has been shown in primates that are fed a high-fat diet. The obese primates being studied demonstrated an increased rate of placental insufficiency and increased stillbirth.[11] Pregnancy induces a pro-inflammatory, hyperlipidemic, insulin-resistant state, and these responses are exaggerated in obese women. These women will exhibit abnormal vascular function and changes to inflammatory mediators that lead to placental inflammation. This inflammation exacerbates insulin resistance and leads to fetal overgrowth, as insulin is the primary growth hormone in the fetus. These inflammatory and vascular changes are also seen within the placenta and will interfere with nutrient and metabolic waste exchange and cause atherosclerotic changes in the placental and fetal vasculature. The inflammation and atherosclerosis in vessels may contribute to the increased rate of stillbirth in pregnancies complicated by maternal obesity.

There is a national movement to decrease maternal morbidity and mortality, both antepartum and postpartum, in the United States. The program designed to decrease these risks is being piloted in New York as the Safe Motherhood Initiative and is supported by the American Congress of Obstetricians and Gynecologists. This program, which is being promoted in almost every hospital in New York that provides maternity care, will be implementing best practices in obstetrical care to screen for, prevent, and treat postpartum hemorrhage, severe hypertension, and venous thromboembolism. Obesity confers a higher risk of all of these maternal complications, and the implementation of these safety bundles is a critical and timely way to minimize pregnancy complications given the rising rates of maternal obesity. Discussion of these risks prior to conception and early in pregnancy allows the patient to understand the issues that may arise in a pregnancy, including embolic phenomena and anesthesia concerns.

Obesity increases the risk of venous thromboembolism, particularly around delivery and for 6 weeks postpartum. If an obese woman has additional risk factors, then antepartum thromboprophylaxis should be used and continued for 6 weeks postpartum. Whether prophylactic versus therapeutic dosing of thromboprophylaxis is used should be based on existing guidelines. All obese patients undergoing cesarean section should have thromboprophylaxis with sequential pneumatic compression devices at a minimum, and these should be continued until the patient is ambulatory.

Anesthesia poses a significant challenge for some patients, and an antepartum consultation with the anesthesia service is suggested. These patients often have difficult airways, and intubation in an emergent situation is a potential complication. They may have excessive soft tissue around their airways, and full extension of the neck may pose difficulties. In addition, swelling of the mucous membranes is normal during pregnancy, and this may pose yet another challenge when trying to secure the airway. Ideally, this evaluation will be considered early in pregnancy.

Ventilatory support can also be a particular issue, particularly in patients with class III obesity. Some obese women may have pendulous breast tissue, and further breast enlargement and engorgement occurs during the last half of pregnancy. When lying supine, this large volume of breast tissue may place significant weight onto the chest wall and increase chest and airway pressures. Some ventilation machines may not be able to generate enough air pressure and will subsequently "pop off" and stop the ventilatory cycle. Our anesthesia colleagues will also need to account for the increased volume of distribution in large patients and compensate for certain anesthetics that may be used. Some inhaled anesthetic agents are fat stored, and this will also need to be taken into account with prolonged periods of inhaled anesthesia. This may prolong the time necessary to wean a patient off the ventilator and safely extubate.

Careful determination of maternal weight is also necessary when planning for admission, as standard operating room tables may not be able to support of some of these women, and a bariatric operating table may needed. Large beds and wheelchairs may also be necessary for some patients with class II or III obesity, and pre-arrangements should be made. Prelabor planning is essential for these patients to ensure necessary equipment is available and so that any extra personnel are available if needed. Induction of labor at term may be considered in certain extreme circumstances to ensure a controlled environment in which all personnel and equipment are readily available.

Regional analgesia and anesthesia are recommended for these patients. This is often problematic due to obscured landmarks, difficulty in patient positioning, and excessive layers of adipose tissue. The last issue may necessitate using special instruments, including extra-long spinal needles to reach the epidural or intrathecal space. Ultrasound guidance may also be used to help proper placement of the needle during anesthesia administration.

PRENATAL SCREENING

Serum screening for aneuploidy, trisomy 21 in particular, has been around for decades in various forms. Serum screening in the second trimester is also employed for NTDs, and the impact of maternal weight on the interpretation of these screening tests has been known since the inception of maternal serum screening. The biochemical markers used in these tests arise either by transplacental passage from the fetus into the maternal serum or from the placenta itself. As such, markers undergo a dilutional effect to a greater degree in obese women due to a greater volume of distribution of these analytes. Reporting of actual measured maternal weight at the time of blood draw is important to be able to correct for this volume of distribution in the calculation of risk.

Each serum analyte is first converted into a multiple of the expected median (MoM) concentration, based on gestational age, obstetric history, number of fetuses, and presence of diabetes. The MoM values are then adjusted for maternal weight based on an assumed linear relationship between the log of the MoM marker level and weight. Several studies have examined whether this should be a log linear relationship or an inverse linear relationship.[12] It appears that either is an acceptable method for correction of maternal weight in the calculation for most analytes examined, across a wide range of maternal weights. The association for an inverse relationship appears to break down with serum human chorionic gonadotropin (hCG) and extreme obesity (>120 kg) and is significantly affected above this weight. However, this is a small impact as it is a relatively small percentage of the population, and hCG is not considered a strong analyte in the detection of trisomy 21.

The analytes utilized in first-trimester screening, free β-hCG and PAPP-A (pregnancy-associated plasma protein A), are decreased with increasing maternal weight,[13] but after correction for maternal weight, the rate of false-positive results for trisomy 21 is no higher than in nonobese individuals. However, false-positive rates for trisomy 18 are significantly increased in obese individuals. There is a 15%–18% decrease in MoM of free β-hCG for each 30-pound increase in maternal weight. There is a 25%–30% reduction in PAPP-A MoM for each 30-pound increase in maternal weight, and the greater the maternal weight, the greater the decrease in PAPP-A MoM. Trisomy 18 risks are greater with lower hCG and PAPP-A levels, and greater maternal weight will result in higher false-positive rates. Reporting of actual maternal weight at the time of testing is crucial to compensate for the decrease in MoM levels. The rate of false-positive results in obese women remains significant even after adjustment for maternal weight but is minimized to an acceptable level to remain useful as a screening tool in obese women.

CELL-FREE FETAL DNA

Use of noninvasive prenatal testing (NIPT) has increased exponentially for prenatal screening of aneuploidy due to its high degree of sensitivity and low false-positive rate when used in the appropriate obstetric population. NIPT can detect fetal trisomy 21 with an up to 99% sensitivity and trisomy 18 with 95%–98% sensitivity, with a false-positive rate of less than 5% depending on the population studied. There have been several different methods developed to test for aneuploidy using cell-free fetal DNA (cffDNA). There is variability in the types of aneuploidy detected depending on the method used, but the sensitivity and false-positive rates of the various methods do not appear to be affected by maternal weight.

Noninvasive prenatal testing may be obtained as early as 10 weeks, and there is no upper gestational age range above which the test may not be obtained, dependent on the patient's wishes for pregnancy outcomes or possible termination in cases of aneuploidy. The amount of cffDNA required for most tests is between 3% and 5% of free fetal DNA per sample, and this level is reached after 10 weeks' gestation. Previous reports[14] have shown no statistically significant difference in the percentage of cffDNA from week to week in maternal plasma, with an average of 11%–13%. High-risk pregnancies between 11 and 13 weeks' gestation show no correlation between percentage fetal cffDNA and fetal karyotype, crown-rump length, or maternal characteristics other than weight. However, the fetal percentage of cffDNA is increased with increased serum PAPP-A and free β-hCG; conversely, the percentage of cffDNA has been shown to decrease with increasing maternal weight.

Wang et al.,[15] in an industry-sponsored evaluation, studied 22,384 maternal plasma samples obtained between July and December 2012 from singleton pregnancies at 10 weeks' gestation and greater. The aim was to evaluate the percentage fetal DNA based on gestational age and compare this to maternal body weight. They found that there was an increase in cffDNA of 0.10% between weeks 10 and 21, with a more rapid increase of 1.0% from weeks 22 onward. There was also a decreasing proportion of patients who had the minimum of 4% of cffDNA fraction with increasing maternal weight, and that this trend was statistically significant ($p < .0001$). There was a 1.9% redraw request rate among the study patients, and the average rate of redraw was associated with lower gestational ages (initial draw 13.9 weeks vs. initial draw 15.8 weeks; $p < .0001$), and higher mean maternal weights (mean 103 kg redraw vs. mean 73 kg no redraw; $p < .0001$). In addition, the proportion of redrawn samples with sufficient cffDNA fraction decreased with increasing maternal body weight. This association began to disappear with later initial samples of cffDNA in women with higher maternal weights, suggesting that delay in drawing of the initial samples in these patients may overcome the issue of insufficient cffDNA.

There were several significant limitations to this study. The first is that not all pregnancies had dating confirmed by ultrasound. As such, there may have been confounding issues in relation to gestational age at the first draw, and as a consequence, the test was obtained too early. Another limitation is that the height of the patients was not recorded, and the data were presented only by maternal weight, as BMI could not be calculated. In obese women, there is a higher rate of adipose tissue turnover, which increases the fraction of maternal cell-free DNA and can affect the proportion of cffDNA. In addition, calculation of BMI tends to overestimate the amount of body fat compared to lean muscle mass in very muscular persons and can underestimate body fat in patients who have low amounts of lean muscle mass.

It appears from this information that there is most likely a dilutional effect of cffDNA based on maternal weight, and that this correlation is linear as maternal weight increases above 130 kg. What is not clear presently is if delay in obtaining cffDNA should be advocated in women who are heavier, at what weight this threshold should exist, and how long the delay should be. Other unknown variables are to obtain the cffDNA per usual guidelines and advise heavier patients that a redraw of the sample may be required if the fraction of cffDNA is not sufficient. There does not appear to be an upper limit BMI "cutoff" above which the test is no longer accurate.

INVASIVE PRENATAL TESTING

Poor ultrasound visualization is a known complication for obese patients, and the rates of nonvisualization of fetal structures and incomplete ultrasound studies increase proportionally with increasing BMI (see next section). The recommendations for invasive prenatal testing for obese patients, based on weight, adequate visualization of fetal structures, and results of noninvasive screening tests, are no different than for the nonobese population. However, maternal weight is correlated with more complicated diagnostic procedures due to increased adiposity, difficulty with visualization with ultrasound guidance, and difficulty in reaching the target area for sampling (placenta or amniotic fluid).

In a study by Harper et al.,[16] rates of loss after chorionic villi sampling (CVS) and amniocentesis were compared in nonobese and obese women and were stratified into class I through class III obesity. There were no differences in loss rates within 14 days of the procedure or prior to 24 weeks' gestation with either procedure or with increasing body mass. The majority of CVS procedures were transcervical as visualization was better with this approach. An important finding was a significantly increased proportion of patients with increased BMI who required a second attempt at amniocentesis due to poor visualization ($p < .02$). This is a common observation, as there is more difficulty in visualization of the needle tip with increased depth of penetration, and the increased tissue may cause the needle to become deflected as it traverses the layers, necessitating a repeat attempt.

ULTRASOUND LIMITATIONS

First-trimester ultrasound for the measurement of nuchal translucency has become commonplace for aneuploidy screening. Obesity has been shown to affect the ability to obtain these measurements. The First and Second Trimester Evaluation of Risk (FaSTER) trial[17] found that maternal BMI significantly affected the ability to obtain the nuchal translucency (NT) measurement, typically assessed by transabdominal ultrasound. The ability to obtain the measurement significantly decreased as the BMI increased, with the rate of unobtainable NT at 1.0% for BMI below 25, 3.2% for class I–II, and 7.8% for class III BMI. There was also a significantly increased amount of time required to obtain measurements. The average was 14 to 17 minutes for patients with class II–III obesity, compared to 9 minutes for normal-weight patients. There was an increased frequency of use of transvaginal ultrasound in the attempts to obtain adequate NT measurements, which also significantly increased the time required during the examination.

Second-trimester ultrasound for the evaluation of fetal anatomy and screening for aneuploidy has also become a mainstay in prenatal care, and obesity significantly affects the ability to obtain measurements and detailed images of the fetus. The FaSTER trial[17] examined a subset of patients who underwent second-trimester genetic sonograms to evaluate for structural anomalies and markers of aneuploidy. The study demonstrated that obesity decreased the sensitivity of markers of aneuploidy, including short humerus, short femur, and pyelectasis, while assessment of other markers such as nuchal fold, echogenic bowel, and echogenic intracardiac focus were not affected. When examining the prenatal detection rate of "any sonographic finding," obese women had lower rates of detection compared to normal-weight women (8.6% vs. 11.9%; $p < .0024$).[17] Overall, there was a higher rate of missed diagnosis for many minor markers of aneuploidy and a lower detection rate for specific congenital anomalies.

In a retrospective study by Dashe et al.,[18] there was a decreased rate of detection of anomalous fetuses with either standard or targeted ultrasound. The rates of detection of major fetal anomalies for standard ultrasound was 66% in normal-weight women, 49% for overweight, 48% for class I obesity, 42% for class II, and 25% for class III obese women ($p < .03$ for the trend). The overall anomaly rate in this study was 1.0% for obese women and 0.4% for normal-weight women ($p < .001$).

The lower detection rates observed was due to suboptimal visualization and decreased rates of complete ultrasound examinations. The anatomical area that is suboptimally visualized most often is the cardiovascular system (18% poorly visualized in normal-weight women vs. 49% in women with class III obesity). Other areas that may be poorly visualized are facial soft tissue (19% for normal-weight vs. 39% for obese women), craniospinal structures (29% in normal weight vs. 49% in obesity) and abdominal wall (<1% in normal weight vs. 3% in obesity).[18]

The rate of completed ultrasound studies also decreases with increasing obesity, and the rate of completion increases with increasing gestational age. Tsai et al.[19] found decreasing rates of completed fetal anatomical evaluations as maternal BMI increased, with 64% of normal-weight women having a completed survey, 61% with class I obesity, 55% with class II, and 47% for class III patients ($p < .0001$). They did find that when comparing only completed studies among all weight categories, the positive screen rate was no different. There was also an increased time required to scan obese patients and an increase in return visits for obese patients to complete the examinations. Overall, 8% of women with class III obesity were unable to have completed examinations during pregnancy despite multiple attempts. The optimal gestational age for performance of the standard ultrasound was about 18–20 weeks for normal-weight women and those with class I obesity; this increased to about 22–24 weeks for patients with class III obesity.

In a study by Handler et al.,[20] the rate of inadequate visualization of cardiac anatomy improved to 80%–90% with repeated ultrasounds, but the rates of persistent suboptimal visualization of the heart in obese women was higher than for normal-weight women (20% for class III obesity vs. 1.5% for normal-weight women). Timing of performance of the scan should be based on institutional guidelines, policies regarding invasive testing, and the legal requirements of pregnancy termination depending on the location of the practice.

Other constraints in the completion of ultrasound examinations include time to perform the exam, level of experience of the sonographer and clinician, and the type of equipment used. On average, there is an increase of anywhere from 10 to 30 minutes in time required to complete an examination. This should be allowed for when scheduling these patients. There is also the well-accepted fact that the rates of completion of studies improves with more senior sonographers and clinicians, with the highest rates of completed studies when performed by senior clinicians who have been practicing for 10 years or more.

High-resolution ultrasound equipment may also aid in the visualization of certain structures. All ultrasound machines have multifrequency ultrasound probes, and the choice of probe should be individualized to patient body habitus when considering. The lower-frequency ultrasound probes have better tissue depth penetration, but with a resultant loss in image resolution. Most machines now also use tissue harmonic imaging (THI), which enhances edge detection and variation in gray scale during real time scanning. Use of THI in combination with lower-frequency probes has allowed for better resolution of fetal structures and may result in higher detection rates of fetal anomalies or aneuploidy markers in obese women.

Size of the image as well as depth and use of focal zones can also have a significant impact on image quality. The smallest possible size image, the least amount of depth, and appropriate adjustment of the focal zone can all aid in improving image quality. In patients with truncal obesity, having the patient roll to one side or using the umbilical window can improve image quality. Often, if the fetus is low in the pelvis, instructing the patient to hold up her pannus or elevating her hips may help with image acquisition.

Third-trimester scans can be an important adjunct in managing pregnancies that are at risk of fetal macrosomia. Identification of these pregnancies may aid in planning for mode of delivery, even in the absence of diabetes. In a prospective study,[7] ultrasound fetal weight estimation was accurate in both obese and nonobese women. It demonstrated that 61% of clinical estimates, 63% of maternal estimates, and 72% of ultrasound estimates were within 10% of actual birth weight.

Umbilical artery Doppler measurements may also be affected by maternal obesity. The pulsatility index (PI) is increased with increasing BMI and is significantly different in patients who are normal weight versus those who are class III obese. This association exists after removal of confounding factors, including presence of diabetes, hypertensive disorders, preeclampsia, and fetal growth restriction. If fetal growth restriction is present, the association of increased PI becomes even stronger. To date, normative data do not exist to correct for maternal BMI when comparing umbilical artery PI; studies in this area would be useful.

PROVIDER ATTITUDES AND IMPACT OF CARE IN OBESE PATIENTS

The prevalence of obesity is rapidly increasing worldwide; yet, there have not been effective countermeasures to date to help decrease these rates. The obstetrician/gynecologist is uniquely situated to help stem the rise in obesity, as we serve as primary caregivers for a large proportion of women, caring for them in adolescence, through their childbearing years, and often beyond menopause. However, there is a disconnect among our specialty regarding counseling these patients and providing effective means to decrease the rise in obesity rates.

A particularly telling study in regard to this issue was published by Herring et al.[21] in 2010. They sent surveys to practicing obstetricians, nurse practitioners, and certified nurse midwives in one multispecialty practice in Massachusetts. The questionnaire contained 26 items, which also included the provider's self-reported weight, sociodemographic characteristics, knowledge, attitudes, and management practices. They created an 8-point scale for adherence to the 8 practices recommended by the American Congress of Obstetricians and Gynecologists.

This study[21] found that 37% of respondents did not correctly identify the BMI definition of obesity, and most (71%) reported weight gain guidelines that were not concordant with the IOM recommendations. However, most respondents (74%) advised regular physical activity and discussed diet (64%). There was a low rate of first-trimester screening for diabetes (26%), planned anesthesia referrals (3%), or referral to a nutritionist (14%). An interesting finding in this study was that the mean self-reported BMI of the providers was 24.3, and 38% were overweight or obese (BMI > 25), but overall only 30% of providers were satisfied with their own body weight. Even among normal-weight providers, only 46% were satisfied with their own body weight. Provider BMI and perception of body weight had a significant impact on counseling, with higher adherence scores in those providers who had lower BMI, and those providers also had better self-perception of body weight compared to obese providers. Self-perception was an independent predictor of self-reported BMI in counseling, and better self-perception was associated with better adherence scores. The association of provider BMI and self-perception of body weight may reflect a greater level of comfort with dealing with these issues and lead to better knowledge and counseling of obese patients.

There is also a certain degree of skepticism among providers regarding patients' attitudes and acceptance of guidelines, and that changing patients' attitudes can be difficult. This may be particularly true in certain regions of the United States, where obesity is seen in much higher rates and may be related to many factors, including race, socioeconomic factors, and attitudes about weight, obesity, and lifestyle.

SUMMARY

In summary, preconception counseling regarding obesity entails many factors to ensure as successful a pregnancy outcome as possible. Counseling regarding weight gain during pregnancy, exercise, and diet choices is critical to good outcomes. Early screening for diabetes is suggested for obese patients, and if negative, follow-up testing early in the third trimester is recommended. Patients should be counseled regarding the increased risks of certain congenital anomalies, and ultrasound should be used liberally to determine if any of these defects are present. Routine prenatal screening is suggested, bearing in mind some of the limitations of these screening and diagnostic tests in this population. Obesity alone is not an indication for induction of labor, and a trial of labor after cesarean should be encouraged if the patient is an appropriate candidate based on current guidelines.

Provider input is important, and repeated counseling and encouragement may be beneficial for these patients, as lifestyle changes may take some time and willpower to implement. It is important to maintain a positive relationship with these patients and to provide information, support, and guidance in a nonjudgmental fashion.

Future directions include the need for a systemic change in lifestyle in the developed world and an attempt to decrease obesity. From a public health perspective, this will greatly decrease rates of complications in pregnancy and improve the health of the population.

REFERENCES

1. Institute of Medicine. *Weight Gain During Pregnancy: Re-examining the Guidelines.* Washington, DC: National Academies Press; 2009.
2. Weiss JL, Malone FD, Emig D, et al. Obesity, obstetric complications and cesarean delivery rate—a population based screening study. *Obstet Gynecol.* 2004;190: 1069–1075.
3. Obesity in Pregnancy. Practice Bulletin 156. *Obstet Gynecol* 2015;126:e112-26.
4. Cnattingius S, Bergstrom R, Lipworth L, Kramer MS. Pre-pregnancy weight and the risk of adverse pregnancy outcomes. *N Engl J Med.* 1998;338:147–152.
5. Hendler I, Goldenberg RL, Mercer BM, et al. The Preterm Prediction Study: association between maternal body mass index and spontaneous and indicated preterm birth. *Am J Obstet Gynecol.* 2005;192: 882–886.
6. Baeten JM, Bukusi EA, Lambe M. Pregnancy complications and outcomes among overweight and obese nulliparous women. *Am J Public Health.* 2001;91:436–440.
7. Tsai P-J, Loichinger M, Zalud I. Obesity and the challenges of ultrasound fetal abnormality diagnosis. *Best Pract Res Clin Obstet Gynaecol.* 2015;29(3):320–327.
8. Freeman DJ. Effects of maternal obesity on fetal growth and body composition: implications for programming and future health. *Semin Fetal Neonatal Med.* 2010;15:113–118.
9. Malcom J. Through the looking glass: gestational diabetes as a predictor of maternal and offspring long-term health. *Diabetes Metab Res Rev.* 2012;28:307–311.
10. Keely EJ, Malcom JC, Lawson M. Glucose tolerance and prevalence of metabolic markers of insulin resistance in offspring of gestational diabetic pregnancies. *Pediatr Diabetes.* 2008;9:53–59.

11. Woolner AM, Bhattacharya S. Obesity and stillbirth. *Best Pract Res Clin Obstet Gynaecol.* 2015;29(3):415–426.

12. Watt HC, Wald NJ. Alternative methods of maternal weight adjustment in maternal serum screening for Down syndrome and neural tube defects. *Prenat Diagn.* 1998;18:842–845.

13. Krantz DA, Hallahan T, Macri VJ, Macri J. Maternal weight and ethnic adjustment within a first-trimester Down syndrome and trisomy 18 screening program. *Prenat Diagn.* 2005;25:635–640.

14. Norton ME, Brar H, Weiss J, et al. Non-Invasive Chromosomal Evaluation (NICE) Study: results of a multicenter prospective cohort study for detection of fetal trisomy 21 and trisomy 18. *Am J Obstet Gynecol.* 2012;207(2):137.e1-8.

15. Wang E, Batey A, Struble C, Musci T, Song K, Oliphant A. Gestational age and maternal weight effects on fetal cell-free DNA in maternal plasma. *Prenat Diagn.* 2013;33:662–666.

16. Harper LM, Cahill AG, Smith K, Macones GA, Odibo AO. Effect of maternal obesity on the risk of fetal loss after amniocentesis and chorionic villus sampling. *Obstet Gynecol.* 2012;119:745–751.

17. Aagaard-Tillery KM, Flint Porter T, Malone FD, et al. Influence of maternal BMI on genetic sonography in the FaSTER trial. *Prenat Diagn.* 2010;30:14–22.

18. Dashe JS, McIntire DD, Twickler DM. Effect of maternal obesity on the ultrasound detection of anomalous fetuses. *Obstet Gynecol.* 2009;113:1001–1007.

19. Tsai LJ, Ho M, Pressman EK, Thornburg LL. Ultrasound screening for fetal aneuploidy using soft markers in the overweight and obese gravida. *Prenat Diagn.* 2010;30:821–826.

20. Hendler I, Blackwell SC, Bujold E, et al. Suboptimal second-trimester ultrasonographic visualization of the fetal heart in obese women: should we repeat the examination? *J Ultrasound Med.* 2005;24:1205–1209.

21. Herring SJ, Platek DN, Elliot P, Riley LE, Stuebe A, Oken E. Addressing obesity in pregnancy: what do obstetric providers recommend? *J Womens Health.* 2010;19(1):65–70.

Checklists for Care: Care Maps for Pregnancy in the Obese Gravida

Stephen J. Bacak, DO, MPH

Loralei L. Thornburg, MD

INTRODUCTION

Checklists and care pathways (synonymous with care maps, critical pathways, and clinical pathways) are document-based tools that link available evidence to health care practice with the intent to optimize clinical outcomes and patient safety.[1] They provide the foundation for translation of evidence into clinical guidelines and protocols. The World Health Organization (WHO) and Institute of Medicine (IOM) have both advocated of the use of checklists as a key concept in reducing medical errors and improving patient safety.[2,3] Checklists and care pathways have clearly shown improvement in many aspects of medical care and patient care.[1,4,5] In a recent study, the use of crisis checklists in critical processes among operating room teams participating in simulated operating room scenarios showed a 75% reduction in failure to adhere to critical management steps in common intraoperative emergencies.[6] In addition, providers preferred checklists and bundles as memory aids. In the same study, almost all of the study participants ($N = 67$) stated their desire to have the checklist used if they experienced an intraoperative emergency.

This chapter summarizes the important concepts and provides a framework for the development of checklists and care pathways for obese women spanning preconception to the postpartum period. The checklists are based on the evidence presented in other chapters of this text as well as our own review and summary of the literature.

Checklists and Care Pathways in Pregnancy

One of the earliest reports on obstetric checklists was a 1998 article by Ransom et al.[7] A 3-week pilot study was conducted with the implementation of a normal vaginal delivery clinical pathway that included standardized order sets. Despite difficulty with pathway development and implementation across sites, the study showed a decrease in length of hospital stay and an approximate $300 reduction in the cost of a vaginal delivery. In a follow-up study, Ransom et al. suggested that clinical pathways for both vaginal and cesarean delivery may reduce litigation costs.[8] In 2010, the British Columbia Perinatal Health Program disseminated the BC Maternity Care Pathway in an effort to standardize care to pregnant women.[9] Other examples of obstetric checklists include one for management of suspected placenta accreta, an airway checklist for general anesthesia, and a short, evidence-based checklist to reduce complications of cesarean delivery.[10-12]

Clark et al. also credit the use of checklist-based protocols in process standardization as a major component in quality and safety improvements in obstetric care in a large health care system.[13] Furthermore, the implementation of checklists has shown improved communication among obstetric teams.[14,15] In 2011, Fausett et al. published an article in the *American Journal of Obstetrics and Gynecology*'s Patient Safety Series on developing and implementing an effective checklist.[16] Key concepts in checklist development included careful selection of the clinical process underlying the checklist, multidisciplinary representation, brevity, and ongoing review of the evidence to ensure current standards of care are being met.

The American College of Obstetricians and Gynecologists (ACOG) recently released a statement encouraging the use of protocols and checklists.[17] These checklists have served as the backbone of "bundle" development to standardize obstetric care across health care systems and improve quality of care. Since 2010, ACOG has published nine Patient Safety Checklists, including induction of labor, magnesium sulfate for neuroprotection in the preterm infant, trial of labor after caesarean delivery, and management of postpartum hemorrhage (http://www.acog.org/Resources-And-Publications/Patient-Safety-Checklists, accessed April 2, 2015). The Society for Maternal Fetal Medicine (SMFM) has also published two checklists related to management of monochorionic twin pregnancies (https://www.smfm.org/mfm-practice/checklists-and-safety-bundles, accessed April 2, 2015). While these documents were developed to help in the standardization of health care processes and reduce variation in patient care, both ACOG and SMFM affirmed that these checklists should serve as a foundation rather than as an exclusive management plan. As stated by SMFM, "The regular use of checklists—standardized, validated, evidence- or consensus-based processes—promotes consistency in obstetrical care and helps provide safe, efficient, high-quality patient care" (https://www.smfm.org/mfm-practice/checklists-and-safety-bundles; accessed April 2, 2015).

Checklists and Care Pathways in Obese Pregnant Women

As discussed throughout this book, obesity and morbid obesity are significant contributors to both maternal and neonatal morbidity.[18-20] In addition, data suggest that providers comply less with prenatal care recommendations in obese women, further reiterating the importance of checklists to keep compliance with prenatal care recommendations high for all women.[21] The obstetric literature regarding clinical care pathways in obese women is sparse. Previously, Catalano published a widely use and referenced well-written and thorough expert opinion article on management of the obese pregnant patient.[22] In 2013, ACOG updated its committee opinion regarding obesity in pregnancy.[19] Both of these documents provide a rich discussion of pregnancy complications and offer general recommendations surrounding obesity in pregnancy. However, they fall short of establishing a specific framework or checklists for care of the obese pregnant woman. Two recent review articles offer a more structured model in the management of the obese woman throughout pregnancy.[23,24]

The Royal College of Obstetricians and Gynecologists in collaboration with the Centre for Maternal and Child Enquiries published a joint guideline in 2010, *Management of Women With Obesity in Pregnancy*.[25] Similar to a traditional care pathway, this guideline was developed by a multidisciplinary and evidence-based effort to standardize care and improve patient outcomes. Fealy et al. implemented and evaluated an alternative (addition to routine prenatal care) clinical care pathway for 79 pregnant women with a body mass index (BMI) of 35 kg/m^2 or greater. The pathway consisted of written education on obesity, dietician referral, early gestational diabetes mellitus (GDM) screening, evaluation of renal and liver function, anesthesia consultation, routine growth ultrasound, and patient self-weight recordings. The data on outcome, however, were mixed. No women took advantage of self-weighing, and fewer than 20% of women utilized dietetic counseling. Most women took advantage of early GDM screening and serial ultrasounds.[26] Despite the lack of direct evidence on outcomes, care maps are effective tools for providers to standardize approach and counseling related to high-risk pregnancy practice.

Throughout this chapter, we endeavor to summarize the best evidence on pregnancy and goals of care for obese women, from preconception to the postpartum period through the use of checklists. The checklists should be routinely evaluated and modified as new evidence becomes available. Our intent is that individual institutions and health care systems will not only tailor these care models to meet the needs of their unique patient populations, as determined by local resources, practice patterns, and service availability, but also expand on them in an effort to standardize care and optimize obstetric management of obese women.

PRECONCEPTION VISIT

The preconception visit for the obese patient considering pregnancy represents an ideal opportunity for the patient and provider to enter into a discussion regarding the risks of pregnancy and the ways to maximize health for the mother and potential infant prior to entry into pregnancy. This should be viewed not as a visit to bully or scold a patient into radical weight loss behaviors or surgical options, but instead to provide unbiased counseling in an attempt to have patients engage in behaviors that allow them to be the healthiest that they can be at any weight and to motivate

---

Prior weight reduction interventions:
- ☐ Behavior modification
- ☐ Dietary changes: Which programs? ______________
    - Planning to use in pregnancy? ______________
- ☐ Exercise
- ☐ Pharmacotherapy: Which? ______________
    - ☐ Currently using? ______________
    - ☐ Discuss safety in pregnancy
- ☐ Referral to dietician/nutrition specialist
- ☐ Prior bariatric surgery
    - Type of surgery: ☐ Banding   ☐ Roux-en-Y gastric bypass
    - Total weight lost: ______________
    - Months from surgery: ______________
    - ☐ Discuss that pregnancy should be delayed at least 12–18 months after surgery
    - ☐ Discussion of nutritional deficiencies (iron, B_{12}, folate, vitamin D, calcium)
    - ☐ Pregnancy risks after bariatric surgery

Prior pregnancy complications:
- ☐ Preeclampsia:
    - ☐ Discuss low-dose aspirin therapy (if history of severe preeclampsia)
    - ☐ Discuss long-term risks (e.g., cardiovascular disease)
- ☐ Prior cesarean: Low success with VBAC (vaginal birth after cesarean); high risk of wound complications
- ☐ Prior LGA (large for gestational age): Discussed early glucose testing, ADA (American Diabetes Association) diet for pregnancy
- ☐ Other

Existing medical complications:
- ☐ Hypertension (baseline electrocardiogram, echocardiogram)
- ☐ Joint/mobility challenges (appropriate weight gain, exercise/water therapy options, challenges of labor/delivery
- ☐ Large pannus/apron: Discuss skin breakdown, wound infection risks, skin care regimens
- ☐ Diabetes (last hemoglobin A_{1c})
- ☐ Other

Preconception planning:
- ☐ Institute of Medicine pregnancy weight gain recommendations
- ☐ Folic acid supplementation (minimum 400–800 g)
- ☐ Pregnancy risks associated with obesity
- ☐ Initiate conversation about breastfeeding
- ☐ Baseline laboratory testing (thyroid, liver function, 2-hour glucose tolerance test, iron, vitamin B_{12}, folate, vitamin D, calcium for those with bypass surgeries)
- ☐ Referral for bariatric surgery (BMI $\geq$ 40 kg/m^2 or BMI $\geq$ 35 kg/m^2 with comorbidities)

FIGURE 19-1. Example of a preconception checklist.

patients to begin their weight loss journey as a portion of their preparation for a health pregnancy (Figure 19-1).

The provider should utilize the preconception visit to discuss weight loss methods the patient used in the past, including successes and failures, and discuss the dietary and weight goals for the pregnancy. This should include the IOM weight gain recommendations. It has been shown that a 10% difference in prepregnancy BMI is associated with improved obstetric outcomes.[27] There are data to support that obese women who maintain an active and healthy lifestyle will improve their pregnancy outcomes and can decrease excessive weight gain and reduce the risk of GDM.[28] Avoiding excess weight gain is associated with improve pregnancy outcome and lower rates of macrosomia.[29,30] Therefore, developing a healthy lifestyle even without weight loss should be emphasized during preconception counseling. Dietary evaluation with avoidance of excessive caloric intake and dietary counseling should be a part of the conversation. A dietician referral should be part of the preconception care pathway. Furthermore, the partner should be involved in these discussions, and dietary and lifestyle interventions should be prescribed not only to the patient, but also to the entire family, with discussion of continuation of good habits after pregnancy to minimize risks of childhood obesity and intergenerational obesity.

Providers should pay special attention to a discussion of weight loss options that may have been particularly metabolically active, such as stimulants, and those regimens involving medications with known cardiac risks, rapid-cycling weight loss, or highly restrictive or liquid supplement–based diets, which could increase the risk of vitamin deficiencies. For those patients planning weight loss surgery prior to pregnancy, a discussion of timing the procedure at least 12–18 months prior to pregnancy is recommended. For patients who have previously undergone weight loss surgery, the time interval to delivery, type of procedure, and the risks and benefits of surgery should be an integral part of the preconception discussion. In a recent study, pregnancies after bariatric surgery were associated with decreased GDM and decreased risk for a macrosomic infant. However, there were increased risks of shorter gestation and infants who were small for gestational age.[31] Vitamin deficiencies are more common in malabsorptive-type procedures; therefore, screening and supplementation may be needed. For those with symptoms associated with vitamin deficiencies, such as bruising and hair loss, evaluation for more rare deficiencies such as vitamin K and niacin may be warranted.[32] Patients with a history of banding procedures, especially adjustable banding, may benefit by revision of the band. Although rare, malabsorptive procedures can be associated with volvulus or obstruction during pregnancy, and clinicians should be aware to take seriously any persistent gastrointestinal complaints. A discussion of sugar/glycemic tolerance may reveal an inability to perform glucose tolerance testing due to gastric dumping, which may therefore necessitate nontraditional testing methods such as candy twists.[33,34]

Obese women are known to have a lower intake of recommended amounts of calcium, iron, folate, and vitamin D from diet alone.[35] Studies have repeatedly demonstrated poor prenatal vitamin use in this cohort. When prescribing prenatal vitamins, attention should be on folic acid, especially when there is concurrent diabetes. However, excessive folic acid is also associated with later adult complications in animal studies.[36] Therefore, counseling on prenatal vitamin supplementation with folic acid should be considered of upmost importance for these women. For all women planning pregnancy, the US Preventative Services Task Force currently recommends 400–800 μg of folic acid daily to reduce the risk of neural tube defects.[37] Some groups recommend higher doses of folic acid in obese women.[38] In addition, data suggest that only 15%–22% of pregnant and lactating women receive adequate iodine.[39] Given the importance of this nutrient to both fetal and maternal thyroid health and fetal brain development, the American Academy of Pediatrics recommends that pregnant and lactating women have adequate iodine intake.[40,41] Given the higher processed food intake, obese women may be iodine deficient despite a high total salt intake as the majority of salt used in processed food in the United States is not iodized. Smoking further blocks iodine transport through thiocyanate exposure; therefore, smoking patients may be an area of focus for supplementation,[41,42] as well as counseling regarding the maternal and neonatal benefits of smoking cessation.

Each patient's risk going into pregnancy will be slightly different. A thorough medical and genetic history, including complications not related to obesity, should be addressed, as they would be in any preconception consult. The provider and patient should engage in a discussion related to other comorbidities such as hypertension, diabetes, and mobility issues and how these conditions may be affected by weight gain during pregnancy as well as their effect on pregnancy outcomes. Emphasis should be given to optimization of existing comorbidities for at least 3 months prior to conception. Medications should be reviewed for their safety both during pregnancy as well during breastfeeding.

ANTEPARTUM PREGNANCY CARE

First Trimester

Ideally, the first trimester of pregnancy will have been largely discussed and planned during the preconception consultation. Therefore, the information should simply need review and reiteration, with additional discussions for any health or medication changes. In reality, many women do not present to care until pregnancy is already established; therefore, the first-trimester care pathway may include a number of baseline assessments and determination of risks that ideally should have been accomplished prior to pregnancy and are within the preconception care map. Therefore, depending on the patient and practice setup, preconception and early pregnancy care maps may be used separately or interchangeably (Figure 19-2).

A discussion of the 2009 IOM pregnancy weight gain recommendations is an integral part of care for the obese pregnant woman. The weight gain guidelines should be reviewed, and dietary counseling and adherence should be confirmed. Multiple studies have shown increased maternal, fetal, and neonatal complications in pregnancies with gestational weight gain outside the recommended ranges. A recent study by Swank et al. showed a significant increased risk for pregnancy hypertension, cesarean delivery, and macrosomia among superobese (defined as BMI $\geq$ 50 kg/m^2) who gained more than the IOM guidelines.[43] For women without recent glycemic screening, rescreening in the first trimester can assess for the presence of underlying diabetes, as poor control has known associated increased risks for embryopathy and fetopathy. In addition, assessments of thyroid function, liver function, and urine protein (especially if there is a history of hypertension) can allow risk stratification and provide a baseline for changes in later pregnancy. Now that maternal age at delivery is known, a more detailed discussion of genetic testing and screening options should be reviewed, including the increased failure rates with noninvasive prenatal testing (NIPT) and nuchal translucency (NT) screening among obese women.

For women with underlying medical conditions who have not been treated or have been poorly optimized prior to pregnancy, medication review and adjustment

---

□ Ultrasound for viability/gestational dating ordered
    □ Reason if not ordered_______________________________________

□ Baseline laboratory testing
    □ Liver function
    □ Thyroid-stimulating hormone
    □ Urine protein/creatinine ratio or 24-hour urine protein and creatinine clearance
    □ Early screening for gestational diabetes
    □ Iron, B_{12}, folate, vitamin D, calcium (if history of bariatric surgery)
    □ Hemoglobin A_{1c} (if diabetes)
□ Aneuploidy screening options
    □ Noninvasive prenatal testing
    □ Nuchal translucency
    □ First-trimester screening

□ Discussion of the pregnancy specific obesity risks
□ Addressed comorbidities and referral to consultants
□ Electrocardiogram, echocardiogram (if hypertension)
    □ Consider sleep apnea referral testing
    □ Referral to dietician/nutrition specialist

□ Review pregnancy risks and nutritional deficiencies (if history of bariatric surgery)
□ Institute of Medicine pregnancy weight gain recommendations reviewed
    □ Behavior modification
    □ Dietary changes
    □ Exercise
□ Folic acid supplementation (minimum 400–800 g)
□ Begin conversation about breastfeeding

FIGURE 19-2. Example of a first-trimester checklist.

should be performed. Assessment for obesity-related comorbidities such as hypertension and diabetes is warranted. For those with prior bypass surgery, screening for nutritional deficiencies, including vitamin B_{12}, vitamin D, protein, iron, calcium, and folate should be performed if not recently accomplished. A prenatal vitamin with both iodine and folic acid should be initiated.

Screening for sleep disorders, including sleep apnea, should be considered for obese pregnant women. Maasilta et al. found higher rates of sleep-related disordered breathing compared to pregnant women with a normal BMI.[44] In another study, third-trimester obstructive sleep apnea was significantly associated with increasing baseline BMI.[45] Sleep-related disorders have been associated with adverse perinatal outcomes, including hypertension and GDM; however, the data is primarily retrospective.[46-48] The results of the Sleep-Disordered Breathing Study, a large prospective substudy from the Nulliparous Pregnancy Outcomes Study Monitoring Mothers-to-Be that includes 23% obese women, are anticipated soon.[49]

Second and Third Trimesters

In the second trimester, anatomic assessments of the fetus present particular challenges for the obese gravida. As detailed in Chapter 18, fetal ultrasound in obesity has

☐ Discuss obesity risks (e.g., neural tube defects, cardiac malformations) in the second trimester
☐ Anatomic ultrasound
☐ Fetal echocardiography for diabetes/glucose intolerance

Readdress and discuss weight gain goals and adherence to date
    ☐ Repeat Glucola testing at 24–28 weeks if initial screen negative
    ☐ Daily kick counts
    ☐ Consider antenatal testing (e.g., nonstress test [NST]) if other pregnancy complications
    ☐ Anesthesia consultation
    ☐ Fetal growth and position assessment at 36 weeks
    ☐ Discussion of delivery mode (increased risk of cesarean delivery/dysfunctional labor, increased risk of failed epidural, wound complications, failed vaginal birth after cesarean [VBAC] attempted, anesthesia complications, postpartum thrombophlebitis)
    ☐ Consideration of skin cleansing/prep if scheduled cesarean

☐ Initiate contraceptive counseling
    ☐ Oral contraceptives
    ☐ Long-acting reversible contraceptives (levonorgestrel/copper intrauterine device, etonogestrel implant)
    ☐ Surgical (tubal ligation at time of cesarean, hysteroscopic tubal occlusion, postpartum tubal ligation, and interval laparoscopic tubal ligation)

☐ Conversation about breastfeeding, physical exam of breasts, discussion of challenges
    ☐ Prenatal breastfeeding medicine/lactation referral (prenatally if available)

FIGURE 19-3. Example of second- and third-trimester checklists.

a higher noncompletion rate. In addition, Dashe et al. have shown a high residual risk of major and minor anomalies even after completed assessment and even after targeted assessments for high-risk referrals, such as uncontrolled diabetes.[50] Early anatomic screening by transvaginal ultrasound has been proposed, with some data suggesting improved completion rates.[51] Other data suggest that waiting until later in the second trimester may improve completion rates for anatomic surveys (seeing all required fetal anatomy); additionally, allotting additional time for ultrasound visits, and utilizing more experienced sonographers may improve the rate of completing fetal anatomy in a single visit (Figure 19-3).

Throughout the second and third trimesters of pregnancy, the practitioner should be vigilant for pregnancy complications, including GDM, preeclampsia, and other hypertensive disorders of pregnancy that may arise earlier or in atypical fashions. A Glucola screen for GDM should be repeated if an early screen was negative or not performed. Although spontaneous preterm birth risk is lower in obese women, indicated preterm birth is higher due to pregnancy complications. Prenatal visits should be used to check with the patient on weight gain goals and dietary adherence and to begin the discussions surrounding delivery planning.

As the obese gravida enters the third trimester, the checklist and care pathway become increasingly focused on delivery preparation and planning, as well as postdelivery complications and management. Routine prenatal care should still include not only active vigilance for pregnancy complications but also, for those women for whom fetal growth cannot be assessed, a necessary serial ultrasound assessment. There is an increased risk of fetal demise in obese women, which is higher in African American women than other races.[54–56] Despite this, no well-designed trials have addressed interventions that may be effective for prevention of stillbirth. Data are insufficient to recommend routine nonstress testing in obese women in the absence of underlying pregnancy disorders, but certainly those women with underlying disorders for whom nonstress testing is indicated (those with hypertension, diabetes, etc.) should undergo routine testing. Daily kick counts are a low-risk intervention that should be considered.

Another focus in the second and especially the third trimesters should be on staff and patient preparation for the delivery and planning for contingencies related to labor and delivery complications. A thorough discussion of labor induction and the increased risks of cesarean delivery is warranted. Initiate planning at the delivery facility to ensure adequate nursing and support staff and available hospital resources, including delivery and operating room tools and supplies. If available, anesthesia consultation should be pursued to review the risks of anesthesia and difficulty of obtaining adequate regional anesthesia in obese women.

INTRAPARTUM AND POSTPARTUM CARE

Intrapartum Period

Delivery planning meetings and staff planning checklists may be especially helpful for administering to obese patients. For morbidly obese women, there will likely need to be additional planning and preparation related to delivery, including room logistics, fetal monitoring, staffing, bed and operating table weight capacity, and availability of appropriate equipment for delivery. Some hospitals may not have the personal resources and bariatric equipment to ensure a safe delivery of the morbidly obese patient. In these cases, arrangements should be made for transfer of care to and delivery at a regional perinatal center. As previously stated, this planning should begin in the third trimester, and assurance for a care plan for patients with supermorbid obesity should be available for staff in the event of an unexpected admission. Fetal monitoring can be especially complicated, and plans for monitoring should be reviewed. Care should be taken to have appropriate lengthened monitoring straps , and if this is not possible then avoid placing knots in straps under a patient which may cause skin breakdown issues. Wedges or pillows can also help to optimize patient position, and accessible ultrasound to determine location of fetal heart or uterine fundus may also help to determine optimal locations for osculation.[57] Labor and delivery staff should be appropriately trained in the variety of techniques that may be necessary to maintain good-quality tracings for nonstress testing or labor monitoring (Figure 19-4).

On admission, a physical examination should be performed, and a decision on the best approach to cesarean delivery should have been predetermined in the event of an emergent situation. Surgical approaches to the obese parturient and complications have been reported elsewhere.[23,58] While the details of surgical procedures are beyond the scope of this section (discussed in detail in Chapter 21), the risks and benefits of incision type should be reviewed with the patient beforehand. In addition to

☐ Ultrasound for fetal position at 36 weeks
☐ Early anesthesia consultation
☐ Obtain clear fetal heart tracing and uterine contraction assessment
☐ Informed consent

Confirmation of the following:
    ☐ Adequate anesthesia equipment
    ☐ Adequate labor and delivery room equipment
    ☐ Adequate operating room equipment
    ☐ Placement of sequential compression devices

Discussion/planning for
    ☐ Delivery route
    ☐ Skin cleansing/preparation
    ☐ Antibiotic dosing if cesarean:
    ☐ Consider cefazolin 3 g if weight >120 kg
    ☐ Postpartum thromboembolism prophylaxis (sequential compression devices, low molecular weight heparin)

FIGURE 19-4. Example of an intrapartum checklist.

consideration of supplies for the patient and infant, the needs for family and support people should also be considered, as obesity is often a common problem throughout the entire family.

Postpartum Period

The postpartum period represents a very high-risk time for most women with morbid obesity. The patient will transition out of weekly physician care; therefore, education and guidance regarding how to care for herself and her infant. Minimizing risk prior to and after discharge, are the goals of this care map. Postpartum care can be separated into two critical periods for education and intervention: immediately postpartum and postpartum follow up visit.

The immediate postpartum care map (Figure 19-5) should address potential complications, such as postpartum hemorrhage, endometritis, and increased risk of venous thromboembolism. Obese women should also be educated on perineal and incision care if a cesarean section was performed. Planning should include wound and skin care at home and teaching partners or others at home how to accomplish for those women unable to reach or see their incision. Women should be educated on the signs and symptoms of cellulitis and infection and instructed to call immediately if they develop. Patient follow-up should be scheduled within 2 weeks after discharge for an inspection of the incision.

Immediately postpartum is also the best time to optimize breastfeeding education and support. Postpartum nurses are often skilled with breastfeeding education and techniques; however, data show that many health professionals struggle with obesity-related breastfeeding concerns.[59] Due to delayed lactation and the known difficulty of breastfeeding in this high-risk population, a referral to a lactation specialist

Discussion of the following:
☐ Complications of pregnancy (postpartum hemorrhage, endometritis, etc.)
☐ Venous thromboembolism prophylaxis
☐ Early ambulation
    ☐ Sequential compression devices
    ☐ Anticoagulation (if indicated) (unfractionated heparin, low molecular weight heparin, resuming warfarin)
☐ Perineal laceration or incision care
☐ Address any medical comorbidities (if indicated)
    ☐ Blood pressure goals and monitoring
    ☐ Blood sugar monitoring
    ☐ Mood disorders
☐ Medication adjustments
☐ Contraceptive counseling
    ☐ Oral contraceptives
    ☐ Long-acting reversible contraceptives (levonorgestrel/copper intrauterine device, etonogestrel implant)
    ☐ Surgical (postpartum tubal ligation, interval laparoscopic tubal ligation, and hysteroscopic tubal occlusion)
☐ Breastfeeding discussion
    ☐ Lactation referral

FIGURE 19-5. Example of an immediate postpartum checklist.

or breastfeeding medicine physicians.[60] Obesity is a known risk factor for lower rates of lactation, and should be addressed.[61]

A contraception plan should be implemented prior to discharge from the hospital. Often, medication (e.g., insulin) adjustments are necessary shortly after delivery. Arrangements should be made with the patient's primary care provider or subspecialist to assist in the management of underlying medical comorbidities.

Ideally, an attempt should be made to communicate frequently with the highest-risk obese patients. However, due to new-parent demands as well as the financial and staff limitations of the primary obstetric provider, this is often not realistic. Therefore, patient education is imperative prior to patient discharge. Written materials may also be helpful to serve as reminders after discharge. In addition to routine postpartum counseling and education, the postpartum visit should include a discussion of any pregnancy, delivery, and postpartum complications, as well as how these will affect future pregnancies and medical risks. Women with preeclampsia have an increased risk of cardiovascular disease and diabetes.[62] Any women with a diagnosis of GDM during pregnancy should undergo a 2-hour glucose tolerance test. This visit should also emphasize contraception and provide a discussion of pregnancy interval spacing (Figure 19-6).

The postpartum visit is also an ideal time to address lifestyle changes in obese women. Counseling regarding weight retention and the importance of physical activity and dietary modifications for a lifetime of maternal-child health is important. A referral to a dietician or nutritionist as well as weight loss/obesity physician care may help patients with their long-term health goals.

Discussion of the following:
□ Complications of pregnancy (postpartum hemorrhage, endometritis, etc.) and recurrence risks
□ Contraception
    □ Oral contraceptives
    □ Long-acting reversible contraceptives (levonorgestrel/copper intrauterine device, etonogestrel implant)
    □ Surgical (postpartum tubal ligation, interval laparoscopic tubal ligation, and hysteroscopic tubal occlusion)
□ Breastfeeding
□ Mood assessment
□ Interpregnancy interval
□ Discontinuation of thromboembolism prophylaxis (if indicated)
□ Two-hour glucose tolerance test (if gestational diabetes mellitus during pregnancy)
□ Address medical comorbidities and appropriate referrals
□ Discuss lifestyle intervention and long-term health goals

FIGURE 19-6. Example of a postpartum visit checklist.

REFERENCES

1. Rotter T, Kinsman L, James E, et al. Clinical pathways: effects on professional practice, patient outcomes, length of stay and hospital costs. *Cochrane Database Syst Rev.* 2010;(3):CD006632.

2. Haugen AS, Softeland E, Eide GE, et al. Impact of the World Health Organization's Surgical Safety Checklist on safety culture in the operating theatre: a controlled intervention study. *Br J Anaesth.* 2013;110(5):807–815.

3. Piotrowski MM, Hinshaw DB. The safety checklist program: creating a culture of safety in intensive care units. *Jt Comm J Qual Improv.* 2002;28(6):306–315.

4. Panella M, Marchisio S, Di Stanislao F. Reducing clinical variations with clinical pathways: do pathways work? *Int J Qual Health Care.* 2003;15(6):509–521.

5. Haynes AB, Weiser TG, Berry WR, et al. A surgical safety checklist to reduce morbidity and mortality in a global population. *N Engl J Med.* 2009;360(5):491–499.

6. Arriaga AF, Bader AM, Wong JM, et al. Simulation-based trial of surgical-crisis checklists. *N Engl J Med.* 2013;368(3):246–253.

7. Ransom SB, McNeeley SG, Yono A, et al. The development and implementation of normal vaginal delivery clinical pathways in a large multihospital health system. *Am J Manag Care.* 1998;4(5):723–727.

8. Ransom S. Reduced medicolegal risk by compliance with obstetric clinical pathways: a case-control study. *Obstet Gynecol.* 2003;101(4):751–755.

9. Program BPH. *BCPHP Obstetric Guideline 19: Maternity Care Pathway.* Vancouver, BC, Canada; 2010:1–24.

10. El-Messidi A, Mallozzi A, Oppenheimer L. A multidisciplinary checklist for management of suspected placenta accreta. *J Obstet Gynaecol Can.* 2012;34(4):320–324.

11. Wittenberg MD, Vaughan DJ, Lucas DN. A novel airway checklist for obstetric general anaesthesia. *Int J Obstet Anesth.* 2013;22(3):264–265.

12. Duff P. A simple checklist for preventing major complications associated with cesarean delivery. *Obstet Gynecol.* 2010;116(6):1393–1396.

13. Clark SL, Meyers JA, Frye DK, Perlin JA. Patient safety in obstetrics—the Hospital Corporation of America experience. *Am J Obstet Gynecol.* 2011;204(4):283–287.

14. Mohammed A, Wu J, Biggs T, et al. Does use of a World Health Organization obstetric safe surgery checklist improve communication between obstetricians and anaesthetists? A retrospective study of 389 caesarean sections. *BJOG.* 2013;120(5):644–648.

15. Hullfish KL, Miller T, Pastore LM, et al. A checklist for timeout on labor and delivery: a pilot study to improve communication and safety. *J Reprod Med.* 2014;59(11–12):579–584.

16. Fausett MB, Propst A, Van Doren K, Clark BT. How to develop an effective obstetric checklist. *Am J Obstet Gynecol.* 2011;205(3):165–170.

17. Committee on Patient Safety and Quality Improvement. Committee opinion no. 629: clinical guidelines and standardization of practice to improve outcomes. *Obstet Gynecol.* 2015;125(4):1027–1029.

18. Weiss JL, Malone FD, Emig D, et al. Obesity, obstetric complications and cesarean delivery rate—a population-based screening study. *Am J Obstet Gynecol.* 2004;190(4):1091–1097.

19. American College of Obstetricians and Gynecologists. ACOG Committee opinion no. 549: obesity in pregnancy. *Obstet Gynecol.* 2013;121(1):213–217.

20. Davies GA, Maxwell C, McLeod L, et al. SOGC clinical practice guidelines: obesity in pregnancy. No. 239, February 2010. *Int J Gynaecol Obstet.* 2010;110(2):167–173.

21. Kominiarek MA, Rankin K, Handler A. Provider adherence to recommended prenatal care content: does it differ for obese women? *Matern Child Health J.* 2014;18(5):1114–1122.

22. Catalano PM. Management of obesity in pregnancy. *Obstet Gynecol.* 2007;109(2 Pt 1):419–433.

23. Gunatilake RP, Perlow JH. Obesity and pregnancy: clinical management of the obese gravida. *Am J Obstet Gynecol.* 2011;204(2):106–119.

24. Ghaffari N, Srinivas SK, Durnwald CP. The multidisciplinary approach to the care of the obese parturient. *Am J Obstet Gynecol.* 2015;213(3):318–325.

25. Modder J, Ftzsimons KJ, for the Centre for Maternal and Child Enquiries and the Royal College of Obstetricians and Gynaecologists. *Management of Women With Obesity in Pregnancy: CMACE/RCOG Joint Guideline.* London: Modder J, Ftzsimons KJ, for the Centre for Maternal and Child Enquiries and the Royal College of Obstetricians and Gynaecologists; 2010:1–29.

26. Fealy S, Hure A, Browne G, Prince C. Developing a clinical care pathway for obese pregnant women: a quality improvement project. *Women Birth.* 2014;27(4):e67–e71.

27. Schummers L, Hutcheon JA, Bodnar LM, Lieberman E, Himes KP. Risk of adverse pregnancy outcomes by prepregnancy body mass index: a population-based study to inform prepregnancy weight loss counseling. *Obstet Gynecol.* 2015;125(1):133–143.

28. Russo LM, Nobles C, Ertel KA, Chasan-Taber L, Whitcomb BW. Physical activity interventions in pregnancy and risk of gestational diabetes mellitus: a systematic review and meta-analysis. *Obstet Gynecol.* 2015;125(3):576–582.

29. Nohr EA, Vaeth M, Baker JL, Sorensen T, Olsen J, Rasmussen KM. Combined associations of prepregnancy body mass index and gestational weight gain with the outcome of pregnancy. *Am J Clin Nutr.* 2008;87(6):1750–1759.

30. Durie DE, Thornburg LL, Glantz JC. Effect of second-trimester and third-trimester rate of gestational weight gain on maternal and neonatal outcomes. *Obstet Gynecol.* 2011;118(3):569–575.

31. Johansson K, Cnattingius S, Naslund I, et al. Outcomes of pregnancy after bariatric surgery. *N Engl J Med.* 2015;372(9):814–824.

32. O'Donnell K. Severe micronutrient deficiencies in RYGB patients: rare but potentially devastating. *Pract Gastroenterol.* 2012;35(11):13–27.

33. Racusin DA, Crawford NS, Andrabi S, et al. Twizzlers as a cost-effective and equivalent alternative to the glucola beverage in diabetes screening. *Diabetes Care.* 2013;36(10):e169–e170.

34. Racusin DA, Antony K, Showalter L, Sharma S, Haymond M, Aagaard KM. Candy twists as an alternative to the glucola beverage in gestational diabetes mellitus screening. *Am J Obstet Gynecol.* 2015;212(4):522 e521–e525.

35. Lindsay KL, Heneghan C, McNulty B, Brennan L, McAuliffe FM. Lifestyle and dietary habits of an obese pregnant cohort. *Matern Child Health J.* 2015;19(1):25–32.

36. Keating E, Correia-Branco A, Araujo JR, et al. Excess perigestational folic acid exposure induces metabolic dysfunction in post-natal life. *J Endocrinol.* 2015;224(3):245–259.

37. US Preventive Services Task Force. Folic acid for the prevention of neural tube defects: US Preventive Services Task Force recommendation statement. *Ann Intern Med.* 2009;150(9):626–631.

38. Wilson RD, Johnson JA, Wyatt P, et al. Pre-conceptional vitamin/folic acid supplementation 2007: the use of folic acid in combination with a multivitamin supplement for the prevention of neural tube defects and other congenital anomalies. *J Obstet Gynaecol Can.* 2007;29(12):1003–1026.

39. Gahche JJ, Bailey RL, Mirel LB, Dwyer JT. The prevalence of using iodine-containing supplements is low among reproductive-age women, NHANES 1999–2006. *J Nutr.* 2013;143(6):872–877.

40. Bath SC, Steer CD, Golding J, Emmett P, Rayman MP. Effect of inadequate iodine status in UK pregnant women on cognitive outcomes in their children: results from the Avon Longitudinal Study of Parents and Children (ALSPAC). *Lancet.* 2013;302(9889):331–337.

41. Leung AM, Pearce EN, Braverman LE, Stagnaro-Green A. AAP recommendations on iodine nutrition during pregnancy and lactation. *Pediatrics.* 2014;134(4):e1282.

42. Rogan WJ, Paulson JA, Baum C, et al. Iodine deficiency, pollutant chemicals, and the thyroid: new information on an old problem. *Pediatrics.* 2014;133(6):1163–1166.

43. Swank ML, Marshall NE, Caughey AB, et al. Pregnancy outcomes in the super obese, stratified by weight gain above and below institute of medicine guidelines. *Obstet Gynecol.* 2014;124(6):1105–1110.

44. Maasilta P, Bachour A, Teramo K, Polo O, Laitinen LA. Sleep-related disordered breathing during pregnancy in obese women. *Chest.* 2001;120(5):1448–1454.

45. Pien GW, Pack AI, Jackson N, Maislin G, Macones GA, Schwab RJ. Risk factors for sleep-disordered breathing in pregnancy. *Thorax.* 2014;69(4):371–377.

46. Bourjeily G, Ankner G, Mohsenin V. Sleep-disordered breathing in pregnancy. *Clin Chest Med.* 2011;32(1):175–189.

47. Bourjeily G, Raker CA, Chalhoub M, Miller MA. Pregnancy and fetal outcomes of symptoms of sleep-disordered breathing. *Eur Respir J.* 2010;36(4):849–855.

48. Pamidi S, Pinto LM, Marc I, Benedetti A, Schwartzman K, Kimoff RJ. Maternal sleep-disordered breathing and adverse pregnancy outcomes: a systematic review and metaanalysis. *Am J Obstet Gynecol.* 2014;210(1):52 e51–52. e14.

49. Facco FL, Parker CB, Reddy UM, et al. NuMoM2b Sleep-Disordered Breathing study: objectives and methods. *Am J Obstet Gynecol.* 2015;212(4):542 e541–542. e127.

50. Dashe JS, McIntire DD, Twickler DM. Effect of maternal obesity on the ultrasound detection of anomalous fetuses. *Obstet Gynecol.* 2009;113(5):1001–1007.

51. Chung JH, Pelayo R, Hatfield TJ, Speir VJ, Wu J, Caughey AB. Limitations of the fetal anatomic survey via ultrasound in the obese obstetrical population. *J Matern Fetal Neonatal Med.* 2012;25(10):1945–1949.

52. Fuchs F, Houllier M, Voulgaropoulos A, et al. Factors affecting feasibility and quality of second-trimester ultrasound scans in obese pregnant women. *Ultrasound Obstet Gynecol.* 2013;41(1):40–46.

53. Rossi AC, Prefumo F. Accuracy of ultrasonography at 11–14 weeks of gestation for detection of fetal structural anomalies: a systematic review. *Obstet Gynecol.* 2013;122(6):1160–1167.

54. Nohr EA, Bech BH, Davies MJ, Frydenberg M, Henriksen TB, Olsen J. Prepregnancy obesity and fetal death: a study within the Danish National Birth Cohort. *Obstet Gynecol.* 2005;106(2):250–259.

55. Salihu HM, Dunlop AL, Hedayatzadeh M, Alio AP, Kirby RS, Alexander GR. Extreme obesity and risk of stillbirth among black and white gravidas. *Obstet Gynecol.* 2007;110(3):552–557.

56. Chu SY, Kim SY, Lau J, et al. Maternal obesity and risk of stillbirth: a metaanalysis. *Am J Obstet Gynecol.* 2007;197(3):223–228.

57. Thornburg LL, Glantz JC, Giffi C, Woods J, eds. *Fetal Heart Rate Monitoring: Pathophysiology and Practice.* Rochester, NY: Peri-Facts Academy; 2013.

58. Marrs CC, Moussa HN, Sibai BM, Blackwell SC. The relationship between primary cesarean delivery skin incision type and wound complications in women with morbid obesity. *Am J Obstet Gynecol.* 2014;210(4):319 e311–e314.

59. Garner CD, Ratcliff SL, Devine CM, Thornburg LL, Rasmussen KM. Health professionals' experiences providing breastfeeding-related care for obese women. *Breastfeed Med.* 2014;9(10):503–509.

60. Matias SL, Dewey KG, Quesenberry CP Jr, Gunderson EP. Maternal prepregnancy obesity and insulin treatment during pregnancy are independently associated with delayed lactogenesis in women with recent gestational diabetes mellitus. *Am J Clin Nutr.* 2014;99(1):115–121.

61. Amir LH, Donath S. A systematic review of maternal obesity and breastfeeding intention, initiation and duration. *BMC Pregnancy Childbirth.* 2007;7:9.

62. Bellamy L, Casas JP, Hingorani AD, Williams DJ. Pre-eclampsia and risk of cardiovascular disease and cancer in later life: systematic review and meta-analysis. *BMJ.* 2007;335(7627):974.

Problems in Labor and Adverse Birth Outcomes

CHAPTER 20

Federico G. Mariona, MD, FACOG, FACS

Niamh Condon, DO

BACKGROUND

Obesity is a complex and multifactorial metabolic heterogeneous disorder that chronically affects the individual. The World Health Organization (WHO) characterizes obesity as a pandemic health issue with a higher prevalence in females than males. In the United States, more than 33% of women are obese.[1] Obesity is the second leading cause of preventable deaths. While the complete pathogenesis of obesity is only partly understood, its effects on health are far reaching, with the aggregate cost of obesity in the United States ranging from 5% to 7% of annual medical expenditures.[2] Obesity is defined as 35% or greater total body fat in women.[3]

In 1832, Quetelet proposed an index to characterize human health status (Table 20-1).[4] Keys reaffirmed the validity of this index in 1972 by introducing the concept of the body mass index (BMI) and recommending it as a proxy for measuring body fat.[5] WHO and the National Institutes of Health (NIH) in the United States classify obesity utilizing BMI. This marker is defined as the individual's body weight divided by the square of his or her height, or $BMI = W/H^2$, and is reported as kilograms per square meter (kg/m^2) (Table 20-1). BMI values are age independent and are used for both sexes. Maternal ethnicity is under scrutiny to determine its association with BMI.

TABLE 20-1 Definitions of Obesity[a]

Definitions

The Quételet index (*homme moyen*), 1832; then Keys's 1972 body mass index
World Health Organization/National Institutes of Health: Body mass index
Body Mass Index (BMI) = W/H^2 or kg/m^2

	BMI
Recommended weight	18.5–24.9
Overweight	25.0–29.9
Obesity	≥30
Class I	30–34.9
Class II	35–39.9
Class III (morbid obesity)	≥40
With comorbidities	≥35
Super- (extreme) obesity (2.9%)	**≥35**

[a]Eknoyan G. The average man and indices of obesity. Adolphe Quetelet (1796–1874). *Nephrol Dial Transplant.* 2008;1:47–51.

IMPACT OF OBESITY ON PREGNANCY

Obesity represents increasingly serious maternal and perinatal health concerns when associated with a woman's pregnancy. In 1988, Thomson and Hanley stated that short maternal stature and increased BMI predisposed patients to difficult labor. WHO estimated that 60% of women between the ages of 20 and 40 years are overweight or obese, as classified by their BMI. In the United States, more than 50% of pregnant women are overweight or obese, and 8% of reproductive-age women are extremely obese, with a BMI greater than 50 kg/m^2, a group that is rapidly increasing,[1] as reaffirmed by the National Health and Nutrition Examination Survey (NHANES).

Women suffering from obesity are at an increased risk for delayed conception.[6] In the preconception period, obstetricians have an opportunity to counsel obese women. Timing of these efforts is critical to pre-date the pregnancy and decrease, or eliminate, the fetal exposure to in utero triggers that will affect the fetuses' life in the long term.

It has been demonstrated by a number of studies that 25%–35% of children from obese mothers are obese by 11 years of age. They have an increased risk of developing metabolic syndrome (MS), defined as the presence of obesity, hypertension, dyslipidemia, and glucose intolerance.[7] Once pregnant, they have an increased risk for multiple morbidities. The Barker hypothesis[8] clearly expresses the need to understand the origins of common complex adult-onset medical disorders, obesity among them. Parental obesity changes the molecular composition of the sperm and the oocyte, and it modifies the epigenetic reprogramming that occurs at the time of conception, both of which negatively affect embryonic and fetal development.[9] In our study of 228 pregnant women with a BMI higher than 50 kg/m^2 (extreme obesity), we found a prevalence of 31.8% for carbohydrate intolerance (pregestational or gestational diabetes) and 46.3% for hypertensive diseases (chronic, gestational, or preeclampsia).

Early prenatal care is not frequent in this population because irregular menses or a false sense of inability to conceive makes early pregnancy detection an infrequent clinical event. The use of pelvic ultrasound is impaired by the maternal body habitus. The use of invasive transvaginal evaluation becomes necessary, as early pregnancy prior to 18 weeks may be compromised. Complete fetal surveys are frequently difficult, and repeated exams do not improve the exploration. Often, some fetal segments are suboptimally visualized during the entire pregnancy. The practice of bariatric obstetrics presents a number of challenges to the clinicians. As obese women approach the third trimester, they are at an increased risk for intrauterine fetal death and altered fetal growth.

The use of serial fetal ultrasound evaluations late in pregnancy in the obese is hindered by excessive acoustic shadowing, rendering the exams inaccurate and of little clinical use. Occasionally, the vaginal transducer is occasionally placed in the maternal navel, the area where the abdominal wall is thinner and allows for increasing ease in the examination. Changes in the maternal position on the examining table or combined transvaginal-transabdominal access may be necessary to complete the fetal evaluation.

During labor, obese women often experience abnormal labor patterns, complications with anesthesia management, or complicated and emergent cesarean deliveries. Their neonates are at risk for needing neonatal resuscitation and admission to the neonatal intensive care unit. The maternal complications extend to the postpartum period, with postpartum hemorrhage (PPH), surgical site infections (SSIs), and abnormal clotting events. These issues prolong the maternal recovery period and negatively affect her ability to care for her newborn infant. Further, obesity and its ongoing metabolic consequences, represented by a chronic inflammatory condition, may affect the proper function of the placenta, with possible dire consequences on fetal growth, development, and maturity. These effects, if not corrected early in the gestational period by appropriate interventions, will influence placental function and gene expression, and therefore negatively affect maternal and perinatal outcomes.[10]

TERM LABOR

It is beyond the scope of this chapter to provide a comprehensive review and bibliography associated with human parturition, human labor, and our understanding of its clinical evolution through the last decades. The definitions of normal and abnormal labor present a challenge to investigators and clinicians. Since the work of Samuel Reynolds,[11] arguably considered the "father of the uterus," and others,[12] investigators have attempted to provide a plausible physiologic explanation for the onset of spontaneous term labor in the human,[13] yet this has proven to be difficult to determine.

Labor is defined as the physiologic process that occurs from the onset of regular uterine contractions until the expulsion of the placenta. This tight definition implies that uterine contractions cause demonstrable and progressive cervical changes.[14] At the myometrial site, the interaction between calcium and the calmodulin-myosin light-chain kinase sequence is critical for normal uterine contractions to occur. Clinicians use frequency of uterine contractions, maternal discomfort generated during these contractions, cervical effacement, and cervical dilation to mark the beginning of active labor.

Progress of labor was made objective in 1954 by Friedman[15] when he described a characteristic pattern of cervical dilation, time, and the descent of the fetal presenting part. In 1972, Friedman defined protraction disorders of labor as either when the cervix stops dilating or when the fetus stops descending, per unit time (1 hour).[16] This approach not only allowed obstetricians to make a diagnosis of abnormal labor but also allowed them to understand that several factors influence labor progression or lack thereof, and that at certain times active interventions may be required.

In the last decade, efforts have been made to reevaluate the original labor curve in view of evolving demographics and changes in obstetrical care. In 2004, half a century after Friedman's original publication, Cesario conducted a multi-institutional international survey of maternity units providing labor care. This study included nulliparous and multiparous women aged 14 to 44 with a single, live, vertex fetus, in spontaneous labor without the use of synthetic oxytocin or labor analgesia. Over 400 patients were involved; 23% were nulliparous. The average length of labor was similar to that described by Friedman; however, a wider range of "normal" was found in the new study.[17] This finding emphasizes the clinical importance of differentiating normal from abnormal labor beyond subjectivity. In 2002, Zhang et al. again challenged Friedman's concepts, and while they uncovered differences from the original Friedman labor curve,[18] maternal BMI was not included as a variable.

The beginning of normal labor is difficult to establish accurately, and the progress of normal labor is subject to considerable biologic variation. This clinical debate continues in association with the new consensus for the safe reduction of primary cesarean deliveries, released by the American College of Obstetricians and Gynecologists (ACOG) and the Society for Maternal Fetal Medicine.[19] This consensus is based on the findings of newer research that focuses on patterns of spontaneous labor. Study methodologies and labor analysis techniques that have evolved over the past half-century were questioned,[20] and it was determined that, in the absence of obvious maternal-fetal complications, the treatment of labor abnormalities and dystocia secondary to "failure to progress" must extend beyond immediate performance of a cesarean delivery.[21]

Dystocia, defined as an abnormal uterine contractility pattern, a fetal structural or positional anomaly, a maternal pelvic anatomic anomaly, or some combination thereof, is the leading indication for cesarean operative delivery, accounting for approximately 50% of the cesareans performed in the United States. Clinical criteria needed to establish the diagnosis of dystocia are multiple. In 2009, cesarean delivery prevalence in the United States was 32.9%, with an average mean prevalence of 22.0% in women with no previous cesarean section.[22,23] In our study group of 228 extremely obese parturients, BMI of 50 kg/m^2 or greater, the cesarean delivery prevalence was 63% for nulliparous patients and 19.2% for multiparous patients, with a vaginal delivery occurring in only 22.4% of cases. This information demonstrates the difficulty of accurately reporting the prevalence of term, spontaneous labor and delivery in obese women and comparing this to the prevalence of labor in nonobese women with singleton, cephalic fetuses without other labor abnormalities.

OBESITY AND MATERNAL COMPLICATIONS DURING LABOR AND DELIVERY

For over a decade, it has been postulated that the course of labor in overweight and obese women differs from that in normal weight women, and that elevated maternal BMI is associated with dysfunctional labor. Maternal obesity may be an independent or a synergistic factor for uterine contraction dysfunction.[24,25] One area of research focuses on cholesterol and its effect on labor because increased BMI and hypercholesterolemia often coexist. Cholesterol, an essential component of the cell membrane in humans, has been reported to be an important factor in the control of smooth muscle contractility. In animal studies, increased cholesterol is associated with a decrease in myometrial activity; cholesterol may be related to uterine quiescence.[26]

Efforts are ongoing to elucidate the basic physiologic causes of this myometrial dysfunction and its association with maternal obesity in humans. For example, investigators are exploring the role of caveolae.[25] Caveolae are the invaginations of the cell membrane of myometrial cells, and they are stabilized by the cholesterol-binding protein caveolin. This area of the myometrial cell membrane may be involved in the excitation-contraction phase of myometrial cells and may be influenced by hormone levels, specifically of estrogens. The increase in cholesterol and triglycerides in normal human pregnancies maintains the nutrient supply needed by the growing fetus and may be necessary to maintain uterine quiescence in the early weeks of pregnancy, yet high levels of cholesterol, often present in obese patients, may hinder normal uterine contractility during labor.[26] Changes in lipid metabolism during pregnancy may lead to abnormal labor in obese women. Evidence has also been offered linking stress and maternal obesity to labor dysfunction, wherein increased levels of leptin, a hormone secreted by adipose tissue and uterine tissue and believed to increase in times of stress, synergistically impair the contractile mechanisms of the myometrium and lead to abnormal labor and increased cesarean rate.[27]

Adipose tissue in the visceral compartments has been considered an active endocrine organ that produces and releases biologically active elements, such as adipocytokines or adipokines. One of these elements is apelin, an adipocytokine expressed in several tissues, including the placenta, but primarily in adipose tissue. Apelin levels are increased in the obese population. In vitro studies have demonstrated a relaxing effect of apelin on smooth muscle, such as the myometrium, the mechanism of which has not been completely elucidated. The adipokine ghrelin has also been reported to have a potential role in metabolic modulation of uterine contractility in the obese parturient. In addition, the chronic low-grade inflammatory state characterized by obesity increases oxidative stress, and this effect is responsible for an irregular production of adipokines, which have adverse systemic effects.[27,28]

One of these systemic effects may be a higher concentration of maternal serum lactic acid, secondary to increased acidosis.[29,30] In vitro studies have demonstrated that this metabolic change may affect the myometrium in the human, specifically by reducing contraction amplitude and decreasing response to oxytocin.

Evidence is also accumulating that demonstrates the independent influence of maternal obesity on the progress of labor. The myometrium of obese women in labor contracts with less power and less frequency and has less calcium transmembrane flux than that of the nonobese pregnant women.[31]

TABLE 20-2 Labor Definitions

Latent Phase: From *onset of labor* until acceleration in dilation at the *onset of active phase*
- Prolonged latent phase: >20 h in nulliparas, >14 h in multiparas

Active Phase: From the *end of latent phase* to full cervical dilation
- Protracted active phase: Linear dilation <1.2 cm/h in nulliparas, <1.5 cm/h in multiparas
- Arrest of dilation: No progress ≥2 h

Deceleration Phase: Between 8 cm and full cervical dilation
- Prolonged deceleration phase: 3 h in nulliparas, 1 h in multiparas

Failure to Descend: No descent of vertex from "early labor" to deceleration phase or second stage
- Protracted descent in second stage: <1 cm/h in nulliparas, 2 cm/h in multiparas

In the obese patient, the first stage of labor is often characterized by slow progress, unrelated to fetal size,[32] resulting in dysfunctional patterns of dilation, the mechanism of which may be mediated by any of the factors discussed previously. A recent study revealed a 3-fold increase in the rate of arrest of dilation during the first stage of spontaneous labor in obese women when compared to nonobese women with otherwise-uncomplicated term pregnancies. Specifically, arrest of dilation was diagnosed in 5.5% of the lean women and in 18.8% of the obese women ($p = .002$). Intensity of contractions was not reported. The difference in neonatal weights in the two groups was not statistically significant and did not explain the dystocia diagnosed in the obese group. The diagnosis of arrest of labor was made by utilizing Friedman's definitions and laborgram[22] (Table 20-2). These definitions have been utilized in the training of obstetricians and clinically applied for the last 50 years. A revision of this classical approach, with the objective of safely preventing a primary cesarean to meet the goal of Healthy People 2020, has been published, yet the labor patterns specific to the obese parturient were not addressed by Friedman's database, Zhang's studies, or the consensus documents.

A recent large study conducted by the Swedish registry reviewed over 50,000 nulliparous women with singleton pregnancies and spontaneous labor onset and documented BMI.[33] Time in labor was reported. Oxytocin for augmentation was utilized in 45% of normal-weight women and in 55.1% of class III obese women ($p < .001$). The emergency cesarean rate, defined as a cesarean performed while in active labor, was 5.1% in normal-weight women and 15.6% in obese parturients ($p < .001$). There was a significant association between BMI and length of labor, with BMI less than 18.5 and BMI greater than 40, $p < .001$. In the obese population, prolonged labor was confined to the first stage of labor. While the predominant etiology of this dysfunction is unclear, an additional factor considered was increased maternal intrapelvic soft tissue.[34]

Understanding the physiology of labor in the obese parturient is critical to improve the clinical management of labor in this population. Further supportive evidence was provided by Vahratian et al. in the observational study of 612 term nulliparous obese patients: Obese women were more likely to have an inadequate contraction pattern during the first stage of labor, requiring oxytocin for induction or augmentation. The authors showed a trend to slower progress from 4 to 6 cm of cervical dilation and a

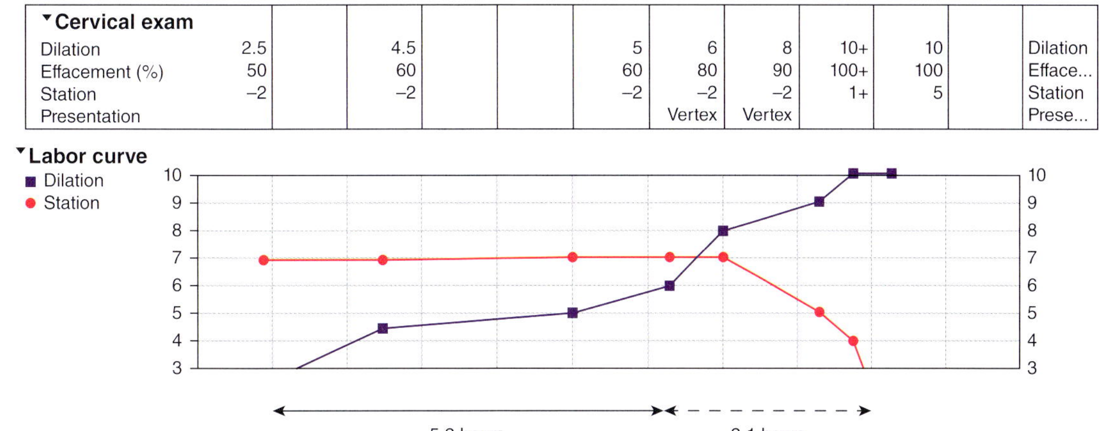

FIGURE 20-1. Gravida 6, para 3. Bishop score 6. BMI 35 kg/m^2. 39 weeks 6/7. Single fetus, vertex presentation. Induced labor. Spontaneous vaginal delivery.

longer median duration from 4 to 10 cm of cervical dilation (7.0 vs. 5.4 hours, $p < .001$). It was again demonstrated that labor progression in obese women, when compared to normal-weight women, is significantly slower prior to 7 cm of cervical dilation (Figure 20-1). This is a consistent clinical finding in various obese patient populations, and it must be noted before interventions are performed (Figure 20-2).[35]

Fyfe et al. performed a prospective study of 1800 nulliparous term patients whose BMI was recorded in early pregnancy, and they reported an association between elevated BMI and first-stage dysfunction. This study demonstrated that, among overweight and obese women, the risk for cesarean delivery occurred during the first stage of labor, when abnormal uterine contraction patterns are common. Obese women

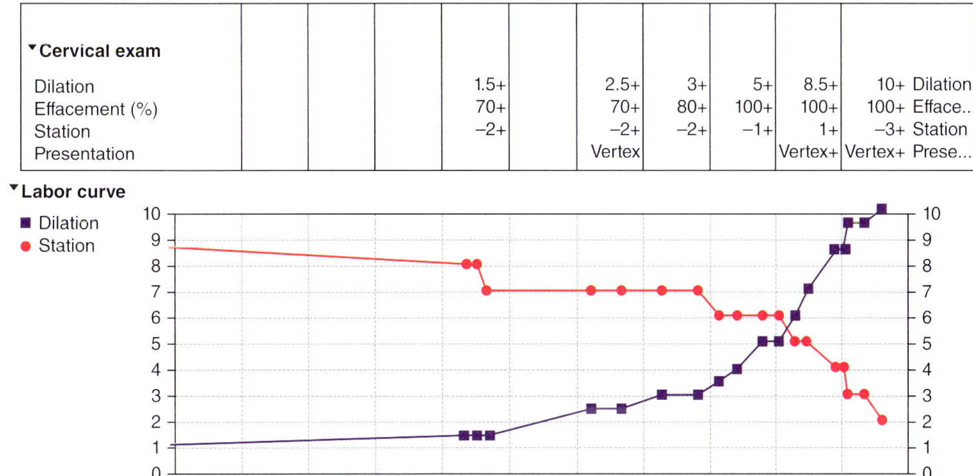

FIGURE 20-2. Nulliparous. 39 weeks 4/7. Spontaneous labor. BMI 42 kg/m^2. Meconium-stained amniotic fluid. Primary cesarean. Apgar 2(1′), 8(5′).

who reached the second stage of labor had a higher rate of spontaneous vaginal deliveries than did those women in the control population who had normal BMIs.[36] Bergholt reported that over 80% of cesarean deliveries in patients with elevated BMIs are performed during the first stage of labor.[37] To avoid or decrease early interventions, this information is critical for the obstetrician to keep in mind when confronted with an obese term patient in labor who has slow, protracted cervical dilation in the absence of fetal or maternal deleterious clinical conditions.

Monitoring obese pregnant women in labor presents a significant challenge for maternity units. Both spontaneous and induced labor can, at times, demand one-on-one obstetrical care at the bedside. After arrival in the obstetric triage area, gestational age, most recent estimated fetal weight, presenting part, any prenatally detected fetal structural anomalies, fetal heart rate, Bishop score, uterine contraction frequency and duration, group B β-strep status, full review of prenatal records, current medications, time and content of maternal last full meal, delivery plan, and labor pain treatment plans must all be reviewed with the patient and documented in detail. Appropriate laboratory tests include blood type and screen.

In diabetic patients, point-of-care blood glucose should be obtained on arrival according to the local protocol and usually every hour during active labor. In insulin-dependent patients, last dose of insulin and amount and type of insulin must be reviewed and documented. Preferably, 2 large-bore venous accesses should be placed.

Frequently, it is practically impossible to ascertain the time of onset of labor, and to obtain appropriate detection of uterine contractions and fetal heart rate by external cardiotocography, the woman is kept in a nonphysiological dorsal supine position. This must be avoided. Until combined or direct monitoring can be implemented, the use of abdominal fetal electrocardiogram and electrohysterography for external monitoring utilizing the Monica™ AN24 device (Norgenix, Spartanburg, SC) interconnected with the existing bedside fetal monitoring equipment has been found to be unaffected by maternal obesity and provides clinically useful information.[38,39] At an appropriate time, and prior to intense discomfort making the catheter placement difficult, an indwelling epidural anesthetic can be started, initially without the use of the full analgesic doses. The patient's cervical dilatation and station, and the position of the presenting part should be evaluated before the full anesthetic is initiated. Intravenous crystalloid should be infused prior to the anesthetic to prevent sudden drops in maternal blood pressure that occur as a result of vasodilation caused by the anesthetic agent. The fetal heart rate and the patient's blood pressure should be monitored immediately following the anesthetic test dose injection. Any significant drop in maternal blood pressure must be rapidly corrected to decrease or avoid the need for an emergent delivery second to maternal hypotension and subsequent fetal bradycardia. The dorsal supine position should be avoided because it reduces the inferior vena cava volume return and therefore decreases uteroplacental blood flow and perfusion. Strict monitoring of fluid intake and output must be maintained until the mother has completed labor and delivery and is in the postpartum unit.

Maternal obesity can be a serious obstetric risk factor, and a hospital unit providing maternity services must be prepared to respond to these patient's needs to decrease maternal and neonatal morbidities. Rapid clinical changes may occur to the obese mother or fetus during labor. The care team must maintain constant preparedness to act swiftly, efficiently, and effectively. The maternal-fetal dyad safety is imperative. The patient must be evaluated in established intervals to enable appropriate action in the presence of a clinically abnormal labor. As fetal descent progresses, neonatology should be alerted for timely arrival in the delivery room. Even in the exceptional case where maternal obesity may be diagnosed as an "isolated" issue, this may not be deemed a normal spontaneous vaginal delivery until every step is completed and the mother and newborn are stable.

Occasionally, an obese pregnant woman may be transported to the obstetrics unit without previous warning. All the preventive elements previously mentioned must be activated in short order. The patient may present with diabetic ketoacidosis, preterm labor, hypertensive crisis, eclampsia, abruptio placenta, severe vaginal bleeding, deep persistent fetal bradycardia, fetal malpresentation, preterm premature rupture of membranes, an upper respiratory infection, a urinary tract infection, a viral illness, motor vehicle accident sequelae, or any combination of common or puzzling clinical conditions with or without prenatal care. The obstetrics care team must act expeditiously to gather all pertinent information and promptly proceed with the indicated approach, with no hesitation in seeking assistance from an appropriate specialist. After clearing the obstetrical issues, any needed diagnostic testing or critical treatment should be provided and not withheld merely because the patient is pregnant. The condition of the patient and the treatment plans should be discussed with the patient and pertinent family members in clear and understandable language, and the scenario should be well documented.

As a vaginal delivery approaches, all care plans should be in place. Additional support personnel must be at the bedside. The dorsal lithotomy position in patients of significantly elevated BMI is not easy to obtain. The patient's upper thighs may need additional equipment and personnel to obtain adequate abduction to safely allow a vaginal delivery. The need to perform an operative vaginal delivery; manage a shoulder dystocia; repair cervical, vaginal, or perineal lacerations; remove a retained placenta; or evaluate and treat a postpartum hemorrhage may arise.

In cases of an operative vaginal delivery, we favor the divergent forceps with double pelvic and perineal curvatures (Laufe type) or the modern-style portable vacuum extractor. These instruments must be available in the delivery room once a vaginal delivery is expected. Recently, a modified fetal extractor has been studied in simulators and in a limited number of patients (Odon device, Becton Dickinson, Franklin Lakes, New York). The device is considered safe, easy to use, accepted by patients, and with the possibility of expanded use in low-cost settings. As of this writing, the product was not commercially available for use outside the research protocol. Readers who practice obstetrics in low-cost settings are encouraged to follow the development of the device. WHO is conducting a 3-phase study with the objective of bringing the device into the obstetrical armamentarium.

We describe the device as a "hoodie puller" once it is applied around the fetal head and inflated. Specific indications and contraindications are established.[40] Elevating the entire bed should be avoided in case suprapubic pressure is needed to assist in the delivery of the fetal shoulders. In extremely obese parturients with significant redundant abdominal pannus, suprapubic pressure needs additional personnel to lift the pannus to gain access to the suprapubic area. Removal of the frame of the bed head is recommended in case emergency maternal intubation becomes necessary. In such a scenario, the rapid response team should be called to provide additional expert support. Proper lighting, additional personnel, and adequate instruments are necessary to obtain adequate exposure in case a birth canal laceration needs repair.

The third stage of labor is actively managed by utilizing intravenous infusion of oxytocin, preferably at the time of the first fetal shoulder delivery, and maintained for at least 1 hour or longer after the placenta has been expelled or removed. A hemostatic balloon must be available in the room in case of postpartum hemorrhage second to uterine atony or lower segment overdistention. The type of balloon used depends on the institution's policy or the operator's preference. Sudden catastrophic events may ensue with little or no warning, such as maternal respiratory failure or cardiac arrest secondary to amniotic fluid infusion (see Chapter 13). For these cases, periodic drills and simulation are of great clinical importance. We encourage any institution providing maternity care to practice safety drills and to be up to date on literature, as a culture of safety becomes increasingly imperative. Recently, the Joint Commission (JC) and the National Safety Council proposed "bundles of care" to be standardized in all institutions providing maternity services.[41]

Given the potentially complicated nature of surgery on the obese patient, the obstetrician must plan in advance for these procedures. As the frequency of obese patients increases, it behooves maternity units to proactively implement bariatric obstetric protocols. These protocols should include a multidisciplinary approach, including but not limited to expert obstetric anesthesia coverage; customized operating room tables and transport equipment, including lateral transfer devices; additional personnel; bariatric instruments; timely preoperative prophylactic antibiotic utilization; neonatal support at the time of the birth; massive transfusion protocols; and the ability to rapidly refer a patient to an adult intensive care unit when necessary. In cases of an unfavorable cervix and an expected prolonged period of cervical ripening, we recommend apply automatic inflatable sequential venous compression devices (SCD, Kendall, Medtronic-Covidien, Mansfield, MA, 02048) on the parturient's legs.

Informed consent, specifically tailored to the obese pregnant woman, must include all the known events surrounding labor and delivery, and it should be obtained during a prenatal visit or on arrival to the maternity unit before any medication is initiated. Individual consideration should be given to some special groups of women (Jehovah Witnesses, patients who require only female attendants, etc.).

In the obese population, the reports regarding intrauterine pressure generated by myometrial contractility during labor and the forces generated during active maternal pushing are conflicting.[38,39] Therefore, the obstetrical team must be prepared to perform operative vaginal deliveries, including vacuum or forceps deliveries, and manage shoulder dystocias and the third stage of labor with possible postpartum hemorrhage or rapid change to a major surgical event.

A cesarean delivery may become indicated. With respect to the specifics of the surgery, in cases of elective cesarean we recommend the patient shower using a chlorhexidine scrub daily for 3 days prior to the planned procedure. Individual institutions implement nursing policies associated with patient preparation for elective cesarean. All patients receive prophylactic antibiotics, preferably prior to the skin incision. We favor adjusting the antibiotic dose to the patients BMI, starting with additional doses at a BMI of 30 kg/m². Intermittent inflatable SCDs are placed and attached to the power supply after the patient's skin is prepped, the Foley catheter is inserted, and the regional anesthesia is completed. With a stable mother scheduled for a repeat elective cesarean, the patient may ambulate to the operating room. Otherwise, once in the operating room, the laboring patient with an active epidural needs to be transferred to the surgical table. An inflatable lateral transfer device (Hovermatt, Hover Tech International, Bethlehem, PA) for single or multiple use may be of assistance, along with a modified operating room table. We utilize "wings" that are attached to the side of the existing table to accommodate the patient's waist. The Foley catheter may be inserted before or after the patient receives the anesthetic, tailored by the clinical circumstances and the personnel's ability to reach the urethral meatus before the mother is anesthetized. A bariatric instrument box should be available for these cases, along with additional instruments in separate wrappers to be used according to need. The fetal position, estimated fetal weight, and the location of the lowermost placental edge should be located with ultrasound prior to the final decision regarding placement of the skin incision.

This process may be conducted in the days that precede an elective procedure. As the numbers of obese and extremely obese pregnant women continue to increase, many of them with multiple cesarean deliveries, efforts must be made in early pregnancy for the identification of pregnancies implanted in the previous scar area, abnormal placenta location (placenta previa), or abnormal placental attachment (placenta accreta, increta, or percreta) and to plan for these complex cases with an experienced team in a tertiary care center.

We individualize the placement of the skin incision according to the patient's body contour and pannus size. This may be planned in advance with either a cephalad or a caudad pannus displacement or, if necessary, a displacement straight upward to avoid interfering with the patient's breathing. These maneuvers allow the operator to place the skin incision where the lower uterine segment can be reached through the shortest distance from the skin incision to the peritoneal cavity and the lower uterine segment (Figure 20-3). Several devices are adapted to mobilize the abdominal pannus according to the body habitus and the presence of previous abdominal scars. Recently, a commercially available product (Traxi™ panniculus retractor, Clinical Innovations, Murray, UT) has been introduced commercially as a disposable, practical, simple device for pannus retraction.

We use the anterior superior iliac spine (ASIS) as an anatomic landmark to determine the approximate location of the lower uterine segment.[42] We avoid incising the suprapubic area, which is often chronically inflamed or infected in the obese population. In extremely obese patients (BMI > 60 kg/m²), we favor a transverse supra- or subumbilical skin incision.[43] We seldom use a vertical or a classical Pfannenstiel incision. With a markedly redundant abdomen, we displace the pannus toward the patient's feet and enter the abdomen between her navel and the xiphoid, usually landing on the lower uterine segment as the entry maneuvers are oblique toward the symphysis. In these cases, caution must be taken to not "buttonhole," or slice through and through the abdominal wall and pannus, without reaching the peritoneal cavity. We enter the abdominal wall using the least-traumatic dissection to reach the peritoneal cavity,[43] keeping in mind the vascular distribution of the abdominal wall. We avoid the use of small, unmarked gauze sponges during the entire procedure.

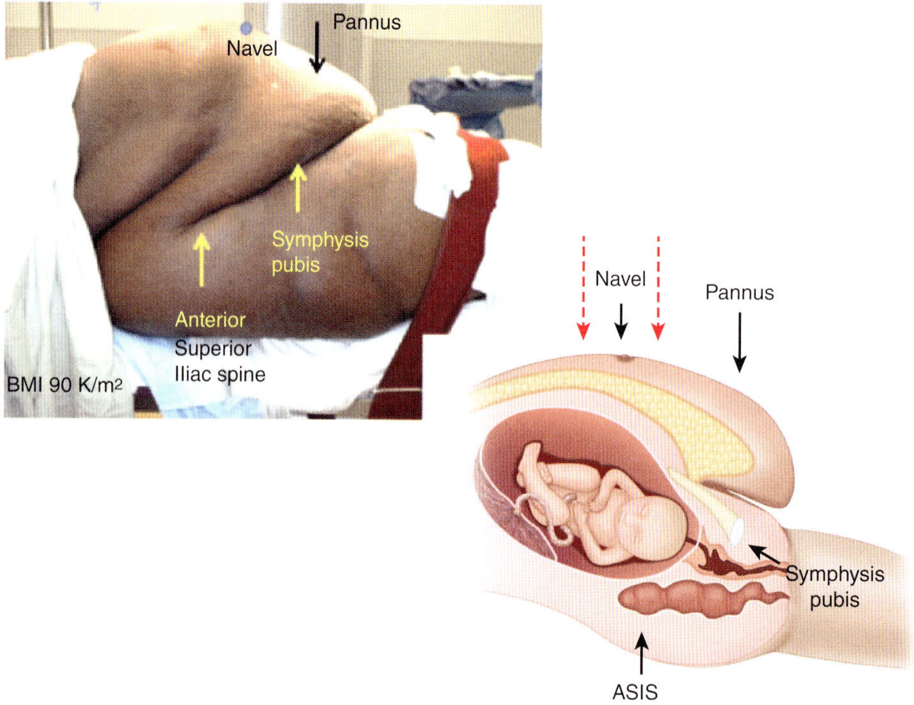

FIGURE 20-3. Preoperative incision planning. Broken arrows represent preferred incision placement to avoid area of potential contamination on the suprapubic area below the pannus.

We utilize a self-retaining wall protector (Alexis "O") of adequate size for the patient's BMI.[44,45] This instrument is useful in reducing the number of operator's hands and instruments needed during the surgery. The device, when fully deployed, creates a 360° surgical field, approximately 17 cm in diameter, which is adequate for the usual hysterotomy incision length whether it is in the low transverse uterine segment or a vertical incision, low or classical. It is important for the surgeon to be familiar with the introduction and deployment technique of this device to avoid excessive prolonged pressure on the abdominal wall by the device's supporting rings. We seldom perform a bladder flap prior to the hysterotomy, which is, in the preponderance of cases, a low segmental transverse incision.

The surgeon should have a mental picture of the fetal position and the placenta location prior to the hysterotomy to plan the maneuvers needed to deliver the fetus. Hydramnios is a frequent occurrence in obese patients with large fetuses, and, if present, obstetricians should anticipate an umbilical cord or fetal small part prolapse at the time of the hysterotomy and be able to proceed to the delivery in an orderly fashion, avoiding excessive manipulation.

Plans should be made to have an assistant gloved hand placed in the vagina to elevate the presenting pole and facilitate the delivery without undue traction on the fetal neck or extension of the uterine incision should the fetal vertex be deeply engaged as a result of prolonged labor. When this maneuver is needed, we prefer to wait until the assistant elevates the presenting part before we perform the hysterotomy.

Once the hysterotomy is performed, the upper uterine segment will contract and may trap the fetal body above the level of the transverse incision and delay the delivery. If the cesarean is performed after prolonged labor and the vertex is deeply engaged or in the occiput posterior position, an alternative is to perform a breech extraction and avoid excessive manipulation of the fetal head. Always follow the cardinal movements for delivery and avoid hectic maneuvers on the fetus or undue traction.

Occasionally, we utilize the portable single-use vacuum extractor to deliver the fetal head. This is most often needed in extremely obese parturients when the depth of the uterus delays the usual manual extraction of the vertex. Most often in these patients, fundal pressure is ineffective to assist in the fetal extraction.

In the presence of multiple fetuses, it is important to have a clear order for the delivery based on preoperative determination of fetal positions and preplanned delivery maneuvers. In cases of monoamniotic twins, rapid removal of the first-delivered co-twin from the field should be avoided until the entangled cords are clearly visualized.

The third stage of labor is usually managed with intravenous oxytocin at the time of the delivery of the first shoulder. Once the delivery and placental extraction are completed, the hysterotomy incision is closed with unlocking continuous suture to avoid excessive tissue strangulation rather than approximation. This suture must avoid the endometrial layer. A second uterine layer is favored by some. Both adnexa should be explored at this time as an integral part of the cesarean procedure and clearly documented. The self-retaining retractor is removed after both lateral gutters are cleared of clots. We do not utilize routine abdominal cavity irrigation, and neither do we exteriorize the uterus for the repair of the incision unless mechanical or other circumstances demand it. For example, we may exteriorize the uterus in the presence of large uterine fibroids; if we need to explore an extended hysterotomy incision; if placement of the uterine incision was in an atypical location, such as fundal or posterior; or to perform additional hemostatic sutures. Permanent sterilization procedures, when planned, are performed following the closure of the hysterotomy incision.

Hemostasis is critical in this area, usually with large venous structures in the mesosalpynx. The peritoneum is not closed. The abdominal wall is closed in layers, using either a Smead-Jones closure or a routine fascial closure.[46] Emphasis is placed on the detailed closure of the fatty layer. We must avoid free unapproximated pockets, which are the source of seromas, hematomas, secondary abscesses, and wound disruptions. We recommend separate stitches of rapid absorbable material in as many layers as needed to provide closure of all pockets. At all levels, hemostasis must be obtained. We avoid the excessive use of Bovie cautery in the fatty layer, especially as it gets closer to the skin. Attention is paid to avoid excessive tissue tension at the skin level, which will militate against proper healing in the days that follow the surgical procedure.

We avoid the use of antiadhesive materials such as sodium hyaluronate and carboxy methyl cellulose. We have found that these materials tend to clump in certain pockets above or below the fascial layer. These areas are frequently diagnosed as hematomas or abscesses should the woman require images during the postpartum period. In addition, there is no substantial evidence that these agents effectively prevent adhesions in obstetric patients.

We favor mattress sutures for the skin closure and keep the stitches in place for approximately 7 days prior to removal. This is especially important for diabetic patients whose blood glucose control has been less that optimal in the weeks that preceded the surgical procedure. If there is clinical evidence of seroma (pink, watery discharge), we periodically drain the incision by placing a sterile probe between stitches and allow for fluid to drain, avoiding retention with secondary infection. This maneuver is usually well tolerated by the patient, especially when a clear explanation for the reason to do it is provided. Some surgeons utilize removable staples or intradermal (subcuticular) continual stitches for the skin closure (see Chapter 22).

Current results indicate that staple closure of the skin is associated with increasing episodes of surgical site infection. We do not use tissue adhesives on the skin. Information is emerging and may be promising regarding the efficacy of incisional negative-pressure therapy in decreasing postoperative wound complications when placed prophylactically at the time of cesarean section in the obese patient. This technique is otherwise used if a surgical site infection or a total disruption of the skin incision occurs. The incision is surgically debrided and primarily repaired to avoid prolonged periods of healing by second intention. Family members are instructed in daily incision cleansing. Incisions in the area under the pannus are particularly troublesome, and we make every effort to avoid them.

The obese parturient is a candidate for prophylactic anticoagulation initiated 12 hours postpartum until she is discharged from the hospital. We favor early maternal feeding and ambulation. We remove the indwelling bladder catheter within 6 hours and encourage the patient to empty her bladder every 2 hours and ambulate as early as possible.

Often, chronic and some acute complications, such as severe preeclampsia, are not immediately resolved with the delivery of the fetus and placenta, and strict bedside care must continue unabated. Monitoring fluid balance, blood glucose levels, blood pressure, amount and characteristics of lochia, pain, peristalsis, breast engorgement, respiratory function, and lung conditions is part of the postpartum care. See more on cesarean alternatives in Chapter 12, especially regarding postpartum hemorrhage and indications for cesarean hysterectomy.

Patient discharge and follow-up vary with the background pathology at the time of the delivery and the events during the postpartum care. Family planning, including pregnancy spacing and avoidance of short interpregnancy interval (IPI) must be included in the discharge counseling. Permanent sterilization plans for those parents still undecided varies according to their desires, medical diagnosis, insurance coverage, and out-of-pocket costs (see Chapter 28).

An independent, however closely related, health care issue is the follow-up mammogram in obese patients. Recent legislative changes created a complex approach for practicing physicians in both primary care and specialties. Hospitals are creating a new service line to counsel patients who have been diagnosed with an abnormal breast ultrasound. All health care workers must remain attentive to the developments created by legislation in their area of practice.

ADVERSE BIRTH OUTCOMES

A birth defect prevalence of greater than 5% is noted in patients with elevated prepregnancy BMIs. This prevalence is 3.9% in women with normal BMIs ($p < .001$) (Table 20-3). The one exception is fetal gastroschisis, which is less prevalent in the offspring of the obese parturient. The detection of fetal structural anomalies via ultrasound is somewhat limited by an elevated maternal BMI, and serial studies may be necessary to complete the fetal anatomic survey. More studies are needed to precisely ascertain which fetal anomalies are more difficult to detect prenatally in this population.

Maternal obesity is associated with an increased risk of suboptimal perinatal outcomes, including stillbirth (adjusted odds ratio [AOR] 2.79, 95% confidence interval [CI] 1.94–4.02); shoulder dystocia (AOR 3.14, 95% CI 1.86–5.31); meconium aspiration (AOR 2.85, 95% CI 1.60–5.07); fetal distress (AOR 2.52, 95% CI 2.12–2.99); and early neonatal death (AOR 3.41, 95% CI 2.07–5.63).[47] Maternal obesity is associated with a more-than-doubled risk of stillbirth (OR 2.8, 95% CI 1.5–5.3) and neonatal death (OR 2.6, 95% CI 1.2–5.8).

There is no single cause to explain these deaths; however, fetoplacental dysfunction appears to be the predominant etiology.[48] Preterm birth deaths are also associated with BMIs greater than 35 kg/m². These deaths are mostly related to spontaneous preterm labor, preterm birth, premature rupture of membranes, and medically indicated preterm delivery. Abnormal birth weight (>90th percentile) triples with the combination of maternal obesity and gestational diabetes (OR 3.62, 95% CI 3.04–4.32). The increase in neonatal weight is associated with failed instrumental delivery (OR 1.75, 95% CI 1.1–2.9), increased maternal blood loss (OR 1.5, 95% CI 1.2–1.9), and increased neonatal intensive care unit admissions. Fetal macrosomia is reported as the single most powerful predictor of shoulder dystocia, especially in diabetic mothers, specifically for fetuses between 4000 and 4999 g (OR 9.0, 95% CI 6.5–12.6). Maternal obesity is not an independent risk factor for shoulder dystocia, yet advanced knowledge of estimated fetal weight is helpful.[48]

Neonatal mortality (deaths in the first 7 days of life per 1000 live births), as defined by the National Center for Health Statistics (NCHS) and the Centers for Disease Control and Prevention (CDC) in the United States, is also increased as maternal BMI increases. Infant mortality rates (equally defined by the NCHS and the CDC as deaths between birth and 12 months per 1000 live births) of 5.8/1000 primarily on term births have been reported in overweight and obese mothers, as opposed to 2.4/1000 in mothers of normal weight.[49] In-depth research associated with specific causes of infant mortality from obese mothers is lacking.

TABLE 20-3 Live Birth Defects Associated With Maternal Obesity

Congenital heart anomalies
Diaphragmatic hernia
Pyloric stenosis
Cleft palate
Hydrocephaly without spina bifida
Rectal and large bowel malformations
Clubbed feet
Limb reduction anomalies

In patients with maternal obesity class II and III, postneonatal mortality is also increased. Primiparous and multiparous mothers are similarly affected. Congenital anomalies, birth asphyxia, and infections are the top three etiologies associated with these deaths.[50] Special attention must be paid to the group of extremely obese mothers (BMI $\geq$ 50 kg/m^2). These fetuses are at increased risk of shoulder dystocia (7.1% vs. 1.4%); birth weight over 4500 g (16.9% vs. 2.1%) and birth weight over 4000 g (38.0% vs. 11.9%); neonatal metabolic abnormalities (8.5% vs. 2.0%); and increased need for neonatal intensive care unit admissions (16.9% vs. 7.8%).[51,52] Obese mothers are at an increased risk of a composite adverse outcome in 81.7% of cases versus 41.5% in a mother at the recommended BMI (AOR 1.57, 95% CI 1.35–1.83).[57] Newborns from obese mothers are at increased risk of developing MS even from mothers who do not fulfill the criteria for gestational diabetes.[54]

Recent studies have demonstrated that maternal obesity affects fetal neurodevelopmental and metabolic gene expression, and because over 200 genes are highly represented in the central nervous system involving the cerebral cortex, these findings may be implicated in the infant's neurodevelopmental abnormalities described in infants of obese mothers.[49] As the frequency of maternal obesity increases in our population, it is important that all the risks mentioned are addressed prior to conception, and that a strong educational program is initiated early in life to encourage healthier lifestyles before pregnancy is planned.

FUTURE DIRECTIONS

Much has been learned in the recent decades regarding the pathophysiology of obesity. Indeed, much remains poorly understood or unknown. It is time to incorporate maternal BMI in a prominent space at the beginning and at the end of the gestational period as a critical variable of the pregnant woman's medical history. This step should start with the general population clinical record as an integral part of screening and recording reproductive health. Perhaps a new creative person-to-person salutation can be suggested worldwide: Good morning, and how is your BMI today?

The arrival of the exome and genome era brings the opportunity for early recognition of markers related to obesity. This important step allows for the implementation of personalized approaches to the detection, prevention, and treatment of obesity. Women of reproductive age are especially vulnerable to all the negative influences of obesity on themselves and the fetuses they carry. The health of the next generation depends on our ability to learn to identify these factors and act on their avoidance. We must work to fully understand the causes or associations between fetal, neonatal, and infant mortality in obese pregnant and postpartum women.[54]

Health improvements depend on individual personal responsibility to access the health care system on a timely basis. Personal involvement must be demanded as a condition of receiving full benefits of health care insurance benefits. Universal interactive medical records will allow for any woman to move freely while having her up-to-date medical care contained in an "intelligent card" to facilitate the continuity of her care.

Obese pregnant women must be risk screened early in prenatal care; the recent ACOG recommendations referring them to the appropriate level of care institution must be followed.[55] Health care workers and public health officials must work together to implement educational programs beginning in elementary school. Legislators must avoid the temptation to practice medicine from the capitol buildings and instead be well informed on the issues that are germane to a healthy, productive, and responsible population. Legislators at the bedside are not a sign of health care improvement. Funding allocation, a legislative expertise, should be a well-thought-out process for the benefit of most. In a civilized society, the quality of maternity care is a proxy for how the country protects its future generation.

SUMMARY

Obesity is often glossed over by physicians when counseling patients or either is treated like the proverbial elephant in the room and not addressed at all or is addressed, but in a lighthearted manner that treats it as though it is a mere nuisance. These approaches have evolved over the years as the obese population grew because physicians either fear that talking about a patient's size will offend and embarrass the patient or think that patients will feel criticized and become defensive once their body mass is addressed. Due to the major negative health consequences that obesity poses on the human body, physicians need to undergo a paradigm shift wherein they think of obesity as a medical illness that the patient has and then treat it as such. Maternal obesity affects the health of the pregnant women and that of her fetus, newborn, and child for years to come. A clear understanding of the physiopathologic influence of obesity during and after the gestational period is imperative.

This chapter brought attention to the multiple facets of this serious and increasing clinical problem in prenatal care. The practice of bariatric obstetrics offers the opportunity to understand all issues related to obesity in the maternal-fetal dyad. With obesity now reaching epidemic proportions worldwide, it is the responsibility of physicians to make their patients aware of just how dangerous their weight can be and to educate them on lifestyle changes that they can make that will help them lose weight. The term *globesity* clearly reflects the gravity and pervasiveness of this contemporary health care challenge, the effects of which will last for generations.

REFERENCES

1. American College of Obstetricians and Gynecologists. Obesity in pregnancy. Committee opinion no. 549. *Obstet Gynecol*. 2013;121:213–217.
2. Agency for Health Care Research and Quality (NCQA) http://circ.ahajournals.org/lookup/doi/10.1161/CIR.Ob013e31828124ad. Accessed September 24, 2016.
3. Hall JE, Guyton AC. Obesity. Unit XIII metabolism and temperature regulation. In *Guyton and Hall, Textbook of Medical Physiology*. 12th ed. Philadelphia: Saunders Elsevier; 2011:850.
4. Eknoyan G. The average man and indices of obesity. Adolphe Quetelet (1796–1874). *Nephrol Dial Transplant*. 2008;1:47–51.
5. Apell SP, Wahlsten O, Gawlitza H. Body mass index: a physics perspective. Chalmers University of Technology, Göteborg, Sweden. arXiv:1109.0296 (2011).
6. Satpathy HK, Fleming A, Frey D, Barsoom M, Satpathy C, Kahndalavala J. Maternal obesity and pregnancy. *Postgrad Med*. 2008 Sep 15;120(3):EO1–EO9.
7. Boney CM, Verma A, Tucker R, Vohr BR. Metabolic syndrome in childhood: association with birth weight, maternal obesity and gestational diabetes mellitus. *Pediatrics*. 2005 Mar;115(3):e290–e296.
8. Dover GJ. The Barker hypothesis: how pediatricians will diagnose and prevent common adult onset diseases. *Trans Am Clin Climatol Assoc*. 2009;120:199–207.
9. Lane M, Zander-Fox DL, Robker RL, McPherson NO. Peri-conception parental obesity, reproductive health, and transgenerational impacts. *Trends Endocrinol Metab*. 2014 Dec 15;26(2):S1043–S2760.
10. Resi V, Basu S, Haghiac M, et al. Molecular inflammation and adipose tissue matrix remodeling precede physiological adaptations to pregnancy. *Am J Physiol Endocrinal Metab*. 2012 Oct 1;303(7):E832–E840.

11. Reynolds SR, Heard OO, Bruns P. Recording uterine contraction patterns in pregnant women; application of the strain gage in a multichannel tocodynamometer. *Science.* 1947 Oct 31;106:427–428.

12. Csapo A, Sauvage J. The evolution of uterine activity during human pregnancy. *Acta Obstet Gynecol Scand.* 1968;47(2):181–212.

13. Karolczak-Bayatti M, Sweeney M, Cheng J, et al. Acetylation of heat shock protein 20 (Hsp20) regulates human myometrial activity. *J Biol Chem.* 2011 Sep 30; 286(39):34346–34355.

14. Fitzpatrick RJ. Changes in cervical function at parturition. *Ann Rech Vet.* 1977;8(4):438–449.

15. Friedman E. The graphic analysis of labor. *Am J Obstet Gynecol.* 1954 Dec;68(6):1568–1575.

16. Friedman EA. An objective approach to the diagnosis and management of abnormal labor. *Bull NY Acad Med.* 1972;48(6):842–858.

17. Cesario SK. Reevaluation of Friedman's labor curve: a pilot study. *J Obstet Gynecol Neonatal Nurs.* 2004 Nov–Dec;33(6):713–722.

18. Zhang J, Troendle JF, Yancey MK. Reassessing the labor curve in nulliparous women. *Am J Obstet Gynecol.* 2002 Oct;187(4):824–828.

19. ACOG/SMFM Consensus. Safe prevention of the primary cesarean delivery. Am *J Obstet Gynecol.* 2014 March;123:693–711.

20. Zhang J, Landy HJ, Branch DW, et al. Contemporary patterns of spontaneous labor with normal neonatal outcomes; consortium on safe labor. *Obstet Gynecol.* 2010 Dec;116(6):1281–1287.

21. Cohen WR, Friedman EA. Perils of the new labor management guidelines. *Am J Obstet Gynecol.* 2015 Apr;212(4):420–427.

22. Kozhimannil KB, Arcaya MC, Subramanian SV. Maternal clinical diagnosis and hospital variation in the risk of cesarean delivery: analyses of a national US hospital discharge database. *PLOS Med.* 2014 October; 11(10):e1001745.

23. Zhang J, Troendle J, Reddy UM, et al. Contemporary cesarean delivery practice in the United States. *Am J Obstet Gynecol.* 2010 Oct;203(4):326 e1–326.e10.

24. Jensen H, Agger AO, Rasmussen KL. The influence of prepregnancy body mass index on labor complications. *Acta Obstet Gynecol Scand.* 1999 Oct;78(9):799–802.

25. Vahratian A, Zhang J, Troendle JF, Savitz DA, Siega-Riz AM. Maternal prepregnancy overweight and obesity and the pattern of labor progression in term nulliparous women. *Obstet Gynecol.* 2004;104:943–951.

26. Smith RD, Babyichuk EB, Noble K, Draeger A, Wray S. Increased cholesterol decreases uterine activity: functional effects of cholesterol alteration in pregnant rat myometrium. *Am J Physiol Cell Physiol.* 2005;288:C982–C988.

27. Lowe NK, Corwin EJ. Proposed biological linkages between obesity, stress, and inefficient uterine contractility during labor in humans. *Med Hypotheses.* 2011 May;76(5):755–760.

28. Hehir MP, Morrison JJ. The adipokine apelin and human uterine contractility. Clin Key. 2012;206(4):359.

29. Marseglia L, Manti S, D'Angelo G, et al. Oxidative stress in obesity; a critical component in human diseases. *Int J Mol Sci.* 2015;16:378–400.

30. Quenby S, Pierce SJ, Brigham S, Wray S. Dysfunctional labor and myometrial acidosis. *Obstet Gynecol.* 2004 Apr;103(4):718–723.

31. Zhang J, Bricker L, Wray S, Quenby S. Poor uterine contractility in obese women. *BJOG.* 2007 Mar;114(3):343–348.

32. Verdiales M, Pacheco C, Cohen WR. The effect of maternal obesity on the course of labor. *J Perinat Med.* 2009;37(6):651–655.

33. Carhäll S, Källén K, Blomberg M. Maternal body mass index and duration of labor. *Eur J Obstet Gynecol Reprod Biol.* 2013 Nov;171(1):49–53.

34. Kaiser PS, Kirby RS. Obesity as a risk factor for cesarean in a low risk population. *Obstet Gynecol.* 2001:97(1):39–43.

35. Vahratian A, Zhang J, Troendle JF, Savitz DA, Siega-Riz AM. Maternal prepregnancy overweight and obesity and the pattern of labor progression in term nulliparous women. *Obstet Gynecol.* 2004;104:943–951.

36. Fyfe EM, Anderson NH, North RA, et al. Risk of first stage and second stage cesarean delivery by maternal body mass index among nulliparous women in labor at term. *Obstet Gynecol.* 2011;117(6):1315–1322.

37. Bergholt T, Lim LK, Jorgensen JS, Robson MS. Maternal body mass index in the first trimester and risk of cesarean delivery in nulliparous women in spontaneous labor. *Am J Obstet Gynecol.* 2007 Feb;196(2): 163.E1-5.

38. Buhimschi CS, Buhimschi IA, Malinow AM, Weiner CP. Intrauterine pressure during the second stage of labor in obese women. *Obstet Gynecol.* 2004 Feb; 103(2):225–230.

39. Cohen WR, Hayes-Gill B. Influence of maternal body mass index on accuracy and reliability of external fetal monitoring techniques. *Acta Obstet Gynecol Scand.* 2014 Jun;93(6):590–595.

40. World Health Organization Odon Device Research Group. Feasibility and safety study of a new device (Odon device) for assisted vaginal deliveries: study protocol. *Reprod Health.* 2013;10:42. http://www.reproductive-health-journal.com/content/10/1/42.

41. Council on Patient Safety in Women's Health Care. Safe health care for every woman. http://www.safehealthcareforeverywoman.org. Published 2015. Accessed April 14, 2015.

42. Joel-Cohen SJ. The place of the abdominal hysterectomy. *Clin Obstet Gynecol.* 1978;5(3):525–543.

43. Krebs H-B, Helmkamp BF. Transverse periumbilical incision in the massively obese patient. *Obstet Gynecol.* 1984;63(2):241–245.

44. Applied Medical. Alexis "O" ring. Rancho Santa Margarita, CA: Applied Medical.

45. Plymel K, Mariona FG. Use of a self-retaining wall protector in cesarean delivery of extremely obese parturients. 5BIRTH; 2015; abstract 64.

46. Powell JL. Powell's pearls: eponyms in medical and surgical history. The Smead-Jones closure of abdominal wounds. *J Surg Educ.* 2011;01.010:335–337.

47. Blank A, Grave GD, Metzger BE. Effects of gestational diabetes on perinatal morbidity reassessed. Report of the International Workshop on Adverse Perinatal Outcomes of Gestational Diabetes Mellitus. December 3–4, 1992. *Diabetes Care.* 1995 Jan;18(1):127–129.

48. Cedergren M. Maternal morbid obesity and the risk of adverse pregnancy outcomes. *Obstet Gynecol.* 2004 Feb;103(2):219–224.

49. Edlow AG, Vora NL, Hui L, et al. Maternal obesity affects fetal neurodevelopmental and metabolic gene expressions: a pilot study. *PLoS ONE.* 2014 Feb;2(9):1–11.

50. Kristensen J, Vestergaard M, Wisborg K, Kesmodel U, Secher NJ. Prepregnancy weight and the risk of stillbirth and neonatal death. *BJOG.* 2005 Apr; 112(4):403–408.

51. Robinson H, Tkatch S, Mayes DC, Bott N, Okun N. Is maternal obesity a predictor of shoulder dystocia. *Obstet Gynecol.* 2003 Jan;101(1):24–27.

52. Johansson S, Villamor E, Altman M, Edstedt-Bonamy AK, Granath F. Maternal overweight and obesity in early pregnancy and risk of infant mortality: a population based cohort study in Sweden. *BMJ.* 2014 Dec; 349(2):1–12. G6572.

53. Crane JM, Murphy P, Burrage L, Hutchens D. Maternal and perinatal outcomes of extreme obesity in pregnancy. *J Obstet Gynecol Can.* 2013 Jul;35(7):606–611.

54. Boney CM, Verma A, Tucker R, Vohr BR. Metabolic syndrome in childhood: association with birth weight, maternal obesity and gestational diabetes mellitus. *Pediatrics.* 2005 Mar;115(3):e290–e296.

55. Obstetric Care Consensus no. 2. Levels of maternal care. *Obstet Gynecol.* 2015;125:502–515.

Cesarean Section/ Surgical Management

Alexandra C. Spadola, MD

BACKGROUND

Incidence

Cesarean delivery (CD) is the most common surgery for hospitalized women in the United States. From 1970 to 2014, the rate of primary CD in the United States increased from 5.5% to 32.2%.[1,2] The concurrent rise in rates of overweight and obese women, now representing over two-thirds of the population, is one of myriad factors playing a role in this trend.[3] Several studies have reported an association between higher body mass indexes (BMIs) and higher rates of CD.[4-8] In a meta-analysis from 2009, likelihood ratios of undergoing CD were 1.46 (95% confidence interval [CI] 1.34–1.60), 2.05 (95% CI 1.86–2.27), and 2.89 (95% CI 2.28–3.79) in populations of overweight, obese, and severely obese women (BMI > 35–40 depending on the study), respectively, compared with normal-weight pregnant women.[8] One statewide analysis in the United States determined that 1 in 7 CDs was attributable only to being overweight or obese.[9]

Contributing Factors

While higher rates of preexisting and pregnancy-related diabetes and hypertension are seen in the pregnancies of overweight and obese women, the additional risk for CD appears to be independent of the common comorbidities.[4] Many factors may play a role in the obese woman's increased risk for a CD, including, but not limited to, excess weight gain in pregnancy, slower progress in the first stage of labor, differences in myometrial contractility, fetal macrosomia, placental inflammation, inadequate intrapartum fetal monitoring, and soft tissue dystocia.[4,10,11] Iatrogenic causes, such as higher induction rates and provider bias toward CD, may also fuel this trend. The relationship between obesity and CD not only contributes to a rise in health care spending[12] but also affects women's complications in childbirth, postpartum course, future pregnancy care, and her long-term health and potentially that of her offspring.

Surgical Risk

Surgery on obese patients is associated in general with an increase in operative time, cost, and complications, in particular disturbed wound healing.[13] CD in obese women is associated with a higher number of complications, such as blood loss, postoperative infection, readmission, and venous thromboembolism (VTE).[11,14-16] Importantly for obesity research, the American College of Obstetricians and Gynecologists (ACOG) recognizes severe hypertension, VTE, and obstetric hemorrhage as the three top national priorities for prevention of maternal mortality and morbidity,[17] all more commonly diagnosed in the setting of elevated BMI.

With the global focus on patient safety and utilization of quality benchmarks like readmission and surgical site infection, hospitals are increasingly looking to improve intrapartum and postpartum care for this at-risk population. Recognizing the challenges for the growing population of women with class III or "supermorbid" obesity at delivery, often defined as BMI greater than 50, regional high-risk centers increasingly accept these patients for antepartum referral.

ANTEPARTUM CONSIDERATIONS

Prenatal Counseling

All overweight and obese women should be counseled about their increased risk for CD. Reproductive health counseling in the preconception period should emphasize the benefits of weight loss for reducing prepregnancy BMI; even a minimal amount of weight loss can result in improvement in pregnancy outcomes.[18] As the incidence of attempted vaginal birth after cesarean in the United States remains low at 1 in 5 women,[19] there may be greater obstacles for obese women compared to women of normal BMI; avoiding the first CD is always the best strategy when possible and safe.

Risk Reduction

Antepartum risk reduction strategies include counseling about appropriate weight gain, encouraging healthy physical activity and nutritional choices, and optimizing glycemic control if diabetes mellitus is preexisting or diagnosed during pregnancy. As many as 40% of obese women gain more weight than is recommended by the Institute of Medicine guidelines (11–20 lb for women with a BMI > 30).[20] Research on the prevention of excess gestational weight gain has not been promising. One Australian trial of over 2000 overweight and obese pregnant participants that randomized them to continuous advice and behavioral support on issues of nutrition and exercise was unique in looking at outcomes rather than simply at gestational weight gain. It found no significant differences in rates of infants who were large for gestational age or in those of multiple maternal outcomes, including CD (34% control group vs. 37% intervention group, $p = .33$).[21] There is a need for more research into understanding the etiologies of excessive gestational weight gain, why obese women are more at risk, and, more important, evidence-based strategies for prevention, such as intensified lifestyle interventions or pharmaceutical means, such as are being examined in forthcoming trials of metformin in the nondiabetic obese.[22]

Screening

Obese women of reproductive age have higher rates of chronic hypertension, diabetes, asthma, and sleep apnea, not all of which are recognized prior to pregnancy. A screening electrocardiogram or echocardiogram should be considered in patients with a cardiac history, chronic hypertension, pregestational diabetes, or sleep apnea. A routine anesthesia consultation may not be indicated for most obese women, but additional medical comorbidities or a history of anesthesia complications should prompt consideration of this service.

Preoperative Counseling

Women undergoing CDs should be counseled about the increased risks for hemorrhage, infectious morbidity, and VTE. There is not a BMI at which it is universally accepted to perform an elective CD for maternal weight alone, especially in the setting of potential future childbearing and the risks of repeat surgery. However, several series have highlighted the challenges in the smaller population of women with BMIs above 50.[5,6] Obese women are more likely to be induced and require interventions such as internal monitoring.[7] In addition, they have more barriers to emergency CD, including possible delays in securing intravenous access, difficulty with transport, achieving adequate anesthesia, and longer time to delivery.[14]

ANESTHESIA

While a routine consult is not obtained for all obese surgical candidates, the on-staff anesthesiologists should be made aware of any patient admitted with class III obesity. Labor epidurals can be useful for obese women due to the option of employing it later if a CD becomes necessary.[23] There is a lack of evidence suggesting that a labor epidural is a contributing factor in CD in the overweight or obese population, but that topic may warrant further investigation, particularly for nulligravidas. As with patients of normal BMI, spinal anesthesia is preferred for patients undergoing CD, but it is not without technical challenges. Patients should be advised about the higher rate of failed placements of regional anesthesia in some obese women due to soft tissue differences.

For women requiring general anesthesia, airway edema and increased soft tissue may be obstacles to visualization, such that as many as 1 in 3 obese women may have a difficult intubation.[23] Obtaining adequate anesthesia in this population can be particularly challenging in the setting of obstetric emergencies such as cord prolapse or acute high-volume hemorrhage with previa or abruption.

OPERATING ROOM EQUIPMENT

Operating Tables

A CD that is safe for both the obese patient and the operating room team can require the presence of specialized equipment. Surgical staff should be aware of weight limitations of all pieces of equipment, especially operating tables, most of which tolerate 350–500 lb.[24] Special bariatric tables can accommodate up to 600–1000 lb. Additional side extensions allow for patients with wider body habitus and are cushioned to prevent compression injury of soft tissue during surgery. Awareness of the extra risk of special positioning during CD such as leftward tilt or, less commonly, Trendelenburg, is important for preventing falls.

Instruments

Surgical instruments, particularly retractors, come in larger and longer sizes for surgery in the bariatric population. A disposable, self-retaining retractor can be helpful in evenly compressing the subcutaneous adipose tissue, especially in the absence of intra-abdominal adhesive disease or with limited assistants to manually retract soft tissue. Although instruments required during CD are less likely to require modifications for obese patients, in the setting of conversion to hysterectomy or working deeper in the pelvis (i.e., repairing a uterine extension), longer instruments may prove useful.

Transfer Devices

An air-assisted mattress is an inflatable device designed for lateral transport of the obese patient from bed or stretcher to operating table and back. It must be placed below the patient prior to anesthesia and is inflated during transfer. As it is a sliding transfer, it avoids the need to roll the patient to the extreme lateral position needed to place sliding boards, it reduces the need for load-bearing lifting on the part of the staff, thus reducing the risk for patient falls and staff injuries, and can bear up to 1200 lb.

INTRAOPERATIVE CONSIDERATIONS

Antibiotic Prophylaxis

Preoperative antibiotics prior to CD are recommended as it is considered "clean contaminated." Women are at increased risk for surgical site infections compared to other procedures, and CD is the biggest risk factor for postpartum endometritis.[25] For women undergoing CD and not already receiving antibiotics for chorioamnionitis or premature rupture of membranes, an antibiotic such as a first-generation cephalosporin should be administered within 60 minutes of the procedure.[25] Antibiotic dosing is based currently on maternal weight due to preliminary evidence that obesity alters pharmacokinetics; for example, in women with BMI over 30 would receive 2 g of cefazolin instead of the standard 1 g.[25] While evidence exists that women with even higher BMIs may not achieve recommended tissue levels under current guidelines,[26] the clinical impact on infection rates has not been studied. More research is needed to define the best prophylactic dosing for women with class III obesity.

Incision Site

Positioning and prepping the patient in the operating room requires deciding first where to make the skin incision. For the majority of overweight and obese women, a low transverse incision of the Joel-Cohen or Pfannenstiel type is appropriate. However, incision sites described for the obese patient with a large panniculus can be divided into three types: subpannus, suprapannus transverse, and suprapannus vertical.

Advocates of placing the incision above the panniculus have been based on hypotheses that doing so avoids a humid, yeast-prone area potentially more conducive to surgical site infection, obviates the need to retract the panniculus above the operative field during surgery, and offers greater ease for inspecting the healing incision for the patient, her family, and health care professionals (Figure 21-1).

Proponents of the subpannus location cite the generally thinnest adipose layer between skin and fascial planes, closer proximity to the lower uterine segment, greater ease of delivery of the neonate, and less traction by the panniculus on the healing incision line. Patients generally prefer the site with the least risk for complications. For some women, the improved cosmesis of the subpannus incision is an advantage, while others are concerned about their inability to visualize the healing surgical site without assistance.

Techniques to lift the panniculus for a subpannus transverse incision include retraction by assistants or, more practically, with a sling of adhesive silk tape or a Montgomery strap, which then affixes to the operating table[23] (Figure 21-2). Communication with the anesthesia team is important in gauging the effect of additional weight on the upper abdomen and lower chest on the patient's comfort and respiratory mechanics.

With few exceptions,[27] studies of obese women comparing subpannus incisions with the suprapannus vertical type have reported significantly fewer postpartum complications with the subpannus site. Suprapannus vertical incisions are more frequently associated with classical hysterotomies, greater blood loss, and longer operative times.[28,29] Notably, these data are not randomized and are likely confounded by factors that originally drove the surgeons' preoperative decisions.

The suprapannus transverse incision, described in 1 retrospective series of 18 patients, may offer the benefits of avoiding the area beneath the panniculus, but, when well positioned (typically by assessing the patient both standing and supine) provides more direct access to the lower uterine segment than the vertical midline incision.[30] For incisions superior to the panniculus, the relationship between the incision and the umbilicus may vary from patient to patient. This third option may avoid short- and long-term complications of the suprapannus

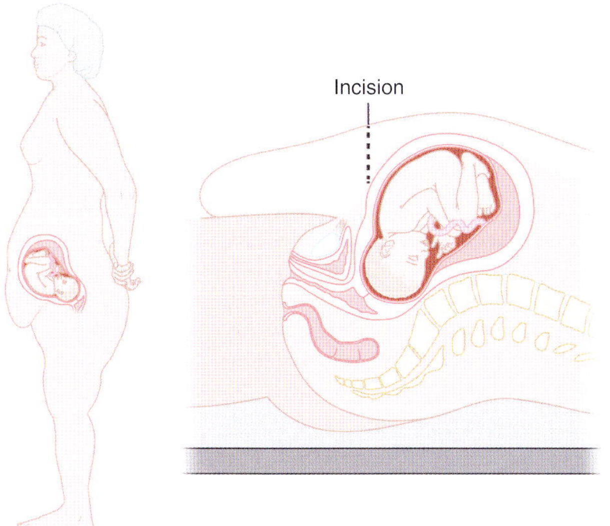

FIGURE 21-1. Obese woman with pannus standing and supine with incision positioned at level of lower uterine segment.

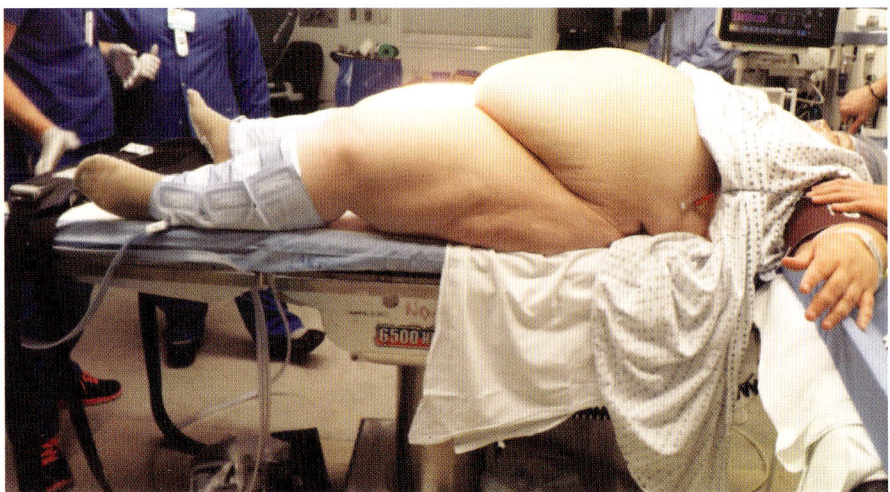

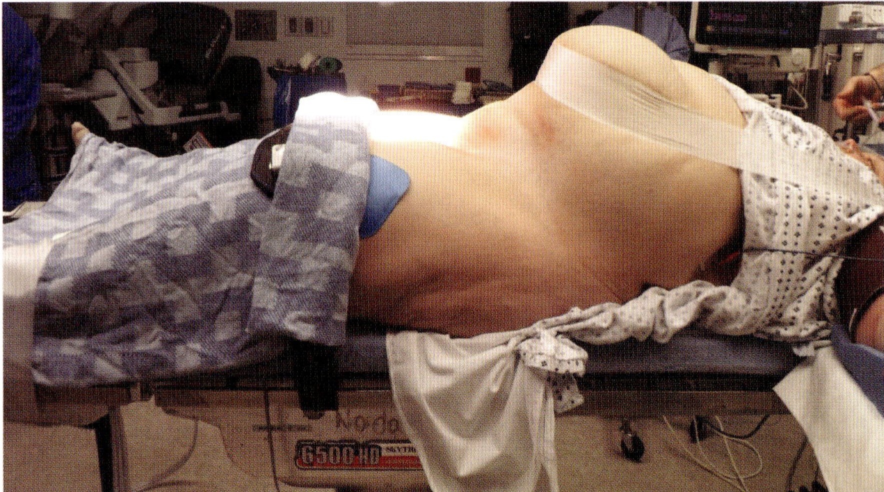

FIGURE 21-2. Supine patient with pannus, before and after retraction of pannus for delivery.

vertical incision, although this has not been studied comparatively. Depending on habitus, it may still require traversing a deep portion of adipose tissue and place the patient at greatest risk for the feared complication of transecting the full thickness of panniculus while attempting to reach the rectus fascia.

Currently, obstetricians make this decision based on patient body habitus, training, and personal bias. Particularly as the population of pregnant women with BMI greater than 50 expands, randomized controlled trials are needed to answer the incision question more systematically.

Wound Closure

Recognizing the greater risk for incisional complications in the obese population, surgeons have experimented with various prevention strategies. Suture closure of the adipose tissue layer greater than 2.0 cm has been found to be beneficial, with a meta-analysis of 5 studies demonstrating a benefit by primarily lowering the rate of wound seroma and reporting a 34% decrease in wound complications with a number needed to treat of 16 to prevent a single wound disruption.[31] In contrast, placement of subcutaneous drains was not found to have a significant difference in wound complications as explored in a Cochrane review of 6 studies.[32]

Mode of skin closure has been a recent topic of interest, with most reports demonstrating significantly lower rates of wound complications with the use of subcuticular sutures versus staples in the general population. In one larger study of 398 women randomized to either sutures or staples, the average BMI was 35–36; however, the primary outcome of wound complications failed to reach statistical significance in women with BMI greater than 30, but did trend toward a benefit (14.1% with staples and 8.2% with sutures, $p = .117$).[33] A meta-analysis of 12 randomized trials reporting on sutures versus staples demonstrated that the positive benefit for patients remained even in the obese population.[34]

The greatest difference has been in the rate of wound separation, and advocates of leaving staples in longer than the manufacturer's suggested time of 3–4 days suggest this discrepancy in outcomes can be remedied by delayed outpatient staple removal. A single randomized study on delayed (days 7–10) versus early (day 3) staple removal after CD failed to show any differences but was ended early due to funding. The authors concluded that delayed removal was favored due to a trend toward non-inferiority.[35] Other outcomes between the two techniques, such as patient satisfaction and cosmesis, appear to be equal, with a small sacrifice of several minutes of operating room time for the suture placement.[33,34]

Negative-pressure wound closure involves a vacuum device placed over an open or closed incision to shorten healing time. Recent evaluations of utilizing negative-pressure wound therapy prophylactically in obese women after CD showed some promise. A pilot study of 63 patients with class III obesity, 21 of whom received the device, reported no wound morbidity in the intervention group.[36] One cost analysis from Australia reported an estimated $50/patient cost savings by using negative-pressure wound closure devices, with a likelihood of cost-effectiveness of 65%.[37] These studies did not address issues surrounding patient acceptance or compliance, and more trials are likely needed prior to incorporating this modality as evidence-based practice.

Hemorrhage

Intrapartum and postpartum hemorrhage in women with obesity may be related to longer operating times, atony related to macrosomia or multiparity, or difficulty in controlling blood loss due to poor visualization. In a study of over 1600 women undergoing CD, those with a weight of greater than 250 lb were more likely to experience significant hemorrhage (odds ratio [OR] 13.1, 95% CI 1.7–102.7).[15]

A Maternal-Fetal Medicine Units study looking at time from incision to delivery found that obesity and morbid obesity were both associated with a significant increase. Time to delivery was greater than 18 minutes in 20% of the morbidly obese women, but only 6% of patients with a normal BMI.[14] Certainly, obesity should be considered in contemplating the need for crossmatching units of blood prior to planned surgery.

POSTOPERATIVE CONSIDERATIONS

Wound Infection/Disruption

Surgical site infections may be divided into early (1–3 days) and late (>3 days). As discussed, ensuring proper preoperative antibiotic coverage adjusted for weight, allowing proper time for skin cleansers to dry, and choice of incision site may influence this outcome. Early complications typically arise from infection preexisting the surgery and are most common in the setting of chorioamnionitis. One meta-analysis examined the benefit of vaginal preparation for prevention and found significant benefit for patients who had ruptured membranes or had been in labor.[38]

Late infections are most commonly discovered after hospital discharge and arise from either intrauterine bacteria or skin flora. They can arise in conjunction with wound seromas or hematomas. Multiple factors outside those in the operating room may influence the increased risk for obese women, including medical comorbidities such as diabetes and hypertension, which may affect the immune system and cause tissue edema, respectively; background chronic inflammation; issues of malnutrition; failed or protracted labor induction; and larger surface area for bacteria to flourish. Studies have reported rates ranging from 3.5% to 30% in the obese population.[39]

One observational study of 2444 women demonstrated a dose effect of obesity on the rate of wound complications, with nonobese women's rate of 6.6% in contrast to 9.2% in women with BMI 30–39.9 (adjusted odds ratio [aOR] 1.4, 95% CI 0.99–2.0, $p =$ .06); 16.8% in women with BMI 40–49.9 (aOR 2.6, 95% CI 1.7–3.8, $p < .01$); and 22.9% in women with BMI ≥50 (aOR 3.0, 95% CI 1.9–4.9, $p < .01$), and a p value less than .01 for test of trend.[39] While routine incision exams the week following discharge are not universally performed, they should be considered strongly in this high-risk group.

Wound infections are typically polymicrobial. Treatment is a combination of complete drainage of any purulence or fluid collection, which may require reopening the entire incision, culture of the fluid, copious irrigation, exploration and determination of the integrity of the fascial planes, packing to prevent fluid reaccumulation, and broad-spectrum antibiotic coverage, especially in the setting of accompanying cellulitis. Necrotizing fasciitis, a true surgical emergency, and fascial dehiscence are both rare after CD but may be more difficult to diagnose and detect in obese patients due to body habitus. Imaging with ultrasound or computed tomographic scan may be indicated in more complicated late infection, especially in a completely healed incision. Negative-pressure wound devices may be employed to assist in improving closure time with resolution of clinically evident infection.

Venous Thromboembolism

Venous thromboembolism is a leading cause of mortality and readmission after childbirth in the developed world.[17] Obesity and CD appear synergistic in increasing this complication for postpartum women. While early ambulation and mechanical compression devices have been shown to be beneficial, there is a growing trend toward pharmaceutical prophylaxis in all obese women after CD. The ACOG District II Safe Motherhood Initiative in New York State advocates for prophylaxis with low molecular weight heparin, unless contraindicated, for all obese parturients following CD at greater than 6 hours.[40] If VTE is diagnosed, weight-based low molecular weight heparin twice daily is typically used for the treatment, with the option of transitioning to warfarin, which is acceptable even in the setting of lactation.

Breastfeeding

Breastfeeding is especially recommended to improve the short- and long-term health outcomes for overweight/obese women and their offspring. Unfortunately, both maternal obesity and CD are associated with delayed onset of lactogenesis II and have been reported as negative factors in rates of breastfeeding initiation and breastfeeding at 6 months, with a 20% decreased likelihood in the obese population.[41] While reduced breastfeeding is a multifactorial issue, breastfeeding within the first hour of life to improve lactation initiation is recommended by the World Health Organization and American Academy of Pediatricians. Thus, providing the same level of immediate postdelivery bonding and breastfeeding support for women undergoing CD as for those experiencing vaginal delivery is both medically indicated and ethical. Hospitals without protocols, personnel, or a culture prioritizing the importance of the mother-infant dyad in the postoperative period contribute to the decreased success in breastfeeding initiation.

RISKS TO THE SURGEON AND TEAM

Ergonomic Concerns in CD

While the operating room environment is designed with the patient's safety as top priority, the well-being of the surgeons and surgical staff should not be ignored. Obesity can complicate even the routine tasks of the surgical team, primarily posing risks to them for musculoskeletal injuries during transport and surgery. Movement of the obese parturient after placement of anesthesia can be difficult. In addition, leftward tilt may decrease access for the primary operating surgeon; if right handed, the surgeon is operating typically from the patient's right side. Both the width and the depth of the operative field may be increased, especially in the setting of class III obesity. As the typically upright operating stances may not allow for sufficient visualization, leaning postures from higher vantage points on raised stepstools may create additional strain on the surgeon's back and legs. The changes in upper body and core muscle mechanics required in delivering an often-macrosomic neonate, usually with less-effective fundal pressure if the abdominal wall is substantially thicker, have not been described well in the obstetrical literature.

There are few data on the topic of musculoskeletal injuries to the surgeon and fewer on the effects of chronic strain over years of treating obese patients. In one study of young surgeons, more than half stated they had no official training in handling patients.[42] A recent opinion piece in the *New York Times* on the dangers of obesity in pregnancy offered an anecdote of an obstetrician who dislocated his shoulder during a CD on a patient weighing over 400 lb.[43] While the surgical literature contains several studies on the ergonomics of laparoscopy, there are almost none describing the side effects of the potential contortions necessary for the successful completion of a CD. One study surveying obstetrician/gynecologists practicing in the United Kingdom reported 2 times the rate of surgeon injury from CD than from operative laparoscopy, although the unspecified category was the most common.[44]

Pregnant Surgeons

An additional consideration in the operating room should be the pregnant surgeon. The majority of residents graduating in the United States are female, and a study from a decade ago reported a 15% pregnancy rate during residency alone.[45] Among obstetricians in their first decade of practice, a significant proportion are likely to experience pregnancy and will continue to practice during most of the gestation period. Ergonomic strategies, such as stools to lean against during surgery, more frequent position changes, and greater utilization of self-retaining retractors, may help avoid musculoskeletal injuries while operating on obese patients during advanced months of pregnancy. Strategies for injury prevention in pregnant obstetricians should be evaluated by outcomes such as work-related pain and antepartum work absences that may detract from planned maternity leave.

Infectious Exposures

Obesity may also increase opportunities for infectious exposures due to suboptimal visualization of the operative field. Studies evaluating percutaneous exposures for surgical staff via needlesticks during CD have been mixed in their conclusions. A Cochrane review that included 10 randomized controlled trials of multiple varied surgical procedures covering 2961 surgeries concluded that blunt needles resulted in significantly fewer exposures, reporting that blunt needles will prevent 1 glove perforation in every 6 operations employed.[46] Although this has not been studied exclusively in the setting of obesity, blunt needles should be considered a reasonable change of practice for safety.

TRIAL OF LABOR AFTER CESAREAN DELIVERY

Success and Risks

Given the higher incidence of CD in the obese population, providers should anticipate discussions regarding a trial of labor after cesarean (TOLAC). Attempting a vaginal birth after cesarean (VBAC) in the setting of obesity remains controversial. Published success rates of a trial of labor are consistently lower in this population, ranging from 39% to 64%,[47] but may be even lower in women with BMI greater than 50.[48]

One of the largest multicenter studies from the Maternal-Fetal Medicine Units Network reported on over 14,000 patients undergoing a trial of labor. Both maternal and neonatal complications rose along with body mass. Compared to those with normal BMI, women with a BMI greater than 40 had a higher failure rate (39.3% vs. 15.2%), uterine rupture/dehiscence (2.1% vs. 0.4%), and composite maternal morbidity (7.2% vs. 3.8%), which included transfusion, uterine infection, surgical injury, rupture/dehiscence, hysterectomy, thromboembolic disease, and length of stay longer than 3 days. In addition, the risk for neonatal injury was higher (1.1% vs. 0.2%), which included fractures, brachial plexus injuries, and lacerations. No differences in neonatal encephalopathy were seen[47] (see Table 21-1).

Obesity-Specific Counseling

While the increased failure rate may be related to the same factors implicated in the higher rate of CD overall in this population, additional safety concerns include challenges of continuous fetal monitoring due to abdominal girth, higher rates of uterine

TABLE 21-1 Risks of TOLAC in Obese Women Compared to Women With a Normal BMI[a]

Risks	Nonobese (%)	Morbid Obese (%)
Successful VBAC	84.8	60.7
Uterine rupture/dehiscence	0.4	2.1
Composite maternal morbidity	3.8	7.2
Neonatal injury	0.2	1.1

[a]From Hibbard JU, Gilbert S, Landon MB, et al. National Institute of Child Health and Human Development Maternal-Fetal Medicine Units Network. Trial of labor or repeat cesarean delivery in women with morbid obesity and previous cesarean delivery. *Obstet Gynecol.* 2006;108(1):125–133.

rupture, and, most commonly, the technical challenges associated with attempting emergency repeat CD once an acute fetal concern is recognized and has not resolved with intrauterine resuscitation. Given the potential for physician bias affecting lack of access to trial of labor for all women, it is important to be transparent and evidence based with any stated recommendations. Being specific about obesity-related concerns, discussing future childbearing plans, and utilizing tools such as the online calculator based on the National Institute of Child Health Data (https://mfmu.bsc.gwu.edu/PublicBSC/MFMU/VGBirthCalc/vagbirth.html) are all suggested in the shared decision-making process surrounding TOLAC.

MODE OF DELIVERY AND OBESITY IN OFFSPRING

Although discussion of the risks of CD in the obese population has centered primarily on the woman's perioperative complications and her own future health risks, a growing body of research examines the effects of mode of delivery on the health of her offspring. As the rate of childhood obesity has accelerated globally over recent generations, epidemiologists have looked for environmental or epigenetic causes for this phenomenon.

Several articles have associated CD is with differences in health outcomes for offspring, such as increased asthma and atopy.[49] Differences in intestinal flora in infants and children, noted by some authors to vary in composition depending on vaginal versus CD, have been hypothesized to be a mechanism for the development of obesity.[49] In one prospective study of 1244 mother-child pairs, CD was associated with an increased risk of obesity at age 3 (OR 2.10, 95% CI 1.36–3.23), even while adjusting for maternal BMI, birth weight, maternal age, education, race/ethnicity, and child age and sex.[50] A meta-analysis of 28 studies showed this effect to be modest, RR 1.34 (CI 1.18–1.51) and likely affected by heterogeneity of studies and how confounding variables were addressed.[50] While this line of inquiry is still in its infancy, it provides further motivation to avoid the unnecessary CD and to search for possible methods to duplicate the benefits of vaginal delivery for children born by CD.

SUMMARY

Obesity in pregnancy is associated with an increased risk of cesarean delivery and greater perioperative complications with potential consequences for the lifelong health of mother and child. Awareness of these risks is important first step for both patients and medical staff. The historically recent rise in overweight and obesity in reproductive age women is a challenging hurdle in the effort to lower overall cesarean rates. Further research is needed to evaluate strategies to optimize preconceptual and antepartum care to avoid possibly preventable cesarean deliveries. Ultimately, there is a need for well-designed studies of perioperative care and surgical techniques in the obese population to achieve further improvements in birth outcomes.

REFERENCES

1. Placek PJ, Taffel SM. Trends in cesarean section rates for the United States, 1970–78. *Public Health Rep.* 1980 Nov–Dec;95(6):540–548.
2. Hamilton BE, Martin JA, OstermanMJ, Curtin SC. Births: preliminary data for 2014. *Natl Vital Stat Rep.* 2015;64(6):1–19.
3. National Center for Health Statistics. Obesity and overweight. http://www.cdc.gov/nchs/fastats/obesity-overweight.htm. Accessed June 10, 2015.
4. Weiss JL, Malone FD, Emig D, et al. FASTER Research Consortium. Obesity, obstetric complications and cesarean delivery rate—a population-based screening study. *Am J Obstet Gynecol.* 2004 Apr;190(4):1091–1097.
5. Crane JM, Murphy P, Burrage L, Hutchens D. Maternal and perinatal outcomes of extreme obesity in pregnancy. *J Obstet Gynaecol Can.* 2013 Jul;35(7):606–611.
6. Stamilio DM, Scifres CM. Extreme obesity and postcesarean maternal complications. *Obstet Gynecol.* 2014 Aug;124(2 Pt 1):227–232.
7. El-Chaar D, Finkelstein SA, Tu X, et al. The impact of increasing obesity class on obstetrical outcomes. *J Obstet Gynaecol Can.* 2013 Mar;35(3):224–233.
8. Chu SY, Kim SY, Schmid CH, et al. Maternal obesity and risk of cesarean delivery: a meta-analysis. *Obes Rev.* 2007 Sep;8(5):385–394.
9. LaCoursiere DY, Bloebaum L, Duncan JD, Varner MW. Population-based trends and correlates of maternal overweight and obesity, Utah 1991–2001. *Am J Obstet Gynecol.* 2005;192:832–839.
10. Cedergren MI. Non-elective caesarean delivery due to ineffective uterine contractility or due to obstructed labour in relation to maternal body mass index. *Eur J Obstet Gynecol Reprod Biol.* 2009 Aug;145(2):163–166.
11. Mission JF, Marshall NE, Caughey AB. Pregnancy risks associated with obesity. *Obstet Gynecol Clin N Am.* 2015;42:335–353.
12. Scott-Pillai R, Spence D, Cardwell CR, Hunter A, Holmes VA. The impact of body mass index on maternal and neonatal outcomes: a retrospective study in a UK obstetric population, 2004–2011. *BJOG.* 2013 Jul;120(8):932–939.
13. Pierpont YN, Dinh TP, Salas RE, et al. Obesity and surgical wound healing: a current review. *ISRN Obes.* 2014 Feb 20;2014:638936.
14. Girsen AI, Osmundson SS, Naqvi M, Garabedian MJ, Lyell DJ. Body mass index and operative times at cesarean delivery. *Obstet Gynecol.* 2014 Oct;124(4):684–689.
15. Naef RW 3rd, Chauhan SP, Chevalier SP, Roberts WE, Meydrech EF, Morrison JC. Prediction of hemorrhage at cesarean delivery. *Obstet Gynecol.* 1994;83:923–926.
16. James AH, Jamison MG, Brancazio LR, Myers ER. Venous thromboembolism during pregnancy and the postpartum period: incidence, risk factors, and mortality. *Am J Obstet Gynecol.* 2006;194:1311–1315.
17. Committee on Patient Safety and Quality Improvement. Committee Opinion No. 629: Clinical guidelines and standardization of practice to improve outcomes. *Obstet Gynecol.* 2015 Apr;125(4):1027–9.
18. Nelson SM, Fleming RF. The preconceptual contraception paradigm: obesity and infertility. *Hum Reprod.* 2007 Apr;22(4):912–915.
19. Curtin SC, Gregory KD, Korst LM, Uddin SF. Maternal morbidity for vaginal and cesarean deliveries, according to previous cesarean history: new data from the birth certificate, 2013. *Natl Vital Stat Rep.* 2015;64(4):1–13.
20. Thangaratinam S, Jolly K. Obesity in pregnancy: a review of reviews on the effectiveness of interventions. *BJOG.* 2010 Oct;117(11):1309–1312.
21. Dodd JM, Turnbull D, McPhee AJ, et al. LIMIT Randomised Trial Group. Antenatal lifestyle advice for women who are overweight or obese: LIMIT randomised trial. *BMJ.* 2014 Feb 10;348:g1285.
22. Dodd JM, Grivell RM, Deussen AR, Dekker G, Louise J, Hague W. Metformin and dietary advice to improve insulin sensitivity and promote gestational restriction of weight among pregnant women who are overweight or obese: the GRoW Randomised Trial.BMC Pregnancy Childbirth. 2016 Nov 21;16(1):359.
23. Tan T, Sia AT. Anesthesia considerations in the obese gravida. *Semin Perinatol.* 2011;35(6):350–355.
24. Johnson D. Management of cesarean delivery in the morbidly obese woman. *Contemp Obstet Gynecol.* 2012 Oct 21.
25. American College of Obstetricians and Gynecologists. ACOG Practice Bulletin No. 120: Use of prophylactic antibiotics in labor and delivery. *Obstet Gynecol.* 2011 Jun;117(6):1472–83.

26. Pevzner L, Swank M, Krepel C, Wing DA, Chan K, Edmiston CE Jr. Effects of maternal obesity on tissue concentrations of prophylactic cefazolin during cesarean delivery. *Obstet Gynecol.* 2011;117(4):877–882.

27. Marrs CC. Moussa HN, Sibai BM, Blackwell SC. The relationship between primary cesarean delivery skin type and wound complications in women with morbid obesity. *Am J Obstet Gynecol.* 2014 Apr;210(4):319.

28. Alanis MC, Villers MS, Law TL, Steadman EM, Robinson CJ. Complications of cesarean delivery in the massively obese parturient. *Am J Obstet Gynecol.* 2010;203(3):271.e1–271.e7.

29. Brocato BE, Thorpe EM Jr, Gomez LM, Wan JY, Mari G. The effect of cesarean delivery skin incision approach in morbidly obese women on the rate of classical hysterotomy. *J Pregnancy.* 2013;2013:890296.

30. Tixier H, Thouvenot S, Coulange L, et al. Cesarean section in morbidly obese women: supra or subumbilical transverse incision? *Acta Obstet Gynecol Scand.* 2009;88(9):1049–1052.

31. Chelnow D, Rodriguez EJ, Sabatini MM. Suture closure of subcutaneous fat and wound disruption after cesarean delivery: a meta-analysis. *Obstet Gynecol.* 2004;103(5 Pt 1):974–980.

32. Gates S, Anderson ER. Wound drainage for caesarean section. *Cochrane Database Syst Rev.* 2005;(1):CD004549.

33. Figueroa D, Chapman Jauk V, Szychowski JM, et al. Surgical staples compared with subcuticular suture for skin closure after cesarean delivery: a randomized controlled trial. *Obstet Gynecol.* 2013 Jan;121(1):33–38.

34. Mackeen AD, Schuster M, Berghella V. Suture versus staples for skin closure after cesarean: a metaanalysis. *Am J Obstet Gynecol.* 2015 May; 212(5):621.e1–10.

35. Nuthalapaty FS, Lee CM, Lee JH, Kuper SG, Higdon HL 3rd. A randomized control trial of early versus delayed skin staple removal following cesarean section in the obese patient. *J Obstet Gynaecol Can.* 2013 May;35(5):426–433.

36. Mark KS, Alger L, Terplan M. Incisional negative pressure therapy to prevent wound complications following cesarean section in morbidly obese women: a pilot study. *Surg Innov.* 2014 Aug;21(4):345–349.

37. Tuffaha HW, Gillespie BM, Chaboyer W, Gordon LG, Scuffham PA. Cost-utility analysis of negative pressure wound therapy in high-risk cesarean section wounds. *J Surg Res.* 2015 May 15;195(2):612–622.

38. Haas DM, Morgan S, Contreras K. Vaginal preparation with antiseptic solution before cesarean section for preventing postoperative infections. *Cochrane Database Syst Rev.* 2014 Dec 21;(12):CD007892.

39. Conner SN, Verticchio JC, Tuuli MG, Odibo AO, Macones GA, Cahill AG. Maternal obesity and risk of postcesarean wound complications. *Am J Perinatol.* 2014 Apr 3;31(4):299–304.

40. American College of Obstetricians and Gynecologists. Safe Motherhood Initiative venous thromboembolism risk assessment and prophylaxis. https://www.acog.org/-/media/Districts/District-II/Public/SMI/v2/VTESlideSetNov2015.pdf?dmc=1&ts=201611 29T1753496911. Accessed February 15, 2015.

41. Bever Babendure J, Reifsnider E, Mendias E, Moramarco MW, Davila YR. Reduced breastfeeding rates among obese mothers: a review of contributing factors, clinical considerations and future directions. *Int Breastfeed J.* 2015;10:21.

42. De Bono JP, Hudsmith LE, de Bono AM. Back pain in preregistration house officers. *Occup Med.* 2001;51:62–65.

43. Putnam CA. Pregnant, obese . . . and in danger. *New York Times.* 2015 Mar 28.

44. Yoong W, Sanchez-Crespo J, Rob J, et al. Sticks and stones may break my bones: work-related orthopedic injuries sustained during obstetrics and gynecology training. *J Obstet Gynecol.* July 2008;28(5):478–481.

45. Finch SJ. Pregnancy during residency: a literature review. *Acad Med.* 2003;78:418–428.

46. Parantainen A, Verbeek JH, Lavoie MC, Pahwa M. Blunt versus sharp suture needles for preventing percutaneous exposure incidents in surgical staff. *Cochrane Database Syst Rev.* 2011 Nov 9;(11):CD009170.

47. Hibbard JU, Gilbert S, Landon MB, et al. National Institute of Child Health and Human Development Maternal-Fetal Medicine Units Network. Trial of labor or repeat cesarean delivery in women with morbid obesity and previous cesarean delivery. *Obstet Gynecol.* 2006;108(1):125–133.

48. Chauhan SP1, Magann EF, Carroll CS, Barrilleaux PS, Scardo JA, Martin JN Jr. Mode of delivery for the morbidly obese with prior cesarean delivery: vaginal versus repeat cesarean section. *Am J Obstet Gynecol.* 2001 Aug;185(2):349–354.

49. Huh SY, Rifas-Shiman SL, Zera CA, et al. Delivery by caesarean section and risk of obesity in preschool age children: a prospective cohort study. *Arch Dis Child.* 2012 Jul;97(7):610–616.

50. Kuhle S, Tong OS, Woolcott CG. Association between caesarean section and childhood obesity: a systematic review and meta-analysis. *Obes Rev.* 2015 Apr;16(4):295–303.

CHAPTER 22

Endocrine Disorders in Pregnancy

Alan D. Bolnick, MD

Satinder Kaur, MD

Elizabeth E. Puscheck, MD

INTRODUCTION

Pregnancy results in multiple normal physiologic changes, and these changes may have an impact on the diagnosis, evaluation, or treatment of endocrine disorders. Pregnancy itself is the result of, and maintained by, a well-choreographed set of endocrine signaling. Ovulation results from the orchestration of signaling from the hypothalamus, pituitary, ovary, and uterus axis. Pregnancy occurs when the ovulated egg is fertilized and implants in the previously prepared endometrium. Pregnancy continues through the first half of the first trimester dependent on the corpus luteum. The rest of pregnancy is maintained by placental hormonal support.

A clinical challenge occurs in the diagnosis and treatment of endocrine disorders during pregnancy because many of the symptoms of the endocrine diseases are common symptoms in pregnancy. Physiologic changes of pregnancy affect the chemistry and biology of the pituitary, thyroid, and adrenal hormones, which hampers the identification of these endocrine dysfunctions and their treatment. A deep understanding of the biology of pregnancy and endocrinology is needed to diagnose and treat these patients well.

Endocrine disorders may be affected by the gestational state, with its large quantities of pregnancy-secreted hormones, increased overall plasma volume, hypermetabolic state, and altered hormonal feedback mechanisms. This chapter reviews the impact of pregnancy on endocrine diseases with the exception of diabetes, which is discussed separately in a different chapter because it is the most prevalent endocrinopathy. Thyroid disorder is the next most frequent endocrinopathy of reproductive-aged women. Our chapter starts with thyroid disease, followed by parathyroid disease, adrenal disorder, and finally by pituitary disorders.

THYROID PHYSIOLOGY IN PREGNANCY

Pregnancy alters both normal thyroid function and thyroid diseases in 3 main ways: changes in iodine physiology; increases in pregnancy hormone (human chorionic gonadotropin, hCG), which simulates thyroid hormone; and increases in thyroxine-binding globulin (TBG) affect the amount of free hormone.

Brief Review of the Normal Hypothalamic-Pituitary-Thyroid System

The thyroid gland is located in the lower front of the neck, just below the larynx; it comprises two lobes connected by the isthmus. The lobes are divided into lobules containing follicular cells, which produce a glycoprotein material called colloid into the follicular lumen. The thyroid gland extracts iodine from dietary intake to incorporate into the thyroid hormone to produce two hormones: thyroxine (T_4, which has 4 iodine molecules) or triiodothyronine (T_3, which has 3 iodine molecules). These hormones are stored in the thyroid until needed. T_3 is made from T_4 by cleaving 1 iodine molecule.

Regulation of thyroid function occurs through the hypothalamic-pituitary-thyroid axis. Within the paraventricular nucleus of the hypothalamus, thyrotropin-releasing hormone (TRH) is created and is regulated by tonic stimulation in response to positive/negative feedback (Figure 22-1). TRH is secreted via the pituitary portal circulation, where it acts as an agonist on anterior pituitary thyrotrope cells. It modulates the

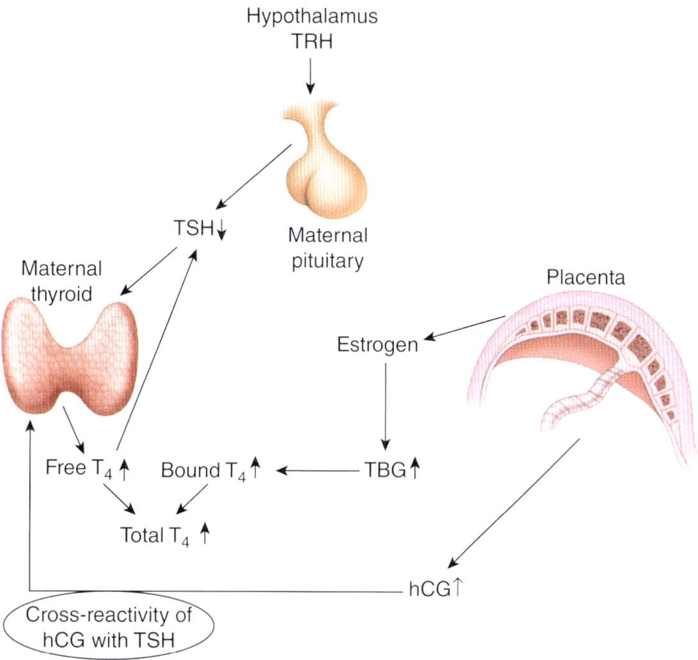

FIGURE 22-1. Thyroid releasing hormones.

manufacture and distribution of thyrotropin (also known as thyroid-stimulating hormone, TSH). This glycoprotein, like all anterior pituitary hormones, is composed of α and β subunits. The unique β subunits of anterior pituitary hormones are exploited in developing specific chemical assays to differentiate endocrine hormones. In particular, the measurement of TSH is critical because it acts as a master regulator of the thyroid gland in both normal physiology and its disease states. TSH is secreted from the anterior pituitary into the peripheral circulation, where it reaches its target organ, the thyroid gland.

TSH regulates thyroid function. In addition, TSH is regulated by a negative-feedback loop, not only from circulating thyroid hormone, but also by somatostatin and dopamine. In this way, TSH acts as a master regulator. TSH mediates thyroid gland production of T_4 and T_3. TSH induces thyroid growth and differentiation, as well as modulates iodine metabolism. Ingested iodine is condensed to iodide, which is absorbed and cleared by the kidney (80%) and thyroid (20%). Iodide is the rate-limiting step in thyroid hormone biosynthesis. Thyroid peroxidase (TPO), an enzyme produced by the thyroid gland, oxidizes iodide, converting it back to iodine, and facilitates its attachment to tyrosyl residues located on the glycoprotein, thyroglobulin. Iodination of thyroglobulin gives rise to monoiodotyrosine or di-iodotyrosine; by coupling these molecules, either T_3 or T_4 is formed.

Thyroid-stimulating hormone regulates hormone secretion by thyroid cells, with degradation of thyroglobulin and extrusion of T_4 and T_3 into the capillaries. Both are distributed to target organs tightly bound to the protein TBG. Removal of an iodine by 5′-monodeiodination from the outer ring of T_4 results in T_3, which is metabolically active. Unbound hormone (or the free form of the thyroid hormone) is the active state and can enter cells. Thyroxine (T_4) completely originates in the thyroid gland, while only 20% of T_3 originates in the thyroid and 80% is derived from peripheral conversion. Thyroxine is metabolized in most tissues (particularly in the liver and kidneys) to T_3 by deionization. In a normal situation, approximately 35% of T_4 is converted to T_3, and 40% is converted to reverse T_3. Some disorders favor the metabolically inert reverse T_3, such as generalized illnesses, starvation, or other catabolic states.[1]

The half-life of T_4 is 1 week. Typically, 3 to 4 half-lives are needed prior to reaching a steady state in the circulation. This information is important when monitoring and treating thyroid disorders. Any change in dose for T_4 therapy will require at least a month to reach a steady state in T_4 values. Free thyroid hormone, particularly T_3, has greater biologic activity and binds to intracellular nuclear receptors, which turn on downstream genes.[2,3] These intracellular nuclear receptors that are affiliated with the active thyroxine hormone are part of a large group of steroid-hormone receptors that includes other endocrine steroid hormones, vitamin D, and retinoic acid receptors.

Maternal Physiologic Changes in Thyroid Function

Pregnancy has a major impact on maternal thyroid physiology (Table 22-1). There is a 30% increase in thyroid gland size by the end of the pregnancy.[4] This change in size occurs mainly by glandular hyperplasia; in addition, there is increased vascularity of the thyroid gland.[4] The thyroid reverts to its baseline size in the postpartum period.[4] During pregnancy, the thyroid gland produces up to double the normal thyroxine amount to meet the requirements of the maternal and fetal unit.[5] Approximately 0.2%–5% of pregnancies will be affected by a thyroid disorder. In 10%–20% of these pregnancies, TPO antibodies form, and about half of these patients will develop autoimmune thyroiditis, which may result in permanent thyroid failure.

Pregnancy significantly increases the production of thyroglobulin (TBG) and its serum concentrations. Thus, laboratory assays reflect these chemistry alterations influenced by increased serum TBG concentration, which include total thyroxine (TT_4), total triiodothyronine (TT_3), and resin triiodothyronine uptake (RT_3U). Although the increased TBG concentrations increase the overall total serum thyroxine

TABLE 22-1 Changes in Thyroid Function Parameters in Normal Pregnancy and in Thyroid Endocrinopathies

Maternal Status	TSH (Initial Screening Test)	Free T_4	Free Thyroxine Index (FTI)	Total T_4	Total T_3	Resin Triiodo-Thyronine Uptake (RT3U)
Pregnancy	No change	No change	No change	Increase	Increase	Decrease
Hyperthyroidism	Decrease	Increase	Increase	Increase	Increase or no change	Increase
Hypothyroidism	Increase	Decrease	Decrease	Decrease	Decrease or no change	Decrease
Subclinical hypothyroidism	Increase	Normal	Normal	Increase	Increase	Decrease

and triiodothyronine, the concentrations of serum free T_4 and T_3 are not significantly different. Total T_4 concentrations reach the highest levels at 18 weeks. Free thyroxine (FT_4) and free thyroxine index (FTI) tend to have transient changes that reflect hCG stimulation.[6]

Thyroid function is altered during the antenatal period. Inadequate maternal adaptations to these changes result in thyroid dysfunction and pregnancy complications. With an enhanced excretion based on the kidney glomerular filtration rate (GFR) changes during pregnancy, iodine is more rapidly metabolized, so there is less iodine available. Iodide levels reflect the fetal usage and increased maternal renal clearance of iodide.[6] Fetal cord T_4 levels at delivery are 20% of maternal origin.[7]

Pregnancy establishes a milieu that enhances TBG production, reaching its zenith at 20 weeks, which doubles the baseline levels and remains at this level during the rest of the pregnancy,[8] because of both the higher hepatic synthesis from the estrogen stimulus and diminished metabolic rate due to elevated TBG sialylation and glycosylation. Elevated levels of total serum T_4 and T_3 are ultimately reflected by these hormonal changes, with increased TBG binding sites incorporating additional T_3. There are fewer to bind to resin, which results in diminished T_3 resin uptake (indirect laboratory measure of available TBG) in the gravid state. The FTI (calculated as the product of the total T_4 and T_3 resin uptake) is unchanged in pregnancy. The normal reference range for total T_4 should be adjusted by a factor of 1.5 for pregnant patients.

The highly sensitive TSH and FT_4 laboratory assessments are the most widely used chemistries to appraise thyroid function in pregnancy. The American Thyroid Association (ATA) guidelines provide trimester-specific reference ranges for TSH, as described in populations with adequate iodine intake, as follows: 0.1 to 2.5 mIU/L in the first trimester, 0.2 to 3.0 mIU/L in the second trimester, and 0.3 to 3.0 mIU/L in the third trimester.[9] The results of the analysis of measuring FT_4 by equilibrium dialysis showed that FT_4 is not affected by the protein changes seen with pregnancy.

Free T_3 (FT_3) levels are informative. Elevated FT_3 will result in suppressed TSH, suggesting overproduction of thyroid hormones. The third-generation TSH assays are sensitive to differentiate both thyroid overactivity (low TSH) and suppression (high TSH). With the dominance of hCG agonist effects seen early in the pregnancy, FT_3 and T_4 concentrations can be elevated. The levels of FT_4 tend to fall through the rest of pregnancy to the lower limits of normal.

Increased quantities of FT_4 in the gravid state can mitigate the hypothalamic TRH and diminish pituitary TSH secretion. Total or bound thyroid hormone values parallel the rising maternal serum concentration of TBG. Early in the pregnancy, there is an elevation of hCG, which is a weak TSH agonist and results in increased thyroxine production.[10] Then, the increased thyroxine provides negative feedback to the pituitary, with subsequent lowering of TSH. The addition of about 10,000 IU/L of hCG results in the homologous binding to TSH receptors and increased production of thyroxine, which lowers the basal TSH level by 0.1 mU/L and has little ramification on the pregnancy.[11]

The level of hCG peaks at the end of the first trimester. The alterations in concentrations of TSH and hCG are interdependent due to the homology of the α subunits, and these concentrations depend on gestational age Consequently, hCG has intrinsic thyrotropic activity, which causes thyroid hormone activation. The subsequent rise in the serum FT_4 level then has an antagonist effect on the pituitary TSH secretion and the hypothalamus TRH results through negative feedback. TSH tends to have a modest rise after the first trimester and gradually rises further in the third trimester, which is stimulated by placental growth and production of placental deiodinase.[12] Normal hormonal changes during pregnancy result in elevation thyroxine (T_4) and triiodothyronine (T_3) levels.

Early in the pregnancy, thyroxine demands increase based on the increased plasma volume changes, thyroid hormone metabolism, and stimulatory effects of estrogen on hepatic production of the TBG.[13] By the beginning of the second trimester of pregnancy, total T_4 and T_3 concentrations have reached their peaks, which reflects stimulatory effects of high amounts of TBG.[8] TBG increases by 3-fold during pregnancy, which mirrors the influence of rising circulating estrogen concentrations and subsequent reduction of hepatic clearance along with a change in its half-life (15 minutes to 3 days) during pregnancy.[8] There are rising values of the total T_4 and T_3 due to increases in TBG and a parallel rise in FT_4, reflecting both the increase in TBG and the functioning fetal thyroid in the second part of the pregnancy.

Modifications in the peripheral metabolism of thyroid hormones occur throughout pregnancy but are more prominent in the second half of gestation. Three enzymes result in the deiodinization of thyroid hormones: types I, II, and III deiodinases. Of these three, types II and III iodinases are particularly important. Type II deiodinases are expressed in the placenta and can maintain T_3 production locally. Type III deiodinases, also produced by the placenta, are noted to be cytoprotective of the gestation by converting T_4 to biologically inert reverse T_3 in the periphery[14] and altering T_3 to T_4.[8]

Thyroid hormone and its metabolic pathways are instrumental in fetal central nervous system development. Rodent studies illustrate abnormal neuronal migration and behavioral dysfunction associated with a maternal hypothyroidism state.[15] Although histological maturity of the fetal thyroid gland is documented by the beginning of the second trimester, fetal thyroid hormone levels do not increase significantly until later in the pregnancy.[16] Research suggests that maternal hypothyroidism early in the pregnancy can have an impact on cerebral delays when the infant is 1 and 2 years.[13]

THYROID DISORDERS AND RELATED PHYSIOLOGY IN PREGNANCY

Thyroid disorders can cause adversities in pregnancy, in both the maternal and the fetal components. Surplus production of thyroid hormones results in the biochemical condition denoted as thyrotoxicosis. Thyrotoxicosis is caused by an overactive thyroid gland, which is also referred to as hyperthyroidism. Graves disease is an autoimmune disorder portrayed by a production of thyroid-stimulating immunoglobulin (TSI) and thyroid-stimulating hormone-binding inhibitory immunoglobulin (TBII), which modulate the TSH mechanism to facilitate thyroid stimulation or inhibition, respectively. A significant complication of hyperthyroidism is thyroid storm. An insufficient state of thyroid hormone production is described as hypothyroidism. Autoimmune inflammation of the thyroid may cause hypothyroidism or may initially cause thyrotoxicosis followed by hypothyroidism existing within a year following delivery, the last is commonly referred to as postpartum thyroiditis (PPT).[17] Polyendocrinopathies are unique autoimmune disorders that increase the risk of developing other endocrine diseases. For example, there is 25% chance of PPT in patients with type 1 diabetes.[18]

The presence of a maternal endocrinopathy is important information for the pediatrician to have at the time of delivery.

Frequent monitoring (i.e., every 4–6 weeks) of thyroid function in patients with thyroid disorders is particularly important during the gestational period and allows for meticulous regulation of the pharmaceuticals given to the maternal component and promotes the well-being of the fetus. Uncontrolled endocrinopathies in pregnancy, including thyrotoxicosis and hypothyroidism, have been associated with adverse outcomes. Thyroid disorders, both overt and subclinical, may have an impact on fetal development. Thyroid medications can cross the placenta barrier and thus can influence the fetal thyroid.[17]

Iodine Deficiency and Goiter in Pregnancy

In the gravid state, there are significant alterations in iodine metabolism. A deficiency in iodine may be manifested by low thyroxine and elevated TSH values. Goiter is produced due to iodine deficiency or other thyroid abnormality. There are 1 to 1.5 billion people in the world at risk of iodine deficiency, and 500 million live in areas of overt iodine deficiency. The World Health Organization recommends 150 µg of iodine per day for adults and 250 µg for pregnant and lactating women which is also endorsed by the Endocrine Society.[18,19]

Increased requirements for iodine in the gravid patient are heightened by increased thyroid hormone production, increased renal losses, and fetal demands. Pregnancy is associated with doubling of renal iodine clearance and a 50% increase in GFR secondary to the changes in renal blood flow and a significant amount of iodine being utilized by the fetus to produce its own thyroid hormones. Iodine deficiency is seen with further changes associated with hypothyroxinemia, which increases TSH and thyroglobulin levels and produces thyroid hypertrophy. Mild decreases in iodine have not been associated with cranial abnormalities. Goiter associated with iodine deficiency is preventable with adequate supplies of this substance.[20]

Significant shortage of iodine in pregnancy has been associated with adverse disorders and with endemic cretinism.[21] Studies have implicated abnormal levels of iodine with central nervous system (CNS) irregularities; as such, iodine deficiency is an important etiology for preventable causes of disrupted neurological development after food shortage periods.[22] Neurological studies showed improvement in newborns exposed to iodine deficiencies in underdeveloped countries when pregnant mothers received iodine supplementation early in gestation.[23]

In addition to iodine deficiency, goiter in pregnancy can be related to the following conditions: Graves disease, Hashimoto thyroiditis, excessive iodine intake, lymphocytic thyroiditis, and thyroid cancer. Pregnancy does not appear to increase the risk for the development of goiters.[24] Excessive ingestion of iodine has been associated with hypothyroidism and autoimmune thyroiditis.[25] The fetus relies on maternal thyroid hormone prior to 12 weeks; thus studies showed the importance of thyroxine for neurodevelopment in offspring, especially in iodine-shortage pregnancies.[3]

Placental-Fetal Thyroid Physiology

The thyroid gland in the fetus forms as a midline outpouching of the anterior pharyngeal floor and reaches its final position by 7 weeks' gestation. Iodine trapping is recognized by week 12, and T_4 production is noted by week 14. The pituitary portal circulation is functional by 10 weeks, and hypothalamic TRH is produced 1–2 weeks earlier. The fetal thyroid gland's iodine uptake and serum T_4 concentrations begin to increase at midgestation.[3] The measurable concentrations of fetal T_4 and FT_4 are at 10 µg/dL and 1.5 ng/dL at term, respectively. Increases in T_3 and FT_3 are smaller, presumably because of the availability of placental type III deiodinase; thus, most fetal T_4 is inactivated to reverse T_3. Fetal tissues that depend on T_3 for development (e.g., brain structures) are supplied by local T_4-to-T_3 conversion by type II deiodinase.[26] Concentrations of fetal TSH, TBG, FT_4, and FT_3 rise throughout gestation analogous to maternal levels, with the peak reported at approximately 36 weeks of gestation.[27]

There are physiological separations between fetal and maternal units that protect the fetus from hormonal excess, keeping the milieu in a euthyroid environment.[13] The placenta acts as a barrier to maternal hormones such as TSH and only warrants passage of minimal quantities of T_4 and T_3. The placenta is porous to TRH, iodine, and TSH receptor immunoglobulins along with thioamides (propylthiouracil [PTU] and methimazole).

Analysis of coelomic and amniotic fluid indicated total T_4 and T_3 are significantly lower than maternal serum levels, whereas FT_4 levels in the fetus are comparable to the mother's concentrations, reflecting the lower amount of T_4-binding proteins in the fetus.[28] Maternal TSH has no influence on the fetus because it is not able to cross the placenta. Maternal thyroxine is transported to the fetus throughout the entire gestational period.[14] Fetal brain development is dependent on maternal thyroxine distribution through the placenta prior to the autonomy of the fetal thyroid gland mechanism, which typically occurs at the end of the first trimester.[29] Fetal thyroxine concentrations in the third trimester remain dependent on maternal levels of the thyroid hormone.[30] The maintenance of maternal thyroid hormones crossing the placenta enables newborns with congenital hypothyroidism (CH) to thwart overt stigmata of hypothyroidism at birth despite cord blood thyroid hormone levels at approximately half of normal concentrations.[31]

Autoimmunity and Thyroid Disease

The TSIs attach to the TSH receptor and stimulate its mechanism to cause hyperactivation of the thyroid gland. Neonatal Graves disorder can be seen secondary to TSIs crossing the placenta. Overproduction of TBIIs can cause maternal and neonatal hypothyroidism.[32] Antithyroid antibodies of this autoimmune disorder occur most often to thyroglobulin and to TPO (anti-TPO).[33] The incidence of these antibodies identified in pregnancy ranges from 5% to 15%.[34] Controversy remains whether miscarriages and preterm delivery (PTD) can be attributed to these antibodies.[35] Postpartum thyroiditis is seen frequently in gravid women who develop positive anti-TPO early in the pregnancy.[36,37] There is up to a 20% incidence of autoantibodies to the thyroid gland and TPO in the reproductive-age women even though most of these women are euthyroid.[35] There is a paucity of reports regarding pregnancies being treated for this disorder and whether improvements in outcome occur. Thus, there are no recommendations for universal screening of thyroid autoimmune antibodies.[38] Mothers with Graves disease treated surgically or with radioactive iodine 131 prior to gestation[39] still tend to have increased frequency of newborns diagnosed with Graves disease due to crossing of antibodies and the lack of mitigating factors associated with a thioamide regimen. Conversely, Graves disease originating in the newborn does not affect the thyroid status of the mother.

Laboratory Testing of Thyroid Disease in Pregnancy

Laboratory assays used to diagnose thyroid disease in pregnancy should include third-generation TSH and FT_4 values. The third-generation TSH assay uses monoclonal antibodies for detection; this TSH assay is the gold standard in screening for thyroid function.[40] Pregnancy does not alter the free component of the thyroid hormone, which is the biologically active portion. FT_4 can be measured by either direct immunoradiometric or chemiluminescent methods and is readily available. Measurement of FT_3 usually is only pursued in patients with thyrotoxicosis with suppressed TSH but normal FT_4 measurements. T_3 toxicosis presents with excessive FT_3, which can precede FT_4 abnormalities.[41]

Typically, there is an inverse log-linear connection between serum TSH and serum thyroid hormone, assuming an intact and functioning hypothalamic-pituitary-thyroid axis. The third-generation TSH values are the most consistent gauge of the thyroid status because it is accurate for detecting both under- and overactive thyroid hormone production. FT_4 should be evaluated when the TSH values are outside the normal range. Pregnancy-specific normal ranges exist but are not referenced in many laboratories where FT_4 is assayed. Equilibrium dialysis for total T_4 measurements are most revealing in a gravid state. The measurement of T_4 in the dialysate or ultrafiltrate of serum samples incorporating tandem mass spectrometry liquid chromatography is the most reliable testing for thyroid dysfunction in pregnancy. In lieu of such specialized testing, serum TSH is more informative of thyroid function in pregnancy compared to any indirect FT_4 analysis.[42] Routine testing of antithyroid antibodies has not been recommended by most research studies and professional societies.[17]

HYPERTHYROIDISM IN PREGNANCY

Hyperthyroidism is seen in 0.2% of pregnancies. Graves disease is the etiology in over 95% of these cases.[6] This disorder is an organ-specific autoimmune disease associated with TSH receptor antibodies.[43] Assays for these antibodies have been suggested as part of the assessment for hyperthyroidism.[43] Elevated FT_4 or FTI levels with a low TSH level and the lack of a nodular goiter are generally the criteria used for the diagnosis of Graves disease. Documenting TSH receptor, antimicrosomal, or anti-TPO antibodies are accessary values that are not required for the diagnosis.[44] Excess production of TSH resulting in thyrotoxicosis can be caused by any of the following: gestational trophoblastic neoplasia, hyperfunctioning thyroid adenoma, toxic multinodular goiter, subacute thyroiditis, and extrathyroid source of thyroid hormone. Diagnostic chemistry values are consistent with elevation of T_4 and markedly depressed TSH in hyperthyroidism seen with pregnancy. With subnormal TSH values, it is recommended that Graves disease is clinically differentiated from gestational hyperthyroidism. Early in the pregnancy, a low TSH should alert the medical provider to perform a thorough history and physical examination and obtain a value for FT_4. Evaluating thyroid antibody assays and FT_3 may be beneficial in narrowing the differential diagnosis.[42] High thyroid-stimulating antibodies are seen in thyrotoxic individuals. Thyroid receptor antibodies freely cross the placenta. These antibodies should be evaluated in the second trimester if there is a maternal history of Graves disease, previous iodine 131 treatment, a prior pregnancy complicated by a fetus affected with Graves disease, and documented antibodies to the thyroid receptor.

During the second half of the pregnancy, symptoms generally lessen with lowering of the receptor antibody concentrations as a reflection of the stabilization of hCG stimulus.[45] Common symptoms associated with hyperthyroidism include nervousness, tremors, tachycardia, heat intolerance, goiter, weight loss, and hypertension. Normal pregnancies typically have an increase in heart rate over baseline (by about 10 beats per minute) and heat intolerance—so these symptoms may make it difficult to distinguish between mild hyperthyroidism disease and normal pregnancy symptoms. Unique features diagnostic of Graves disease include ophthalmopathy (signs include lid lag and lid retraction so the eye looks like it is bulging out) and dermopathy (signs include localized or pretibial myxedema). Thyroid function tests (TFTs) are used to discriminate between thyroid disease and nonthyroid disorders. Laboratory confirmation illustrates a significantly reduced TSH concentration with increased FT_4 levels.

Fetal, Obstetrical, and Neonatal Effects

In cases of thyrotoxicosis, both the disease and the treatment can complicate the course and outcome of pregnancy. Obstetric abnormalities associated with poorly controlled maternal thyrotoxicosis include PTD, low birth weight (LBW), preeclampsia, heart arrhythmias, and heart failure.[46] Studies have been inconsistent concerning the association with miscarriages.[44]

Pregnancies that do not maintain euthyroid status have a substantial risk for newborns. One study noted neonatal hearing loss in pregnancies associated with subclinical hyperthyroidism.[47] Another prospective study was conducted on 600 singleton pregnant women to investigate the ramifications of thyroid dysfunctions in women. It revealed that thyroid abnormalities during pregnancy were associated with intrauterine growth restriction (IUGR) and low Apgar scores. Further studies are required to determine whether early diagnosis and treatment of thyroid diseases, even in subclinical form, can prevent possible adverse effects on the fetus.[48] Miscarriages have been associated with excessive thyroxine.[49] In a large retrospective Danish study, both early (spontaneous abortion) and late (stillbirth) pregnancy losses were more common in women with hyperthyroidism.[50] Another study again confirmed that poorly controlled hyperthyroidism was associated with an increase in medically indicated preterm deliveries, LBW, preeclampsia, heart failure, adverse perinatal outcomes, and possibly fetal loss.[51]

The fetus is at risk for thyrotoxicosis in women with Graves disease.[6] There is documentation of transient hypothyroidism and hyperthyroidism or neonatal Graves disease secondary to transplacental passage of maternal TBII and TSI, respectively.[44,52] It is suggested that the ideal predictor of perinatal thyrotoxicosis is the presence of TSH receptor antibodies in pregnancies complicated by Graves disease, especially ones with levels 3-fold higher than normal.[43] The occurrence is relatively limited due to the balance of stimulatory and inhibitory antibodies as well as maternal pharmaceutical treatment.[39] Routine evaluation of TSH receptor antibodies in the second trimester of the pregnancy is not endorsed by the American College of Obstetricians and Gynecologists (ACOG) (practice bulletin #148, April 2015).

Maternal thyroid function does not alter the presence of neonatal Graves disease. Patients who have been treated surgically or with radioactive iodine 131 prior to pregnancy, which destroys the function of the thyroid gland and results in a hypothyroid state, are still at risk for neonatal Graves disease because the TSH receptor antibodies may persist in the maternal bloodstream and cross the placenta. Nonimmune hydrops and fetal demise have been seen with fetal thyrotoxicosis.[53] Perinatal thyrotoxicosis should be suspected with the presence of a 3-fold increase in values over baseline of TSH receptor antibodies in pregnancies associated with Graves disease.[43]

With a differential diagnosis of a fetal endocrinopathy, experts advocate increased radiological surveillance and possible umbilical blood sampling when signs of hydrops, growth restriction, goiter, or fetal tachycardia occur.[33] Thioamides are cleared more efficiently than maternal antibodies, and subsequently there may be a hiatus prior to the appearance of neonatal Graves disease. Due to a stabilization of the stimulatory and inhibitory antibodies with treatment, there is limited exposure to these newborns.[39] There has been recent research in fetal-to-maternal transfusion, which may be the etiology of the increase in autoimmune endocrinopathy documented in the female gender.[36] The ATA and the American Association of Clinical Endocrinologists in 2011 recommended universal testing of TSH receptor antibodies between 22 and 26 weeks in pregnancies complicated with Graves disease, whereas ACOG (2013) did not suggest routine screening because positive results would not significantly alter the patient's previous treatment plans.

Universal screening, especially radiological and umbilical cord procedures, for fetal thyroid function is not recommended.[37] With the possibility of a maternal endocrinopathy as a culprit for fetal hydrops, IUGR, goiter, and tachycardia, fetal thyrotoxicosis should be in the differential diagnosis[54] and should be managed appropriately. In gravid women with uncontrolled hyperthyroidism or high thyroid antibody levels, there should be increased surveillance with ultrasound evaluation for fetal growth and cardiac function, amniotic fluid, and fetal goiter evaluation.[42] The Endocrine Society suggests consideration of umbilical blood sampling when the diagnosis of fetal thyroid disease cannot be ruled out by conventional chemistry and radiological studies.[55]

Subclinical Hyperthyroidism

Subclinical hyperthyroidism is associated with normal T_4 and decreased TSH levels.[56] Infrequently, this endocrinopathy can be associated with elevated T_3 levels, described as T_3 toxicosis. Typically, low TSH levels will be seen in conjunction with normal thyroxine hormone values.[56] Potential complications secondary to this disorder are seen in 1.7 % of pregnancies[57] and include bone abnormalities, cardiovascular dysfunction, and progression to clinical hyperthyroidism.[58] Studies have not correlated the presence of subclinical hyperthyroidism with increased risk for adverse pregnancy outcomes, and there is no evidence that medical treatment will benefit these pregnancies.[56,59] Elevated FT_4 levels can be seen in molar pregnancies, reflecting the high hCG levels that stimulate the TSH receptors.[60] Molar pregnancies must be treated surgically, and then these thyroid dysfunctions resolve.

Hyperemesis Gravidarum and Hyperthyroidism

Hyperemesis gravidarum is associated with biochemical hyperthyroidism (3%–15% of early pregnancies) but rarely with clinical hyperthyroidism. This disorder is largely temporary and usually requires no intervention besides adequate hydration.[61] Supportive therapy, supplementation with vitamin B_6 and doxylamine, and hydration are recommended, but occasionally the management of dehydration may require hospitalization. Thyroid function analysis in hyperemesis gravidarum is typically not needed unless there are other explicit signs of hyperthyroidism. Gastrointestinal (GI) disturbances, such as nausea and vomiting, have been ascribed to the high hCG levels in the first trimester, which increases the likelihood for the development of subclinical hyperthyroidism secondary to stimulation of the TSH receptor. Studies with singleton pregnancies and hyperemesis have shown that biochemical hyperthyroidism can be noted in 2 of 3 patients with an undetectable level of TSH, elevated FTI, or both. After 18 weeks of gestation, the hyperthyroidism of hyperemesis gravidarum usually will be mitigated without medication in the patients, although TFT abnormalities reflect more severe hyperemesis.[62]

Gestational transient hyperthyroidism has been described, and these mostly asymptomatic patients typically do not need any pharmaceutical intervention.[57] ACOG does not recommend treatment. Occasionally, treatment may be needed and continued throughout the balance of a pregnancy, although these patients typically show symptoms of thyroid disease, including thyroid enlargement (goiter), persistent tachycardia despite fluid replacement, and abnormal response to TRH stimulation.[63] As a matter of fact, there are currently no recommendations to measure TFTs routinely in women with hyperemesis unless these other thyroid symptoms and signs are present.

Thyroid Storm and Heart Failure

Thyroid storm is a hypermetabolic state that is seen in 1% of pregnancies associated with hyperthyroidism. Thyroid storm is an emergency situation with a high risk of maternal cardiac dysfunction and morbidity.[51] Abnormalities seen include fever, tachycardia, neurological irregularities, GI dysfunction, and cardiac arrhythmias.[64] Pulmonary hypertension and heart failure are common secondary to the myocardial ramifications of thyroxine.[65] Cardiomyopathy, seen in up to 8% of pregnancies with thyrotoxicosis, is associated with a high-output state secondary to minimal cardiac reserve and cardiac decompensation precipitated by preeclampsia, anemia, and sepsis.[66] Expedient treatment is required to avoid the untoward consequences of untreated thyroid storm, which includes shock, stupor, and coma. Serum FT_4, FT_3, and TSH levels should be acquired to help solidify this diagnosis.

The standard protocol in treating thyroid storm consists of utilizing pharmaceuticals to block thyroid function. Thioamides block the synthesis of thyroid hormone, and PTU specifically inhibits peripheral conversion of T_4 to T_3. A saturated solution of potassium iodide or sodium iodide will obstruct the release of thyroid hormones from the gland, both T_4 and T_3. It can be prescribed either parenterally (sodium iodide) or by mouth (saturated solution of potassium iodide or Lugol's solution). Lithium carbonate, 300 mg every 6 hours, is utilized in cases of significant allergies to iodine. Dexamethasone further decreases thyroid hormone release and peripherally inhibits the conversion of T_4 to T_3. Dexamethasone is usually given as a 2-mg dose every 6 hours. A β-blocker impedes the adrenergic effects of excessive thyroid hormone, and one must be careful using this medication in patients with cardiac problems.

A phenobarbital can reduce agitation or restlessness and may increase the catabolism of thyroid hormone.[64] Resuscitative efforts include oxygen, maintenance of intravascular volume and electrolytes, and an intensive care setting with central monitoring capabilities available.

Coincident with treating the thyroid storm, the underlying cause of the storm should be identified and treated. Testing is needed to determine fetal status. Typically, the goal is to avoid delivery while aggressively treating the mother for any coexisting infection, preeclampsia, or anemia, unless a scenario develops that compromises the well-being of the fetus or is an imminent threat to the fetus and outweighs the maternal hazards of the thyroid storm.

Pharmaceuticals to Treat Hyperthyroidism in Pregnancy

The mainstay of hyperthyroidism treatment in pregnancy is thionamides. The most commonly used medications include PTU and methimazole. PTU blocks the peripheral conversion of T_4 to T_3 and thus may have a more rapid suppressant effect than methimazole. PTU was reported to have less drug crossing the placenta than methimazole, though this statement is debatable. Methimazole downregulates thyroid hormone synthesis by inhibiting the organification of iodide. Reports of teratotoxicity are associated with first-trimester exposure to methimazole, namely, esophageal or choanal atresia and possibly aplasia cutis congenita.[38,67,68] On the other hand, PTU is associated with hepatotoxicity, resulting in liver failure in rare cases (0.1%–0.2%); this finding resulted in a black box warning from the Food and Drug Administration (FDA) in 2009 regarding PTU. Despite this black box warning, both the ATA and the American Association of Clinical Endocrinologists recommend treatment with PTU in the first trimester of pregnancy to avoid the teratogenicity risk from methimazole, then switching to methimazole in the second trimester of pregnancy for the duration and postpartum.

Other side effects of thionamides include thrombocytopenia, transient leukopenia, hepatitis, and vasculitis, which are seen in less than 1% of patients.[44] Antineutrophil cytoplasmic antibodies develop in 20% of these pregnancies treated by PTU, but only a fraction of individuals subsequently will develop significant vasculitis.[69] Agranulocytosis is a rare response, occurring in 0.1%–0.4% of pregnancies.[67] Symptoms associated with agranulocytosis include fever and sore throat. There should be a high index of suspicion when these symptoms occur in close proximity to starting the thionamide; the medication should be discontinued while evaluating the patient hematologically.[67]

Recent rebuttals referring to the premise that PTU crosses the placenta less efficiently compared to other thionamides and methimazole's adverse association with fetal aplasia cutis have risen in the literature. A retrospective study that contrasted pregnancies exposed to PTU to women treated with methimazole conveyed no cases of aplasia cutis, and comparable rates of fetal anomalies with both the drugs was 3%.[70] One study looked at FT_4 and TSH in newborn umbilical cord blood tests of women treated with PTU compared with those of women prescribed methimazole and discovered no significant difference in mean FT_4 or TSH levels. There was also no association between maternal dosage of thionamide and umbilical cord blood levels of TSH or FT_4.[71] Currently, no change in medical approach is recommended.

The ATA has reported guidelines on thionamide treatment in pregnancy complicated with hyperthyroidism. The association recommended a total daily dose of 300 to 450 mg PTU given in divided doses and 5 to 10 mg daily for methimazole.[72] Ideal management during pregnancies complicated by hyperthyroidism is to achieve levels of FT_4 or FTI in the upper end of the normal range by using the least amount of medications possible to reduce the exposure risk to the fetus. Maternal thyroid levels should be monitored monthly to maintain the FT_4 or FTI within the ideal range, which will result in slightly suppressing the TSH level.[72] Thionamides may be used with women who are breastfeeding. Studies have implemented methimazole in producing higher concentrations of the thionamide in breast milk compared to PTU.[73]

Thioamide therapy for Graves disease can suppress fetal and neonatal thyroid function, although it is usually transient and rarely requires therapy. The fetuses of pregnancies affected by Graves disease should be monitored regularly for appropriate growth. Doppler examinations of fetal vessels or fetal echocardiographs may be recommended. In some cases, fetal thyrotoxicosis results from exposure to maternal antibodies. The pediatrician should be notified when there is a maternal history of Graves disease.

In addition to thionamide therapy, patients with hyperthyroidism may need medical therapy to control symptoms until the thionamide reaches steady state and optimal control of thyroid hormones is obtained. The β-blockers are usually the first line of therapy used during pregnancy to ameliorate these symptoms of thyrotoxicosis. Surgical intervention with a thyroidectomy is rarely indicated unless pharmaceuticals are not effective.

When medical therapy fails or is not tolerated, surgical intervention needs to be considered. The surgical intervention is a partial thyroidectomy; it can be performed in the second or third trimester of the pregnancy, preferably.[74] Surgery is usually well tolerated. Complications associated with these surgical procedures performed in the gravid state, although uncommon, include iatrogenic parathyroid gland removal and damage to the recurrent laryngeal nerve.[61]

Although radiation treatment with iodine 131 is one of the most common treatments of hyperthyroidism, it is contraindicated in pregnancy because of the risk of radioactive iodine 131 concentrating not only in the maternal thyroid but also in the fetal thyroid, resulting in its ablation. It is recommended to avoid pregnancy for 4–6 months after radioactive iodine treatment.[67,75] Prior to 10 weeks of gestation, exposure to iodine 131 most likely has little consequence; however, contact after 10 weeks is associated with a risk for iatrogenically induced fetal CH. Fetuses exposed to radioactive iodine should be evaluated appropriately, and the risk for fetal endocrinopathy depends on gestational age of exposure and dosage given.[76] Avoidance of breastfeeding for 4 months is a standard precaution after treatment with iodine 131.[77]

HYPOTHYROIDISM IN PREGNANCY

Maternal hypothyroidism occurs in about 0.2%–1% of pregnancies.[57] Elevated thyroid replacement is required due to inability for the thyroid gland to respond to the greater demands from the fetus.[78] Common complaints accompanying hypothyroidism are fatigue, constipation, intolerance to cold, muscle cramps, hair loss, dry skin, prolonged relaxation phase of deep tendon reflexes, and weight gain. Again, many of these complaints are similar to pregnancy symptoms. In general, the biochemical markers for diagnosing hypothyroidism are a clinically abnormally high TSH and low FT_4. The suggested goal of treatment will be to maintain the TSH levels at slightly less than 2.5 mIU/L in the first trimester and 3.0 mIU/L in the remainder of the pregnancy.

Iodine deficiency may be a confounding factor in this disorder. Significant hypothyroidism can be seen in pregnancies that are complicated by diminished thyroid reserve, such as women with previous thyroidectomy, status after radioiodine ablation, and those undergoing in vitro fertilization.[79]

Hypothyroidism in pregnancy and postpartum is associated in the majority of clinical situations with Hashimoto disease (chronic thyroiditis or chronic autoimmune thyroiditis), subacute thyroiditis, thyroidectomy, radioactive iodine treatment, and iodine deficiency. The most commonly seen hypothyroidism is Hashimoto thyroiditis. This autoimmune thyroid disease is associated with glandular inflammation and destruction by autoantibodies (especially antithyroid antibodies). Whether this disorder is associated with an enlarged thyroid gland is subject to the etiology of the disorder (e.g., Hashimoto thyroiditis) and is a sign of compensatory TSH production.[80] Severe hypothyroidism in a gravida is relatively uncommon due to its association with infertility and miscarriages.[19]

Fetal, Obstetrical, and Neonatal Effects

Low birth weight, PTD, preeclampsia, and abruption have been seen in pregnancies with poorly treated hypothyroidism.[81] Uncontrolled hypothyroidism is associated with a higher risk of adverse obstetric and neonatal outcomes. Some studies suggested an increasing miscarriage rate in women with positive TPO antibodies and TSH levels between 2.5 and 5 mIU/L.[82] Also, a 2- to 3-fold increased risk of obstetrical complications in pregnancies is associated with subclinical hypothyroidism.[83] Many studies have shown no significant adverse outcomes when the disorder is managed appropriately with replacement pharmaceuticals.[84,85] Maternal TSH receptor blocking antibodies can cross the placenta and cause fetal thyroid abnormalities. Fetal hypothyroidism is seen in only 1 in 180,000 neonates from pregnancies complicated by maternal Hashimoto thyroiditis due to the rare scenario of thyroid inhibitory antibodies crossing the placenta.[86]

The ATA and the Endocrine Society recommend the daily iodine intake should be 250 μg of iodine for pregnant women.[42] Women with iodine-deficient hypothyroidism are at significant risk of having babies with congenital cretinism (growth failure, mental retardation, and other neurophysiologic deficits), which can be mitigated by iodine treatment in the first and second trimesters of pregnancy.[87]

A French study investigated pregnancy outcomes in a population-based registry of young adult women with CH. In both the overall and prospective analyses, CH was associated with higher percentages of pregnancies associated with gestational hypertension, emergency cesarean delivery, induced labor for vaginal delivery, and prematurity. These nationwide data illustrate that better thyroid disease control is a necessity for better outcomes, particularly during the first 2 trimesters of pregnancy, together with vigilant monitoring.[88]

Untreated CH also results in cretinism. The incidence of CH is 1 per 4000 newborns, and only 5% of neonates are identified by clinical symptoms at birth, likely because of the ameliorative effects of maternal thyroid hormone.[8] Fetal hypothyroidism seen in pregnancies associated with Hashimoto thyroiditis has an incidence of 1 in 180,000 neonates.[89]

Adequate thyroid replacement in pregnancy mitigates most of the adverse obstetrical outcomes and newborn complications.[61] Recent studies indicated neonates born from pregnancies associated with autoimmune thyroiditis have a significant risk for TPO antibodies and elevated TSH,[90] although despite the transient chemistry findings, there is minimal effect on fetal thyroid function.[91] Screening of newborns for CH is state mandated. Clinical signs are problematic because of the difficulty in categorizing them secondary to the suppressive effects of maternal thyroid hormone. Normal growth and neurological development are generally obtained with treatment protocols implemented early in life.[92] Decreased school performance, impaired reading, lower IQ scores, and adverse outcomes in the maternal and fetal components have been associated with this endocrinopathy.

Subclinical Hypothyroidism

Subclinical hypothyroidism is found in asymptomatic patients and is based on chemical values indicating the TSH level above the standard range for the general population (>2.5 or 3.5 mIU/mL, depending on the lab) and the FT_4 level within normal limits.[93] The incidence of this disorder appears to be approximately 2%–5% of pregnancies.[94] Estrogen-mediated increases in maternal thyroid-binding protein, physiological similarities between TSH and hCG, and a deficiency of iodine during pregnancy are potential etiologies for subclinical hypothyroidism and make gravidas more prone for this disorder.[3]

Controversy exists whether subclinical hypothyroidism should be screened and treated. Initial reports of a mild decrease in IQ points in school-aged children who were exposed to mothers with untreated subclinical hypothyroidism started the inquiry. Research involves assessing fetal neurodevelopment and its relationship to thyroid irregularities in pregnancies.[80] Up to 5% of pregnancies screened could be associated with subclinical hypothyroidism with routine thyroid function testing.[83] The US Preventive Services Task Force recommends screening of asymptomatic individuals *only* when treatment results in improvement in health outcomes.[95] Currently, there is a lack of evidence demonstrating improvements in maternal or newborn medical conditions when treating gravidas with subclinical hypothyroidism.

A number of studies reported mixed findings regarding the prognosis of subclinical hypothyroidism. A study following nonpregnant women with previous subclinical hypothyroidism for a duration of 5 years showed one-third of the women reverted to normal TFTs. In the other two-thirds, women with a TSH level above 10 mU/L had a 19% chance of developing overt hypothyroidism compared to 2% of women with a TSH level below 10 mU/l.[96] The US Preventive Services Task Force on screening for subclinical hypothyroidism also reported a low rate of development to overt hypothyroidism with TSH levels below 10 mU/L. Another researcher showed a 17% risk for hypothyroidism over a period of 20 years, but most of these pregnancies were associated with TPO or thyroglobulin (TG) antibodies.[97,98] In 2012, Lazarus et al refuted an earlier article regarding subclinical hypothyroidism in pregnancy being associated with cognitive impairment of exposed offspring and Lazarus showed that cognition was not altered with diagnosis or treatment.[86,99] General screening for subclinical hypothyroidism is not currently advocated by the Endocrine Society, ATA, or American Association of Clinical Endocrinologists unless there is a significant risk during the gravid state.[55]

Placenta-mediated disorders such as preeclampsia have been associated with untreated hypothyroidism, although no absolute risk factors have been associated with subclinical hypothyroidism.[100] Some small studies suggested there is an increased risk for miscarriage in pregnancies associated with subclinical hypothyroidism and negative TPO antibodies, but there is not enough proof to propose levothyroxine therapy. However, in pregnancies with TPO antibody positivity, studies have shown an association with increased spontaneous miscarriage, recurrent abortion, PTD, and abnormal thyroid test results (elevated TSH and low FT_4). Therefore, women who test positive for TPO antibody and have subclinical hypothyroidism may be treated with levothyroxine.[9] Others reported the chance of progression from subclinical hypothyroidism to overt hypothyroidism when diagnosed during pregnancy or postdelivery is approximately a 15% lifelong risk of having a true endocrinopathy.[98] There are few good studies indicating any clinical benefit in the identification or treatment of subclinical hypothyroidism during pregnancy and resulting in improvement in adverse obstetrical or neonatal outcomes.[94] Until proven clinical benefit, either obstetrically or pediatrically, routine testing for the thyroid autoantibodies is not advocated by any major professional organization at this time.[19]

Pharmaceuticals Utilized to Treat Hypothyroidism

Implementing thyroid replacement for hypothyroidism in pregnancy is the same as in the nongravid state. Pharmaceutical replacement of thyroid hormone in pregnancies associated with true hypothyroidism has been shown to mitigate adverse obstetrical outcomes.[101] Pregnancy is associated with a 30% increase in thyroxine requirement in pregnancy.[102] Increased thyroxine requirements are seen in one-third of supplemented pregnancies and it is thought to be related to the increase in estrogen production; thus, this increase in thyroxine replacement should be anticipated, especially in women without thyroid reserve (e.g., history of thyroidectomy).[103,104] The ATA (2011) suggested pharmaceutical replacement of 1 to 2 µg/kg/d of the thyroid supplement. Primary quantities of thyroxine replacement drugs empirically should be started at 50 to 100 µg/d, with levels adjusted based on surveillance of TFTs every 4 to 6 weeks. The goal is to normalize the TSH levels. Women on levothyroxine who are newly pregnant should increase the dosage by 30%, and maternal serum TSH should be monitored every 4 weeks during the first half of pregnancy.[19] Pregnancy causes intrinsic demands on the maternal thyroid and subsequent increased demands for replacement in patients with prepregnancy endocrinopathy.

Pregnancies in women with previous thyroidectomies or prior radioiodine ablation have minimal thyroid reserve and should be counseled prior to conception that their levothyroxine replacement dose will need to be increased when pregnant to reduce the chance of problems from the development of subsequent significant hypothyroidism.[79] Elevated TSH and lower FTI levels are seen in these women, necessitating a change in mean thyroxine dosage baseline from 0.1 µg/d before pregnancy to 0.148 µg/d during gestation.[105]

OTHER THYROID DISEASES IN PREGNANCY

Thyroid Nodule or Thyroid Cancer Management

Nodules in the thyroid gland are seen in 1%–2% of reproductive-aged females. A thyroid nodule in pregnancy should be evaluated in a similar manner as in a nonpregnant state, with a thorough examination along with TSH and ultrasound testing. Fine-needle aspiration is a reliable method to assess for thyroid cancer during pregnancy, using standard histologic tumor markers and immunostaining.[106] Thyroid cancer can be seen in 0.1% of thyroid nodules identified in pregnancies, and it behooves the medical provider to meticulously evaluate all thyroid nodules. Pregnancy itself does not appear to alter the course of thyroid cancer. In a cohort study contrasting thyroid cancer in pregnant and postpartum women with nonpregnant women with thyroid cancer, there were no dissimilarities in the presenting physical findings, tumor type, tumor size, presence of metastases, time between diagnosis and treatment, recurrence rates, or death rates. Outcome findings did not waiver from each group despite surgical interventions occurring in some cases months to up to a year after diagnosis.[107]

One study looked at pregnancy outcomes in women who had thyroid cancer and compared obstetrical disorders to pregnancies before or after treatment with surgical and iodine intervention; they found no significant differences in outcomes.[108] Thyroid cancer requires a multidisciplinary treatment plan, incorporating discussions contrasting pregnancy termination, treatment during pregnancy, and preterm or term delivery with treatment after delivery. Gestational age at diagnosis and the tumor characteristics potentially may modify the recommendations. Definitive treatment, such as surgical interventions, can be performed during pregnancy, preferably in the second trimester. On the other hand, radiation treatment should be deferred until after delivery.[77]

Postpartum Thyroiditis

Postpartum thyroiditis can be seen within 12 months of parturition and can be associated with clinical evidence of hyperthyroidism, hypothyroidism, or a combination of both entities.[17] PPT is a transient, autoimmune inflammatory disorder of the thyroid, caused by changes in humoral and cell-mediated immune response. It is the most prevalent thyroid disorder in the postpartum period, with incidence ranging between 5% and 9% of pregnancies.[109] In 5% of pregnancies without a history of any endocrinopathy, PPT will be seen.[110] PPT has a unique biphasic course, with an episode of transient thyrotoxicosis followed by transient or permanent hypothyroidism. The disease course may manifest itself by precipitating other hormonal disorders and producing significant subjective consequences. Hypothyroid complications of fatigue, constipation, or depression may be seen or symptoms of hyperthyroid may manifest with irritability, weight loss, palpitations, or heat intolerance.[111] It is imperative to identify at-risk groups early for prophylaxis and to provide adequate therapy for thyroid dysfunction in the postpartum period.

Close to a half of pregnancies complicated with PPT have hypothyroidism, while the remaining women are evenly split between thyrotoxicosis and thyrotoxicosis followed by hypothyroidism.[112] An acute change illustrating abnormal levels of TSH or FT_4 along with the presence of positive titers of TPO antibodies are the most common precipitating factors for the initiation of this syndrome. In a large, prospective study, only 11% of asymptomatic gravid or postpartum women diagnosed with PPT developed permanent hypothyroidism. With a low prevalence of this abnormality and the finding that pharmaceuticals are mostly not indicated, inspection for adverse TFTs and antimicrosomal antibodies in asymptomatic women is not cost effective.[113]

There is an increased propensity (up to 50% risk) for postpartum thyroiditis in pregnancies associated with autoimmune thyroid antibodies.[74] Thyroid antimicrosomal or anti-TPO antibodies along with TSH and FT_4 levels are warranted for women with the development of a goiter or other signs of an endocrinopathy. Because some of these symptoms are common in the postpartum state, clinicians must use their judgment to determine whether the symptoms merit evaluation. The highest levels of TSH and anti-TPO antibodies have the most significant risk for developing permanent hypothyroidism.[110] Execution of mass screening programs remains controversial. Implementation of studies can be used to introduce targeted and cost-effective screening for early detection of at-risk patients and prevention of morbidity and complications of PPT.[114] ACOG, the Endocrine Society, the American Association of Clinical Endocrinologists, and the ATA are in agreement regarding not endorsing widespread screening for thyroid autoantibodies in the gravid state.[19]

Screening for Thyroid Abnormalities

Testing for thyroid dysfunction is recommended in pregnancy for individuals with a personal history of thyroid disease or symptoms of a thyroid disorder. Development of a significant goiter or distinct nodules should be evaluated. The efficiency of obtaining TFTs in asymptomatic pregnant women who have a mildly enlarged thyroid has not been proven. Studies showing no benefit in screening and intervention for subclinical hypothyroidism in pregnancy (based on cognitive function analysis of children at age 3)[86] have been the clinical infrastructure for the recommendations by the ACOG, Endocrine Society, and American Association of Clinical Endocrinologists against universal screening for thyroid disease in the gravida.[115]

In a research analysis of 25,216 pregnancies undergoing prenatal laboratory baselines, only 75 women had TSH levels above the 99.7th percentile. These research scientists then looked at the results of neuropsychologic testing for 62 children of hypothyroid women with those of 124 children of matched women with normal thyroid function when the children were approximately 8 years of age. There was no significant difference in mean IQ scores between the children of women who were hypothyroid and those of controls.

However, there remains controversy regarding whether maternal hypothyroidism is associated with a decline in some neuropsychologic testing. A study of over 21,000 pregnant women who were seen for antenatal screening at gestational age of 11 to 14 weeks documented that treatment of maternal hypothyroidism did not result in improved cognitive function in children at the age of 3 years.[86] Another research project came to the same conclusion: Children born either to mothers who were treated for hypothyroidism and had normal TSH during pregnancy or to mothers who had hypothyroidism with inadequate levothyroxine replacement (i.e., elevated TSH) during pregnancy had children similar IQ levels and cognitive performance.[116]

Because a large study illustrated that there was no rise in adverse pregnancy outcomes or neurodevelopment improvements with pharmaceutical treatment with isolated hypothyroxinemia (low T_4 and normal values of TSH), routine screening is not indicated.[86] The professional societies—ACOG (2012), Endocrine Society, ATA, and American Association of Clinical Endocrinologists—all concur that there is insufficient evidence to condone routine screening of asymptomatic pregnant women for TFTs, and screening should be limited to those at high risk for thyroid disease.[115]

PARATHYROID PHYSIOLOGY AND DISEASE

The parathyroid hormone (PTH) is a 85 amino acid hormone that acts on bone, kidney, and intestine to maintain extracellular fluid calcium concentrations.[117] Plasma levels remain low in the first trimester but rise throughout the pregnancy. PTH is involved in the production of vitamin D ($1,25\text{-OH}_2\text{D}_3$), and both PTH and vitamin D are responsible for maintaining calcium homeostasis. Concentrations are regulated by a negative-feedback mechanism. Lowering of the concentrations of calcium and magnesium activate PTH, which in turns alters bone resorption, intestinal absorption, and kidney resorption and subsequently elevates extracellular fluid calcium levels and decreases phosphate values. Maternal PTH-related protein (PTHrP) is supplied by multiple sources, including both fetal and maternal components: placenta, myometrium, breast, and fetal parathyroid glands. PTHrP is also involved in altering $1\text{-}\alpha$-hydroxylase activity, with a subsequent rise in 1,25-hydroxy vitamin D; altering the placental calcium transport mechanism; and protecting the maternal skeleton during gestation by inhibiting osteoclastic bone resorption.[118]

Calcium regulation occurs in collaboration with magnesium, phosphate, PTH, vitamin D, and calcitonin physiology. One study showed that all markers of bone turnover became elevated during the gravid state and did not return to a normal status until about 12 months postpartum.[119] Half of the serum calcium is protein bound (mostly to albumin), and about 40% circulates free as ionized calcium. Calcitonin is a powerful chemical that acts as a PTH antagonist. Agonists include calcium and magnesium. The gravid state has a significant impact on calcium and stimulates calcitonin.[120] Its levels are higher in pregnancy compared to a nongravid state. Calcitonin is produced in the thyroidal C cells, breast, and placenta. Its role in pregnancy has not been identified, yet it appears to be cytoprotective of the maternal skeleton from the risk of extreme resorption of calcium.

Normally, the skeleton responds to various stressors, resulting in new bone formation by osteoblasts in some areas while resorbing bone with osteoclasts in other, less-stressed, areas. Osteoblasts produce osteocalcin, which is a bone-specific protein that, when measured, parallels the rate of new bone formation. During pregnancy, osteocalcin tends to be low in midgestation but rises postpartum.[121] Bone resorption increases during pregnancy, with markers indicating twice the normal rate of resorption at the end of gestation, which goes along with the rise in bone turnover at the time of maximal transfer of maternal calcium to the fetus.

Fetal demand for calcium reaches a total of 30 g over the course of the pregnancy, with the greatest demands in the third trimester, when calcium is deposited into the fetal skeleton. The maternal system modifies its physiology by increasing the GFR, increasing intestinal calcium absorption, and increasing bone resorption. Ionized calcium levels remain constant, but both total serum calcium and serum albumin concentrations decrease during pregnancy.[122] Decreases in albumin, which occur naturally in pregnancy, results in freeing more calcium to the bioactive, ionized form into the bloodstream.

Other notable values in pregnancy include serum phosphate (and renal tubular reabsorption of phosphorus), which is unchanged, and PTH levels, which are lower in the first half of pregnancy and readjust to normal by the end of the second trimester. Levels of vitamin D (1,25-OH$_2$D$_3$ or calcitriol) are increased 2-fold in pregnancy, which most likely is influenced by the decidua and the placenta because maternal PTH levels are usually normal.[123] Also, this rise in calcitriol reflects the agonistic effect of maternal renal 1-α-hydroxylase activity by estrogen, placental lactogen, and PTH on calcitriol manufactured by the placenta. Levels of both free and total calcitriol rise in gestation mainly due to the increase in vitamin D–binding protein.[124]

Hyperparathyroidism

The incidence of primary hyperparathyroidism (PHP) in pregnancy is unknown (estimated at 1 in 5000 women of childbearing age), and it is fairly uncommon. Most cases (80%) are associated with a single parathyroid adenoma, and most of the rest with primary hyperplasia of the 4 parathyroid glands (15%). Hyperparathyroidism symptoms include malaise, renal calculi, behavior changes, and occasional pancreatitis.[123,125] This disorder tends to improve with pregnancy due to the calcium shunting from the fetus and maternal renal exchange.[126] Fetal complications of hyperparathyroidism include fetal demise, preeclampsia, IUGR, preterm labor, and neonatal abnormalities.[125,127]

In review of the literature (1976–1990) regarding maternal morbidity associated with hyperparathyroidism,[3,128] there were only 2 perinatal deaths (5%) among 37 infants born of mother with hyperparathyroidism. The most common symptoms of these women included nausea, vomiting, anorexia, weakness, and fatigue, which were present in 36% of patients. Some gravida experienced nephrolithiasis, acute pancreatitis, and hypertension. Parathyroid cancer is a sporadic cause of hyperparathyroidism, with only a couple of cases occurring during pregnancy and documented in the literature. Serum calcium levels are extraordinarily elevated, with high mortality and morbidity.

Hyperparathyroid crisis is a serious complication of PHP and has been described with pregnancy. Symptoms of hyperparathyroid crisis include generalized malaise, neurological changes, hypertension, and severe dehydration. The serum calcium level is frequently higher than 14 mg/dL; hypokalemia and elevation in serum creatinine can also be seen. If not identified and corrected, hyperparathyroid crisis may progress to uremia, coma, and death. The two most common causes of neonatal morbidity are prematurity and neonatal hypocalcemia, the latter related to levels of maternal hypercalcemia.

Based on multiple reports, PHP should be considered a risk factor for preeclampsia.[129] The diagnosis of PHP is identified with documentation of persistent hypercalcemia in the presence of increased serum PTH levels.[8,130] A recurrent serum calcium value higher than 9.5 mg/dL is suspicious of hypercalcemia. Serum phosphorus is decreased in about 50% of pregnant women with PHP. Radiological studies with sonography of the neck can detect parathyroid masses in a significant percentage of affected patients.

Hypercalcemia during pregnancy can be associated with other endocrine disorders (thyrotoxicosis and adrenal insufficiency), vitamin D or vitamin A overdose, diuretic use, or granulomatous diseases.

Acute pancreatitis can be seen with PHP, with an incidence of less than 1% of normal pregnancies. This scenario, if found, in the gravid state can be associated with neonatal and maternal morbidity; it behooves the clinician to obtain calcium levels in pregnancy associated with persistent nausea, vomiting, and abdominal pain.[131]

Surgery is the usually the only effective treatment of PHP. Symptomatic parathyroid adenomas are treated by surgical excision in all trimesters. Exploration of the maternal neck is typically tolerated without major complications.[125] Because most of the neonatal complications have been reported in patients with symptomatic disease, a surgical approach is indicated in such patients, as well as in those with complications such as nephrolithiasis, bone disease, or persistent hypercalcemia (above 1 mg of the normal range). Although surgery can be done in any trimester, surgical intervention is best scheduled in the second trimester of pregnancy.[132] In cases complicated by postsurgical hypocalcemia, intravenous calcium should be initiated to normalize these values.

Medical therapy has been attempted in nonsurgical candidates with significant hypercalcemia. Oral phosphate therapy (1.5 to 2.5 g/d) has been shown to ameliorate some of the symptoms these patients experience.

The incidence of excessive calcium concentrations in association with cancer is as high as 1.4% when asymptomatic cases are incorporated in the analysis.[133] A solitary adenoma is most likely the culprit, and in 15% of the cases, multiple glands are involved. PTH maintained in carcinoma differs from the natural hormone. Most patients are asymptomatic and have only slight increases in serum calcium levels.[134] Symptoms of significantly elevated calcium levels include stupor, vomiting, and dehydration. These symptoms should alert one regarding this hypercalcemic crisis. Treatment with a parathyroidectomy is recommended after pregnancy for symptomatic hyperparathyroidism, with calcium levels 1.0 mg/dL above the upper normal range, creatinine clearance less than 60 mL/min, osteopenia, or age younger than 50.[135] Elevated maternal and fetal levels of calcium suppress fetal PTH, which subsequently contributes to decrease newborn calcium levels. The pediatrician should be alerted to this history because neonates may have severe hypocalcemia and the possibility of tetany.[136] The neonatal hypoparathyroidism caused by maternal hyperparathyroidism is transient and is treated with calcium and calcitriol. In preterm infants, the intestine lacks sufficiently expressed vitamin D receptor. Consequently, calcitriol is suboptimal therapy for these patients.[127]

Vitamin D shortage historically was known for its association with rickets and its negative impact on maternal, fetal, and neonate health.[137] Elevation of vitamin D with pregnancy seems to reflect the placental production of either PTH or PTHrP. One study showed an association with fetal growth due to elevated PTH and vitamin D deficiency, which suggested this finding was consistent with the effect on maternal calcium homeostasis.[138] Other reports, involving pregnancies with maternal deficiency in vitamin D, showed elevated risks for preeclampsia, gestational diabetes, operative deliveries, and poor fetal and neonatal outcomes.[139,140]

Hypoparathyroidism

Hypoparathyroidism is usually associated with surgical interventions of the parathyroid or thyroid. Symptoms include facial muscle spasms and cramps and generalized paresthesias. History of previous thyroid surgery, abnormal chemistry (low serum calcium and high phosphate levels), and radiological documentation can be the incentive for investigation of this disorder. Reports of improper management of hypoparathyroidism in pregnancy can be associated with miscarriages, stillbirths, and neonatal deaths. Hypocalcemia in pregnant patients may result in a fetus with demineralization of the skeletal system.[141]

Treatment of pregnancies associated with hypoparathyroidism is similar to the nongravid state. Calcitriol levels of 1 to 3 μg/d or large vitamin D dosages of 50,000 IU/wk to 150,000 IU/d are advocated. Calcium values are monitored closely to maintain them in the low normal ranges. Because of maternal reabsorption and fetal demands, serial calcium testing is done on a monthly basis.

ADRENAL GLAND DISORDERS IN PREGNANCY

The adrenal gland is composed of 3 main structures: zona glomerulosa, which produces mainly aldosterone; zona fasciculata, which produces mainly cortisol; and zona reticulata, which produces mostly androgens and some estrogens. Of all of the adrenal hormones, cortisol is the main product; it is found in 2 main forms: bound to protein (either corticosteroid-bound globulin [CBG] or albumin) or unbound (free hormone). The free form is the biologically active form and accounts for about 10%–15% of total cortisol; about 80% is bound. During pregnancy, the total cortisol level increases about 3-fold by the end of the third trimester, with only about a 1.5-fold increase in free cortisol. During pregnancy, the cortisol clearance rate is decreased.

Besides the increase in cortisol, pregnancy influences the rise in plasma renin activity, angiotensin II, and aldosterone. Renin is manufactured by the ovaries, kidney, and decidua, with a significant rise noted in the first trimester. Estrogen stimulates plasma angiotensinogen volumes, especially in the first half of the pregnancy, with a parallel rise in the angiotensin II concentration. Rising aldosterone levels mirror the urinary aldosterone values, correlating with the gravida's elevation in GFR and progesterone levels. Progesterone inhibits sodium retention at the distal renal tubules and illustrates an antikaliuretic effect.[142,143]

Congenital Adrenal Hyperplasia

Congenital adrenal hyperplasia (CAH) is a genetic defect of adrenal steroid biosynthesis and is most often associated with 21-hydroxylase (*CYP21* gene) deficiency (90%). This autosomal recessive disorder has been associated with ambiguous genitalia, virilization, reduced fertility rate, and salt wasting.[144] The carrier status of the father should be evaluated. If the father is not a carrier, then there is no risk to the fetus. A positive carrier status in the father confers a potential risk associated with virilization occurring in a female fetus with classic 21-hydroxylase deficiency unless fetal adrenal androgen production is adequately suppressed.[145] Dexamethasone crosses the placenta because it is not bound to CBG and is not metabolized by placental 11β-hydroxysteroid dehydrogenase. Hydrocortisone is metabolized by this enzyme and can be given to the patient with little harm to the fetus. Maternal monitoring of androstenedione and testosterone values is recommended during the gestational period.[146]

There is some controversy associated with antenatal steroid use in pregnancies that are at risk for congenital CAH. A suppressive regimen incorporates dexamethasone at doses of 20 μg/kg maternal body weight per day to a maximum of 1.5 mg daily in 3 divided doses starting at the time of pregnancy. Suppressive treatment, if used, should be given before the 9th week of gestation to effectively reduce the risk of virilization in the affected female fetus.[144,145]

Monitoring of maternal estriol levels will estimate fetal adrenal synthesis, and cortisol and DHEA-S (dehydroepiandrosterone sulfate) values will characterize maternal adrenal suppression. Historically, chorionic villus sampling and amniocentesis were used for gender determination at 10 and 15 weeks, respectively. Cell-free fetal DNA can now be used at 10 weeks or later for fetal diagnosis. Most recently, a case report of the successful determination of fetal gender through testing fetal cells obtained from the cervix, like a Papanicolaou test; this noninvasive experimental technique is called trophoblast retrieval and isolation from the cervix (TRIC).[117] Therapeutically, we want to limit maternal exposure to high-dose steroids because there are side effects, including gestational diabetes, edema, and weight gain. Dexamethasone levels can be decreased in affected pregnancies in the second half of the pregnancy of female fetuses. Stress dosage of steroids (i.e., hydrocortisol) should be used during labor and delivery in these patients because maternal adrenals would be suppressed.[147–149]

Pheochromocytoma

Pheochromocytoma is seen in 1 per 10,000 pregnancies and has been documented in 0.1% of hypertensive, gravid patients.[150] These tumors secrete catecholamines and are most commonly identified in the adrenal medulla. Of these, 10% are bilateral, 10% are extraadrenal, and 10% become malignant. There is an association of these tumors with multiple endocrine neoplasia (MEN) syndromes, medullary thyroid carcinoma, and hyperparathyroidism. Worsening hypertension is commonly seen with pregnancy and may be mistakenly diagnosed as gestational hypertension or preeclampsia instead of pheochromocytoma. Differentiating these disorders may be difficult.[151] Nonspecific findings include headache, seizures, flushing, and GI complaints. Studies have documented worsening mortality if the tumor is not diagnosed in the antepartum time period.[152]

Catecholamines are associated with minimal transfer through the placenta, which is likely due to the high placental concentrations of catechol-*O*-methyltransferase and monoamine oxidase.[153] Fetal hypoxia and other fetal adversities are associated with catecholamine-induced uteroplacental vasoconstriction and placental insufficiency or maternal vascular abnormalities. Case studies have shown fetal demise with presumed severe preeclampsia, but subsequent diagnosis of postpartum pheochromocytoma may be associated symptoms of cardiomyopathy, paroxysmal hypertension, and von Hippel–Lindau disease.[154,155]

Pheochromocytoma is usually a diagnosis of exclusion and requires an elevated index of suspicion. Interest in this diagnosis should be increased with pregnancies associated with hypertension, palpitations, and other signs of cardiac dysfunction. The challenge occurs when trying to differentiate preeclampsia from the hypertensive crisis caused by pheochromocytoma. Edema, proteinuria, and hyperuricemia may help differentiate the diagnosis of preeclampsia from pheochromocytoma. Another confounder is that there may be a slight rise in plasma and urinary catecholamines seen with severe preeclampsia.[156]

The diagnosis of pheochromocytoma in the gravid state is made similar to that for the nonpregnancy state: elevated 24-hour urine collection for catecholamine metabolites, such as metanephrines and vanillylmandelic acid (VMA).[150,151] VMA quantification may be the most sensitive metabolite to measure in pregnancy.[157] Magnetic resonance imaging (MRI) tumor localization is the preferred radiological testing with the highest sensitivity, without exposing the fetus to ionizing radiation.

Initially, control of hypertension is paramount in treating this disorder. An α-adrenergic blocker (phenoxybenzamine, 10 to 30 mg three times daily) is the first line of therapy. A β-blocker may also be prescribed to counter the tachycardia or arrhythmias that persist after full α blockade and volume repletion.[151]

Definitive treatment of pheochromocytoma is surgical removal of the tumor. Laparoscopy is typically the modality of choice, especially in the nonpregnant state.[158] Surgical resection can be performed in the first half of the pregnancy once adequate α blockade has been implemented. Case reports of successful second-trimester surgical intervention have been described utilizing a laparoscopic approach.[159] Third-trimester intervention can be accompanied by a planned cesarean section. Cesarean section is the modality of choice in the third trimester to avoid unpredictable volumes of catecholamine release associated with labor pains and contractions of the vaginal delivery process.[160] Alternatively, a postpartum procedure can be performed. Recurrent pheochromocytoma is possible and may be suspected if symptoms recur despite adequate hypertensive control medically.

Cushing Syndrome

In the nonpregnant state, the incidence of Cushing syndrome about 2 to 3 per million annually. Only 150 cases of Cushing syndrome have been reported in pregnancy.[161] One of the most common etiologies of this disorder is the iatrogenic form, secondary to chronic corticosteroid treatment. Cushing disease is an endogenous disorder involving bilateral adrenal hyperplasia stimulated by a small (<1-cm) pituitary adenoma producing ACTH (corticotropin). Rare cases of hypothalamic corticotropin-releasing factor secretion may cause corticotropic hyperplasia resulting in Cushing syndrome.

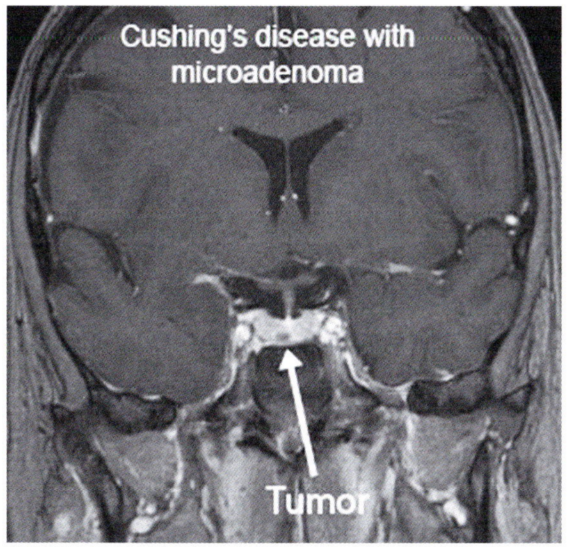

FIGURE 22-2. Cushing disease. In pregnant women, the pregnancy may worsen symptoms of Cushing disease. The MRI test indicates Cushing disease.

The cushingoid body habitus appears with the adipose tissue deposition resulting in moon facies, buffalo hump, and truncal obesity. Other symptoms commonly encountered include hypertension, hirsutism, glucose intolerance, and malaise. Androgen excess may lead to virilization.[162]

Screening tests for Cushing syndrome are positive when plasma cortisol levels are not suppressed by dexamethasone or the presence of elevated 24-hour urine free cortisol.[163] Radiological testing with computed tomography (CT) or preferably MRI in pregnancy can identify pituitary and adrenal tumors or hyperplasia.

Cushing syndrome is much less frequent in pregnancy due to the elevated androgen levels of this disease causing subsequent menstrual irregularities and anovulation (Figure 22-2). One-third of

Cushing cases result from pituitary adenomas, and approximately 10% are associated with adrenal carcinoma.[145] Hypercortisolism may initially become obvious during the gravid state, with resolution possible after delivery.[164] There is minimal alteration of the maternal adrenal glands throughout pregnancy. Circulating cortisol levels are elevated, with most bound to CBG. Glucocorticoid secretion is not affected by the gestation, although the metabolic clearance rate is lower, reflecting the change in the half-life (doubling) with the pregnancy.[165]

Diagnosis of Cushing syndrome is difficult during pregnancy because many of the common Cushing symptoms are also common in the normal gravid state, such as weight gain, glucose intolerance, hypertension, and edema. Measurement of 24-hour urinary free cortisol levels will also be associated with elevations of plasma cortisol, corticotropin, and corticotropin-releasing factors in both pregnancy and Cushing syndrome. Diagnosing Cushing syndrome during pregnancy thus may be difficult. ACTH levels become elevated with gestational age. It has been proposed that this paradoxical change in ACTH concentrations may be a result of the antagonistic action of progesterone on mineralcorticoids.[166] ACTH values are normal to elevated even with adrenal adenomas reflecting placenta production of ACTH, possibly due to the nonsuppressible activation of pituitary ACTH by placental corticotropin releasing hormone (CRH).

The overnight dexamethasone test remains a relatively reliable procedure in illustrating inadequate suppression during a normal pregnancy to make the diagnosis. Circadian variation of the high levels of total and free serum cortisol during normal pregnancy may be the most promising chemistry finding in the differential diagnosis identifying Cushing syndrome from the hypercortisolism of pregnancy because this finding is characteristically absent in all forms of Cushing syndrome.[167] Radiological evaluation of the pituitary with an MRI (without contrast) or CT may be beneficial for the diagnosis because CRH stimulation testing and petrosal venous sinus sampling have not been adequately analyzed in pregnancy.[161] MRI may be less risky for the fetus and is usually the technique most favored by radiologists for documenting the mass associated with Cushing syndrome. There is no evidence of toxicity with contrast during pregnancy, but few medical providers will request this adjunctive procedure.[168]

Cardiac dysfunction, osteoporotic fractures, and emotional changes are seen commonly during pregnancy with this endocrine abnormality.[169] Adverse obstetrical outcomes and elevated risk for fetal mortality may occur with uncontrolled Cushing syndrome during pregnancy, including those caused by hypertension, gestational diabetes, preeclampsia, myopathy, and prematurity.[170] The pregnancy loss rate is 25% and may include spontaneous abortion, stillbirth, and early neonatal death due to PTD associated with this disorder. Recent reports advocated treatment in pregnancy, starting in the second trimester of the pregnancy, because medical treatments improve live birth rates.[171] Occasionally, this syndrome is diagnosed in pregnancies, and its manifestations are thought to be due to the unregulated placental CRH, resolving in the postpartum time period.[169]

Definitive surgical intervention with resection of pituitary or adrenal adenoma or bilateral adrenalectomy for hyperplasia is usually required for long-term management.[172] Pharmaceutical intervention in pregnancy is commonly effective. Metyrapone is most commonly used to control hypertension prior to postpartum surgical modalities. Pasireotide is a new somatostatin that may be helpful in this disorder; yet, there is little experience in pregnancy, and there is a side effect of hyperglycemia.[173] Pituitary resection has been successfully treated in the pregnancy via a transphenoidal approach[171] as well as adrenalectomy in the latter part of pregnancies.[150]

Adrenal Insufficiency: Addison Disease

Autoimmune adrenalitis (also known as Addison Disease) and tuberculosis are associated more commonly with adrenal insufficiency than primary adrenocortical insufficiency. The last requires over 90% of total gland volume to be destroyed prior to developing symptoms.[174] Incidence of primary adrenal insufficiency has been reported as high as 1 in 3000 births in Norway.[145] Symptoms generally include weakness, GI issues, hyponatremia, CNS abnormalities, and anorexia. Morning plasma cortisol values of 3 µg/dL or less are diagnostic of adrenal insufficiency, and a laboratory reading higher than 19 µg/dL (fasting, morning) rules out an adrenal suppressive disorder.[175]

An ACTH stimulation test to illustrate the lack of response to corticotropin is suggested when low cortisol values are found in pregnancy.[176] ACTH levels above 100 pg/mL are characteristic of primary adrenal insufficiency, although values in secondary forms will not be low due to the placental contribution to its production.[177]

Retrospective studies indicated the increase risk for PTD, IUGR, and operative deliveries in women diagnosed with adrenal insufficiency within 3 years of pregnancy. Abnormal fetal development is usually not a characteristic of this disorder because the fetoplacental unit typically independently regulates its own steroid environment. Adverse outcomes have been attributed to maternal hyponatremia or metabolic acidosis.[178]

Cortisol therapy should be held prior to pregnancy and given as needed during the antenatal period. Replacement of mineralocorticoids is similar during pregnancy as in the nonpregnant state. Some medical providers have advocated lowering third-trimester dosages that develop preeclampsia or worsening hypertension.[179] Stress dosages of steroids are required during the peripartum, delivery, and postpartum periods for patients receiving glucocorticoids as anti-inflammatory therapy and assumed to have adrenal axis suppression. A steroid dosage equivalent to 100 mg hydrocortisone every 8 hours for 3 dosages is required for the stress doses.[180]

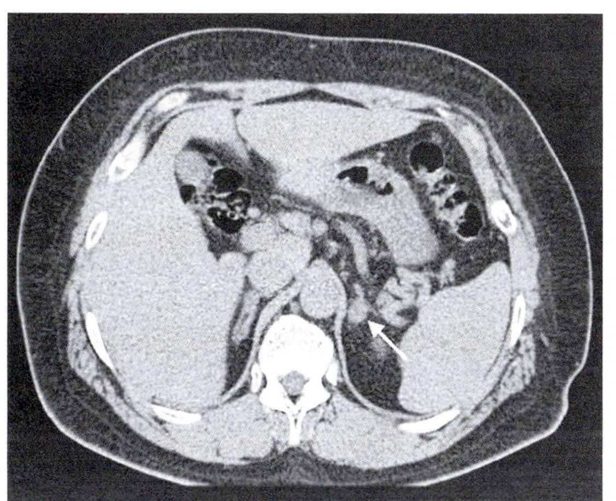

FIGURE 22-3. Magnetic resonance imaging to indicate primary aldosteronism.

Primary Hyperaldosteronism

Most cases of hyperaldosteronism are associated with adrenal adenomas and infrequently as a result of idiopathic bilateral adrenal hyperplasia or carcinoma of the adrenals (Figure 22-3).[15] Concentrations of aldosterone, the primary mineralocorticoid, are elevated by the second trimester. With limiting sodium intake, there is increasing levels of the steroid hormone.[181] During the end of the gravid state, renin and angiotensin II are elevated, which has an effect on the glomerulosa of the adrenal glands and is responsible for the high aldosterone secretion. This hormone may have an importance in the modulating properties in the pathway involving trophoblast growth and placenta size.[182]

Pregnancy adverse outcomes have been associated with primary hyperaldosteronism.[183] Maternal complications associated with this disease include hypertension, muscle weakness, and chemistry (hypokalemia and proteinuria) abnormalities.[184]

Diagnosis is made by elevated serum or urine aldosterone values. Difficulty arises in detection of abnormal levels of aldosterone in pregnancy because progesterone blocks aldosterone, and the values are high in pregnancy. The aldosterone/renin ratio may contribute to the diagnosis as renin levels are diminished in pregnancies associated with hyperaldosteronism.

Therapy includes potassium replacement and hypertension management. Drugs utilized with success for this disorder in pregnancy include calcium channel blockers, β-blockers and amiloride.[185] A laparoscopic approach for resection of the adrenal gland has been reported in pregnancy.[159] With the lower levels of progesterone during the postpartum period, hypertension and hypokalemia may be aggravated.[142]

PITUITARY DISORDERS IN PREGNANCY

Anatomical changes in the pituitary gland during pregnancy include the enlargement of the pituitary gland volume to greater than 120% over the nonpregnant state. Within 6 months postpartum, the gland involutes to its original size.[186] Pituitary gland enlargement is a radiological dilemma in pregnancy because MRI does not have the sensitivity to differentiate pregnancy enlargement from other pituitary tumors. Asymmetrical enlargement and deviation of the stalk is of concern because it is not ordinarily seen in a normal gestation. Physicians should be alerted to the possibility of pituitary tumors in women with headaches and visual problems in pregnancy. Surgical intervention may be required to treat pituitary adenomas with symptoms of compression or pituitary apoplexy on MRI.[187] MRI without contrast is recommended in pregnancy. For definitive diagnosis, intravenous contrast is suggested after the first trimester, although the FDA-approved gadolinium chelates belong to the pregnancy category C category.[188]

Anterior Pituitary

In pregnancy, the pituitary gland undergoes hypertrophic changes associated with lactotrophic cellular enhancement induced by estrogen stimulation.[189] Hormonal levels are altered throughout the gestational period. In anticipation of lactation, prolactin values increase during each trimester of pregnancy.[190] With respect to growth hormone (GH), there are two forms with a dichotomy in its concentrations: one GH variant produced by the placental syncytiotrophoblasts, which increases during gestation, and the other GH produced by the pituitary, which decreases in secretion due to negative feedback from insulinlike growth factor 1 (IGF-1) dominance in pregnancy.[191] There is a steady rise throughout the pregnancy of cortisol values, which reflects an estrogen-induced increase in CBG and a rise in cortisol production, which is reflected with a subsequent rise in the bioactive "free" fraction, urinary free cortisol and salivary cortisol volumes.[167]

Hypopituitarism

Hypopituitarism is usually associated with the loss of some (partial) or all (complete) of pituitary hormone secretion. This disorder is associated commonly with neoplastic, vascular, traumatic, or infiltrative disorders and causes gonadotropin abnormalities and infertility. It may originate with pregnancy or postpartum, likely associated with enlargement of an adenoma, lymphocytic hypophysitis, and infarction of the pituitary gland. Pregnancies associated with hypopituitarism have elevated risks for operative delivery, miscarriages, and growth restriction without a statistically increased malformation rate.[192] In light of the fact that patients with hypothalamic/pituitary dysfunction may not compensate for the increased requirements for thyroxine (normally regulated by elevations in TSH), it may be prudent to prophylactically raise the pharmaceutical dosages of levothyroxine in these pregnancies.[105]

A study of 25 pregnancies of patients with GH deficiency and in which the hormone was not given, there were no reported significant adverse outcomes.[193] Stress doses of steroids are recommended during labor and delivery (e.g., 75–100 mg of hydrocortisone every 8 hours for 3 dosages).[167]

Prolactinomas

Prolactinomas comprise 25%–35% of all pituitary tumors, and 25% of hyperprolactinemic patients will have prolactin-secreting adenomas (Figure 22-4).[194,195] Pregnancy is usually not obtainable in women with untreated prolactinomas. The rise in prolactin from the prolactinoma influences the pulsatility of gonadotropin releasing hormone, which diminishes follicle-stimulating hormone and luteinizing hormone production, lowering the estrogen level so ovulation typically does not occur. As a consequence, amenorrhea, infertility, and hypogonadism are seen.[196] Hyperprolactinemia is the etiology of over 30% of infertile patients.[197] Fertility rates have been documented in up to 80% after successful pharmaceutical treatments with dopamine agonists.[198]

Hyperprolactinemia has multiple potential etiologies. Physiological culprits include pregnancy, breastfeeding, stress, exercise, sleep, and eating. Pharmacologic causes entail use of antipsychotics (dopamine receptor blockers), antidepressants (dopamine receptor blockade), antihypertensives, opiates, medicinal herbs, GI medications (dopamine modulators), hormones, and antiepileptic and TB drugs. Other etiologies include pituitary disorders such as adenomas, hypophysitis, empty

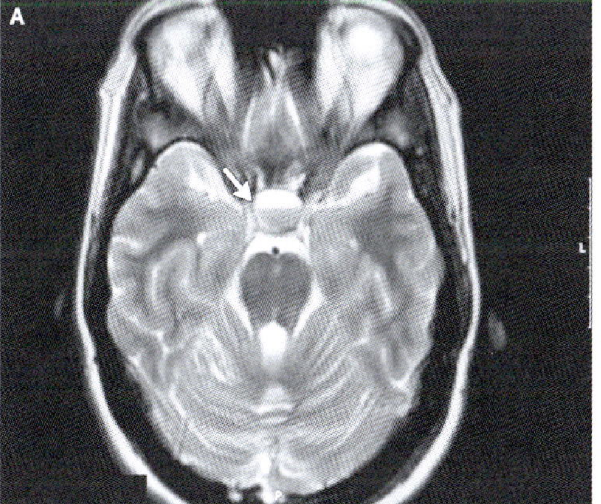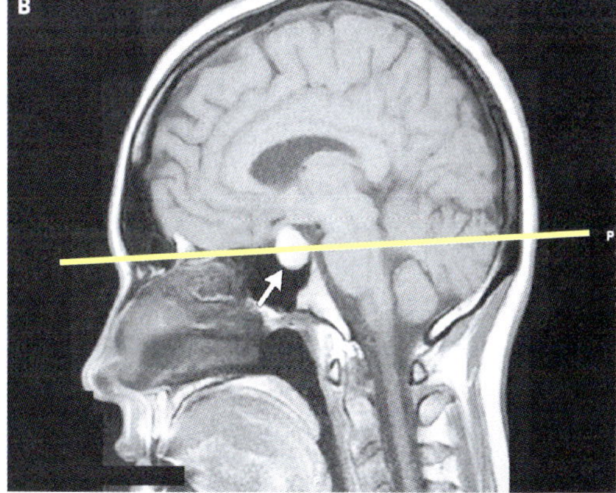

FIGURE 22-4. A. MRI of the head in the axial view. The arrow points to the pituitary which has both hyperintense and hypointense areas. B. MRI of the head showing a mid-saggital section. The pituitary gland is enlarged and the arrow is pointing to it.

sella syndrome, Rathke cyst, infiltrative disorders (TB and sarcoidosis), and some cancers, particularly certain metastases. Also, elevation of the prolactin can be attributed to hypothalamic entities that disrupt dopamine distribution, including tumors and granulomas, radiation treatment, and hypothyroidism.[199]

Symptoms of prolactinomas include bleeding abnormalities, headaches, and galactorrhea. Pituitary adenomas are subdivided into 2 categories based on size: Microadenomas are less than 1 cm or 10 mm; a macroadenoma is defined as an adenoma larger than 10 mm seen on either CT or MRI imaging. MRI is a better way to image the pituitary because there is less artifact from the bony sella, which distorts imaging via CT. Microadenomas rarely undergo symptomatic growth during pregnancy.[136] With the unique hormonal milieu of pregnancy along with the withdrawal of dopamine pharmaceuticals, there tends to be a stimulatory effect on the size of prolactinomas. Studies showed only 15%–35% change in size for macroadenomas that cause visual disturbance, headaches, and diabetes insipidus (DI).[200]

Based on expert opinion, it is suggested that dopamine agonists be discontinued in pregnancy to limit fetal exposure, except in selected macroadenomas (large or compressing optic chiasm). In a review of over 6000 pregnancies in which either bromocriptine or cabergoline was implemented only as needed, there were no changes over the normal rates of spontaneous abortions, ectopic pregnancies, trophoblastic disease, or anomalies found in the general population.[201] The pharmaceutical treatment regimen for prolactinomas in pregnancy is similar to the nonpregnant state. Bromocriptine or cabergoline may be used; both are dopamine agonists. These medications may produce a significant reduction in the volume of macroadenomas. Cabergoline has a longer half-life compared to other agonists and has been shown to restore menses (nongravid state) and decrease tumor size in approximately 90% of patients.[202] Bromocriptine does cross the placenta[203]; thus, use in patients with microadenomas is not needed. This will mitigate exposure during organogenesis and will restrict medication during a time when tumor changes are less likely.[202] Long-term analysis of infants up to 9 years of age has confirmed the safety of these drugs in pregnancy.[204] Information on pregnancy outcomes after exposure to this medication from the first trimester did not show any increased risk of complications compared to the general population.[204] There have been isolated cases of neurological issues in children followed up to 12 years postdelivery, but these have not been of statistical significance.[205]

Prolactin levels and routine visual field testing are not recommended. However, regular macroadenoma evaluation of the patient along with trimester visual field examinations is recommended during pregnancy.[206] Assessments of prolactin levels are not indicated due to elevation in pregnancy and the fact that they may not rise with tumor enlargement.[207] Radiological studies using unenhanced MRI should be scheduled with the onset of symptoms representing adenoma growth, especially headaches or visual abnormalities.[208] Enlargement of microprolactinomas is occasionally noticed, although symptomatic growth is documented in 2% of pregnancies.[187] Tumor growth may be seen in up to 30% of macroprolactinomas with subsequent complications in 5% of these gravida women. It is critical to implement visual field assessment in these patients frequently.[209] With evidence of tumor advancement, dopamine agonist pharmaceuticals should be immediately restarted, and therapeutic levels may shrink the tumor and improve visual fields. Alternatively, transsphenoidal surgery may be considered or even delivery if the gestation length is acceptable. Pregnancies involving macroprolactinomas with no surgical or radiological intervention prior to conception are at the highest risk for tumor enlargement.[202] Breastfeeding may be encouraged for women after pregnancy despite this disorder.[199]

Acromegaly

Acromegaly is an endocrine disorder associated with elevated GH levels and is often associated with large pituitary tumors. The symptoms are typically coarse features of the face and hands. It is a difficult disorder to diagnose in general because the symptoms typically emerge slowly over time. In a third of acromegaly cases, there is an association with hyperprolactinemia due to the mass effect on the pituitary or stalk. Some patients are identified with elevated prolactin levels and associated anovulation during an infertility workup. These patients are then treated with dopamine agonist therapy, and they are typically responsive, with ovulation and conception.[210] Infertility is commonly seen with acromegaly due to a high incidence of anovulation associated with hyperprolactinemia, but they are also at risk for hypopituitarism secondary to the tumor mass effects and other hormonal abnormalities in conjunction with elevated GH/IGF-1 levels, so it is imperative that an MRI be performed to diagnose any tumor that may be present.[211] Surgical intervention is the mainstay of treatment for these patients. If a complete cure is not obtained by the surgical approach, then medical treatment with somatostatin analogues (octreotide and lanreotide) and possibly dopamine agonists (e.g., bromocriptine, cabergoline) may be beneficial.[212,233]

In the healthy individual, GH secretion by the mother during pregnancy increases around week 10 of gestation and plateaus about 28 weeks. The placenta provides a majority of GH, which then reduces maternal production by the pituitary. Stimulation testing such as insulin-induced hypoglycemia or arginine stimulation results in a blunted maternal response during pregnancy.

Diagnosis of an abnormality such as acromegaly during pregnancy can be determined by the failure of an oral glucose tolerance test to suppress pituitary GH.[213] It is possible to differentiate the GH produced by the mother from that produced by the placenta by assaying special epitopes, but not by the normal commercial GH assays.[214] In acromegaly with pregnancy, IGF-1 levels are affected by pituitary and placental GH, but they are restricted by the estrogen levels and may only be slightly elevated.[83]

Those with acromegaly may be observed during pregnancy similar to patients with prolactinomas, depending on their symptoms and tumor size. Excess GH acts as an insulin antagonist and may result in hyperglycemia and diabetes during pregnancy.[215] Hormonal assessments of GH or IGF-1 are not necessary or useful. It is recommended that the patient have formal visual field screening and neurological evaluation each trimester. Changes in findings suspicious for adenoma enlargement would warrant an enhanced MRI. Hemorrhage into the tumor with subsequent neurological symptoms and visual changes during pregnancy can occur acutely.[216] Rapid evaluation would be needed in this last case. Otherwise, treatment of those with acromegaly during pregnancy may include dopamine agonists (bromocriptine, cabergoline), octreotide, or transphenoidal surgery.[172] There have been successful pregnancies using GH analogue and a somatostatin receptor ligand.[217] Surgical intervention along with GH receptor drugs have also been used to treat this disorder. Typically, definitive surgery is usually deferred until after delivery.

Acromegaly typically does not adversely affect the pregnancy or the fetus unless there are complications either with pituitary tumor enlargement or with the medications. Some women have had an increased risk for metabolic, cardiovascular, and skeletal compliations.[215,218] Rare pregnancies treated with somatostatin analogues have had notable Doppler changes, described as increased resistance during diastolic flow of fetal vessels and associated with fetal growth restriction.

The major issue concerning acromegaly in pregnancy is associated with rapid, significant tumor growth. Surgical intervention is a consideration with symptomatic compression of the optic chiasm as well as the occurrence of pituitary apoplexy, although most pregnancies are without significant complications.[220–222] Apoplexy is a rare emergency associated with hemorrhagic infarction of the pituitary. Symptoms include central nervous entities, including cranial nerve palsy and chemistry findings associated with hypopituitarism. This is a life-threatening problem. Treatment is centered on high-dose steroids.

Sheehan Syndrome

Sheehan syndrome results from pituitary ischemia and necrosis associated with obstetrical blood loss. It is assumed that the pituitary changes during the gravid state with its increased size and influences the chance for ischemia with occlusive spasm of the arteries to the anterior pituitary and stalk.[223] Women may experience persistent hypotension, tachycardia, and hypoglycemia; the diagnosis may be missed for years due to heterogenicity of the disorder.[224] These individuals may have menstrual abnormalities, decreased libido, failure to lactate, hair loss, generalized malaise, and secondary adrenal insufficiency signs and symptoms. MRI scans may be informative, showing empty sellae.[225,226] If this abnormality is suspected, the adrenal insufficiency is the most critical aspect and should be addressed with glucocorticoid replacement, subsequent analyses, and replacement of thyroid and gonadal hormones and GHs.[227] Cases of DI have been attributed to vascular occlusion with atrophy and scarring of the neurohypophysis.[228]

Lymphocytic Hypophysitis

Lymphocytic hypophysitis is a rare disorder, and it is thought to be an autoimmune disorder.[229] Serum antipituitary antinuclear antibodies and antimitochondrial antibodies have been detected in some cases. Massive infiltration by lymphocytes and plasma cells are seen with this autoimmune pituitary anomaly. This disorder is mainly seen in the third trimester of pregnancy or postpartum.[230] Symptoms include headaches, visual field defects, and cranial palsy. MRI of the pituitary will detect a diffusely symmetric enlarged pituitary, rather than a focal lesion. It is associated with elevated prolactin levels, low TSH, and adrenal insufficiency. Therapy is conservative and includes mitigating any pituitary deficits, especially adrenal deficits.[230] Coexisting autoimmune disorders (such as Addison disease, DI, hyperprolactinemia, and pernicious anemia) are seen in 33% of cases. Hormonal replacement is required.[230] High dose glucocorticoid therapy may be needed. In situations with severe chiasm compression that occurs during pregnancy despite high-dose steroid therapy, surgical consideration is offered.[231] Most of these patients will progress to a state of chronic panhypopituitarism with a delayed discovery of an empty sella on MRI.[232]

TSH-Secreting Adenomas and Gonadotropin-Secreting Adenomas

The TSH-secreting pituitary adenomas are rare. According to case reports, octreotide has been used successfully in pregnancy to treat these tumors. The critical issue of the tumors is regulation of the hyperthyroidism during the gravid state.[233] Thionamide treatment can be utilized to control the symptoms of hyperthyroidism.[233]

Nonfunctioning adenomas are usually gonadotropin adenomas. There have only been a couple of cases of tumor enlargement in clinically nonfunctioning adenomas (CNFAs) during pregnancy. Intervention with a dopamine agonist has been successful because pregnancy does not have an impact on these adenomas.[234]

Posterior Pituitary and Diabetes Insipidus

The supraoptic and paraventricular nuclei of the hypothalamus have neurosecretory neurons that extend their axons into the neurohypophysis or posterior pituitary and secrete arginine vasopressin–antidiuretic hormone (AVP-ADH), a cyclic nonapeptide. This hormone is the key regulator responsible for maintaining blood osmolality within a narrow range (±1.8%). It does this by increasing osmotic pressures or decreasing hydrostatic pressures, which results in the kidney adjusting the amount of water retention at the level of the tubules and initiating thirst stimulation. During pregnancy, there is normally a decrease in plasma osmolality by about 10 mOsm/kg, which occurs within the first trimester and continues throughout gestation; it is thought to be related to elevated levels of hCG.[233,235] Interestingly, this change in osmolality during pregnancy does not affect the level of AVP-ADH; the posterior pituitary acts as if the set point for osmolality regulation has been changed and maintains AVP-ADH at the same level.

Diabetes insipidus is a disorder involving the inappropriate loss of water due to the kidney tubules not reabsorbing water sufficiently. The causes of DI are usually described as either central or peripheral (nephrogenic). In pregnancy, we may add a third grouping: transient DI. Pregnancy-related causes of DI may result from increased vasopressinase production by the placenta or decreased breakdown by the liver due to preeclampsia or acute fatty liver. Symptoms of DI include polydipsia due to excessive thirst, polyuria, and dehydration.[234]

The central form is caused by decreased production of vasopressin. The differential diagnoses include infiltrating tumors or inflammatory cells in the neurohypophysis, pituitary surgery/trauma, or infection. Some examples of specific causes during pregnancy are an expanding pituitary adenoma with lymphocytic hypophysitis or disorders such as histiocytosis X. DI is a rare complication of pregnancy in which the vasopressin deficiency is mainly associated with a hypothalamic or a pituitary stalk disorder.[235] Symptoms may result in the acute onset of polyuria, which can be massive (i.e., up to 15 L/d). In this central disorder, the level of AVP-ADH is low. Pregnancy usually worsens central DI, which appears to be associated with the low AVP-ADH becoming even lower with an increase in vasopressinase produced by the placenta or reduced vasopressinase clearance.[234]

Pharmaceutical management for this abnormality is with an analogue to vasopressin, desmopressin, which is L,deamino-8-D-arginine vasopressin (DDAVP). DDAVP is given intranasally, 2–20 μg twice daily. With this regimen, there have been no significant complications for either the mother or the fetus. Only minimal amounts of DDAVP reach breast milk, and it has no negative effects on infants. So, breastfeeding is not contraindicated when treating DI with DDAVP. Vasopressinase-induced DI is seen in 3 per 100,000 pregnancies.[236]

CONCLUSION

Endocrine disorders in pregnancy can pose a diagnostic challenge, primarily due to the fact that pregnancy itself has symptoms that overlap those seen with certain endocrine disorders. Clinical symptoms presented by some of these endocrine disorders include hypertension and headaches in pheochromocytomas, and these symptoms may mimic preeclampsia or gestational hypertension. Likewise, heat intolerance, warm skin, and tachycardia of hyperthyroidism may sometimes be confused with the hypermetabolic state of pregnancy.

Diabetes is the most common endocrinopathy in pregnancy, followed by thyroid disorders. Pituitary, adrenal, and parathyroid disorders are relatively less common, with only a few cases reported. Despite the fact that studies have linked the endocrine disorders with adverse outcomes in both the mother and the fetus, routine screening is not recommended during pregnancy except for diabetes.

Screening for pregnant women is emphasized by ACOG and ATA only when the women have a personal history of thyroid diseases or present with clinical symptoms of thyroid disease. Once diagnosed, overt hypothyroidism should always be treated in pregnancy even if FT_4 is normal and the TSH levels are above 10 mIU/L. No treatment is, however, recommended for isolated hypothyroxinemia and subclinical hypothyroidism. Similarly, other endocrine disorders, once identified, should be managed first with medical therapy as indicated, and if no improvement, surgery is recommended in the second or early third trimester preferably.

In pregnancy, when the index of suspicion is high for endocrinopathies based on family or personal history or clinical symptoms, testing should be initiated early. A multidisciplinary approach should be used in the diagnosis and management of these conditions; once identified, treatment should be started immediately to reduce the maternal or fetal adverse outcomes. Because there are few large studies regarding the evaluation and the management of these relatively infrequent endocrine disorders in pregnancy, it is paramount that treatments be individualized based on patient needs.

REFERENCES

1. Brennan MD, Bahn RS. Thyroid hormones and illness. *Endocr Pract*. 1998;4(6):396–403.
2. Brent GA. The molecular basis of thyroid hormone action. *N Engl J Med*. 1994;331(13):847–853.
3. Glinoer D, de Nayer P, Bourdoux P, et al. Regulation of maternal thyroid during pregnancy. *J Clin Endocrinol Metab*. 1990;71(2):276–287.
4. Fister P, Gaberscek S, Zaletel K, Krhin B, Gersak K, Hojker S. Thyroid volume changes during pregnancy and after delivery in an iodine-sufficient Republic of Slovenia. *Eur J Obstet Gynecol Reprod Biol*. 2009;145(1):45–48.
5. Smallridge RC, Glinoer D, Hollowell JG, Brent G. Thyroid function inside and outside of pregnancy: what do we know and what don't we know? *Thyroid*. 2005;15(1):54–59.
6. Ecker JL, Musci TJ. Treatment of thyroid disease in pregnancy. *Obstet Gynecol Clin North Am*. 1997;24(3): 575–589.
7. Leung AM. Thyroid function in pregnancy. *J Trace Elem Med Biol*. 2012;26(2–3):137–140.
8. Burrow GN, Fisher DA, Larsen PR. Maternal and fetal thyroid function. *N Engl J Med*. 1994;331(16): 1072–1078.
9. Azizi F. Early detection and optimized management of thyroid disease in pregnancy. *Int J Endocrinol Metab*. 2015;13(1):e25728.

10. Krajewski DA, Burman KD. Thyroid disorders in pregnancy. *Endocrinol Metab Clin North Am*. 2011;40(4): 739–763.

11. Grun JP, Meuris S, De Nayer P, Glinoer D. The thyrotrophic role of human chorionic gonadotrophin (hCG) in the early stages of twin (versus single) pregnancies. *Clin Endocrinol*. 1997;46(6):719–725.

12. Huang SA. Physiology and pathophysiology of type 3 deiodinase in humans. *Thyroid*. 2005;15(8):875–881.

13. Williams GR. Neurodevelopmental and neurophysiological actions of thyroid hormone. *J Neuroendocrinol*. 2008;20(6):784–794.

14. Calvo RM, Jauniaux E, Gulbis B, et al. Fetal tissues are exposed to biologically relevant free thyroxine concentrations during early phases of development. *J Clin Endocrinol Metab*. 2002;87(4):1768–1777.

15. Auso E, Lavado-Autric R, Cuevas E, Del Rey FE, Morreale De Escobar G, Berbel P. A moderate and transient deficiency of maternal thyroid function at the beginning of fetal neocorticogenesis alters neuronal migration. *Endocrinology*. 2004;145(9):4037–4047.

16. Vulsma T, Gons MH, de Vijlder JJ. Maternal-fetal transfer of thyroxine in congenital hypothyroidism due to a total organification defect or thyroid agenesis. *N Engl J Med*. 1989;321(1):13–16.

17. Practice bulletin no. 148: thyroid disease in pregnancy. *Obstet Gynecol*. 2015;125(4):996–1005.

18. Alvarez-Marfany M, Roman SH, Drexler AJ, Robertson C, Stagnaro-Green A. Long-term prospective study of postpartum thyroid dysfunction in women with insulin dependent diabetes mellitus. *J Clin Endocrinol Metab*. 1994;79(1):10–16.

19. De Groot L, Abalovich M, Alexander EK, et al. Management of thyroid dysfunction during pregnancy and postpartum: an Endocrine Society clinical practice guideline. *J Clin Endocrinol Metab*. 2012;97(8):2543–2565.

20. Stagnaro-Green A, Sullivan S, Pearce EN. Iodine supplementation during pregnancy and lactation. *JAMA*. 2012;308(23):2463–2464.

21. Delange F. Iodine deficiency as a cause of brain damage. *Postgrad Med J*. 2001;77(906):217–220.

22. Kennedy RL, Malabu UH, Jarrod G, Nigam P, Kannan K, Rane A. Thyroid function and pregnancy: before, during and beyond. *J Obstet Gynaecol*. 2010;30(8): 774–783.

23. Pearce EN. What do we know about iodine supplementation in pregnancy? *J Clin Endocrinol Metab*. 2009;94(9):3188–3190.

24. Levy RP, Newman DM, Rejali LS, Barford DA. The myth of goiter in pregnancy. *Am J Obstet Gynecol*. 1980;137(6):701–703.

25. Teng W, Shan Z, Teng X, et al. Effect of iodine intake on thyroid diseases in China. *N Engl J Med*. 2006;354(26):2783–2793.

26. LaFranchi S. Thyroid function in the preterm infant. *Thyroid*. 1999;9(1):71–78.

27. Thorpe-Beeston JG, Nicolaides KH, Felton CV, Butler J, McGregor AM. Maturation of the secretion of thyroid hormone and thyroid-stimulating hormone in the fetus. *N Engl J Med*. 1991;324(8):532–536.

28. Contempre B, Jauniaux E, Calvo R, Jurkovic D, Campbell S, de Escobar GM. Detection of thyroid hormones in human embryonic cavities during the first trimester of pregnancy. *J Clin Endocrinol Metab*. 1993;77(6):1719–1722.

29. Bernal J. Thyroid hormone receptors in brain development and function. *Nat Clin Pract Endocrinol Metab*. 2007;3(3):249–259.

30. Thorpe-Beeston JG, Nicolaides KH, Snijders RJ, Felton CV, McGregor AM. Thyroid function in small for gestational age fetuses. *Obstet Gynecol*. 1991;77(5):701–706.

31. Utiger RD. Maternal hypothyroidism and fetal development. *N Engl J Med*. 1999;341(8):601–602.

32. McKenzie JM, Zakarija M. Fetal and neonatal hyperthyroidism and hypothyroidism due to maternal TSH receptor antibodies. *Thyroid*. 1992;2(2):155–159.

33. Kilpatrick S. Umbilical blood sampling in women with thyroid disease in pregnancy: Is it necessary? *Am J Obstet Gynecol*. 2003;189(1):1–2.

34. Abbassi-Ghanavati M, Casey BM, Spong CY, McIntire DD, Halvorson LM, Cunningham FG. Pregnancy outcomes in women with thyroid peroxidase antibodies. *Obstet Gynecol*. 2010;116(2 Pt 1):381–386.

35. Thangaratinam S, Tan A, Knox E, Kilby MD, Franklyn J, Coomarasamy A. Association between thyroid autoantibodies and miscarriage and preterm birth: meta-analysis of evidence. *BMJ*. 2011;342:d2616.

36. Greer LG, Casey BM, Halvorson LM, Spong CY, McIntire DD, Cunningham FG. Antithyroid antibodies and parity: further evidence for microchimerism in autoimmune thyroid disease. *Am J Obstet Gynecol*. 2011;205(5):e471–474.

37. Luton D, Le Gac I, Vuillard E, et al. Management of Graves' disease during pregnancy: the key role of fetal thyroid gland monitoring. *J Clin Endocrinol Metab*. 2005;90(11):6093–6098.

38. Stagnaro-Green A. Overt hyperthyroidism and hypothyroidism during pregnancy. *Clin Obstet Gynecol*. 2011;54(3):478–487.

39. Laurberg P, Nygaard B, Glinoer D, Grussendorf M, Orgiazzi J. Guidelines for TSH-receptor antibody measurements in pregnancy: results of an evidence-based symposium organized by the European Thyroid Association. *Eur J Endocrinol*. 1998;139(6):584–586.

40. Ladenson PW, Ewertz ME, Dickey RA. Practical application of recombinant thyrotropin testing in clinical practice. *Endocr Pract*. 2001;7(3):195–201.

41. Gittoes NJ, Franklyn JA. Hyperthyroidism. Current treatment guidelines. *Drugs*. 1998;55(4):543–553.

42. Stagnaro-Green A, Abalovich M, Alexander E, et al. Guidelines of the American Thyroid Association for the diagnosis and management of thyroid disease during pregnancy and postpartum. *Thyroid*. 2011;21(10):1081–1125.

43. Barbesino G, Tomer Y. Clinical review: clinical utility of TSH receptor antibodies. *J Clin Endocrinol Metab*. 2013;98(6):2247–2255.

44. Weetman AP. Controversy in thyroid disease. *J R Coll Physicians Lond*. 2000;34(4):374–380.

45. Mestman JH. Hyperthyroidism in pregnancy. *Curr Opin Endocrinol Diabetes Obes*. 2012;19(5):394–401.

46. Millar LK, Wing DA, Leung AS, Koonings PP, Montoro MN, Mestman JH. Low birth weight and preeclampsia in pregnancies complicated by hyperthyroidism. *Obstet Gynecol*. 1994;84(6):946–949.

47. Su PY, Huang K, Hao JH, et al. Maternal thyroid function in the first twenty weeks of pregnancy and subsequent fetal and infant development: a prospective population-based cohort study in China. *J Clin Endocrinol Metab*. 2011;96(10):3234–3241.

48. Saki F, Dabbaghmanesh MH, Ghaemi SZ, Forouhari S, Ranjbar Omrani G, Bakhshayeshkaram M. Thyroid function in pregnancy and its influences on maternal and fetal outcomes. *Int J Endocrinol Metab*. 2014;12(4):e19378.

49. Anselmo J, Cao D, Karrison T, Weiss RE, Refetoff S. Fetal loss associated with excess thyroid hormone exposure. *JAMA*. 2004;292(6):691–695.

50. Andersen SL, Olsen J, Wu CS, Laurberg P. Spontaneous abortion, stillbirth and hyperthyroidism: a danish population-based study. *Eur Thyroid J*. 2014;3(3):164–172.

51. Davis LE, Lucas MJ, Hankins GD, Roark ML, Cunningham FG. Thyrotoxicosis complicating pregnancy. *Am J Obstet Gynecol*. 1989;160(1):63–70.

52. Matsuura N, Harada S, Ohyama Y, et al. The mechanisms of transient hypothyroxinemia in infants born to mothers with Graves' disease. *Pediatr Res*. 1997;42(2):214–218.

53. Nachum Z, Rakover Y, Weiner E, Shalev E. Graves' disease in pregnancy: prospective evaluation of a selective invasive treatment protocol. *Am J Obstet Gynecol*. 2003;189(1):159–165.

54. Brand F, Liegeois P, Langer B. One case of fetal and neonatal variable thyroid dysfunction in the context of Graves' disease. *Fetal Diagn Ther*. 2005;20(1):12–15.

55. Garber JR, Cobin RH, Gharib H, et al. Clinical practice guidelines for hypothyroidism in adults: cosponsored by the American Association of Clinical Endocrinologists and the American Thyroid Association. *Thyroid*. 2012;22(12):1200–1235.

56. Surks MI, Ortiz E, Daniels GH, et al. Subclinical thyroid disease: scientific review and guidelines for diagnosis and management. *JAMA*. 2004;291(2):228–238.

57. Casey BM, Leveno KJ. Thyroid disease in pregnancy. *Obstet Gynecol*. 2006;108(5):1283–1292.

58. Casey BM, Dashe JS, Wells CE, McIntire DD, Leveno KJ, Cunningham FG. Subclinical hyperthyroidism and pregnancy outcomes. *Obstet Gynecol*. 2006;107(2 Pt 1):337–341.

59. Wilson KL, Casey BM, McIntire DD, Halvorson LM, Cunningham FG. Subclinical thyroid disease and the incidence of hypertension in pregnancy. *Obstet Gynecol*. 2012;119(2 Pt 1):315–320.

60. Hershman JM. Physiological and pathological aspects of the effect of human chorionic gonadotropin on the thyroid. *Best Pract Res Clin Endocrinol Metab*. 2004;18(2):249–265.

61. Fitzpatrick DL, Russell MA. Diagnosis and management of thyroid disease in pregnancy. *Obstet Gynecol Clin North Am*. 2010;37(2):173–193.

62. Goodwin TM, Montoro M, Mestman JH. Transient hyperthyroidism and hyperemesis gravidarum: clinical aspects. *Am J Obstet Gynecol*. 1992;167(3):648–652.

63. Shulman A, Shapiro MS, Bahary C, Shenkman L. Abnormal thyroid function in hyperemesis gravidarum. *Acta Obstet Gynecol Scand*. 1989;68(6):533–536.

64. Molitch ME. Endocrine emergencies in pregnancy. *Baillieres Clin Endocrinol Metabol*. 1992;6(1):167–191.

65. Sheffield JS, Cunningham FG. Thyrotoxicosis and heart failure that complicate pregnancy. *Am J Obstet Gynecol*. 2004;190(1):211–217.

66. Siu CW, Zhang XH, Yung C, Kung AW, Lau CP, Tse HF. Hemodynamic changes in hyperthyroidism-related pulmonary hypertension: a prospective echocardiographic study. *J Clin Endocrinol Metab*. 2007;92(5):1736–1742.

67. Brent GA. Clinical practice. Graves' disease. *N Engl J Med*. 2008;358(24):2594–2605.

68. Yoshihara A, Noh J, Yamaguchi T, et al. Treatment of Graves' disease with antithyroid drugs in the first trimester of pregnancy and the prevalence of congenital malformation. *J Clin Endocrinol Metab*. 2012;97(7):2396–2403.

69. Kimura M, Seki T, Ozawa H, et al. The onset of anti-neutrophil cytoplasmic antibody-associated vasculitis immediately after methimazole was switched to propylthiouracil in a woman with Graves' disease who wished to become pregnant. *Endocr J*. 2013;60(3):383–388.

70. Wing DA, Millar LK, Koonings PP, Montoro MN, Mestman JH. A comparison of propylthiouracil versus methimazole in the treatment of hyperthyroidism in pregnancy. *Am J Obstet Gynecol*. 1994;170(1 Pt 1):90–95.

71. Momotani N, Noh JY, Ishikawa N, Ito K. Effects of propylthiouracil and methimazole on fetal thyroid status in mothers with Graves' hyperthyroidism. *J Clin Endocrinol Metab*. 1997;82(11):3633–3636.

72. Bahn RS, Burch HB, Cooper DS, et al. Hyperthyroidism and other causes of thyrotoxicosis: management guidelines of the American Thyroid Association and American Association of Clinical Endocrinologists. *Endocr Pract.* 2011;17(3):456–520.

73. Briggs GG. Medication use during the perinatal period. *J Am Pharm Assoc.* 1998;38(6):717–726; quiz 726–717.

74. Stagnaro-Green A, Pearce E. Thyroid disorders in pregnancy. *Nat Rev Endocrinol.* 2012;8(11):650–658.

75. Ayala C, Navarro E, Rodriguez JR, Silva H, Venegas E, Astorga R. Conception after iodine-131 therapy for differentiated thyroid cancer. *Thyroid.* 1998;8(11):1009–1011.

76. Berlin L. Iodine-131 and the pregnant patient. *AJR. Am J Roentgenol.* 2001;176(4):869–871.

77. McClellan DR, Francis GL. Thyroid cancer in children, pregnant women, and patients with Graves' disease. *Endocrinol Metab Clin North Am.* 1996;25(1):27–48.

78. Yassa L, Marqusee E, Fawcett R, Alexander EK. Thyroid hormone early adjustment in pregnancy (the THERAPY) trial. *J Clin Endocrinol Metab.* 2010;95(7):3234–3241.

79. Loh JA, Wartofsky L, Jonklaas J, Burman KD. The magnitude of increased levothyroxine requirements in hypothyroid pregnant women depends upon the etiology of the hypothyroidism. *Thyroid.* 2009;19(3):269–275.

80. Haddow JE, Palomaki GE, Allan WC, et al. Maternal thyroid deficiency during pregnancy and subsequent neuropsychological development of the child. *N Engl J Med.* 1999;341(8):549–555.

81. Davis LE, Leveno KJ, Cunningham FG. Hypothyroidism complicating pregnancy. *Obstet Gynecol.* 1988;72(1):108–112.

82. Negro R, Formoso G, Mangieri T, Pezzarossa A, Dazzi D, Hassan H. Levothyroxine treatment in euthyroid pregnant women with autoimmune thyroid disease: effects on obstetrical complications. *J Clin Endocrinol Metab.* 2006;91(7):2587–2591.

83. Casey BM, Dashe JS, Wells CE, et al. Subclinical hypothyroidism and pregnancy outcomes. *Obstet Gynecol.* 2005;105(2):239–245.

84. Matalon S, Sheiner E, Levy A, Mazor M, Wiznitzer A. Relationship of treated maternal hypothyroidism and perinatal outcome. *J Reprod Med.* 2006;51(1):59–63.

85. Tan TO, Cheng YW, Caughey AB. Are women who are treated for hypothyroidism at risk for pregnancy complications? *Am J Obstet Gynecol.* 2006;194(5):e1–e3.

86. Lazarus JH, Bestwick JP, Channon S, et al. Antenatal thyroid screening and childhood cognitive function. *N Engl J Med.* 2012;366(6):493–501.

87. Cao XY, Jiang XM, Dou ZH, et al. Timing of vulnerability of the brain to iodine deficiency in endemic cretinism. *N Engl J Med.* 1994;331(26):1739–1744.

88. Leger J, Dos Santos S, Larroque B, Ecosse E. Pregnancy outcomes and relationship to treatment adequacy in women treated early for congenital hypothyroidism: a longitudinal population-based study. *J Clin Endocrinol Metab.* 2015;100(3):860–869.

89. Brown RS, Bellisario RL, Botero D, et al. Incidence of transient congenital hypothyroidism due to maternal thyrotropin receptor-blocking antibodies in over one million babies. *J Clin Endocrinol Metab.* 1996;81(3):1147–1151.

90. Rovelli R, Vigone MC, Giovanettoni C, et al. Newborn of mothers affected by autoimmune thyroiditis: the importance of thyroid function monitoring in the first months of life. *Ital J Pediatr.* 2010;36:24.

91. Fisher DA. Fetal thyroid function: diagnosis and management of fetal thyroid disorders. *Clin Obstet Gynecol.* 1997;40(1):16–31.

92. US Preventive Services Task Force. Screening for congenital hypothyroidism. In: *US Preventive Services Task Force. Guide to Clinical Preventive Services.* 2nd ed. Baltimore: Williams & Wilkins, 1996:503–507.

93. Surks MI. Response to position statement on subclinical thyroid dysfunction. *Endocr Pract.* 2004;10(6):513–514.

94. Cleary-Goldman J, Malone FD, Lambert-Messerlian G, et al. Maternal thyroid hypofunction and pregnancy outcome. *Obstet Gynecol.* 2008;112(1):85–92.

95. Gharib H, Tuttle RM, Baskin HJ, et al. Consensus Statement #1: subclinical thyroid dysfunction: a joint statement on management from the American Association of Clinical Endocrinologists, the American Thyroid Association, and the Endocrine Society. *Thyroid.* 2005;15(1):24–28; response 32–23.

96. Diez JJ, Iglesias P. Spontaneous subclinical hypothyroidism in patients older than 55 years: an analysis of natural course and risk factors for the development of overt thyroid failure. *J Clin Endocrinol Metab.* 2004;89(10):4890–4897.

97. Karmisholt J, Andersen S, Laurberg P. Variation in thyroid function tests in patients with stable untreated subclinical hypothyroidism. *Thyroid.* 2008;18(3):303–308.

98. Mannisto T, Vaarasmaki M, Pouta A, et al. Thyroid dysfunction and autoantibodies during pregnancy as predictive factors of pregnancy complications and maternal morbidity in later life. *J Clin Endocrinol Metab.* 2010;95(3):1084–1094.

99. Lazarus J, Okosieme OE. Hypothyroidism in pregnancy. In: De Groot LJ, Beck-Peccoz P, Chrousos G, et al., eds. *Endotext.* South Dartmouth, MA: MDText.com; 2000. www.endotext.org.

100. Leung AS, Millar LK, Koonings PP, Montoro M, Mestman JH. Perinatal outcome in hypothyroid pregnancies. *Obstet Gynecol.* 1993;81(3):349–353.

101. Abalovich M, Gutierrez S, Alcaraz G, Maccallini G, Garcia A, Levalle O. Overt and subclinical

hypothyroidism complicating pregnancy. *Thyroid.* 2002;12(1):63–68.

102. Abalovich M, Alcaraz G, Kleiman-Rubinsztein J, et al. The relationship of preconception thyrotropin levels to requirements for increasing the levothyroxine dose during pregnancy in women with primary hypothyroidism. *Thyroid.* 2010;20(10):1175–1178.

103. Alexander EK, Marqusee E, Lawrence J, Jarolim P, Fischer GA, Larsen PR. Timing and magnitude of increases in levothyroxine requirements during pregnancy in women with hypothyroidism. *N Engl J Med.* 2004;351(3):241–249.

104. Arafah BM. Increased need for thyroxine in women with hypothyroidism during estrogen therapy. *N Engl J Med.* 2001;344(23):1743–1749.

105. Mandel SJ, Larsen PR, Seely EW, Brent GA. Increased need for thyroxine during pregnancy in women with primary hypothyroidism. *N Engl J Med.* 1990;323(2):91–96.

106. Bartolazzi A, Gasbarri A, Papotti M, et al. Application of an immunodiagnostic method for improving preoperative diagnosis of nodular thyroid lesions. *Lancet.* 2001;357(9269):1644–1650.

107. Vini L, Hyer S, Pratt B, Harmer C. Management of differentiated thyroid cancer diagnosed during pregnancy. *Eur J Endocrinol.* 1999;140(5):404–406.

108. Schlumberger M, De Vathaire F, Ceccarelli C, et al. Exposure to radioactive iodine-131 for scintigraphy or therapy does not preclude pregnancy in thyroid cancer patients. *J Nucl Med.* 1996;37(4):606–612.

109. Amino N, Tada H, Hidaka Y, Izumi Y. Postpartum autoimmune thyroid syndrome. *Endocr J.* 2000;47(6):645–655.

110. Lucas A, Pizarro E, Granada ML, Salinas I, Foz M, Sanmarti A. Postpartum thyroiditis: epidemiology and clinical evolution in a nonselected population. *Thyroid.* 2000;10(1):71–77.

111. Muller AF, Drexhage HA, Berghout A. Postpartum thyroiditis and autoimmune thyroiditis in women of childbearing age: recent insights and consequences for antenatal and postnatal care. *Endocr Rev.* 2001;22(5):605–630.

112. Lazarus JH, Ammari F, Oretti R, Parkes AB, Richards CJ, Harris B. Clinical aspects of recurrent postpartum thyroiditis. *Br J Gen Pract.* 1997;47(418):305–308.

113. Gerstein HC. How common is postpartum thyroiditis? A methodologic overview of the literature. *Arch Intern Med.* 1990;150(7):1397–1400.

114. Argatska AB, Nonchev BI. Postpartum thyroiditis. *Folia Med.* 2014;56(3):145–151.

115. Garber JR, Cobin RH, Gharib H, et al. Clinical practice guidelines for hypothyroidism in adults: cosponsored by the American Association of Clinical Endocrinologists and the American Thyroid Association. *Endocr Pract.* 2012;18(6):988–1028.

116. Behrooz HG, Tohidi M, Mehrabi Y, Behrooz EG, Tehranidoost M, Azizi F. Subclinical hypothyroidism in pregnancy: intellectual development of offspring. *Thyroid.* 2011;21(10):1143–1147.

117. Bolnick JM, Kilburn BA, Bajpayee S, Reddy N, Jeelani R, Crone B, et al. Trophoblast retrieval and isolation from the cervix (TRIC) for noninvasive prenatal screening at 5 to 20 weeks of gestation. *Fertil Steril.* 2014 Jul;102(1):135–142.e6. doi: 10.1016/j.fertnstert.2014.04.008. Epub 2014 May 10.

118. Kovacs CS, Kronenberg HM. Maternal-fetal calcium and bone metabolism during pregnancy, puerperium, and lactation. *Endocr Rev.* 1997;18(6):832–872.

119. More C, Bhattoa HP, Bettembuk P, Balogh A. The effects of pregnancy and lactation on hormonal status and biochemical markers of bone turnover. *Eur J Obstet Gynecol Reprod Biol.* 2003;106(2):209–213.

120. Weiss M, Eisenstein Z, Ramot Y, Lipitz S, Shulman A, Frenkel Y. Renal reabsorption of inorganic phosphorus in pregnancy in relation to the calciotropic hormones. *Br J Obstet Gynaecol.* 1998;105(2):195–199.

121. Dahlman T, Sjoberg HE, Bucht E. Calcium homeostasis in normal pregnancy and puerperium. A longitudinal study. *Acta Obstet Gynedol Scand.* 1994;73(5):393–398.

122. Vargas Zapata CL, Donangelo CM, Woodhouse LR, Abrams SA, Spencer EM, King JC. Calcium homeostasis during pregnancy and lactation in Brazilian women with low calcium intakes: a longitudinal study. *Am J Clin Nutr.* 2004;80(2):417–422.

123. Cooper MS. Disorders of calcium metabolism and parathyroid disease. *Best Pract Res Clin Endocrinol Metab.* 2011;25(6):975–983.

124. Seely EW, Brown EM, DeMaggio DM, Weldon DK, Graves SW. A prospective study of calciotropic hormones in pregnancy and post partum: reciprocal changes in serum intact parathyroid hormone and 1,25-dihydroxyvitamin D. *Am J Obstet Gynecol.* 1997;176(1 Pt 1):214–217.

125. Schnatz PF, Thaxton S. Parathyroidectomy in the third trimester of pregnancy. *Obstet Gynecol Surv.* 2005;60(10):672–682.

126. Power ML, Heaney RP, Kalkwarf HJ, et al. The role of calcium in health and disease. *Am J Obstet Gynecol.* 1999;181(6):1560–1569.

127. Kovacs CS. Calcium and bone metabolism disorders during pregnancy and lactation. *Endocrinol Metab Clin North Am.* 2011;40(4):795–826.

128. Kelly TR. Primary hyperparathyroidism during pregnancy. *Surgery.* 1991;110(6):1028–1033; discussion 1033–1024.

129. Hultin H, Hellman P, Lundgren E, et al. Association of parathyroid adenoma and pregnancy with preeclampsia. *J Clin Endocrinol Metab.* 2009;94(9):3394–3399.

130. Ficinski ML, Mestman JH. Primary hyperparathyroidism during pregnancy. *Endocr Pract.* 1996;2(5):362–367.

131. Dahan M, Chang RJ. Pancreatitis secondary to hyperparathyroidism during pregnancy. *Obstet Gynecol.* 2001;98(5 Pt 2):923-925.

132. Pothiwala P, Levine SN. Parathyroid surgery in pregnancy: review of the literature and localization by aspiration for parathyroid hormone levels. *J Perinatol.* 2009;29(12):779-784.

133. Farford B, Presutti RJ, Moraghan TJ. Nonsurgical management of primary hyperparathyroidism. *Mayo Clin Proc.* 2007;82(3):351-355.

134. Bilezikian JP, Silverberg SJ. Clinical practice. Asymptomatic primary hyperparathyroidism. *N Engl J Med.* 2004;350(17):1746-1751.

135. Bilezikian JP, Khan AA, Potts JT Jr; Third International Workshop on the Management of Asymptomatic Primary Hypoparathyroidism. Guidelines for the management of asymptomatic primary hyperparathyroidism: summary statement from the third international workshop. *J Clin Endocrinol Metab.* 2009;94(2):335-339.

136. Molitch ME. Pituitary tumors and pregnancy. *Growth Horm IGF Res.* 2003;13(Suppl A):S38-S44.

137. Barrett H, McElduff A. Vitamin D and pregnancy: an old problem revisited. *Best Pract Res Clin Endocrinol Metab.* 2010;24(4):527-539.

138. Brunvand L, Quigstad E, Urdal P, Haug E. Vitamin D deficiency and fetal growth. *Early Hum Dev.* 1996;45(1-2):27-33.

139. Bodnar LM, Catov JM, Simhan HN, Holick MF, Powers RW, Roberts JM. Maternal vitamin D deficiency increases the risk of preeclampsia. *J Clin Endocrinol Metab.* 2007;92(9):3517-3522.

140. Merewood A, Mehta SD, Chen TC, Bauchner H, Holick MF. Association between vitamin D deficiency and primary cesarean section. *J Clin Endocrinol Metab.* 2009;94(3):940-945.

141. Alikasifoglu A, Gonc EN, Yalcin E, Dogru D, Yordam N. Neonatal hyperparathyroidism due to maternal hypoparathyroidism and vitamin D deficiency: a cause of multiple bone fractures. *Clin Pediatr.* 2005;44(3):267-269.

142. Escher G. Hyperaldosteronism in pregnancy. *Ther Adv Cardiovasc Dis.* 2009;3(2):123-132.

143. Ehrlich EN, Lindheimer MD. Effect of administered mineralocorticoids or ACTH in pregnant women. Attenuation of kaliuretic influence of mineralocorticoids during pregnancy. *J Clin Investig.* 1972;51(6):1301-1309.

144. Speiser PW, Azziz R, Baskin LS, et al. A summary of the Endocrine Society clinical practice guidelines on congenital adrenal hyperplasia due to steroid 21-hydroxylase deficiency. *Int J Pediatr Endocrinol.* 2010;2010:494173.

145. Lekarev O, New MI. Adrenal disease in pregnancy. *Best Pract Res Clin Endocrinol Metab.* 2011;25(6):959-973.

146. Merke DP. Approach to the adult with congenital adrenal hyperplasia due to 21-hydroxylase deficiency. *J Clin Endocrinol Metab.* 2008;93(3):653-660.

147. Coleman MA, Honour JW. Reduced maternal dexamethasone dosage for the prenatal treatment of congenital adrenal hyperplasia. *BJOG.* 2004;111(2):176-178.

148. Pang S, Clark AT, Freeman LC, et al. Maternal side effects of prenatal dexamethasone therapy for fetal congenital adrenal hyperplasia. *J Clin Endocrinol Metab.* 1992;75(1):249-253.

149. Pang SY, Pollack MS, Marshall RN, Immken L. Prenatal treatment of congenital adrenal hyperplasia due to 21-hydroxylase deficiency. *N Engl J Med.* 1990;322(2):111-115.

150. Abdelmannan D, Aron DC. Adrenal disorders in pregnancy. *Endocrinol Metab Clin North Am.* 2011;40(4):779-794.

151. Sarathi V, Lila AR, Bandgar TR, Menon PS, Shah NS. Pheochromocytoma and pregnancy: a rare but dangerous combination. *Endocr Pract.* 2010;16(2):300-309.

152. Sarathi V, Bandgar TR, Menon PS, Shah NS. Pheochromocytoma and medullary thyroid carcinoma in a pregnant multiple endocrine neoplasia-2A patient. *Gynecol Endocrinol.* 2011;27(8):533-535.

153. Harper MA, Murnaghan GA, Kennedy L, Hadden DR, Atkinson AB. Phaeochromocytoma in pregnancy. Five cases and a review of the literature. *Br J Obstet Gynaecol.* 1989;96(5):594-606.

154. Desai AS, Chutkow WA, Edelman E, Economy KE, Dec GW Jr. Clinical problem-solving. A crisis in late pregnancy. *N Engl J Med.* 2009;361(23):2271-2277.

155. Grimbert P, Chauveau D, Remy SR, Grunfeld JP. Pregnancy in von Hippel-Lindau disease. *Am J Obstet Gynecol.* 1999;180(1 Pt 1):110-111.

156. Pedersen EB, Rasmussen AB, Christensen NJ, et al. Plasma noradrenaline and adrenaline in pre-eclampsia, essential hypertension in pregnancy and normotensive pregnant control subjects. *Acta Endocrinol.* 1982;99(4):594-600.

157. Boyle JG, Davidson DF, Perry CG, Connell JM. Comparison of diagnostic accuracy of urinary free metanephrines, vanillyl mandelic acid, and catecholamines and plasma catecholamines for diagnosis of pheochromocytoma. *J Clin Endocrinol Metab.* 2007;92(12):4602-4608.

158. Lal G, Duh QY. Laparoscopic adrenalectomy--indications and technique. *Surg Oncol.* 2003;12(2):105-123.

159. Miller MA, Mazzaglia PJ, Larson L, Ankner GM, Bourjeily GR, Curran P. Laparoscopic adrenalectomy for phaeochromocytoma in a twin gestation. *J Obstet Gynaecol.* 2012;32(2):186-187.

160. Schenker JG, Granat M. Phaeochromocytoma and pregnancy—an updated appraisal. *Aust N Z J Obstet Gynaecol.* 1982;22(1):1-10.

161. Vilar L, Freitas Mda C, Lima LH, Lyra R, Kater CE. Cushing's syndrome in pregnancy: an overview. *Arq Bras Endocrinol Metabol.* 2007;51(8):1293–1302.

162. Danilowicz K, Albiger N, Vanegas M, Gomez RM, Cross G, Bruno OD. Androgen-secreting adrenal adenomas. *Obstet Gynecol.* 2002;100(5 Pt 2):1099–1102.

163. Boscaro M, Barzon L, Fallo F, Sonino N. Cushing's syndrome. *Lancet.* 2001;357(9258):783–791.

164. Guilhaume B, Sanson ML, Billaud L, Bertagna X, Laudat MH, Luton JP. Cushing's syndrome and pregnancy: aetiologies and prognosis in 22 patients. *Eur J Med.* 1992;1(2):83–89.

165. Migeon CJ, Bertrand J, Wall PE. Physiological disposition of 4-C14-cortisol during late pregnancy. *J Clin Investig.* 1957;36(9):1350–1362.

166. Keller-Wood M, Wood CE. Pregnancy alters cortisol feedback inhibition of stimulated ACTH: studies in adrenalectomized ewes. *Am J Physiol.* 2001;280(6): R1790–R1798.

167. Lindsay JR, Nieman LK. The hypothalamic-pituitary-adrenal axis in pregnancy: challenges in disease detection and treatment. *Endocr Rev.* 2005;26(6):775–799.

168. De Wilde JP, Rivers AW, Price DL. A review of the current use of magnetic resonance imaging in pregnancy and safety implications for the fetus. *Prog Biophys Mol Biol.* 2005;87(2–3):335–353.

169. Kamoun M, Mnif MF, Charfi N, et al. Adrenal diseases during pregnancy: pathophysiology, diagnosis and management strategies. *Am J Med Sci.* 2014;347(1):64–73.

170. Monticone S, Auchus RJ, Rainey WE. Adrenal disorders in pregnancy. *Nat Rev Endocrinol.* 2012;8(11):668–678.

171. Lindsay JR, Jonklaas J, Oldfield EH, Nieman LK. Cushing's syndrome during pregnancy: personal experience and review of the literature. *J Clin Endocrinol Metab.* 2005;90(5):3077–3083.

172. Motivala S, Gologorsky Y, Kostandinov J, Post KD. Pituitary disorders during pregnancy. *Endocrinol Metab Clin North Am.* 2011;40(4):827–836.

173. Colao A, Petersenn S, Newell-Price J, et al. A 12-month phase 3 study of pasireotide in Cushing's disease. *N Engl J Med.* 2012;366(10):914–924.

174. Kamoun M, d'Herbomez M, Lemaire C, et al. Coexistence of thyroid-stimulating hormone-secreting pituitary adenoma and Graves' hyperthyroidism. *Eur Thyroid J.* 2014;3(1):60–64.

175. McKenna DS, Wittber GM, Nagaraja HN, Samuels P. The effects of repeat doses of antenatal corticosteroids on maternal adrenal function. *Am J Obstet Gynecol.* 2000;183(3):669–673.

176. Salvatori R. Adrenal insufficiency. *JAMA.* 2005; 294 (19):2481–2488.

177. Grinspoon SK, Biller BM. Clinical review 62: laboratory assessment of adrenal insufficiency. *J Clin Endocrinol Metab.* 1994;79(4):923–931.

178. Ambrosi B, Barbetta L, Morricone L. Diagnosis and management of Addison's disease during pregnancy. *J Endocrinol Investig.* 2003;26(7):698–702.

179. Albert E, Dalaker K, Jorde R, Berge LN. Addison's disease and pregnancy. *Acta Obstet Gynecol Scand.* 1989;68(2):185–187.

180. Schlaghecke R, Kornely E, Santen RT, Ridderskamp P. The effect of long-term glucocorticoid therapy on pituitary-adrenal responses to exogenous corticotropin-releasing hormone. *N Engl J Med.* 1992;326(4): 226–230.

181. Watanabe M, Meeker CI, Gray MJ, Sims EA, Solomon S. Secretion rate of aldosterone in normal pregnancy. *J Clin Investig.* 1963;42:1619–1631.

182. Gennari-Moser C, Khankin EV, Schuller S, et al. Regulation of placental growth by aldosterone and cortisol. *Endocrinology.* 2011;152(1):263–271.

183. Neerhof MG, Shlossman PA, Poll DS, Ludomirsky A, Weiner S. Idiopathic aldosteronism in pregnancy. *Obstet Gynecol.* 1991;78(3 Pt 2):489–491.

184. Okawa T, Asano K, Hashimoto T, Fujimori K, Yanagida K, Sato A. Diagnosis and management of primary aldosteronism in pregnancy: case report and review of the literature. *Am J Perinatol.* 2002;19(1): 31–36.

185. Cabassi A, Rocco R, Berretta R, Regolisti G, Bacchi-Modena A. Eplerenone use in primary aldosteronism during pregnancy. *Hypertension.* 2012;59(2): e18–e19.

186. Dinc H, Esen F, Demirci A, Sari A, Resit Gumele H. Pituitary dimensions and volume measurements in pregnancy and post partum. MR assessment. *Acta Radiol.* 1998;39(1):64–69.

187. Karaca Z, Tanriverdi F, Unluhizarci K, Kelestimur F. Pregnancy and pituitary disorders. *Eur J Endocrinol.* 2010;162(3):453–475.

188. Kanal E, Barkovich AJ, Bell C, et al. ACR guidance document for safe MR practices: 2007. *AJR Am J Roentgenol.* 2007;188(6):1447–1474.

189. Cunningham FG, Leveno KJ, Bloom SL, et al. *Williams Obstetrics.* 24th ed. New York: McGraw-Hill; 2014.

190. Rigg LA, Lein A, Yen SS. Pattern of increase in circulating prolactin levels during human gestation. *Am J Obstet Gynecol.* 1977;129(4):454–456.

191. Eriksson L, Frankenne F, Eden S, Hennen G, Von Schoultz B. Growth hormone 24-h serum profiles during pregnancy—lack of pulsatility for the secretion of the placental variant. *Br J Obstet Gynaecol.* 1989;96(8):949–953.

192. Kubler K, Klingmuller D, Gembruch U, Merz WM. High-risk pregnancy management in women with hypopituitarism. *J Perinatol.* 2009;29(2):89–95.

193. Curran AJ, Peacey SR, Shalet SM. Is maternal growth hormone essential for a normal pregnancy? *Eur J Endocrinol.* 1998;139(1):54–58.

194. Berinder K, Stackenas I, Akre O, Hirschberg AL, Hulting AL. Hyperprolactinaemia in 271 women: up to three decades of clinical follow-up. *Clin Endocrinol*. 2005;63(4):450–455.

195. Biller BM. Hyperprolactinemia. *Int J Fertil Womens Med*. 1999;44(2):74–77.

196. Kaiser UB. Hyperprolactinemia and infertility: new insights. *J Clin Investig*. 2012;122(10):3467–3468.

197. Kredentser JV, Hoskins CF, Scott JZ. Hyperprolactinemia—a significant factor in female infertility. *Am J Obstet Gynecol*. 1981;139(3):264–267.

198. Ono M, Miki N, Amano K, et al. Individualized high-dose cabergoline therapy for hyperprolactinemic infertility in women with micro- and macroprolactinomas. *J Clin Endocrinol Metab*. 2010;95(6):2672–2679.

199. Koch L. New Endocrine Society guidelines for hyperprolactinemia-piecing together the pituitary puzzle. *Nat Rev Endocrinol*. 2011;7(5):247.

200. Schlechte JA. Long-term management of prolactinomas. *J Clin Endocrinol Metab*. 2007;92(8):2861–2865.

201. Molitch ME. Prolactinomas and pregnancy. *Clin Endocrinol*. 2010;73(2):147–148.

202. Melmed S, Casanueva FF, Hoffman AR, et al. Diagnosis and treatment of hyperprolactinemia: an Endocrine Society clinical practice guideline. *J Clin Endocrinol Metab*. 2011;96(2):273–288.

203. Bigazzi M, Ronga R, Lancranjan I, et al. A pregnancy in an acromegalic woman during bromocriptine treatment: effects on growth hormone and prolactin in the maternal, fetal, and amniotic compartments. *J Clin Endocrinol Metab*. 1979;48(1):9–12.

204. Molitch ME. Prolactinoma in pregnancy. *Best Pract Res Clin Endocrinol Metab*. 2011;25(6):885–896.

205. Stalldecker G, Mallea-Gil MS, Guitelman M, et al. Effects of cabergoline on pregnancy and embryo-fetal development: retrospective study on 103 pregnancies and a review of the literature. *Pituitary*. 2010;13(4):345–350.

206. Molitch ME. Management of medically refractory prolactinoma. *J Neurooncol*. 2014;117(3):421–428.

207. Divers WA Jr, Yen SS. Prolactin-producing microadenomas in pregnancy. *Obstet Gynecol*. 1983;62(4):425–429.

208. Chrisoulidou A, Boudina M, Karavitaki N, Bili E, Wass J. Pituitary disorders in pregnancy. *Hormones*. 2015;14(1):70–80.

209. Gillam MP, Molitch ME, Lombardi G, Colao A. Advances in the treatment of prolactinomas. *Endocr Rev*. 2006;27(5):485–534.

210. Herman-Bonert V, Seliverstov M, Melmed S. Pregnancy in acromegaly: successful therapeutic outcome. *J Clin Endocrinol Metab*. 1998;83(3):727–731.

211. Grynberg M, Salenave S, Young J, Chanson P. Female gonadal function before and after treatment of acromegaly. *J Clin Endocrinol Metab*. 2010;95(10): 4518–4525.

212. Melmed S, Colao A, Barkan A, et al. Guidelines for acromegaly management: an update. *J Clin Endocrinol Metab*. 2009;94(5):1509–1517.

213. Melmed S. Medical progress: Acromegaly. *N Engl J Med*. 2006;355(24):2558–2573.

214. Beckers A, Stevenaert A, Foidart JM, Hennen G, Frankenne F. Placental and pituitary growth hormone secretion during pregnancy in acromegalic women. *J Clin Endocrinol Metab*. 1990;71(3):725–731.

215. Caron P, Broussaud S, Bertherat J, et al. Acromegaly and pregnancy: a retrospective multicenter study of 59 pregnancies in 46 women. *J Clin Endocrinol Metab*. 2010;95(10):4680–4687.

216. Cheng S, Grasso L, Martinez-Orozco JA, et al. Pregnancy in acromegaly: experience from two referral centers and systematic review of the literature. *Clin Endocrinol*. 2012;76(2):264–271.

217. Brian SR, Bidlingmaier M, Wajnrajch MP, Weinzimer SA, Inzucchi SE. Treatment of acromegaly with pegvisomant during pregnancy: maternal and fetal effects. *J Clin Endocrinol Metab*. 2007;92(9):3374–3377.

218. Melmed S, Casanueva FF, Klibanski A, et al. A consensus on the diagnosis and treatment of acromegaly complications. *Pituitary*. 2013;16(3):294–302.

219. Maffei P, Tamagno G, Nardelli GB, et al. Effects of octreotide exposure during pregnancy in acromegaly. *Clin Endocrinol*. 2010;72(5):668–677.

220. Cozzi R, Attanasio R, Barausse M. Pregnancy in acromegaly: a one-center experience. *Eur J Endocrinol*. 2006;155(2):279–284.

221. Atmaca A, Dagdelen S, Erbas T. Follow-up of pregnancy in acromegalic women: different presentations and outcomes. *Exp Clin Endocrinol Diabetes*. 2006;114(3):135–139.

222. Koshy TG, Rajaratnam S, Mathews JE, Rajshekhar V. Acromegaly in pregnancy. *Indian J Endocrinol Metab*. 2012;16(6):1029–1031.

223. Feinberg EC, Molitch ME, Endres LK, Peaceman AM. The incidence of Sheehan's syndrome after obstetric hemorrhage. *Fertil Steril*. 2005;84(4):975–979.

224. Tessnow AH, Wilson JD. The changing face of Sheehan's syndrome. *Am J Med Sci*. 2010;340(5):402–406.

225. Kelestimur F. Sheehan's syndrome. *Pituitary*. 2003;6(4):181–188.

226. Bakiri F, Bendib SE, Maoui R, Bendib A, Benmiloud M. The sella turcica in Sheehan's syndrome: computerized tomographic study in 54 patients. *J Endocrinol Investig*. 1991;14(3):193–196.

227. Gei-Guardia O, Soto-Herrera E, Gei-Brealey A, Chen-Ku CH. Sheehan syndrome in Costa Rica: clinical experience with 60 cases. *Endocr Pract*. 2011;17(3):337–344.

228. Sheehan HL, Whitehead R. The neurohypophysis in post-partum hypopituitarism. *J Pathol Bacteriol*. 1963;85:145–169.

229. Caturegli P, Newschaffer C, Olivi A, Pomper MG, Burger PC, Rose NR. Autoimmune hypophysitis. *Endocr Rev*. 2005;26(5):599–614.
230. Foyouzi N. Lymphocytic adenohypophysitis. *Obstet Gynecol Surv*. 2011;66(2):109–113.
231. Lee MS, Pless M. Apoplectic lymphocytic hypophysitis. Case report. *J Neurosurg*. 2003;98(1):183–185.
232. Carpinteri R, Patelli I, Casanueva FF, Giustina A. Pituitary tumours: inflammatory and granulomatous expansive lesions of the pituitary. *Best Pract Res Clin Endocrinol Metab*. 2009;23(5):639–650.
233. Blackhurst G, Strachan MW, Collie D, Gregor A, Statham PF, Seckl JE. The treatment of a thyrotropin-secreting pituitary macroadenoma with octreotide in twin pregnancy. *Clin Endocrinol*. 2002;57(3): 401–404.
234. Masding MG, Lees PD, Gawne-Cain ML, Sandeman DD. Visual field compression by a non-secreting pituitary tumour during pregnancy. *J R Soc Med*. 2003; 96(1):27–28.
235. Lindheimer MD, Davison JM. Osmoregulation, the secretion of arginine vasopressin and its metabolism during pregnancy. *Eur J Endocrinol*. 1995;132(2): 133–143.
236. Ananthakrishnan S. Diabetes insipidus in pregnancy: etiology, evaluation, and management. *Endocr Pract*. 2009;15(4):377–382.
237. Lamberts SW, de Herder WW, van der Lely AJ. Pituitary insufficiency. *Lancet*. 1998;352(9122): 127–134.
238. Wallia A, Bizhanova A, Huang W, Goldsmith SL, Gossett DR, Kopp P. Acute diabetes insipidus mediated by vasopressinase after placental abruption. *J Clin Endocrinol Metab*. 2013;98(3):881–886.

Pregestational and Gestational Diabetes

CHAPTER 23

Serdar H. Ural, MD, FACOG

INTRODUCTION
PREGESTATIONAL DIABETES MELLITUS
  · Management of Pregestational Diabetes
  Mellitus Types 1 and 2

GESTATIONAL DIABETES
  · Management of Gestational Diabetes
  Mellitus

INTRODUCTION

Pregestational diabetes, based on literature, appears to be present in approximately 1% of all pregnancies.[1] Type 1 diabetes mellitus tends to occur early in human life and appears to be associated with an autoimmune disorder that alleviates pancreatic β cells. This generally leads to a requirement for insulin replacement. Type 2 pregestational diabetes mellitus is associated with obesity, insulin deficiency, insulin resistance, and development of certain complications, such as neurologic, renal, and vascular issues. Type 2 diabetes has increased significantly in number due to the obesity epidemic in the United States.[2] Of diabetic cases in pregnancy, 90% are related to gestational diabetes mellitus. Over 50% of such patients will eventually develop type 2 pregestational diabetes. Obesity, along with diabetes, has many negative consequences during pregnancy, to the mother, to the fetus, to the newborn, or to all.

PREGESTATIONAL DIABETES MELLITUS

Type 1 diabetes mellitus accounts for about 5%–7% of diabetes in the United States. This subclass develops as a result of an autoimmune disorder that is usually directed against insulin-producing β cells in the pancreas. Destruction of such cells leads to the requirement for insulin replacement. Usually, onset occurs before age 30 and can affect about 0.5% of all pregnancies in the United States. Prior to insulin therapy, infertility was the most common consequence of diabetes mellitus for reproductive-age women. Mortality rates in neonates could have been as high as 60%.[1-3] Advances in insulin therapy and improvements in neonatal care have decreased this mortality rate to 2%. All risks associated with diabetes are increased once obesity is factored in as well.

All of the causes of this disorder are still not clear. Some suggest that there is a general inflammatory state called insulinitis that may lead to this type of diabetes. Macrophages, B lymphocytes, and CD[+] T lymphocytes may be able to infiltrate the Langerhans islets in the pancreas. A complex cycle generally leads to accumulation of CD[+] lymphocytes, therefore leading to gradual destruction of insulin-producing β cells.[3-5] Ultimately, insulin deficiency that causes hyperglycemia occurs. In general, pregnancy itself is a diabetogenic state in which postprandial glucose levels are already elevated and insulin sensitivities are decreased.[4] This has been associated with an increase in hormones, including cortisol, progesterone, estrogen, prolactin, and human placental lactogen.[6] Recently, there have been other molecules that have been associated with this entity as well. The literature has been supportive of the need for an overall increase in insulin requirement during advancing gestational weeks. This increase is even greater if obesity is a factor as well.

This especially has been noted to happen beginning near the second trimester and for the rest of the pregnancy. It is known that those with pregestational diabetes show increasing insulin requirements throughout pregnancy. A Danish prospective study showed an increase in C-peptide during pregnancy in such diabetic moms.[7] This report showed an association between the variability of insulin requirements throughout the progression of pregnancy, as have several other recent reports.

Hypoglycemia, particularly during the nighttime, is a common complication.[3] Hypoglycemia warning signs include tachycardia, sweating, and weakness that can occur due to this effect. If low blood glucose is evident, a glass of milk or juice is the first step in alleviating the symptoms and correcting the blood glucose values.[8] Hypoglycemia, if untreated, is the leading cause for maternal mortality.

Diabetic ketoacidosis (DKA) may occur due to insulin deficiency that is seen as starvation by the body (Table 23-1).[15] There is a decreased intracellular glucose concentration. Fatty acids are tapped into so energy can be provided for the body. This leads to ketone generation. When this occurs, energy from fatty acids is directed to the brain and heart, which are essential for survival.

Hyperglycemia may actually worsen the insulin-deficiency state by dehydration. As plasma osmolarity increases with glucose increase (Table 23-2),[8] diuresis occurs that may be at the level of polyuria. This prevents bicarbonate from being reabsorbed. This is turn increases glucose and ketones in the body.

Diabetic ketoacidosis is more commonly seen when compared to hypoglycemic episodes during pregnancy. This issue occurs in about 2% of pregnancies with pregestational diabetes. Decreased levels of bicarbonate may be associated with the physiologic response to increased minute ventilation, which may further decrease

TABLE 23-1 Treating DKA in Pregnancy

1. Obtain arterial blood gas, blood glucose, electrolyte, and ketone values.
2. If pH is 7 or less, give an ampule of bicarbonate.
3. Fluid replacement: 4–6 L over 24 hours.
4. Start 5% dextrose/normal saline when blood glucose is below 250 mg/dL.
5. Intravenous insulin: 0.2–0.4 U/kg loading dose, then 2–10 U/h.
6. Potassium replacement: 15–20 mEq/h.

TABLE 23-2 Blood Glucose Levels and Glycosylated Hemoglobin Levels (Hb A_{1C}) as Percentages

mg/dL	%
126	6.0
140	6.5
154	7.0
169	7.5
183	8.0
197	8.5
212	9.0
240	10.0

the body's capability of buffering. DKA can develop faster in patients who have urinary tract infections or upper respiratory infections or are on tocolytics or corticosteroids. Intrauterine fetal demise can be seen in about 30% of patients with DKA.[9] This is increased in obesity, and although the exact numbers and percentages are not known for certain and are debatable, there clearly is an association with more and increased risks.

Diabetes is associated with shoulder dystocia during vaginal delivery, and some reports suggested that the risk can be doubled in such patients.[10] When obesity is involved in those with diabetes, the risks and outcomes in preeclampsia, preterm labor, malformations, urinary tract infections, overdue gestations, labor problems, and cesarean rates all increase, and their outcomes worsen as well. These patients have a higher rate of urinary tract infections and other infections overall. Pyelonephritis, asymptomatic bacteriuria, and preeclampsia could be manifestations of glucose intolerance leading to infections, thus aiding with diagnosing diabetes.

The rate of fetal congenital malformations is approximately 8% in those with pregestational diabetes. The spontaneous abortion rate is approximately 4%. One study showed a direct relationship between hemoglobin A_{1C} and the rate of fetal malformation.[11] When hemoglobin A_{1c} levels were between 5% and 6%, normal pregnancy outcomes and no major malformations could be expected. Whereas if the levels were above 10%, the malformation rate could be as high as 25%. The risk of macrosomia in a large group of those with diabetes showed a high prevalence.

A recent cohort study[12] that had demonstrated preterm delivery rates as high as 24% in women with pregestational diabetes, there is increased risk for preterm delivery. Spontaneous preterm deliveries were also elevated.

Preeclampsia, characterized by gestational hypertension, systolic and diastolic blood pressures above 140/90 mm Hg, and with onset after 20 weeks of gestation is associated with diabetes mellitus in pregnancy. Pregestational diabetes mellitus is a well-known risk factor for preeclampsia.[13] The risk is about 15%, compared to about 7% in the general population.[3]

Diabetic nephropathy affects the interstitial and glomerular compartments of the kidney. Ultimately, end-stage renal disease can occur. Collagen, laminin, and fibronectin can accumulate in such areas and affect clinical and physiologic performance. Due to a heightened risk of preeclampsia in diabetic pregnancies, renal damage can worsen in a shorter amount of time. If patients already have a creatinine level greater than 1.5 mg/dL, end-stage disease progression can occur. Methyldopa can be used for antihypertensive and renoprotective properties. A recent study has shown an improved outcome with such medications.[14]

Diabetic retinopathy is the leading cause of blindness in the United States in the reproductive age group.[8] Glucose permeates into sensitive endothelial cells that line capillaries and blood vessels in the retina. Pericytes are susceptible to high glucose levels and may lead to continuous damage to the endothelial cells, eventually effecting vascular sclerosis and edema. In subsequent response to this environment, retinal tissue secretes proangiogenic growth factors. This neovascularity leads to proliferative diabetic retinopathy. This leads to blindness, retinal detachment, and hemorrhages.[15] New insulin analogues have been associated with increased levels of insulin growth factor, which can negatively affect retinal health. Laser therapy during pregnancy for the treatment of proliferative retinopathy is an appropriate option and actually may cure the pathology that has taken place.

Management of Pregestational Diabetes Mellitus Types 1 and 2

Preconception management can be associated with successful pregnancy outcomes in those with pregestational diabetes even before conception. Strict glycemic control, especially before and throughout pregnancy, has been shown to reduce the rate of perinatal mortality and malformations.[16] It is up to health care providers and physicians to counsel patients and guide them to achieve glycemic control goals as this is the single most important factor associated with a healthy pregnancy outcome. It is also important to uncover any underlying disorder that may be associated with diabetes. For example, vascular damage can be evaluated by a retinal examination, renal function can be evaluated by 24-hour urine protein and creatinine clearance, and cardiac function by electrocardiography.

Dietary recommendations associated with carbohydrate limitations should be reviewed, and bedtime snacks given to prevent nocturnal hypoglycemia.[8] This will allow for an increase of caloric consumption by up to 300 kcal/day. Caloric requirements during pregnancy should be restricted to 24 kcal/kg/d. The majority of the diet needs to be composed of complex, high-fiber foods.[15] Premeal plasma glucose levels of less than 100 mg/dL, 1-hour postprandial levels less than 140 mg/dL, and 2-hour levels of less than 120 mg/dL should be the goals if Coustan/Carpenter criteria are to be used. Hemoglobin A_{1c} values can be obtained every month or two if diet control is required.

Insulin management is the proven standard to maintain the pregnancy with pregestational diabetes. Certain literature compared daily regimens of twice-daily insulin versus insulin given 4 times daily. The regimen given 4 times daily does appear to have a better association with decreased complications during pregnancy.[17]

Recent options seen in insulin formulations have increased the choices for patients. Regular human insulin still is the benchmark and gold standard, especially for mealtime boluses. The rapid onset of insulin analogues such as lispro aspart are causing them to become the drugs of choice. Clinical retrospective trials have shown no difference in perinatal outcomes between regimens that use human insulin or lispro. In actuality, rapid onset formulations have been shown to lead to better postprandial glucose control.[18] Lispro aspart in combination with NPH (neutral protamine Hagedorn) or isophane insulin has been shown to have similar results. Long-acting insulin formulations are also options. These are peakless formulations, and initial studies looking at them demonstrated no difference in glycemic control.[19] One study looking at 56 patients with pregestational diabetes showed improved maternal and perinatal outcomes when compared to the patients receiving NPH. In this study, all patients received insulin lispro as their prandial bolus insulin.[20] There have been some recent concerns over the safety of certain insulins due to mitogenic properties (insulin glargine).

Overall titration of glucose levels in labor can be managed with intravenous regular insulin and 5% dextrose. In labor, if values are above 110 mg/dL, regular insulin should be given at a dose of 1.25 U/h. If less than 70 mg/dL, 5% dextrose at 125 mL/hour needs to be given. Hourly blood glucose checks are recommended while in labor.[8] Improving compliance and adherence to a regimen are key for successful outcomes. In the postpartum period, insulin can be restarted at half the rate.

GESTATIONAL DIABETES

Pregnancy creates a state of insulin resistance and hyperinsulinemia that is a predisposition to diabetes and perhaps obesity. When a pregnant woman's pancreatic function is not sufficient then gestational diabetes may occur. Glucose intolerance that was not present prior to pregnancy is defined as gestational diabetes. In the United States, certain ethnic groups, such as African Americans, Hispanics, and American Indians, have higher rates. The incidence is about 3%–12%. Gestational diabetes does affect about 3%–4% of pregnant women.[21] There are 2 different methods of classification of diabetes in pregnancy. The first is the White classification, and the second is the American Diabetes Association classification.

The White classification is used to assess maternal and fetal risk. It distinguishes between gestational diabetes (type A) and diabetes that existed before pregnancy (pregestational diabetes). These two groups are further subdivided according to their associated risks and management.[4]

There are 2 classes of gestational diabetes:

- Class A: gestational diabetes; diet controlled
- Class A: gestational diabetes; medication controlled

The second group of diabetes was present prior to pregnancy:

- Class B: onset at age 20 or older or with duration of less than 10 years
- Class C: onset at age 10–19 or duration of 10–19 years
- Class D: onset before age 10 or duration greater than 20 years
- Class E: overt diabetes mellitus with calcified pelvic vessels
- Class F: diabetic neuropathy
- Class R: proliferative retinopathy

- Class RF: retinopathy and nephropathy
- Class H: ischemic heart disease
- Class T: kidney transplant

The American Diabetes Association classification is as follows[28]:

I. Type 1 diabetes
   A. Immune mediated
   B. Idiopathic
II. Type 2 diabetes
III. Other specific types
   A. Genetic defects of β-cell function
   B. Genetic defects in insulin action
   C. Diseases of the exocrine pancreas
   D. Endocrinopathies
   E. Drug or chemical induced
   F. Infections
   G. Uncommon forms of immune-mediated diabetes
   H. Other genetic syndromes sometimes associated with diabetes
IV. Gestational diabetes mellitus

Insulin resistance increases due to growth hormone, cortisol secretion, insulin antagonists, human placental lactogen secretion, and insulinase secretion imbalances. Lactogen is produced by the placenta and affects fatty acids and glucose metabolism lipolysis occurs and glucose uptake slows down. Insulinase facilitates metabolism of insulin. Estrogen and progesterone also cannot be left out of the picture as imbalances may contribute to the disruption of this delicate balance.[22] In addition, decreasing exercise, increasing adipose intake, and overall caloric intake may lead to glucose intolerance and eventually obesity. The most common risk factors associated with gestational diabetes are macrosomia, polycystic ovary syndrome, hypertensive disorders, intrauterine fetal death, and miscarriages. Having a first-degree relative with a history of diabetes also has a strong association. Unfortunately, 50% of patient cases are related to unknown risk factors.[23]

Universal screening of pregnant women may be beneficial as not all women who develop gestational diabetes may have risk factors. The American Diabetes Association states that low-risk women may not need to be screened. Low risk is identified as being younger than 25 years of age; having a body mass index (BMI) less than 25 prior to pregnancy; not being of Hispanic, African American, American Indian, South or East Asian, or Pacific Islander descent; and having no history of prior glucose intolerance or prior poor obstetric outcome. There is still a debate about whether to universally screen. The decision is usually dependent on clinical judgment. Obese patients have a higher inclination toward developing gestational diabetes. Therefore, in such a group, screening would likely be more beneficial.

Screening entails a 1-hour glucose test, also called a glucose challenge test, to be performed between 24 and 28 weeks of gestation. If patients have known or higher risk factors, this test can be performed much earlier, prior to 24 weeks, and repeated at 24 to 28 weeks during prenatal care. If at this early gestational age the initial screen is normal, then the test is again repeated at the usual time of 24 to 28 weeks.[22] The patient receives 50 g of oral glucose, and 1 hour later blood is drawn to assess plasma glucose levels. A glucose value above 130 to 140 mg/dL is considered abnormal, and when necessitated, a second test is suggested. Some centers use 130, 140, or another number in between. It is useful to pick one cutoff number to avoid confusion. The higher the number you choose, the more false negatives will appear. On the other hand, if the lower cutoff number is used, the more false positives that will be obtained. If the general idea is not to miss any diabetic mother, then to use a lower cutoff, such as 130 mg/dL, is the obvious choice.

If the screening test is abnormal, which occurs in about 15% of patients, these patients will go on to have a 3-hour screening test, by which 15% will be diagnosed with gestational diabetes. The 3-hour glucose tolerance test is begun by drawing a fasting glucose sample and then administrating 100 g of oral glucose. Blood for glucose values is drawn at 1, 2, and 3 hours. Some centers do perform a 75-g 2-hour glucose tolerance test; however, the most traditional option has been the 3-hour test. In the Carpenter/Coustan conversion analysis, diagnosis of gestational diabetes is based on the presence of 2 or more of the following abnormal factors[29]:

- Fasting glucose more than 95 mg/dL
- 1-hour serum glucose above 180 mg/dL
- 2-hour serum glucose over 155 mg/dL
- 3-hour serum glucose over 140 mg/dL[24]

Some centers also may apply the National Diabetes Data Group criteria.[25] If these are to be used, the abnormal values are as follows:

- Fasting: 105 mg/dL
- 1-hour serum glucose concentration: 190 mg/dL
- 2-hour serum glucose concentration: 165 mg/dL
- 3-hour serum glucose concentration: 145 mg/dL.[25]

The Hyperglycemic and Adverse Pregnancy Outcomes study showed that higher plasma glucose results have a correlation with birth weight above the 90th percentile, cord blood serum C-peptide levels above the 90th percentile, and to a small degree, increase in primary cesarean section rates, and neonatal hypoglycemia.[22] Maternal hyperglycemia itself can have correlation with perinatal disorders and problems. This ultimately may be more challenging in obese patients.

Management of Gestational Diabetes Mellitus

The key is to control glucose levels. Blood glucose levels need to be monitored about 4 times a day, in general on awakening for a fasting level and a 2-hour blood glucose after breakfast, lunch, and dinner. The morning fasting glucose blood level needs to be 70 to 90 mg/dL. The postprandial goal is below 120 mg/dL. The patient should truly try to maintain the cutoff of 120 mg/dL if she is to get full benefit. Quality nutritional intake is also helpful in maintaining normal glucose levels. This is based on ideal body weight.

Having a nutrition, and a dietician consult would be beneficial for all of these patients. The overall caloric intake recommendations are 30 kcal/kg for a woman with a BMI of 23 to 25 and 24 kcal/kg for a woman with a BMI of 26 to 29. If the BMI is above 30, then it would be 12 to 15 kcal/kg. The overall dietary ratio of complex carbohydrates is about 35%. This is a normal finding based on eating healthy and a regular diet. In general, the patients with this type of diet enhancement may become normoglycemic . Obesity will alter the approach to achieve such a goal. One must keep this issue in mind when counseling these types of patients.

Obviously, if diet cannot afford this level of control, then these patients will require insulin therapy.

The main goal of insulin therapy is to be able to minimize the risk of macrosomia and its associated risks to the infant and pregnant mother. Insulin can be initiated if the fasting blood glucose concentration is greater than 90 mg/dL on 2 or more occasions during a 2-week period or when the 2-hour postprandial blood glucose concentration is above 120 mg/dL. The most common insulin types used include NPH and regular insulin. This is the most traditionally used regimen. NPH is an intermediate-acting insulin,[22] and regular insulin is short acting. NPH has an onset of action of 2 to 4 hours, with peak effect up to 12 hours from administration; overall duration of action could be as much as 16 hours. Regular insulin has an onset of action within 30 to 60 minutes, a peak effect up to 3 hours later, and a duration total of up to 6 hours.[22] Human insulin appears to be the least immunogenic and should be used exclusively.

Oral hypoglycemic agents are still in the discussion phase, although there are reports that show that they can be used in pregnancy. However, this has not been approved by the US Food and Drug Administration at this juncture. A substantial amount of patients may require insulin therapy even if oral hypoglycemic agents are begun. Metformin is an oral hypoglycemic agent, and when compared to insulin in one study, neonatal complications did not appear to vary between the 2 groups. There was less-severe hypoglycemia in infants with metformin use, preterm birth was more common in the metformin group, but there was no increase in other complications. As mentioned, of women who have been on metformin, less than half will need to switch to insulin. A trial compared glyburide, which is another oral agent, to metformin and was able to show that blood glucose levels were better. Exercise has been shown to improve glucose control by decreasing insulin resistance.[26] A typical recommendation is to exercise 3 or more times a week for at least 15 to 30 minutes each time. It also is suggested that this may protect against developing gestational diabetes.[26]

Diabetic moms have a higher risk for developing preeclampsia.[22] A baseline preeclampsia workup is recommended to be able to compare results later if actual preeclampsia does develop. Antepartum fetal monitoring can begin at 32 weeks in patients who have diabetes. The nonstress test is the most commonly used antenatal test method and can be performed twice a week.

The ideal way to deliver a woman with gestational or pregestational diabetes is vaginally. There appear to be no contraindications for anesthesia. It is rare that insulin is required during labor and delivery; a normal saline infusion is adequate at this point.

Once a woman with gestational diabetes is delivered, there are no further insulin requirements in the postpartum period, majority will return to a completely normal glucose status postpartum. If glucose tolerance screening is to be performed in the postpartum, it can be done months after delivery using a 75-g glucose tolerance test.[22]

This will detect roughly 4% of women who will remain diabetic and require further treatment. The number for obese patients is much lower.

There is about a 10% per year risk of developing type 2 diabetes after the pregnancy in which gestational diabetes occurred. Macrosomia is associated with complications such as fetopelvic disproportion, operative delivery, shoulder dystocia, and neonatal hypoglycemia. There is also an increased risk for hyperbilirubinemia, hypocalcemia, respiratory distress syndrome, polycythemia, and polycythemia in the neonate. Long-term complications can include hyperactivity, impaired motor function, diabetes, and obesity.[22]

In summary gestational diabetes is a significant issue in the 21st century. The main reason is that not much has been accomplished other than the ability to control blood glucose levels. All of our effort needs to be directed toward maintaining normal glucose levels. Gestational diabetes can have lasting health defects; therefore, it is important to face this disorder seriously and take the appropriate steps to ensure there is a high quality of care for these patients.[27-29]

Future studies are needed to enhance the screening methods, efficacious treatments, and guidance regarding what the optimal management should be for insulin use and other types of modalities. This will also be important not only for better diabetic management but also for significant reduction of complications that arise from being obese and diabetic.

REFERENCES

1. Centers for Disease Control. *National Diabetes Fact Sheet: General Information and National Estimates on Diabetes in the United States, 2007*. Atlanta, GA: Centers for Disease Control and Prevention, Department of Health and Human Services; 2008.

2. Gibbs RS, Danforth DN. *Danforth's Obstetrics and Gynecology*. 10th ed. Philadelphia: Wolters Kluwer Lippincott Williams & Wilkins; 2008.

3. Garner P. Type I diabetes mellitus and pregnancy. *Lancet*. 1995;346:157–161.

4. White P. Pregnancy complicating diabetes. *Am J Med*. 1949;7:609–616.

5. Atkinson MA, Eisenbarth GS. Type I diabetes: new perspectives on disease pathogenesis and treatment. *Lancet*. 2001;358:221–229.

6. Gabbe SG, Niebyl JR, Simpson JL. *Obstetrics: Normal and Problem Pregnancies*. 5th ed. Philadelphia: Churchill Livingston/Elsevier; 2007.

7. Nielsen LR, Rehfeld JF, Pedersen-Bjergaard U, et al. Pregnancy-induced rise in serum C-peptide concentrations in women with type I diabetes. *Diabetes Care*. 2009;32:1052–1057.

8. Vargas R, Repke JT, Ural SH. Type I diabetes mellitus and pregnancy. *Rev Obstet Gynecol*. 2010;3(3): 92–100.

9. Reece EA, Coustan DR, Gabbe SG. *Diabetes in Women: Adolescence, Pregnancy, and Menopause*. 3rd ed. Philadelphia: Lippincott Williams & Wilkins; 2004.

10. ACOG Committee on Practice Bulletins. ACOG practice bulletin. Clinical management guidelines for obstetrics-gynecologists. Number 60, March 2005. Pregestational diabetes mellitus. *Obstet Gynecol*. 2005;105:675–685.

11. Hanson U, Persson B, Thunell S. Relationship between haemoglobin A1C in early type I (insulin-dependent) diabetic pregnancy and the occurrence of spontaneous abortion and fetal malformation in Sweden. *Diabetologia*. 1990;33:100–104.

12. Lepercq J, Coste J, Theau A, et al. Factors associated with preterm delivery in women with type I diabetes: a cohort study. *Diabetes Care*. 2004;27:2824–2828.

13. Sibai BM, Caritis SN, Hauth JC, et al. Preterm delivery in women with pregestational diabetes mellitus or chronic hypertension relative to women with uncomplicated pregnancies. The National Institute of Child Health and Human Development Maternal-Fetal Medicine Units Network. *Am J Obstet Gynecol*. 2000;183:1520–1524.

14. Nielsen LR, Damm P, Mathiesen ER. Improved pregnancy outcome in type I diabetic women with microalbuminuria or diabetic nephropathy: effect of intensified antihypertensive therapy? *Diabetes Care*. 2009;32:38–44.

15. Kronenberg H, Williams RH. *Williams Textbook of Endocrinology*. 11th ed. Philadelphia: Saunders/ Elsevier; 2008.

16. McElvy SS, Miodovnik M, Rosenn B, et al. A focused preconceptional and early pregnancy program in women with type I diabetes reduces perinatal mortality and malformation rates to general population levels. *J Matern Fetal Med.* 2000;9:14–20.

17. Nachum Z, Ben-Shlomo I, Weiner E, Shalev E. Twice daily versus four times daily insulin dose regimens for diabetes in pregnancy: randomized controlled trial. *BMJ.* 1999;319:1223–1227.

18. Torlone E, Di Cianni G, Mannino D, Lapolla A. Insulin analogs and pregnancy: an update. *Acta Diabetol.* 2009;46:163–172.

19. Imbergamo MP, Amato MC, Sciortino G, et al. Use of glargine in pregnant women with type I diabetes mellitus: a case-control study. *Clin Ther.* 2008;30:1476–1484.

20. Negrato CA, Rafacho A, Negrato G, et al. Glargine vs. NPH insulin therapy in pregnancies complicated by diabetes: an observational cohort study. *Diabetes Res Clin Pract.* 2010;89:46–51.

21. American College of Obstetricians and Gynecologists Committee on Practice Bulletins—Obstetrics. ACOG practice bulletin. Clinical management guidelines for obstetrician-gynecologists. Number 30, September 2001 (replaces Technical Bulletin Number 200, December 1994). Gestational diabetes. *Obstet Gynecol.* 2001;98:525–538.

22. Gilmartin AH, Ural SH, Repke JT. Gestational diabetes mellitus. *Rev Obstet Gynecol.* 2008;1(3):129–134.

23. Proceedings of the 4th International Workshop-Conference on Gestational Diabetes Mellitus. Chicago, Illinois, USA. 14–16 March 1997. *Diabetes Care.* 1998;21(suppl 2):B1–B167.

24. National Institute of Health, US Department of Health and Human Services. *Diabetes in America.* 2nd ed. Bethesda, MD: National Diabetes Data Group of the National Institute of Diabetes and Digestive and Kidney Diseases, National Institutes of Health; 1995. NIH publication 95–1468.

25. Classification and diagnosis of diabetes mellitus and other categories of glucose intolerance: National Diabetes Data Group. *Diabetes.* 1979;28:1039–1057.

26. Gavard JA, Artal R. Effect of exercise on pregnancy outcome. *Clin Obstet Gynecol.* 2008;51:467–480.

27. Metzger BE, Lowe LP, Dyer AR, et al; for HAPO Study Cooperative Research Group. Hyperglycemia and adverse pregnancy outcomes. *N Engl J Med.* 2008;358:1991–2002.

28. American Diabetes Association. Diagnosis and classification of diabetes mellitus. *Diabetes Care.* 2005;29;542–548.

29. Carpenter MW, Coustan DR. Criteria for screening tests for gestational diabetes. *Am J Obstet Gynecol* 1982;144;768–773.

CHAPTER 24

Hypertensive Disorders

John J. Folk, MD, FACOG

INTRODUCTION

> We believe that there is little to support the prevailing concept that a true caloric gain of weight during pregnancy predisposes to toxemia. Pre-existing obesity is quite a different problem.
>
> Ernest W. Page, MD[1]

The incidence of hypertension among adults in the United States has been estimated at between 29% and 31%. Obesity is commonly associated with treatment-resistant hypertension or hypertension that requires 3 or more antihypertensive agents to achieve blood pressure control by established guidelines.[2] Among obese individuals, the incidence of hypertension has been reported as high as 50%.[3] In the United States, over one-half of reproductive-age women are overweight or obese. More than one-third of these women are obese, with about 8% classified as extremely obese. During pregnancy, these women are expected to be at increased risk for pregnancy complications related to obesity.[4] Maternal obesity and morbid obesity have been reported to be strongly associated with elevated blood pressure readings during the 3 trimesters of pregnancy, as well as with an increased risk for gestational hypertensive disorders.[5] To further establish the importance of obesity as a risk factor for hypertensive disorders during pregnancy, one study clearly demonstrated that obesity is a dose-dependent variable: Women with a body mass index (BMI) range of 25–30 kg/m^2 demonstrated a relative risk (RR) for preeclampsia of 1.88 (with a 95% confidence interval [CI] of 1.34–2.62), while women with BMI greater than 40 kg/m^2 had a RR of 7.17 with a CI of 5.06–10.16.[6]

The objectives of this chapter include a review of the underlying pathophysiology that predisposes obese women to develop hypertensive disorders, particularly during pregnancy. A review of the definitions of hypertensive disorders occurring during pregnancy is undertaken, as well as the management of mild-to-severe hypertensive disease, including life-threatening complications.

PATHOPHYSIOLOGY OF HYPERTENSION RELATED TO OBESITY AND PREGNANCY

Pathophysiology of Hypertension Related to Obesity

The pathophysiology of hypertension in obesity is complex and multifactorial. Prior to the onset of clinically overt hypertension, there is an increase in cardiac output considered to be a response to the increased demand for peripheral tissue oxygen delivery. The clinical normotensive state is maintained by a compensatory reduction in systemic vascular resistance. Among nulliparous women at risk for development of preeclampsia with marked increase in cardiac output with reduction in systemic vascular resistance, one subgroup at increased risk comparable to women with diabetes mellitus were women with overall increased weight of 14 kg compared to controls not at increased risk.[7] Over time, an increase in the activation of the renin-angiotensin-aldosterone axis gradually increases systemic vascular resistance, resulting in a rise in blood pressure and the development of clinical hypertension.

Early hypertension among obese individuals is characterized by increased cardiac output and increased systemic vascular resistance.[8,9] The process of moving from clinically normotensive to hypertensive among obese individuals is highly complex and largely speculative. Multiple pathophysiologic pathways have been proposed and have varying relevance depending on patient population characteristics.[10] The end results of these pathophysiologic pathways include increased sympathetic tone, expanded intravascular volume, and endothelial dysfunction. Increased insulin resistance resulting in hyperinsulinemia has been recognized since 1989 as potentially associated with hypertension among obese individuals.[11] Increased plasma insulin levels stimulate sympathetic neuron firing, resulting in an increase in sympathetic tone and systemic vascular resistance.[12]

Leptin is a circulating protein that increases in concentration with increasing adipose tissue formation and acts as negative feedback at the level of neurons within the brain. Neurons that are receptive to insulin are also receptive to leptin, resulting in increased expression of melanocortin receptors that participate in the control of energy stores as well as sympathetic tone. With an abnormal response to increasing leptin, there is a disproportionate increase in sympathetic tone in what has been described as the leptin-melanocortin pathway. The effect of increased insulin and leptin is an increase in sympathetic tone and systemic vascular resistance.[13–15]

Among obese individuals with sleep apnea, episodic hypoxia results in endothelial stress, which increases release of endothelins, a class of proteins with vasoconstrictive properties, resulting in an additional increase in systemic vascular resistance.[16] Increased systemic vascular resistance usually results in diuresis and a reset of the intravascular volume to a point at which overall blood pressure is normalized.

With obesity, hyperinsulinemia contributes to direct renal endothelial injury and overall endothelial dysfunction, which result in upregulation of angiotensin II receptors and decreased production of cardiac-derived natriuretic peptides and a resultant increase in sodium retention and expansion of the intravascular volume.[17-19] The combination of increased systemic vascular resistance and expanded intravascular volume act to synergistically increase measurable blood pressure.

Pathophysiology of Hypertension Related to Pregnancy

Hypertensive disorders during pregnancy are described as the result of the interaction of factors derived from maternal as well as uteroplacental/fetal origins. Pregnancy-related hypertensive disorders such as preeclampsia begin with conception and the earliest stages of placental vascular development. Instead of placental vasculature, where blood moves through a high-flow, low-resistance circuit as seen in normal placental development, vasculature develops with a low-flow, high-resistance state that results in placental hypoperfusion, which leads to placental hypoxemia and ultimately placental ischemia.

In a normal pregnancy, trophoblastic invasion results in extensive remodeling of maternal spiral arterioles, which produce wide-open vascular channels within the placenta. In the abnormal state that results in a pregnancy-related hypertensive disorder, trophoblastic remodeling of the spiral arterioles is suboptimal in producing the wide-open vascular channels observed in the normal placenta. Placental tissue ischemia results in the release of antiangiogenic factors, which are distributed in the maternal circulation and negatively affect maternal endothelial cell function, resulting in the classic microscopic ultrastructural triad of arteriolar constriction, endothelial cell damage, and tissue hypoxemia.

Pregnancy-related hypertensive disorders are described as a 2-stage process, with the first stage involved with abnormal placental development and the second stage involved with the clinical manifestations of the disorder, including hypertension, proteinuria, and a wide spectrum of organ system issues (e.g., dysfunction of the central nervous, renal, hepatic, or hematologic/coagulation systems).[20] Obesity remains a major risk factor for the development of preeclampsia and other hypertensive disorders of pregnancy.[21]

DEFINITIONS: HYPERTENSION SPECTRUM DISORDERS OF PREGNANCY

In 2013, the American College of Obstetricians and Gynecologists (ACOG) Task Force on Hypertension in Pregnancy published recommendations based on the available evidence related to hypertension and pregnancy, taking the implications and the confidence in estimates of effect utilizing the strategy developed by the Grading of Recommendations Assessment, Development, and Evaluation (GRADE) Working Group. In this report, the task force made the decision to continue using the classification schema for hypertensive disorders of pregnancy introduced in 1972 by ACOG and modified in 1990 and 2000 by the Working Group of the National High Blood Pressure Education Program.[22] The definitions include four broad categories:

1. Preeclampsia-eclampsia
2. Gestational hypertension
3. Chronic hypertension of any cause
4. Chronic hypertension with superimposed preeclampsia

The definition of preeclampsia includes the following:

- New-onset elevated blood pressure after 20 weeks' gestation in a woman with normal blood pressure readings prior to pregnancy
- Systolic blood pressure (SBP) of 140 mm Hg or higher or diastolic blood pressure (DBP) of 90 mm Hg or higher on 2 occasions at least 4 hours apart
- New-onset proteinuria determined by 1 of the following:
  ◦ 24-hour urine collection with 300 mg or more of protein or an equivalent amount extrapolated from a shorter, timed collection
  ◦ Ratio of urine total protein to total creatinine 0.3 or greater (each measured as milligrams/deciliter)
  ◦ Urine dipstick reading of 1+ or higher (only to be used if other methods are not available)
- In the absence of proteinuria, new-onset hypertension as defined previously with new onset of any one of the following:
  ◦ Blood platelet count 100,000 or fewer platelets/microliter
  ◦ Blood creatinine concentration greater than 1.1 mg/dL or doubling of baseline creatinine concentration in the absence of any other renal disease
  ◦ Elevated blood transaminase concentrations twice the upper limit of normal range for assay employed

Features consistent with preeclampsia exhibiting severe features include any one of the following:

- SBP of 160 mm Hg or higher or DBP of 110 mm Hg or higher on two occasions at least 4 hours apart while the patient is at bed rest (note that this is also the definition for severe acute hypertension; blood pressure reading should be repeated within 15 minutes and if persistently elevated in the severe range should be followed immediately by antihypertensive therapy[23])
- Thrombocytopenia (blood platelet count of 100,000 or fewer platelets/microliter)
- Impaired liver function:
  ◦ Elevated blood transaminase concentrations twice the upper limit of normal range for assay employed
  ◦ Right upper quadrant or epigastric pain not responsive to medication and not attributable to another cause
- Progressive renal insufficiency (blood creatinine concentration greater than 1.1 mg/dL or doubling of baseline creatinine concentration in the absence of any other renal disease)
- New-onset pulmonary edema
- New-onset cerebral or visual disturbances

The definition of gestational hypertension is elevation of blood pressure after 20 weeks' gestation without proteinuria or other systemic findings.

CONTROLLING HYPERTENSION DURING PREGNANCY AND POSTPARTUM

The ACOG Task Force on Hypertension in Pregnancy defined the goals of treatment for hypertension during pregnancy to include prevention of acute complications of hypertension while maintaining the pregnancy in a state of health for as long as possible safely. These goals include the recognition and reduction of risks to the pregnant woman and her fetus attributable to hypertension and related vascular compromise. For the fetus, this approach also includes the recognition and reduction of adverse risk potentially attributable to the effects of antihypertensive agents on maternal hemodynamics, uteroplacental perfusion, and potential to cross the maternal-placental interface. Presently, the anticipated long-term benefit of antihypertensive management on maternal cardiovascular morbidity and mortality is not a primary concern during pregnancy.[22]

Nonpharmacological Interventions

Many nonpharmacological interventions and strategies have been utilized to reduce blood pressure in nonpregnant hypertensive patients; these interventions and strategies include regular aerobic exercise, attaining/maintaining ideal body weight; moderating alcohol intake; and modifying the diet to include such things as abundant fruits and vegetables, low-fat dairy products, high-fiber items, and reduced sodium, such as what constitute the Dietary Approaches to Stop Hypertension (DASH) diet. These interventions have appeal for use during pregnancy due to their nonpharmacological basis; however, most are not appropriate for pregnancy or have not been evaluated during pregnancy.[22] Strategies and interventions that are potentially applicable during pregnancy due to supporting evidence include the following:

- Weight loss and diets with less than 100 mEq/d (extremely low) sodium are not recommended.
- Moderate-level physical activity is recommended.
- Home blood pressure monitoring is recommended.

Weight loss and extreme sodium restriction are not recommended; however, the quality of the evidence is reported as low and the recommendation is qualified in scope. The recommendation regarding moderate-level physical activity is also reported as having low-quality evidence.[24,25] Exercise during pregnancy may reduce the risk of developing preeclampsia.[26] Obese women are considered at extraordinarily high risk for developing severe hypertension, which often requires multiple antihypertensive agents to achieve control.[27]

Home blood pressure monitoring for this group is reasonable, with the quality of the evidence described as low. Despite recognized advantages of ambulatory blood pressure monitoring and home blood pressure monitoring, it is likely office blood pressure monitoring will remain the most common method to screen and monitor blood pressure in outpatient medicine. This is due to the lack of reimbursement for ambulatory and home monitoring equipment, limited availability of the equipment

TABLE 24-1 Proper Blood Pressure Cuff Size Selection Based on Upper Arm Circumference[a]

Arm Circumference (centimeters)	Cuff Bladder Size (centimeters)	Cuff Size Classification
22–26	12 by 22	Small adult
27–34	16 by 30	Adult
25–44 cm	16 by 36	Large adult
45–52 cm	16 by 42	Adult thigh

[a]From Mancia G, Fagard R, Narkiewicz K, et al. 2013 practice guidelines for the management of arterial hypertension of the European Society of Hypertension (ESH) and the European Society of Cardiology (ESC): ESH/ESC Task Force for the Management of Arterial Hypertension. *J Hypertens.* 2013;31:1925–1938; and Preventative Services Task Force. Screening for high blood pressure: US Preventative Services Task Force reaffirmation recommendation statement. *Ann Intern Med.* 2007;147:783–786.

needed, and a lack of detailed guidelines for monitoring strategies other than office blood pressure monitoring. Attention to the recognized factors that contribute to accurate blood pressure assessment include time of measurement, type of device used, cuff size, patient positioning, cuff placement, technique for obtaining measurement, the number of measurements taken, and recent use of tobacco or caffeine.[28,29] Proper selection of appropriate blood pressure cuff size is an essential component of accurate reproducible measurements. For example, too small a cuff leads to increased pressure within the cuff bladder compared to the occluding pressure of the brachial artery, resulting in overestimation of the patient's blood pressure.[30,31] Please see Table 24-1 for details of blood pressure cuff selection based on a patient's upper arm circumference.

Antihypertensive Agent Management

The ACOG Task Force on Hypertension in Pregnancy provides limited guidance for the use of antihypertensive agents during pregnancy. Oral antihypertensive agents are only indicated for control of chronic hypertension, where the SBP is greater than or equal to 160 or DBP is greater than or equal to 105 mm Hg based on evidence of moderate quality while making a strong recommendation. Meanwhile, if the SBP is less than 160 mm Hg, DBP is less than 105 mm Hg, and evidence for end-organ damage is absent, then antihypertensive medication management is not recommended, a recommendation based on low-quality evidence.

Antihypertensive agents discussed for use during pregnancy include labetalol, nifedipine, methyldopa, and thiazide diuretics. The use of each agent is summarized in a table that lists a dosage range from initial to maximum toxic dose and a few notes.[22] The only classes of agents discussed as second-line therapy for managing chronic hypertension during pregnancy are diuretics, specifically thiazide-class agents.[32,33] Given the difficult and complex nature of controlling hypertension among women with obesity, and the lack of direct evidence to guide more complex management during pregnancy, an approach that extrapolates lessons learned among nonpregnant hypertensive patients can be used to enhance our understanding of how subpopulations respond to specific agents and how the difference between the standard dose and the maximum dose can guide the organization of first-, second-, and third-line management.

When considering and initiating antihypertensive management, an essential component of care is what to select as a target range for blood pressure. The ACOG Task Force on Hypertension in Pregnancy proposed, based on low-quality evidence, a target range for control that includes SBP between 120 and 160 and DBP between 80 and 105 mm Hg.[22] The National Institute for Health and Care Excellence (NICE) in the United Kingdom has published guidelines for the management of chronic hypertension that recommend a target SBP less than 150 and DBP between 80 and 100 mm Hg.[34] The Control of Hypertension in Pregnancy Study (CHIPS) conducted an open, international, multicenter trial that studied two treatment targets for chronic hypertension, with one group having a target DBP at 100 mm Hg and a second group having a target DBP at 85 mm Hg. There was no difference in outcomes, except the group with DBP at 100 mm Hg had an increased frequency of severe maternal hypertension.[35]

Given that severe acute hypertension is associated with serious maternal complications, such as intracranial hemorrhage, congestive heart failure, and acute renal failure, controlling hypertension in a manner that reduces the incidence of severe hypertension is reasonable: target SPB 130–150 and DBP 80–90 mm Hg for uncomplicated hypertension. For obese women with complicated hypertension (1 or more of the following: secondary hypertension, left ventricular hypertrophy, microalbuminuria, retinopathy, dyslipidemia, maternal age greater than 40 years, history of stroke, previous perinatal loss, or diabetes mellitus), target treatment of SBP is lower, at 120–140 mm Hg, while DBP is the same, at 80–90 mm Hg.[36]

Table 24-2 summarizes the antihypertensive agents that can be considered for control of hypertension during pregnancy. The classic agents used during pregnancy as outlined by the ACOG Task Force on Hypertension in Pregnancy are listed first and include labetalol, methyldopa, and nifedipine and hydrochlorothiazide as a representative member of the thiazide diuretic agent category. As older agents, their efficacy and safety during pregnancy have been documented over time. The standard dose is the range where the medication has efficacy with limited side effects. The maximum dose, if exceeded, will result in toxic effects. If the upper limit of the standard dose is exceeded, one can expect little increase in effect while increasing the risk for side effects. The standard dose ranges have not been determined in pregnant women; it would be reasonable to expect, with the physiologic increase in medication clearance, that the standard dose range during pregnancy may be wider for some of these agents. With endothelial dysfunction expected among obese women during pregnancy, it is also possible that medication clearance due to target-organ dysfunction may as likely be compromised.

Once the upper standard dose of an agent is met, it is reasonable to consider adding a second agent to improve hypertensive control as needed. Labetalol remains the overall best choice for initial management of hypertension during pregnancy due to the agent's long history of use during pregnancy, efficacy for most patients, and potential benefit for target-organ protection in complicated hypertension, such as renal protection with renin reduction that leads to reduced afferent glomerular arteriolar hypertension. If a second agent is needed, then it should be medication from a different category that will likely result in a synergistic effect on blood pressure control.

TABLE 24-2 Oral Antihypertensive Medications[a]

Medication	Medication Category	Standard Dose	Maximum Dose
Labetalol	Nonselective β blocker, α blocker, renin reduction	200–600 mg/d	2400 mg/d
Methyldopa	Central α_2-adrenergic agonist	500–3000 mg/d	3000 mg/d
Nifedipine	Calcium channel blocker	30–60 mg/d	120 mg/d
Hydrochlorothiazide	Thiazide diuretic (sodium reuptake inhibitor distal renal tubules)	12.5–50 mg/d	50 mg/d
Hydralazine	Direct peripheral vasodilator	20–250 mg/d	300 mg/d
Clonidine	Central α_2-adrenergic agonist	0.2–0.6 mg/d	2.4 mg/d
Nicardipine	Calcium channel blocker	60–120 mg/d	120 mg/d
Amlodipine	Calcium channel blocker	2.5–10 mg/d	10 mg/d
Carvedilol	Nonselective β blocker, α blocker, renin reduction	6.25–50 mg/d	80 mg/d

[a]From Hamilton RJ, Allen JE, Birtcher KK, et al. *Tarascon Pharmacopoeia 2015 Professional Desk Reference*. 16th ed. Burlington, MA: Jones & Bartlett Learning; 2015:5:126–127, 132, 137, 139–141, 144; Markham KB, Funai EF. Chapter 48: pregnancy-related hypertension. In: Creasy RK, Resnik R, Iams JD, et al., eds. *Creasy & Resnik's Maternal-Fetal Medicine: Principles and Practice*. 7th ed. Philadelphia: Elsevier Saunders; 2014:768–775; Magee LA, Miremadi S, Li J, et al. Therapy with both magnesium sulfate and nifedipine does not increase the risk of serious magnesium-related maternal side effects in women with preeclampsia. *Am J Obstet Gynecol*. 2005;193:153–163; and Emergent therapy for acute-onset, severe hypertension during pregnancy and the postpartum period. Committee Opinion No. 623. American College of Obstetricians and Gynecologists. *Obstet Gynecol*. 2015;125:521–525.

Careful monitoring would be required to follow up a woman on a second or third agent for control of blood pressure.

Methyldopa is an agent with a favorable profile on uteroplacental hemodynamics but is limited in efficacy treating hypertension; this is further complicated by multiple daily doses and a risk for triggering hemolytic anemia with use. Nifedipine can be a first-line agent for women with a history of difficulty with labetalol, or nifedipine can be a second-line agent if needed. As a thiazide category diuretic, hydrochlorothiazide can be used as a second-line agent. Clonidine can be used to enhance central α block as a second- or third-line agent. Hydralazine can also be used as a second- or third-line agent for a limited time as the efficacy of oral hydralazine drops off over time, and there is an increased risk for precipitating systemic lupus erythematosus. Nicardipine is included as an alternative to nifedipine that can be given orally or intravenously that has been used during pregnancy. Finally, amlodipine and carvedilol are included as newer agents that have lower standard dosage ranges, good efficacy, and tolerance in the general nonobstetrical population and can be considered for hypertension refractory to traditional agents.[37]

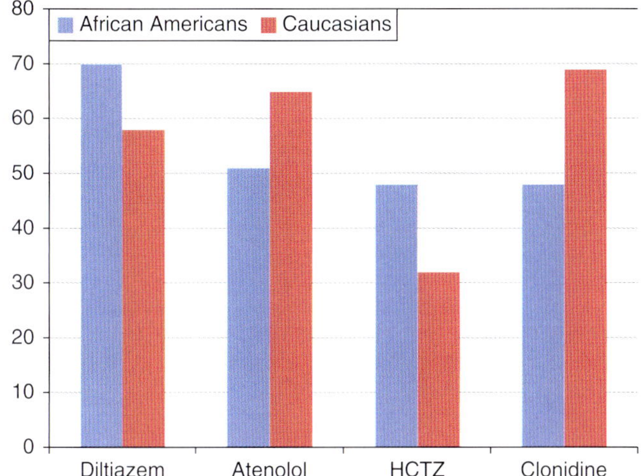

FIGURE 24-1. Response to antihypertensive agents for African American and white patients. HCTZ, hydrochlorothiazide. (From Materson BJ, Reda DJ, Cushman WC, et al. Single-drug therapy for hypertension in men: a comparison of 6 antihypertensive agents with placebo. *N Engl J Med*. 1993;328(13):914–921; and Materson BJ, Reda DJ, Cushman WC. Department of Veterans Affairs single-drug therapy of hypertension study. *Am J Hypertens*. 1995;8:189–192.)

Limited data are available regarding racial differences in patient response to antihypertensive agent management. One case series published by the Department of Veterans Affairs included two groups of male subjects, all less than 60 years of age, who were started on single-agent management for hypertension and followed for a year. Successful management was defined as DBP less than 95 mm Hg. The original study had to be published in two separate articles due to a statistical error in the first article. Figure 24-1 summarizes the results. If the response rates are compared by antihypertensive agent category, white individuals responded most often to clonidine, with β blocker a close second, and responded less well to a thiazide diuretic. African American individuals responded best to a calcium channel blocker and less well to a β blocker, clonidine, and thiazide diuretic.[38,39] These data do not imply that labctalol has no role in the management of hypertensive African American women during pregnancy. After initial treatment with labetalol that results in only a partial response, it is reasonable to consider nifedipine or nicardipine as a second-line agent due to the evidence presented that suggests African American individuals with hypertension may respond better to a calcium channel blocker. See Table 24-3 as one example of a management strategy for control of hypertension during pregnancy and postpartum.

Management Not Directly Related to Control of Hypertension

- To reduce risk for preeclampsia, probable benefit to starting women with obesity and chronic hypertension during pregnancy on low-dose aspirin (81 mg/d orally) from 12 weeks of gestation until delivery.[34]
- To reduce risk for preeclampsia, probable benefit to starting women during pregnancy on high-dose calcium, 1–2 g/d orally, particularly among women with low calcium intake; administration of low-dose calcium, 500–600 mg/d orally, less clear but considered better than no supplementation, particularly among women with low calcium intake.[26]
- Possible benefit of statin agents such as pravastatin for the prevention of preeclampsia in high-risk women.[40]
- Possible benefit of exercise for risk reduction for preeclampsia during pregnancy.[41]
- No demonstrated benefit or insufficient data to conclude the risk of developing preeclampsia is reduced for the following strategies: restricted-sodium diet; fish

TABLE 24-3 Proposed Strategy Oral Agent Hypertension Management[a]

Step 1	Home blood pressure monitoring 1–3 times a day.
Step 2	If SBP ≥ 150 mm Hg or DBP ≥ 100 mm Hg on more than half the readings within previous week, then initiate antihypertensive medication.
Step 3	Start *labetalol* 100–200 mg orally 2 times per day; 3 times per day for underlying renal disease to enhance nephroprotective effect. If African American woman or patient has moderate-to-severe asthma, consider starting *nifedipine* 30 mg extended release once per day.
Step 4	If SBP persists ≥ 150 or DBP persists ≥ 100 mm Hg over next 3 days to 1 week, increase *labetalol* 100–200 mg per dose; continue to monitor each 3 days to 1 week until adequate control of SBP < 150 and DBP < 100 mm Hg is achieved or standard dose is exceeded at 600–800 mg/d. If SBP persists ≥ 150 or DBP persists ≥ 100 mm Hg over next week, increase *nifedipine* 30 mg extended release per dose; continue to monitor each week until adequate control of SBP < 150 and DBP < 100 mm Hg is achieved or standard dose 120 mg/d is reached; may give 30 or 60 mg extended release 2 times per day if needed to control end-of-dose breakthrough hypertension.
Step 5	If *labetalol* does not achieve adequate control as defined in previous steps, consider second agent, such as *nifedipine* 30 mg extended release once per day or *methyldopa* 250 mg 2–3 times per day If *nifedipine* does not achieve adequate control as defined in previous steps, consider second agent, such as *labetalol* 100–200 mg 2–3 times per day or *methyldopa* 250 mg 2–3 times per day.
Step 6	Continue home blood pressure monitoring and review of recorded measurements as in previous steps. Increase second-line agents to achieve control as previously described with *nifedipine* extended release up to 120 mg/d, *labetalol* up to 600–800 mg/d, or *methyldopa* up to 3000 mg/d.
Step 7	If second agent does not control blood pressure as previously described, then consider adding a third agent: *hydrochlorothiazide* 12.5–25 mg once per day or *clonidine* 0.1 mg 2 times per day. *If considering a third agent*: Repeat assessment of activity tolerance and functional status; repeat laboratory assessment of renal function; assess cardiac function with b-type natriuretic peptide level; repeat electrocardiogram and echocardiogram. *If considering a third agent and evaluation is complete*: Consider consultation with maternal-fetal medicine, nephrology (suspect underlying renal contribution to persistent hypertension), or cardiology (suspect underlying cardiac contribution to persistent hypertension).
Step 8	As antihypertensive management increases, begin fetal surveillance at 24–32 weeks' gestational age with patient daily fetal movement monitoring, serial ultrasound evaluation of fetal growth, nonstress testing, biophysical profile.
Step 9	Hospitalize patient and consider consultation as outlined previously if • Severe hypertension is present (SBP ≥ 160 or DBP ≥ 110 mm Hg). • Fetal surveillance is not reassuring or normal. • Concern exists for maternal cardiac or renal dysfunction.
Step 10	Other agents and considerations: • *Hydralazine* 20–250 mg orally per day: Avoid long-term use with risk for triggering systemic lupus erythematosus–like syndrome. • *Methyldopa*: Monitor for rare hemolytic anemia, abnormal liver function studies. • *Hydrochlorothiazide*: Hypokalemia, electrolyte imbalance, bone marrow failure all cell lines, acute angle closure glaucoma, pancreatitis. • *Clonidine*: Monitor for fetal and neonatal effects with placental transfer of agent.

(Continued)

TABLE 24-3 Proposed Strategy Oral Agent Hypertension Management[a] (*Continued*)

- *Nifedipine (immediate release)*: Immediate-release tablets should not be chewed or placed sublingually for severe hypertension or hypertensive emergencies, including ST elevation myocardial infarct (STEMI); avoid grapefruit juice; can be used for a limited time to prevent severe hypertension while extended-release agent comes up to therapeutic level.
- *Nicardipine*: 60–120 mg total per day sustained release; can be used instead of *nifedipine* sustained release.
- *Amlodipine*: Consider if blood pressure control not obtained with *nifedipine* or *nicardipine*.
- *Carvedilol*: Consider if blood pressure control not obtained with labetalol; monitor women with diabetes mellitus for blunted hypoglycemia symptoms, asthma concern regarding bronchoconstriction.

[a]From Hamilton RJ, Allen JE, Birtcher KK, et al. *Tarascon Pharmacopoeia 2015 Professional Desk Reference.* 16th ed. Burlington, MA: Jones & Bartlett Learning; 2015:5:126–127, 132, 137, 139–141, 144.

oil supplementation; antihypertensive agents (as a strategy to reduce preeclampsia risk), antioxidant vitamins C, D, or E; or low-dose aspirin in combination with heparin.

- Detailed initial physical examination with follow-up detailed or focal examination as clinically indicated.
- Scrutiny for important symptoms, such as headache, visual disturbances, epigastric or right upper quadrant abdominal pain, rapid weight gain.
- Baseline urinary protein analysis either as ratio of total protein to creatinine or 24-hour collection, which can be repeated as clinically indicated.
- Monitor weight gain.
- Serial blood pressure determination with the patient in a seated position with an appropriate-size cuff.
- Baseline plasma creatinine and hepatic aminotransferase levels; platelet count and hemoglobin concentration, with repeat analysis as needed.
- Consider baseline plasma uric acid and lactic dehydrogenase levels and coagulation studies if active disease is suspected, with repeat analysis as needed.
- Determination of estimated fetal weight, amniotic fluid volume at baseline with repeat evaluation as needed; ACOG indications for ultrasonography in the second and third trimesters include estimation of gestational age, evaluation of fetal growth every 2–4 weeks, examination of significant discrepancy between uterine size and clinical dating, and evaluation of fetal well-being.[42]
- Fetal surveillance as clinically indicated; ACOG recommends fetal surveillance to begin at 32 weeks' gestation for hypertension, gestational hypertension, and preeclampsia; earlier surveillance is recommended for multiple or particularly serious conditions, starting at the gestational age when delivery would be considered for overall perinatal benefit.[43]
- Fetal delivery and placental evacuation are considered the only intervention that ends the pathophysiological progression of preeclampsia.[44]
- Delivery should be considered after maternal stabilization; undertaking resuscitation, including volume replacement with attention to measured input and output

determinations; particularly in situations involving hemodynamic instability, non-reassuring fetal testing, persistent severe hypertension, persistent central nervous system irritability (headache, visual disturbances, right upper quadrant or epigastric pain), eclampsia, pulmonary edema, renal failure with markedly increased plasma creatinine levels, rapid increase in plasma aminotransferase levels or decrease in platelet count, coagulopathy, or placental abruption.

- Expectant management can be considered in appropriate cases on an in-hospital setting.
- Consider immediate delivery with severe disease at less than 24 weeks or greater than 34 weeks or for women not able to have appropriate maternal and fetal monitoring or not willing to agree to expectant management.
- Consider maternal transport to a regional, tertiary, or quaternary care center capable of management of maternal or fetal complications or for preterm delivery.
- Provide intravenous magnesium sulfate for seizure prophylaxis; an antenatal corticosteroid course for 24–34 weeks' gestational age; initiation or modification of antihypertensive management; monitoring and management for oliguria; and management as needed for coagulopathy and cardiopulmonary dysfunction or failure.[45]
- The combination of calcium channel–blocking agents and magnesium sulfate did not result in hypotension, as had been a concern early in the use of calcium channel–blocking agents.[46]

MANAGEMENT OF SEVERE ACUTE HYPERTENSION

The ACOG Committee on Obstetrical Practice published a committee opinion regarding the management of acute-onset, severe hypertension during pregnancy and postpartum that proposed utilizing evidence-based clinical guidelines that provide a clear, concise, and stepwise checklist approach that allows obstetrical providers and institutions to ensure mechanisms are in place to promptly and effectively address women with hypertensive urgencies or emergencies.[47] Hypertensive urgency is defined as severe acute hypertension with absent or minimal symptoms, such as mild headache.[48] A hypertensive emergency is defined as severe acute hypertension with severe symptom or life-threatening complication or complications that can include hypertensive encephalopathy, retinal hemorrhage, papilledema, acute congestive heart failure, myocardial ischemia, or acute renal injury. In the nonpregnant adult, grade 3 or severe hypertension is defined as SBP greater than or equal to 180 mm Hg or DPB greater than or equal to 110 mm Hg.[38] The obstetrical definition for severe hypertension is SBP greater than or equal to 160 mm Hg, with the same DBP at 110 mm Hg. In one series, SBP elevated at or greater than 160 mm Hg was associated with 96% of cases for which both antepartum and postpartum pregnant women experienced stroke. Arterial hemorrhagic stroke was seen in 93% of women in this series.[49] In contrast to stroke in older individuals, for whom elevated DBP is more likely to cause vessel damage and rupture or thrombosis due to atherosclerotic stiffening of the vessels, stroke among younger pregnant women is more likely to reflect higher levels of wall tension due to increased cardiac output, intravascular volume expansion, and arterial wall connective tissue weakness. This definition of severe hypertension during pregnancy and postpartum has been integrated into the ACOG protocols for management.[47]

Given that obese women are at increased risk for severe hypertension and additional complications related to pregnancy, such as eclampsia, hepatic dysfunction, thrombocytopenia, and coagulation dysfunction, fetal demise, and placental abruption, a lower threshold for severe systolic hypertension is applicable in this population.[36] The ACOG protocols for the management of severe acute hypertension include three strategies based on intravenous labetalol, intravenous hydralazine, or oral nifedipine as the primary agent for management. The document has three boxes, one for each of these agents acting as first-line management. Each box is presented in a stepwise ordered approach that can easily be adapted into protocols for the management of severe acute hypertension, including adaptation into standardized order sets. The boxes can also be copied, cut out, laminated, and provided as rapid reference guides for obstetrical care providers. Each box contains the following elements:

- Notify physician (or other managing obstetrical provider) of a woman with severe acute hypertension.
- Initiate fetal surveillance if appropriate.
- Recheck blood pressure; if severe acute hypertension continues, initiate bolus-dose treatment with first-line agent from one of the three protocols based on medication availability, intravenous access, and obstetrical provider preference as no individual agent has demonstrated superiority.
- Monitor and repeat bolus-dose treatment with first-line agent as indicated.
- If severe acute hypertension persists beyond the first-line agent protocol, then cross over to another first-line agent, such as labetalol or hydralazine; do not continue with initial first-line agent.
- If severe acute hypertension persists after use of the crossover agent, obtain expert consultation with maternal-fetal medicine, anesthesia, internal medicine, or critical care medicine; the process of moving from initial detection of severe acute hypertension to expert consultation or resolution of the severe acute hypertension should not take more than 45–60 minutes.
- Give additional antihypertensive agents to control persistent severe acute hypertension and to prevent rebound hypertension once the short-acting first-line agents are cleared.
- Once severe acute hypertension is controlled, establish a plan for ongoing close blood pressure monitoring, maternal and fetal assessment, and additional management beyond hypertensive treatment; be prepared to reenter the protocol and obtain expert consultation for reoccurring severe acute hypertension.
- If the patient were to develop focal neurologic deficit or is found to have acute retinal changes or papilledema on fundoscopic examination, then bolus therapy should move toward management as outlined for hypertensive emergency.

Please see Table 24-4 for a summary of the antihypertensive agents used for management of severe acute hypertension.

TABLE 24-4 Agents for Severe Acute Hypertension Management[a]

Agent	Dose/Route	Next Agent
Labetalol	• 20 mg IV over 2 min; monitor 10 min, if SBP ≥ 160 or DBP ≥ 110 mm Hg, then • 40 mg IV over 2 min; monitor 10 min, if SBP ≥ 160 or DBP ≥ 110 mm Hg, then • 80 mg IV over 2 min; monitor 10 min, if SBP ≥ 160 or DBP ≥ 110 mm Hg, then • Next agent	• Hydralazine 10 mg IV over 2 min • Monitor 20 min, if SBP ≥ 160 or DBP ≥ 110 mm Hg, then • Manage as hypertensive emergency
Hydralazine	• 5 or 10 mg IV over 2 min; monitor 20 min, if SBP ≥ 160 or DBP ≥ 110 mm Hg, then • 10 mg IV over 2 min; monitor 20 min, if SBP ≥ 160 or DBP ≥ 110 mm Hg, then • Next agent	• Labetalol 20 mg IV over 2 min • Monitor 10 min, if SBP ≥ 160 or DBP ≥ 110 mm Hg, then • Labetalol 40 mg IV over 2 min • Monitor 10 min, if SBP ≥ 160 or DBP ≥ 110 mm Hg, then • Manage as hypertensive emergency
Nifedipine	• 10 mg orally; monitor 20 min, if SBP ≥ 160 or DBP ≥ 110 mm Hg, then • 20 mg orally; monitor 20 min, if SBP ≥ 160 or DBP ≥ 110 mm Hg, then • 20 mg orally; monitor 20 min, if SBP ≥ 160 or DBP ≥ 110 mm Hg, then • Next agent	• Labetalol 40 mg IV over 2 min • Monitor 10 min, if SBP ≥ 160 or DBP ≥ 110 mm Hg, then • Manage as hypertensive emergency

Abbreviations: IV, intravenous; SBP, systolic blood pressure; DBP, diastolic blood pressure; min, minutes.
[a]Markham KB, Funai EF. Chapter 48: pregnancy-related hypertension. In: Creasy RK, Resnik R, Iams JD, et al., eds. *Creasy & Resnik's Maternal-Fetal Medicine: Principles and Practice.* 7th ed. Philadelphia: Elsevier Saunders; 2014:768–775

MANAGEMENT OF HYPERTENSIVE EMERGENCIES

A hypertensive emergency is defined as severe hypertension with either threatened or acute target or end-organ damage, and these are considered by definition to be life threatening; management mandates short-acting intravenous vasodilator therapy with an agent that can be readily titrated to specific parameters in a critical care setting. Hypertensive emergencies are divided into categories that include neurologic, cardiovascular, renal, or catecholamine excess scenarios. Neurologic emergencies include severe hypertension with encephalopathy, subarachnoid hemorrhage, intracranial hemorrhage, or thrombotic stroke. Cardiovascular emergencies include severe hypertension with left ventricular failure, unstable angina, myocardial infarction, or aortic dissection. Renal emergencies include severe hypertension with gross hematuria or acute renal dysfunction to failure.[50]

During pregnancy and postpartum, hypertensive emergencies can range from severe acute hypertension that does not respond to intravenous bolus antihypertensive agent management as outlined previously to the complications described. Consultation should be undertaken with other services, including maternal-fetal medicine, anesthesia, critical care, and neonatal intensive care, when appropriate.[47] When the patient has a persistent or severe headache, focal neurologic deficit or deficits, significant visual disturbances or fundoscopic evidence for retinopathy or papilledema, or a history of chronic hypertension with acute-onset severe hypertension, then a neurologic hypertensive emergency is suspected. In addition to physical examination, brain imaging and lumbar puncture can be undertaken during pregnancy to better define the complication. Intensive care admission with intravenous vasodilator therapy and consultation with additional specialty areas, such as neurology or neurosurgery, should be considered.

The most difficult diagnosis to make is that of hypertensive encephalopathy, as the pathophysiology involves disruption of the blood-brain barrier and loss of cerebral vascular autoregulation, which results in cerebral edema, particularly involving the distribution of the posterior cerebral arteries.[50] The physiologic changes of normal pregnancy enhance the progress of encephalopathy due to increased pulse pressure with increased cardiac output, decreased vessel wall tensile strength with connective tissue laxity, and increased movement of intravascular fluid and proteins into the extravascular space surrounding the vasculature of the brain. The 2010 American Heart Association (AHA) guidelines for adult advanced cardiac life support (ACLS) adult suspected stoke can be followed, including a percutaneous carotid endovascular procedure or thrombolytic therapy when indicated as part of initial evaluation and management of a pregnant or postpartum woman with severe hypertension and suspected neurologic emergency.

Hypertension associated with acute coronary syndrome can occur during pregnancy and is usually the result of physiologic demands for increased cardiac output, enhanced coagulation function, and increased circulating inflammatory mediators that enhance endothelial reactivity. A combination of acute coronary artery spasm, atherosclerotic plaque rupture, and thrombosis formation can occur, as can coronary artery dissection. Management includes reduction of severe hypertension to reduce myocardial ischemia and related symptoms, generally about 20%–30% reduction in mean arterial blood pressure.[50]

Additional management should follow guidelines established by the AHA ACLS for monitoring and management of acute coronary syndromes; when indicated, percutaneous coronary intervention and thrombolytic therapy are not contraindicated by pregnancy. Left heart failure that precipitates pulmonary edema with hypertension should be treated with a vasodilator agent such as nitroglycerin. Aortic dissection can be visualized on echocardiography, computed tomography, or magnetic resonance imaging of the chest and is treated with morphine for pain reduction and titration of β blockade and vasodilator agents, usually in preparation for surgical management. Severe hypertension with gross hematuria generally requires consultation with the urology service once blood pressure is controlled. After initial management, some form of renal replacement therapy (dialysis, hemofiltration) may be needed acutely, with recovery of renal function after a period of support.[50]

One agent of interest for severe hypertension associated with acute renal injury is fenoldopam; this agent is a peripheral dopamine-1 agonist that avoids the toxicity associated with prolonged infusion of agents that release cyanide and thiocyanate while enhancing natriuresis and diuresis and reduces plasma creatinine levels. Large-scale data for the efficacy of fenoldopam for this indication are lacking.[51] There is limited experience in the use of fenoldopam during pregnancy; however, the advantages mentioned combined with data that suggest little effect on vasoconstriction or dilation in isolated human umbilical artery segments.[52] These results, in combination

TABLE 24-5 Agents for Hypertensive Emergency Management[a]

Agent	Dosage	Maximum	Notes
Labetalol	0.5–2 mg/min	300 mg total dose	• Avoid with cocaine intoxication
Esmolol	500 µg/kg load over 1 min; 50 µg/kg/min titrate to effect; repeat bolus as needed	200 µg/kg/min	• Aortic dissection • Avoid with cocaine intoxication
Nicardipine	5 mg/h, increase 2.5 mg/h every 5–15 min	15 mg/h	• Caution with acute heart failure
Diltiazem	5 mg/h, increase 5 mg/h	15 mg/h	• Atrial fibrillation/flutter • Paroxysmal supraventricular tachycardia • Hypertension • Myocardial ischemia
Fenoldopam	0.03 µg/kg/min, titrate every 15 min	1.6 µg/kg/min	• Beneficial effect on renal function with renal hypertensive emergency • May have advantage in hypertension associated with preeclampsia
Nitroglycerin	10 µg/min, titrate every 3–5 min	100 µg/min	• Myocardial ischemia • Cocaine intoxication
Nitroprusside	0.3 µg/kg/min initial; titrate to target	10 µg/kg/min for 10 min	• Monitor thiocyanate level • Last resort during pregnancy

[a]From Hamilton RJ, Allen JE, Birtcher KK, et al. *Tarascon Pharmacopoeia 2015 Professional Desk Reference.* 16th ed. Burlington, MA: Jones & Bartlett Learning; 2015:5:126–127, 132, 137, 139–141, 144; Markham KB, Funai EF. Chapter 48: pregnancy-related hypertension. In: Creasy RK, Resnik R, Iams JD, et al., eds. *Creasy & Resnik's Maternal-Fetal Medicine: Principles and Practice.* 7th ed. Philadelphia: Elsevier Saunders; 2014:768–775; and Boudville N, Ward S, Benaroia M, House AA. Increased sodium intake correlates with greater use of antihypertensive agents by subjects with chronic kidney disease. *Am J Hypertens.* 2004;18:1300–1305.

with the effects on renal function, suggest fenoldopam may have advantages in the management of severe hypertension with target-organ dysfunction over other agents that are more commonly used for women with severe acute hypertension during pregnancy or postpartum.

According to accumulated data regarding the use of antihypertensive agents for severe hypertension, it appears that calcium channel blockers are less likely to have persistent severe hypertension when compared to hydralazine. Until better evidence is available for antihypertensive agent selection, a clinician's experience and familiarity with commonly used agents are still the method used to select these agents for treatment.[53] Clonidine clears more rapidly from circulation in pregnant women compared to nonpregnant controls, with fetal umbilical cord levels at the time of birth similar to maternal clonidine concentrations.[54] Please see Table 24-5 for details regarding agents commonly used during hypertensive emergencies.

FUTURE DIRECTIONS

To reduce the incidence and severity of hypertensive disorders and related complications during pregnancy, we need to investigate strategies such as preconceptual consultation and interventions that will reduce BMI and optimize control of blood pressure as well as end-organ issues prior to conception. Strategies for enhancing diagnosis and monitoring of blood pressure during pregnancy need to be investigated, with creation of specific pregnancy-related guidance if techniques such as ambulatory blood pressure monitoring, home blood pressure monitoring, and ultrasound hemodynamic monitoring is proven to be of clinical utility. Given that obese pregnant women tend to have difficult-to-treat hypertension, research that guides development of medication management strategies employing commonly used medications, investigates the safety and efficacy of more current agents, and thoughtfully assesses the use of agent classes traditionally thought to be contraindicated is in order. Foundational or basic science investigation would be helpful to more thoroughly define the interaction that is occurring between the maternal cardiovascular system, which is primed to display hypertensive pathophysiology, and placental tissue, which is more likely to release oxidative stress mediators and thus produce an excessive hypertensive response that is earlier in onset and more severe in course among obese pregnant women when compared to normal-weight pregnant women. A more detailed understanding of this maternal vascular and placental pathophysiological interaction has the potential to define interventions that will reduce morbidity and mortality for obese pregnant women and their children.

CONCLUSION

Chronic hypertension and the hypertensive disorders of pregnancy are essential considerations in the management of women with obesity during pregnancy and postpartum. The pathophysiology of obesity establishes a baseline prerequisite state of altered hemodynamics and vascular endothelial dysfunction that contributes to the overall increased incidence of hypertension and pregnancy-related hypertensive disorders. Important first steps include establishing a baseline for each pregnant woman with obesity that includes a detailed assessment of underlying comorbidities, such as hypertension, renal disease, and other evidence of target-organ dysfunction. Interventions that may help reduce the risk for developing either primary or superimposed preeclampsia should be considered, preferably prior to a planned pregnancy. Management of hypertension with antihypertensive agents will require careful attention to avoid exposure to contraindicated or otherwise-problematic agents. Ongoing monitoring of blood pressure and urinary protein and assessment of signs or symptoms suggestive of evolving preeclampsia as well as close follow-up for fetal status are strongly recommended.

A detailed plan for management of severe acute hypertension is essential, as is an understanding of the differentiation and management of severe hypertensive urgency and emergency situations. Although there remains a lack of data that renders clear guidance for the selection and use of the various antihypertensive agents prescribed during pregnancy, obstetrical providers should have a working knowledge of the agents that are used commonly and a plan for consultation as indicated for unusual circumstances or complications. Improved maternal and fetal surveillance and timely intervention are the best hope for reducing the morbidity and mortality that can accompany hypertensive disease among women with obesity during pregnancy.

REFERENCES

1. Page EW. Chapter 1: clinical aspects. In: Page EW. *The Hypertensive Disorders of Pregnancy.* Springfield, IL: Thomas, Bannerstone House; 1953:6–7.

2. Egan BM, Zhao Y, Axon RN. US trends in prevalence, awareness, treatment, and control of hypertension, 1988–2008. *JAMA.* 2010;303(20):2043–2050.

3. Sjostrom L, Lindroos AK, Peltonen M, et al. Lifestyle, diabetes, and cardiovascular risk factors 10 years after bariatric surgery. *N Engl J Med.* 2004;351:2683–2693.

4. Obesity in pregnancy. Committee Opinion No. 549. American College of Obstetricians and Gynecologists. *Obstet Gynecol.* 2013;121:213–217.

5. Gaillard R, Steegers EA, Hofman A, Jaddoe VW. Association of maternal obesity with blood pressure and the risk of gestational hypertensive disorders. The Generation R Study. *J Hypertens.* 2011;29:937–944.

6. Pare E, Parry S, McElrath TF, et al. Clinical risk factors for preeclampsia in the 21st century. *Obstet Gynecol.* 2014;124:763–770.

7. Easterling TR, Brateng D, Schmucker B, et al. Prevention of preeclampsia: a randomized trial of atenolol in hyperdynamic patients before onset of hypertension. *Obstet Gynecol.* 1999;93:723–733.

8. Schmieder RE, Messerli FH. Does obesity influence early target organ damage in hypertensive patients? *Circulation.* 1993;87:1482–1488.

9. Ahmed SB, Fisher ND, Stevanovic R, Hollenberg NK. Body mass index and angiotensin-dependent control of the renal circulation in healthy humans. *Hypertension.* 2005;46:1316–1320.

10. Saad MF, Lillioja S, Nyomba BL, et al. Racial differences in the relation between blood pressure and insulin resistance. *N Engl J Med.* 1991;324:733–739.

11. Rocchini AP, Katch V, Kveselis D, et al. Insulin and renal sodium retention in obese adolescents. *Hypertension.* 1989;14:367–374.

12. Rahmouni K, Correia ML, Haynes WG, Mark AL. Obesity-associated hypertension: new insights into mechanisms. *Hypertension.* 2005;45:9–14.

13. Greenfield JR, Miller JW, Keogh JM, et al. Modulation of blood pressure by central melanocortinergic pathways. *N Engl J Med.* 2009;360:44–52.

14. Ward KR, Bardgett JF, Wolfgang L, Stocker SD. Sympathetic response to insulin is mediated by melanocortin 3/4 receptors in the hypothalamic paraventricular nucleus. *Hypertension.* 2011;57:435–441.

15. Aucott L, Rothnie H, McIntyre L, et al. Long-term weight loss from lifestyle intervention benefits blood pressure? A systematic review. *Hypertension.* 2009;54:756–762.

16. Pedrosa RP, Drager LF, Gonzaga CC, et al. Obstructive sleep apnea: the most common secondary cause of hypertension associated with resistant hypertension. *Hypertension.* 2011;58:811–817.

17. Sarzani R, Salvi F, Dessì-Fulgheri P, Rappelli A. Renin-angiotensin system, natriuretic peptides, obesity, metabolic syndrome, and hypertension: an integrated view in humans. *J Hypertens.* 2008;26:831–843.

18. Steinberg HO, Chaker H, Leaming R, et al. Obesity/insulin resistance is associated with endothelial dysfunction. Implications for the syndrome of insulin resistance. *J Clin Invest.* 1996;97:2601–2610.

19. Kincaid-Smith P. Hypothesis: obesity and the insulin resistance syndrome play a major role in end-stage renal failure attributed to hypertension and labelled "hypertensive nephrosclerosis." *J Hypertens.* 2004;22:1051–1055.

20. Lain KY, Roberts JM. Contemporary concepts of the pathogenesis and management of preeclampsia. *JAMA.* 2002;287:3183–3186.

21. Angeli F, Angeli E, Reboldi G, Verdecchia P. Hypertensive disorders during pregnancy: clinical applicability of risk prediction models. *J Hypertens.* 2011;29:2320–2323.

22. American College of Obstetricians and Gynecologists Task Force on Hypertension in Pregnancy. Hypertension in pregnancy. *Obstet Gynecol.* 2013;122(5):1122–1131.

23. Clark SL, Hankins GDV. Preventing maternal death: 10 clinical diamonds. *Obstet Gynecol.* 2012;119:360–366.

24. Haakstad LAH, Bo K. Effect of regular exercise on prevention of excessive weight gain in pregnancy: a randomized controlled trial. *Eur J Contracep Reprod Health Care.* 2011;16:116–125.

25. Martin CL, Brunner Huber LR. Physical activity and hypertensive complications during pregnancy: findings from 2004 to 2006 North Carolina Pregnancy Risk Assessment Monitoring System. *Birth.* 2010;37:202–210.

26. Hofmeyr GJ, Lawrie TA, Atallah AN, Duley L, Torloni MR. Calcium supplementation during pregnancy for preventing hypertensive disorders and related problems. *Cochrane Database Syst Rev.* 2010;(8):CD0015059.

27. Huang Z, Willett WC, Manson JE, et al. Body weight, weight change, and risk for hypertension in women. *Ann Intern Med.* 1998;128(2):81–88.

28. Pickering TG, Hall JE, Appel LJ, et al. Recommendations for blood pressure measurement in humans and experimental animals part 1: blood pressure measurement in humans: a statement for professionals from the Subcommittee of Professional and Public Education of the American Heart Association Council on High Blood Pressure Research. *Hypertension.* 2005;45:142–261.

29. Pickering TG, Miller NH, Ogedegbe G, Krakoff LR, Artinian NT, Goff D. Call to action on use and reimbursement for home blood pressure monitoring:

executive summary: a joint scientific statement from the American Heart Association, American Society of Hypertension, and Preventative Cardiovascular Nurses Association. *J Am Soc Hypertension.* 2008;2(3):192–202.

30. Mancia G, Fagard R, Narkiewicz K, et al. 2013 practice guidelines for the management of arterial hypertension of the European Society of Hypertension (ESH) and the European Society of Cardiology (ESC): ESH/ESC Task Force for the Management of Arterial Hypertension. *J Hypertens.* 2013;31:1925–1938.

31. Preventative Services Task Force. Screening for high blood pressure: US Preventative Services Task Force reaffirmation recommendation statement. *Ann Intern Med.* 2007;147:783–786.

32. Roberts JM, Pearson G, Cutler J, et al. Summary of the NHLBI Working Group on Research on Hypertension During Pregnancy. *Hypertension.* 2003;41:437–445.

33. Churchill D, Beevers GD, Meher S, Rhodes C. Diuretics for preventing pre-eclampsia. *Cochrane Database Syst Rev.* 2007;(1):CD004451.

34. Visitin C, Mugglestone MA, Almerie MQ, et al. Management of hypertensive disorders during pregnancy: summary of NICE guidance. *BMJ.* 2010;341:c2207.

35. Magee LA, von Dadelszen P, Rey E, et al. Less-tight versus tight control of hypertension in pregnancy. *N Engl J Med.* 2015;372(5):407–417.

36. Sibai BM. Chronic hypertension in pregnancy. *Obstet Gynecol.* 2002;100:369–377.

37. Hamilton RJ, Allen JE, Birtcher KK, et al. *Tarascon Pharmacopoeia 2015 Professional Desk Reference.* 16th ed. Burlington, MA: Jones & Bartlett Learning; 2015:5:126–127, 132, 137, 139–141, 144.

38. Materson BJ, Reda DJ, Cushman WC, et al. Single-drug therapy for hypertension in men: a comparison of 6 antihypertensive agents with placebo. *N Engl J Med.* 1993;328(13):914–921.

39. Materson BJ, Reda DJ, Cushman WC. Department of Veterans Affairs single-drug therapy of hypertension study. *Am J Hypertens.* 1995;8:189–192.

40. Costantine MM, Cleary K. Pravastatin for the prevention of preeclampsia in high-risk pregnant women. *Obstet Gynecol.* 2013;121:349–353.

41. Kasawara KT, Nascimento SL, Costa MR, et al. Exercise and physical activity in the prevention of preeclampsia: systemic review. *Acta Obstet Gynecol Scand.* 2012;91:1147–1157.

42. Ultrasonography in pregnancy. ACOG Practice Bulletin No. 101. American College of Obstetricians and Gynecologists. *Obstet Gynecol.* 2009;113:451–461.

43. Antepartum fetal surveillance. Practice Bulletin No. 145. American College of Obstetricians and Gynecologists. *Obstet Gynecol.* 2014;124:182–192.

44. Chapter 40: hypertensive disorders. In: Cunningham FG, Leveno KJ, Bloom SL, et al., eds. *Williams Obstetrics.* 24th ed. New York: McGraw-Hill Education; 2014:748–750.

45. Markham KB, Funai EF. Chapter 48: pregnancy-related hypertension. In: Creasy RK, Resnik R, Iams JD, et al., eds. *Creasy & Resnik's Maternal-Fetal Medicine: Principles and Practice.* 7th ed. Philadelphia: Elsevier Saunders; 2014:768–775.

46. Magee LA, Miremadi S, Li J, et al. Therapy with both magnesium sulfate and nifedipine does not increase the risk of serious magnesium-related maternal side effects in women with preeclampsia. *Am J Obstet Gynecol.* 2005;193:153–163.

47. Emergent therapy for acute-onset, severe hypertension during pregnancy and the postpartum period. Committee Opinion No. 623. American College of Obstetricians and Gynecologists. *Obstet Gynecol.* 2015;125:521–525.

48. Boudville N, Ward S, Benaroia M, House AA. Increased sodium intake correlates with greater use of antihypertensive agents by subjects with chronic kidney disease. *Am J Hypertens.* 2004;18:1300–1305.

49. Martin JN Jr, Thigpen BD, Moore RC, et al. Stroke and severe preeclampsia and eclampsia: a paradigm shift focusing on systolic blood pressure. *Obstet Gynecol.* 2005;105:246–254.

50. Augoustides JGT. Chapter 46: When is hypertension a true crisis and how should it be managed in the intensive care unit? In: Deutschman CS, Neligan PJ, eds. *Evidence-Based Practice of Critical Care.* Philadelphia: Saunders Elsevier; 2010:317–322.

51. Murphy MB, Murray C, Shorten GD. Fenoldopam: a selective peripheral dopamine-receptor agonist for the treatment of severe hypertension. *N Engl J Med.* 2001;345(21):1548–1557.

52. Sato N, Tanaka KA, Szlam F, et al. The vasodilatory effects of hydralazine, nicardipine, nitroglycerin, and fenoldopam in the human umbilical artery. *Anesth Analg.* 2003;96:539–544.

53. Duley L, Meher S, Jones L. Drugs for treatment of very high blood pressure during pregnancy. *Cochrane Database Syst Rev.* 2013;(7):CD001449.

54. Buchanan ML, Easterling TR, Carr PB, et al. Short communication: clonidine pharmacokinetics in pregnancy. *Drug Metab Dispos.* 2009;37:702–705.

CHAPTER 25

Anesthesia and Obesity

Parakulam S. Thomas, MD

Parikshith Sumathi, MBBS, DA, MD

INTRODUCTION

Obesity during pregnancy can be associated with numerous maternal and perinatal risks. These risks may increase proportionately to the level of obesity.[1-3] Therefore, addressing and managing these potential risk factors pose a challenge to the obstetrician and the anesthesiologist.

DEFINITION

Obesity is a multifactor, chronic disease involving social, cultural, physiologic, metabolic, endocrine, genetic, psychological, and behavioral components, resulting in excess adipose and tissue mass.[4] The modern basis of therapy for demographic determination is the body mass index (BMI) or the Quetelet index. It is measured by body weight in kilograms divided by the height in square meters (kg/m^2). The standard for ideal body weight (IBW), the sex-specific desired weight for persons with small-, middle-, and large-build frames, is published in Metropolitan Life Insurance tables.[5]

Anorexia is defined as a BMI of less than 17.5 in both men and women.
Ideal weight is defined as a BMI of 19.1–25.8 in women and 20.7–26.4 in men.
Overweight is defined as a BMI of 27.3–32.3 in women and 27.9–31.1 in men.
Obesity is defined as a BMI of 32.4–34.9 in women and 31.2–34.9 in men.
Morbid obesity is defined as a BMI greater than 40.
Superobesity is defined as BMI greater than 50.

Obesity in pregnancy is defined as prepregnancy BMI of 30 kg/m^2 or greater.[6] The definition of obesity in pregnant women involves issues unique to this population because the pregnant woman's weight increases over a relatively short interval of time, and much of this weight gain is related to accretion of matter that will be lost at delivery: the fetus, amniotic fluid, and blood.

PREVALENCE

The prevalence of obesity in reproductive-aged and pregnant women varies widely depending on the definition used, year, and characteristics of the study population but has increased in concordance with the increased prevalence of obesity in the general population.[7,8] In the 2009–2010 National Health and Nutrition Examination Survey (NHANES), 31.9% of women of reproductive age (20 to 39 years old) were obese (BMI ≥ 30 kg/m^2); the prevalence was highest in non-Hispanic blacks (56.2%).[9] By comparison, in 1980 (before routine calculation of BMI), only 7% of women weighed over 200 pounds at their first prenatal visit.[8]

PATHOPHYSIOLOGY

Central Mechanisms

Regulation of appetite by the hypothalamus involves the collaboration or interaction of the satiety center in the ventromedial hypothalamic nucleus and the feeding center in the lateral hypothalamus.[10] These areas involve numerous neurotransmitters and modulators that regulate appetite. Long-term signals communicating information about the energy stores and endocrine status of the body are mediated predominantly by humoral mechanisms. Short-term signals, mediated by gut hormones and neural signals from the brain and the gut, regulate meal initiation and termination[10] (Figure 25-1). The hypothalamic arcuate nucleus integrates these signals. Energy expenditure, modulated by both long- and short-term signals, is mediated by the actions of the sympathetic nervous system on brown fat.

Neuropeptides expressed in the hypothalamus are classified into anabolic or catabolic peptides. Appetite stimulating, or orexigenic, peptides include neuropeptide Y (NPY), agouti-related peptide (AgRP), melanin-concentrating hormone (MCH), and orexin (ORX).[10] Appetite-inhibiting, or anorexigenic, peptides such as corticotropin-releasing hormone (CRH), alpha-melanocyte-stimulating hormone (α-MSH), and cocaine and amphetamine–regulated transcript (CART) decrease food intake,[10] and selective cannabinoid 1 (CB1) receptor blockade decreases food intake.[11]

FIGURE 25-1. Mediators and pathways in appetite control. CCK, cholecystokinin; GH, growth hormone; PYY, gut hormone fragment peptide YY; +, stimulates appetite; –, inhibits appetite.

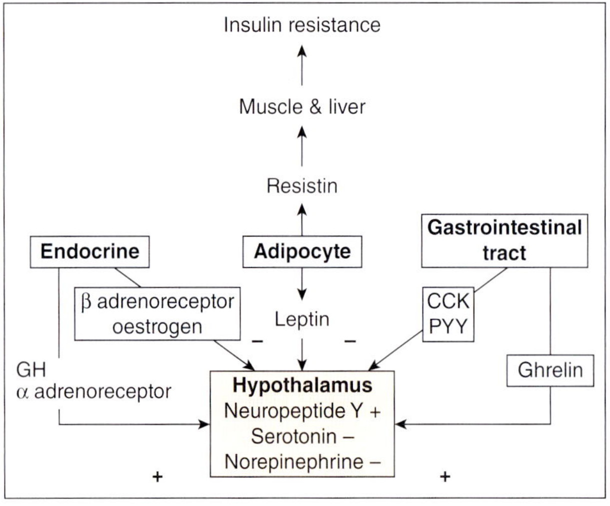

Peripheral Mechanisms

Numerous peripheral factors transmit afferent signals to the central nervous system to control the expression of orexigenic and anorexigenic neurotransmitters that regulate short-term and long-term food intake and expenditure. Short-term signals related to meals, like nutrients (glucose, amino acids, fatty acids) and gastrointestinal hormones (glucagon-like peptide 1 [GLP-1], peptide YY [PYY], cholecystokinin [CCK]), promote the feeling of satiety and limit the size of meals. Gastrointestinal mechanoreceptors and chemoreceptors sense the presence and type (caloric content) of food in the gastrointestinal tract and contribute to the feeling of satiety in the immediate postprandial period. These short-term signals do not produce sustained changes in energy balance and body adiposity.[12]

Long-term regulators of energy homeostasis include insulin, leptin, and possibly ghrelin (an appetite-stimulating gastric peptide). These hormones normally regulate food intake and energy expenditure to ensure that energy homeostasis is maintained so that body weight and adiposity remain relatively constant.[12]

The following are peptides that decrease appetite or increase energy expenditure:

leptin; CCK; insulin; GLP-1; gut hormone fragment PYY; gastrin-releasing polypeptide (GRP); enterostatin; pancreatic hormones (glucagon, amylin, and pancreatic polypeptide); vasopressin; calcitonin; apolipoprotein A-IV; the cyclized form of histidyl-proline, thyrotropin-releasing hormone.[12]

The following are peptides that increase appetite or decrease energy expenditure:

ghrelin, desacetyl melanocyte-stimulating hormone, growth hormone, prolactin.

Hence, it is not clear whether obesity is a direct cause of an adverse pregnancy outcome or whether the association between obesity and adverse pregnancy outcome is due to factors that are shared characteristics of both entities. Adverse outcomes are often attributed to the increased prevalence of diabetes in obese women. However, glucose-tolerant obese women are also at greater risk of adverse outcome; therefore, other pathways are likely to play a role.[13] The pathogenesis of some adverse outcomes may be adipose tissue-related dysregulation of metabolic, vascular, and inflammatory pathways, which can affect many organ systems.[14] The risk of some pregnancy complications rises with increasing obesity, which supports this hypothesis.[15]

In addition, epigenetic changes in response to increased fetal exposure to glucose, lipids, and inflammatory cytokines may result in permanent or transient changes in metabolic programming, leading to adverse health outcomes in adult life.[16]

PHYSIOLOGIC EFFECTS

Both obesity and pregnancy are associated with significant physiologic changes, and many of these changes have similar implications (Tables 24-1 and 24-2).[17,18] In early pregnancy, even before the uterus is large enough to affect respiratory function, women begin to have a sensation of dyspnea. This sensation likely occurs from the increased alveolar ventilation seen in pregnant patients, which is probably secondary to progesterone effects on the respiratory center in the brainstem. By the fifth month of pregnancy, the mechanical effects of the growing uterus begin to produce a progressive decrease in expiratory reserve volume (ERV), residual volume (RV), and

TABLE 25-1 Respiratory Changes in Pregnancy, in Obesity, and in Pregnancy and Obesity Combined

Parameter	Pregnancy	Obesity	Combined
Progesterone level	↑	↔	↑
Sensitivity to CO_2	↑	↓	↑
Tidal volume	↑	↓	↑
Respiratory rate	↑	↔ or ↑	↑
Minute volume	↑	↓ or ↔	↑
Inspiratory capacity	↑	↓	↑
Inspiratory reserve volume	↑	↓	↑
Expiratory reserve volume	↓	↓↓	↓
Residual volume	↓	↓ or ↔	↑
Functional residual capacity	↓↓	↓↓↓	↓↓
Vital capacity	↔	↓	↓
FEV_1	↔	↓ or ↔	↔
FEV_1/VC	↔	↔	↔
Total lung capacity	↓	↓↓	↓
Compliance	↔	↓↓	↓
Work of breathing	↑	↑↑	↑
Resistance	↓	↑	↓
V/Q mismatch	↑	↑	↑↑
DL_{CO}	↑ or ↔	↔	↔
PaO_2	↓	↓↓	↓
$PaCO_2$	↓	↑	↓

Abbreviations: ↑, increase; ↓, decrease; ↔, no change (multiple arrows represent the degree of effect). CO_2, carbon dioxide; DL_{CO}, diffusion capacity of lung for carbon monoxide; FEV_1, forced expiratory volume in 1 s; $PaCO_2$, partial pressure of carbon dioxide; PaO_2, partial pressure of oxygen; VC, vital capacity; V/Q, ratio of ventilation to perfusion.

functional residual capacity (FRC), which at term are about 15%–20% below those of the nonpregnant state.[19]

Several studies[19,20] have shown that obesity in nonpregnant subjects is associated with a decrease in ERV, RV, and FRC, most likely caused by the added weight and decreased compliance of the chest wall. However, obese pregnant women did not

TABLE 25-2 Cardiovascular Changes in Pregnancy, in Obesity, and in Pregnancy and Obesity Combined

Parameter	Pregnancy	Obesity	Combined
Heart rate	↑	↑↑	↑↑
Stroke volume	↑↑	↑	↑
Cardiac output	↑↑	↑↑	↑↑↑
Cardiac index	↑ or ↔	↔	↔ or ↓
Hematocrit	↓↓	↑	↓
Blood volume	↑↑	↑	↑
Systemic vascular resistance	↓↓	↑	↔ or ↓
Mean arterial pressure	↑	↑↑	↑↑
Supine hypotension	Present	Present	↑↑
Left ventricular morphology	Hypertrophy	Hypertrophy and dilation	Hypertrophy and dilation
Sympathetic activity	↑	↑↑	↑↑↑
Systolic function	↔	↔ or ↓	↔ or ↓
Diastolic function	↔	↓	↓
Central venous pressure	↔	↑	↑↑
Pulmonary wedge pressure	↔	↑↑	↑↑
Pulmonary hypertension	Absent	May be present	May be present
Preeclampsia	↔	N/A	↑↑

Abbreviations: ↑, increase; ↓, decrease; ↔, no change (multiple arrows represent the degree of effect). N/A, not applicable.

have an additional significant reduction in FRC, as is the case in normal-weight pregnant patients. It is possible that these findings can be partially explained by the fact that the study was performed with the patients in the sitting position.[19] The supine, especially the Trendelenburg, position worsen lung volumes significantly. Another possible explanation is that the relaxing effect of progesterone on smooth muscle decreases airway resistance, thus reducing some of the negative effects of obesity on the respiratory system.[17,18] Arterial blood gas analysis demonstrates hypoxemia in the obese parturient much more frequently than in the nonobese, which suggests a greater degree of venoarterial shunting.[19] This is especially true when the FRC is further reduced by the induction of general anesthesia or when the patient assumes the supine or the Trendelenburg position.[20] The FRC may fall below the closing capacity, leading to airway closure, especially in the dependent lung regions, thereby causing increased venoarterial shunting.[20]

The work of breathing is increased in obese parturients due to chest wall weight, and they typically show a rapid and shallow breathing pattern.[21] This in turn leads to a higher ventilatory requirement and oxygen cost of breathing.[20,22] Hence, excess body weight increases oxygen consumption and CO_2 production in a linear fashion.[21] These physiologic changes make the obese parturient particularly prone to rapid desaturation, stressing the importance of adequate denitrogenation ("preoxygenation") before induction of general anesthesia.

In nonobese pregnant women, physiologic changes during pregnancy are thought to protect against obstructive sleep apnea due to high circulating levels of progesterone, which is a ventilatory stimulant.[23] However, obesity increases the risk for obstructive sleep apnea significantly, and this is not uncommon in the obese pregnant woman. Obstructive sleep apnea has been associated with increased systemic, and possibly pulmonary, hypertension. In addition, these patients are at an increased risk for coronary artery disease, stroke, and cardiac arrhythmias.[24] Maternal oxygen desaturation, occurring as a result of apnea, may result in fetal hypoxia and poor fetal growth.[25]

Obstructive sleep apnea usually presents clinically as a combination of loud snoring and excessive daytime sleepiness. Because daytime fatigue is common in pregnancy, this disease is often not identified. Recognizing obstructive sleep apnea early in gestation will help dictate treatment options and may prevent adverse maternal fetal outcomes, especially as it relates to postcesarean pain management. Continuous positive airway pressure (CPAP) is a safe treatment with minimal adverse effects and may improve perinatal outcomes.[25]

Both obesity and pregnancy have profound effects on the maternal cardiovascular system. Pregnancy is associated with a significant increase in cardiac output, becoming detectable by the third week of pregnancy, with a 35%–40% increase by the end of the first trimester. Cardiac output continues to rise throughout the second trimester until it reaches a level that is approximately 50% greater than that in the nonpregnant state. For the remainder of the pregnancy, cardiac output remains relatively stable around that level. During labor, cardiac output increases further by approximately 10% in the early first stage, 25% in the late first stage, and 40% in the second stage. Uterine contractions contribute an additional 10%–15% increase, and in the immediate postpartum period the cardiac output peaks at as much as 75% above predelivery values.[26] Obesity increases cardiac output even further because any extra amount of fat deposited in the body demands its share of cardiac output. Every 100 g of fat increases the cardiac output by 30–50 mL/min.[27]

Blood volume is increased in pregnancy and even more when pregnancy is complicated by obesity. In nonobese women, pregnancy is associated with a significant reduction in afterload.[27] In obese pregnant patients, however, afterload reduction may be impaired due to increased peripheral resistance and greater conduit artery stiffness.[28]

In addition, obesity is associated with a higher prevalence of hypertension, diabetes mellitus, hyperlipidemia, and poor cardiac function, and it is one of the leading risk factors for coronary artery disease and cerebrovascular accidents.[29]

During pregnancy, these adverse effects of obesity are exacerbated partially due to the secretion of human placental lactogen, human chorionic gonadotropin, and steroid hormones, which increase the resistance of target tissue to insulin. Estrogen also accelerates the insulin secretion from pancreatic β cells. These changes during pregnancy lead to hyperinsulinemia and fat deposition, very similar to the pathophysiological status of obesity.[29]

The dramatically increased cardiac demands in combination with the potentially decreased functional reserves of the heart in obese patients places the obese parturient at particular risk during the peripartum period. In addition, obesity has been mentioned as a risk factor for peripartum cardiomyopathy, a potentially lethal disease.[30] There have been several reports of cardiac arrest in both pregnant and nonpregnant morbidly obese surgical patients.[31,32] Sudden circulatory changes associated with positional change may have accounted for the sudden death in some of these patients.[31]

During the second half of pregnancy, aortocaval compression by the uterus in the supine position can severely reduce cardiac output and placental perfusion. This problem is greatly exacerbated in the obese parturient, when the large fat panniculus may further compress the great vessels.[32]

Morbidly obese patients are more prone to develop fatal arrhythmias.[33] Even minor or borderline Q-T interval prolongation can result in sudden cardiac death in these patients. Therefore, medications known to prolong the Q-T interval, such as erythromycin, droperidol, granisetron, nicardipine, methadone, and others, are best avoided in these patients.

Both obesity and pregnancy have been associated with an increased risk for aspiration and Mendelson syndrome (chemical pneumonitis associated with the aspiration of gastric acid, first described by Mendelson in 1946).[34,35] In addition, obese patients have a higher incidence of hiatal hernia and elevated intragastric pressures, further increasing the risk of pulmonary aspiration of gastric contents.[32] Obesity is one of the major risk factors for diabetes, which can cause delayed gastric emptying, in turn increasing the risk for aspiration. Also, it is well known that obesity is a predisposition to difficult or failed intubation, both of which are associated with a higher incidence of aspiration.

ANESTHETIC MANAGEMENT OF THE OBESE PARTURIENT FOR CESAREAN DELIVERY

Obesity significantly increases the incidence of cesarean delivery.[36] In addition, obesity is associated with an increase in maternal mortality, morbidity, and operative complications, such as excessive blood loss, increased operative time, and increased incidence of postoperative wound infection and endometritis.[37] Good communication between anesthesiologists, obstetricians, and nursing staff is mandatory on every labor and delivery ward, but even more so when dealing with the morbidly obese parturient. These patients can certainly benefit from antepartum anesthesiology consultation and multidisciplinary meetings with obstetricians, anesthesiologists, and nursing staff in which key points can be discussed beforehand, such as the availability of a suitable bed and operating table, surgical technique and panniculus retraction, thromboembolism prophylaxis, type and cross matching of blood, postoperative care and overnight monitoring in an intensive care unit, and possible comorbidities and their consequences.

An appropriate size operating table is imperative. The use of two operating tables (side by side) has been described.[38] The problem with this technique is that it is impossible to raise, lower, or change the position of the tables in a completely synchronous manner. Another possibility is to use one set of armboards, placed parallel to the operating table, to extend the width of the table, while an extra set of armboards can be used to position the arms of the patient.

When dealing with the morbidly obese parturient, the anesthesiologist should evaluate the patient's ability to lie supine, especially when considering regional anesthesia, because cephalad retraction of a large panniculus can further compromise respiratory function. If the patient suffers from sleep apnea and was using CPAP preoperatively, this modality should be available for intraoperative and postoperative use also. The American Society of Anesthesiologists (ASA) "Practice Guidelines for the Perioperative Management of Patients With Obstructive Sleep Apnea" recommend the preoperative initiation of CPAP in patients with severe obstructive sleep apnea, as this may improve their preoperative condition.[39] Nasal CPAP (n-CPAP) at 10–15 cm of water has been used successfully for such purposes.

Many consider obesity an important risk factor for venous thromboembolism,[40,41] and prophylaxis should be considered with sequential compression stockings started preoperatively at a minimum. Another problem that the anesthesiologist often encounters when dealing with morbidly obese patients is difficulty with noninvasive blood pressure monitoring. Unless the length of the cuff exceeds the circumference of the arm by 20%, systolic and diastolic blood pressure measurements may overestimate true maternal blood pressure. In some cases, the use of a radial intra-arterial catheter may be preferable, especially in patients with comorbidities, such as chronic hypertension and preeclampsia. An intra-arterial catheter also offers the advantage of having the opportunity to perform repeated blood gas sampling, if indicated.

Regional Anesthesia

Many anesthesiologists use decreased amounts of neuraxial local anesthetic in obese patients out of fear for an unpredictable and exaggerated spread with possible high spinal block. These concerns are supported by the findings of an increased cephalad spread of local anesthetics in obese patients. A low average cerebrospinal fluid (CSF) volume in subjects with a high BMI could explain the decreased local anesthetic dose requirements in obese patients due to decreased anesthetic dilution. Because similar changes were noticed with external abdominal compression and abdominal pressure increases linearly with increased body weight, increased abdominal pressure is probably the cause. Others have also attributed the decrease in CSF volume to compression of the dural sac due to engorgement of the epidural venous plexus and increased epidural space pressure, secondary to compression of the inferior vena cava with redistribution of the venous return from the lower limbs and pelvis.

Spinal anesthesia is widely used for elective cesarean delivery. However, in the morbidly obese parturient, this technique may involve additional risks. First, as discussed previously, obesity may result in an unpredictable, exaggerated spread of local anesthetics and may therefore increase the risk of a high spinal block. As a result, it may be difficult to determine the optimal amount of local anesthetic required to produce a sufficient level of anesthesia for cesarean delivery. Moreover, a single-dose spinal injection produces only a finite period of anesthesia, and surgery in these patients may be prolonged, requiring additional anesthesia. Epidural anesthesia via an epidural catheter could overcome this problem; however, an epidural block may be inadequate in more than 25% of these patients, mainly because of difficulty in blocking the sacral roots (secondary to nerve diameter, its distance from the epidural space, number of nodes of Ranvier blocked, concentration of local anesthetic), resulting in visceral pain on stimulation of the bladder.[42]

A combined spinal epidural (CSE) technique for cesarean delivery combines the quality of a spinal block with the flexibility of an epidural catheter. In addition, it has been shown that lower doses of local anesthetics are needed using a CSE technique compared with a single-shot spinal technique, which can possibly be explained by the fact that epidural insertion causes a change in epidural pressure (from subatmospheric to atmospheric) with compression of the lumbar thecal sac. This could possibly enhance the extent and duration of the spinal component when using a CSE technique. This, and the flexibility of epidural supplementation of anesthesia afforded by CSE, may justify using significantly lower doses of local anesthetics, which may reduce the risk of a total spinal block and also possibly reduce side effects, such as hypotension. It produces reliable anesthesia, and the catheter allows incremental dosing and precise extension of the block when greater duration is necessary. Achievement of a surgical anesthetic level can occur within minutes in emergency situations, with small increments of a local anesthetic.

Regardless of the regional technique used, a thorough assessment for the adequacy of the block before surgical incision is even more important in the morbidly obese parturient than in the nonobese one. Inadequate block and the need for conversion to general anesthesia during surgery may result in catastrophic sequelae in these patients.

The anticoagulation status of the patient becomes particularly important for the anesthesiologist when the patient has a spinal or an epidural catheter. According to the American Society of Regional Anesthesia and Pain Medicine guidelines, neuraxial catheters should be removed 2 hours before the first dose, and the first dose should be 24 hours after surgery. The administration of a small dose (5000 U) of subcutaneous heparin has not been considered a contraindication for neuraxial techniques.

General Anesthesia

Prevention of acid aspiration is important in every parturient, but even more so in the obese patient. It is standard practice to administer 30 mL of a nonparticulate antacid (0.3 M sodium citrate or its equivalent) before the initiation of any anesthetic administration to a pregnant patient. This agent will rapidly decrease the acidity of gastric contents and help ameliorate the consequences of aspiration. The optimal time for administration of a nonparticulate antacid is approximately a half hour before the procedure.

For elective cesarean delivery, oral administration of an H_2 antagonist (such as ranitidine) or a proton pump inhibitor (such as omeprazole) the evening before and again 60–90 minutes before the induction of anesthesia may further reduce gastric acidity and volume. However, the addition of a prokinetic agent, such as metoclopramide, may be necessary to maximize the effect. Metoclopramide can be particularly useful for those parturients who have ingested a large meal shortly before arrival and in the diabetic patient, whose disease results in delayed gastric emptying. Obese patients have a higher incidence of both of these conditions.[43]

The obese parturient is particularly prone to rapid desaturation. Preoxygenation (denitrogenation) before induction of general anesthesia is crucial in these patients. Among the different techniques of preoxygenation, the most common method is 3–5 minutes of 100% O_2 breathing. However, in obstetric emergencies, there may not be adequate time for preoxygenation using this technique. The desired level of denitrogenation was obtained more rapidly in the technique of 8 deep breaths compared with the 3 minutes of tidal volume breathing, making the 8 deep breaths method more suitable for obstetric emergencies.[44] Position may also be important. Preoxygenation has been shown to be more effective in the sitting or the 25° head-up position than in the supine position in severely obese patients.

The position of the patient for laryngoscopy is important. It is found that the "ramped" position, accomplished by arranging blankets underneath the patient's upper body and head until horizontal alignment is achieved between the external auditory meatus and the sternal notch, clearly improves the laryngeal view when compared with the standard "sniff" position[45] (Figure 25-2).

Obesity alters the distribution of and response to anesthetic drugs. The elimination half-life, and thus the duration of action, is prolonged, and the administration of a larger dose may be associated with delayed arousal in the event of failed intubation.[46] For propofol, there is no difference in the initial distribution volume between obese and nonobese patients; it has been suggested that the induction dose should be based on lean body weight. Succinylcholine is still the muscle relaxant of choice for intubation in the obstetric patient. The duration of action of succinylcholine is determined by the level of pseudocholinesterase activity and the volume of extracellular fluid.[47,48] Both of these factors are increased in obesity. Therefore, succinylcholine should be administered on the basis of total, rather than lean, body weight in nonpregnant patients.[48] However, pregnancy reduces pseudocholinesterase activity. Hence, a dose of 1.0–1.5 mg/kg (up to a maximum of 200 mg) succinylcholine is reasonable.[46]

The incidence of difficult airway among obese parturients is much higher than among nonobese patients,[49] especially in patients with a large neck circumference or a high Mallampati score of 3 or 4 (Figure 25-3), as they may be difficult to intubate.[50] In addition, there is not only an increased risk of failed intubation, but also increased difficulty in maintaining adequate mask ventilation.[49] Increased risk for failed intubation, the possible difficult mask ventilation, and the need for rapid sequence induction with cricoid pressure highlight the need for an additional pair of experienced hands during the administration of general anesthesia in the obese patient.[46] Awake fiber-optic intubation should be considered in elective cases; however, this is not an ideal technique for emergencies. Although the use of laryngeal mask airway (LMA) in obstetrics cannot prevent gastric content aspiration, it can be lifesaving in case of failed intubations.

The ASA provides a guideline for management of a difficult airway. The guideline was created by a panel of experts under the direction of ASA in 1993, with modifications

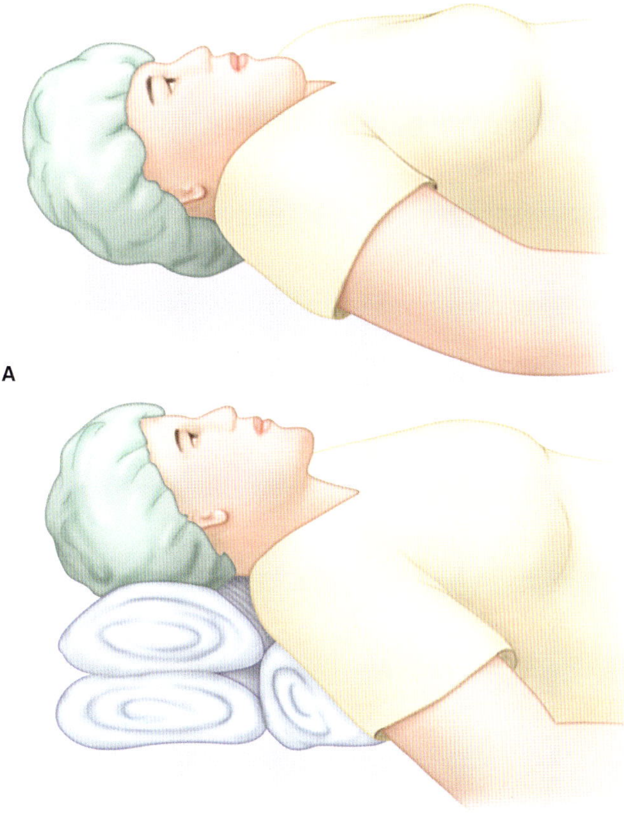

FIGURE 25-2. Optimal positioning for obese patients with a short neck. **A,** The normal supine position often prevents extension of the head and makes endotracheal intubation difficult. **B,** Elevation of the shoulder allows some neck flexion with more optimal extension of the head at the atlantooccipital joint, facilitating intubation. (Copyright © 2006 by The McGraw-Hill Companies, Inc. All rights reserved.)

in both 2003 and 2013. Implementation of algorithms will be altered in different patient populations and are dependent on factors such as patient demographics, comorbidities, surgical requirements, equipment availability, presence of additional personal, and probably most important, the skill set of the anesthesiologist.[51]

Maintenance of anesthesia involves a balanced technique of oxygen, nitrous oxide (contraindicated in the presence of pulmonary hypertension), volatile anesthetics, and muscle relaxant. After delivery, most anesthesiologists will either dramatically decrease or discontinue the administration of volatile halogenated agents to allow for optimal uterine involution and increase the concentration of nitrous oxide. However, in the obese patient, it may not be possible to administer as high a concentration of nitrous oxide as it would be given to a nonobese patient; these patients often require a higher inspired concentration of oxygen. Desflurane has been shown to be a safe supplement to the nitrous oxide–oxygen mixture for cesarean delivery and has been

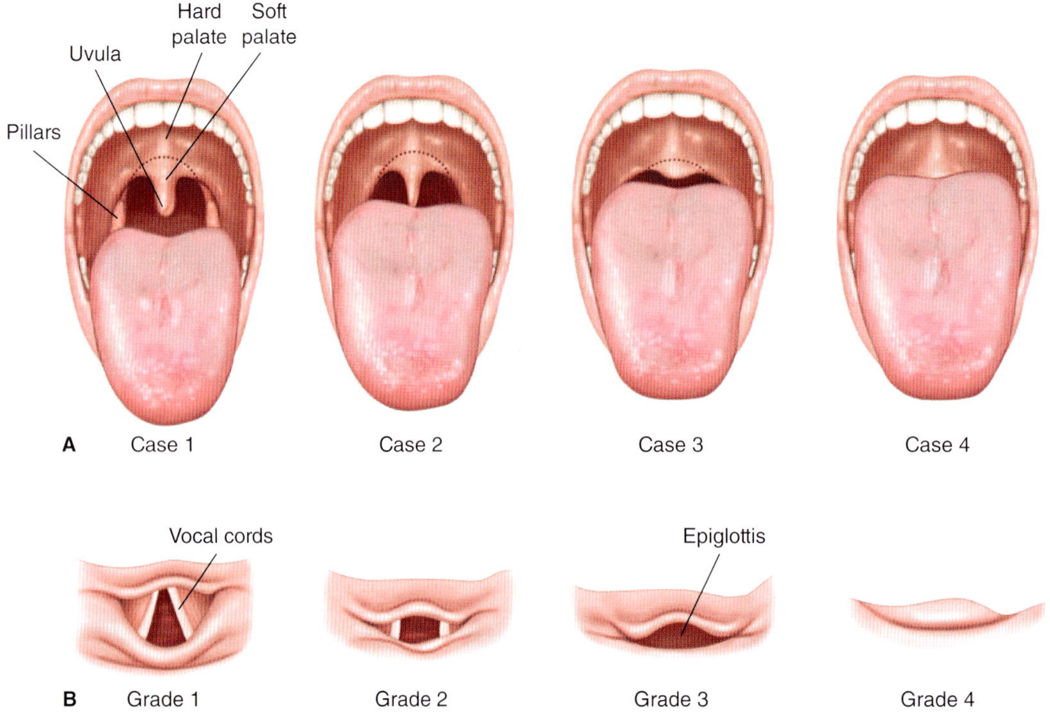

FIGURE 25-3. A. Mallampati classification modified by Samsoon and Young: class 1, visualization of the soft palate; class 2, complete visualization of the uvula; class 3, visualization of the base of the uvula; class 4, soft palate is not visible at all. **B.** Laryngoscopy according to the classification of Cormack and Lehane: grade 1, most of the glottis is visible; grade 2, only the posterior extremity of the glottis is visible; grade 3, only the epiglottis is visible; grade 4, not even the epiglottis is visible.

associated with both faster recovery times and higher oxygen saturations on entry in the recovery room when compared with sevoflurane in morbidly obese patients.[52,53]

Low doses of opioids, as well as midazolam, are usually administered to reduce the risk of intraoperative maternal awareness. In obesity, higher loading doses of midazolam are needed to reach adequate serum concentrations due to the highly lipophilic nature of the drug and the larger volume of distribution. Emptying of the stomach with an orogastric tube before extubation may help prevent gastric content aspiration. Extubation should only be attempted in fully awake patients with adequate reversal of neuromuscular blockade and preferably in the semiupright position, as this minimizes compression of the diaphragm by abdominal contents.[39,54]

Complications

Many postpartum complications, such as hemorrhage, endometritis, wound infection, deep venous thrombosis (DVT), pulmonary embolism (PE), respiratory depression, and hypoxemia occur more frequently in morbidly obese women.[55] Several studies[37,56] have noted an increased risk of endometritis and wound infection after cesarean delivery in the obese patient, and prophylactic antibiotics should be administered prior to the incision or before clamping the umbilical cord, as this has been shown to reduce the incidence of infectious morbidity after cesarean section.[57] Morbidly obese patients are also at an increased risk for serious, potentially life-threatening complications, such as hypoxemia, DVT, PE, and postpartum cardiomyopathy.[55]

General anesthesia in morbidly obese patients produces much more atelectasis than in nonobese patients. A semirecumbent position, early mobilization, and adequate pain control can certainly contribute to the early resolution of atelectasis and faster recovery of pulmonary function. Both systemic and neuraxial opioids are used for postcesarean delivery analgesia; however, neuraxial opioids are more effective than intravenous opioids. In addition, neuraxial opioids, when compared with systemic opioids, have been shown to decrease the incidence of atelectasis and reduce the incidence of pulmonary complications.[58] However, opioids should be used with caution because of the increased risk for respiratory depression, especially in patients with sleep apnea. Vigilant nursing monitoring for signs of respiratory depression (on an hourly basis during the first 24 hours and then every 2 hours for the second 24 hours) postoperatively has been recommended. Because of the increased risk for venous thromboembolism in obese patients, both mechanical and pharmacological measures for thromboprophylaxis should be undertaken.

SUMMARY

Despite increased public awareness and aggressive education, the prevalence of obesity continues to increase in both developed and developing countries. The anesthetic management of the morbidly obese parturient is associated with special hazards. The safe care of these women requires careful planning and preparation, which should ideally begin at the preconception stage. Hence, preconception weight reduction and limitation of maternal weight gain in obese gravidas through diet and exercise have overall health benefits for obese individuals, irrespective of pregnancy.

REFERENCES

1. Torloni MR, Betrán AP, Horta BL, et al. Prepregnancy BMI and the risk of gestational diabetes: a systematic review of the literature with meta-analysis. *Obes Rev.* 2009;10:194.
2. Scott-Pillai R, Spence D, Cardwell CR, et al. The impact of body mass index on maternal and neonatal outcomes: a retrospective study in a UK obstetric population, 2004–2011. *BJOG.* 2013;120:932.
3. Blomberg M. Maternal obesity, mode of delivery, and neonatal outcome. *Obstet Gynecol.* 2013;122:50.
4. Adams JP, Murphy PG. Obesity in anaesthesia and intensive care. *Br J Anaesth.* 2000 Jul;85(1):91–108.
5. Metropolitan Life Insurance Company. Overweight: its prevention and significance. *Stat Bull Metropol Life Insur Co.* 1960;41:6.
6. American College of Obstetricians and Gynecologists. ACOG Committee opinion no. 549: obesity in pregnancy. *Obstet Gynecol.* 2013;121:213.
7. Abrams BF, Laros RK Jr. Prepregnancy weight, weight gain, and birth weight. *Am J Obstet Gynecol.* 1986;154:503.
8. Lu GC, Rouse DJ, DuBard M, et al. The effect of the increasing prevalence of maternal obesity on perinatal morbidity. *Am J Obstet Gynecol.* 2001;185:845.
9. Flegal KM, Carroll MD, Kit BK, Ogden CL. Prevalence of obesity and trends in the distribution of body mass index among US adults, 1999–2010. *JAMA.* 2012;307:491.
10. Druce M, Bloom SR. Central regulators of food intake. *Curr Opin Clin Nutr Metab Care.* 2003;6:361–367.
11. Matteri RL. Overview of central targets for appetite regulation. *J Anim Sci.* 2001;79:E148–E158.
12. Drazen DL, Woods SC. Peripheral signals in the control of satiety and hunger. *Curr Opin Clin Nutr Metab Care.* 2003;6:621–629.
13. Owens LA, O'Sullivan EP, Kirwan B, et al. ATLANTIC DIP: the impact of obesity on pregnancy outcome in glucose-tolerant women. *Diabetes Care.* 2010;33:577.
14. Ramsay JE, Ferrell WR, Crawford L, et al. Maternal obesity is associated with dysregulation of metabolic, vascular, and inflammatory pathways. *J Clin Endocrinol Metab.* 2002;87:4231.

15. Marshall NE, Guild C, Cheng YW, et al. Maternal superobesity and perinatal outcomes. *Am J Obstet Gynecol.* 2012;206:417.e1.

16. Reynolds RM, Allan KM, Raja EA, et al. Maternal obesity during pregnancy and premature mortality from cardiovascular event in adult offspring: follow-up of 1,323,275 person years. *BMJ.* 2013;347:f4539.

17. Saravanakumar K, Rao SG, Cooper GM. Obesity and obstetric anesthesia. *Anaesthesia.* 2006;61:36–48.

18. Unterborn J. Pulmonary function testing in obesity, pregnancy, and extremes of body habitus. *Clin Chest Med.* 2001;22:759–767.

19. Eng M, Butler J, Bonica JJ. Respiratory function in pregnant obese women. Am J *Obstet Gynecol.* 1975;123: 241–245.

20. Øberg B, Poulsen TD. Obesity: an anaesthetic challenge. *Acta Anaesthesiol Scand.* 1996;40:191–200.

21. Dempsey JA, Reddan W, Rankin J, et al. Alveolar arterial gas exchange during muscle work in obesity. *J Appl Physiol.* 1966;21:1807–1814.

22. Cherniak RM. Respiratory effects of obesity. *Can Med Assoc J.* 1959;80:613–616.

23. Lefcourt LA, Rodis JF. Obstructive sleep apnea in pregnancy. *Obst Gynecol Surv.* 1996;51:503–506.

24. Parish JM, Somers VK. Obstructive sleep apnea and cardiovascular disease. *Mayo Clin Proc.* 2004;79: 1036–1046.

25. Roush SF, Bell L. Obstructive sleep apnea in pregnancy. *J Am Board Fam Pract.* 2004;17:292–294.

26. Chang AB. Physiologic changes of pregnancy. In: Chestnut DH, ed. *Obstetric Anesthesia: Principles and Practice.* 3rd ed. Philadelphia: Elsevier Mosby; 2004:15–36.

27. Veille JC, Hanson R. Obesity, pregnancy, and left ventricular functioning during the third trimester. *Am J Obstet Gynecol.* 1994;171:980–983.

28. Vasan RS. Cardiac function and obesity. *Heart.* 2003;89:1127–1129.

29. Tomoda S, Tamura T, Sudo Y, et al. Effects of obesity on pregnant women: maternal hemodynamic change. *Am J Perinat.* 1996;13:73–78.

30. Shnaider R, Tiberiu E, Szmuk P, et al. Combined spinal-epidural anesthesia for cesarean section in a patient with peripartum dilated cardiomyopathy. *Can J Anesth.* 2001;48:681–683.

31. Tseuda K, Debrand M, Zeok S, et al. Obesity supine sudden death syndrome: report of two morbidly obese patients. *Anesth Analg.* 1979;58: 345–347.

32. Cohen SE. Anesthesia for the morbidly obese pregnant patient. In: Hughes SC, Levinson G, Rosen MA, eds. *Shnider and Levinson's Anesthesia for Obstetrics.* 4th ed. Philadelphia: Lippincott Williams & Wilkins; 2002:545–558.

33. Drenick EJ, Fisler JS. Sudden cardiac arrest in morbidly obese surgical patients unexplained after autopsy. *Am J Surg.* 1988;155:720–726.

34. Mendelson CL. The aspiration of stomach contents into the lungs during obstetric anesthesia. *Am J Obstet Gynaecol.* 1945;52:191–204.

35. Olsson GL, Hallen B, Hambraeus-Jonzon K. Aspiration during anaesthesia: a computer-aided study of 185,358 anaesthestics. *Acta Anaesthesiol Scand.* 1986;30:84–92.

36. Machado LS. Cesarean section in morbidly obese parturients: practical implications and complications. *N Am J Med Sci.* 2012 Jan;4(1):13–18.

37. Vincent RD, Chestnut DH. Which position is more comfortable for the parturient during identification of the epidural space? *Int J Obstet Anesth.* 1991;1:9–11.

38. Hamza J, Smida H, Benhamou D, Cohen SE. Parturient's posture during epidural puncture affects the distance from skin to epidural space. *J Clin Anesth.* 1995;7:1–4.

39. Maitra AM, Palmer SK, Bachhuber SR, Abram SE. Continuous epidural analgesia for cesarean section in a patient with morbid obesity. *Anesth Analg.* 1979;58: 348–349.

40. Grau T, Leipold RW, Horter J, Conradi R, Martin E, Motsch J. The lumbar epidural space in pregnancy: visualisation by ultrasonography. *Br J Anaesth.* 2001;86:798–804.

41. Wasson C. Failed epidural in an obese patient—blame it on Pythagoras. *Anaesthesia.* 2000;56:585–610.

42. Thomas TA, Cooper GM. Anaesthesia. In: *Why Mothers Die 1997–99. Fifth Report of Confidential Enquiries into Maternal Deaths in the United Kingdom.* London: RCOG Press; 2001:134–149.

43. Carroll CS Sr, Magann EF, Chauhan SP, Klauser CK, Morrison JC. Vaginal birth after cesarean section versus elective repeat cesarean delivery: weight-based outcomes. *Am J Obstet Gynecol.* 2003;188:1516–1522.

44. Norris MC. Height, weight and spread of subarachnoid hyperbaric bupivacaine in term parturient. *Anesth Analg.* 1988;67:555–558.

45. Kuczkowski KM, Benumof JL. Repeat cesarean section in a morbidly obese parturient: a new anesthetic option. *Acta Anaesth Scand.* 2002;46:753–754.

46. UshaKiran TS, Hemmadi S, Bethel J, Evans J. Outcome of pregnancy in a woman with an increased body mass index. *Br J Obstet Gynaecol.* 2005;112:768–772.

47. Cohn AI, Hart RT, McGraw SR, Blass NH. The Bullard laryngoscope for emergency airway management in a morbidly obese parturient. *Anesth Analg.* 1995;81:872–873.

48. Norris MC, Dewan DM. Preoxygenation for cesearean section: a comparison of two techniques. *Anesthesiology.* 1985;62:827–829.

49. Hawkins JL, Koonin LM, Palmer SK, Susan K, Gibbs CP. Anesthesia-related deaths during obstetric delivery in the United States, 1979–90. *Anesthesiology.* 1997;86:277–284.

50. Hodgkinson R, Husain FJ. Caesarean section associated with gross obesity. *Br J Anaesth.* 1980;52:919–923.

51. Apfelbaum JL, Hagberg CA, Caplan RA, et al. American Society of Anesthesiologists Task Force on Management of the Difficult Airway. Practice guidelines for management of the difficult airway: an updated report by the American Society of Anesthesiologists Task Force on Management of the Difficult Airway. *Anesthesiology.* 2013 Feb;118(2):251–270.

52. Goldberg ME, Norris MC, Larijani GE, Marr AT, Seltzer JL. Preoxygenation in the morbidly obese: a comparison of two techniques. *Anesth Analg.* 1989;68:520–522.

53. Bentley JB, Borel JD, Vaughan RW, et al. Weight, pseudocholine esterase activity and succinylcholine requirement. *Anesthesiology.* 1982;57:48–49.

54. Vaughan RW, Bauer S, Wise L. Effect of position (semi-recumbent versus supine) on postoperative oxygenation in markedly obese. *Anesth Analg.* 1976;55:37–41.

55. Harris HE, Ellison GTH, Richter LM, Wet TD, Levin J. Are overweight women at increased risk of obesity following pregnancy? *Br J Nutr.* 1998;79:489–494.

56. Von Ungern-Sternberg BS, Regli A, Bucher E, Reber A, Schneider MC. Impact of spinal anaesthesia and obesity on maternal respiratory function during elective caesarean section. *Anaesthesia.* 2004;59:743–749.

57. Ballantyne JC, Carr DB, De Ferranti S, et al. The comparative effects of postoperative analgesic therapies on pulmonary outcome: cumulative meta-analyses of randomised, controlled trials. *Anesth Analg.* 1998;86:598–612.

58. Shnaider R, Ezri T, Szmuk P, et al. Combined spinal-epidural anesthesia for cesarean section in a patient with peripartum dilated cardiomyopathy. *Can J Anesth.* 2001;48:681–683.

Gynecology

Bariatric Surgery and Pregnancy

CHAPTER 26

Unzila Ali Nayeri, MD

INTRODUCTION
PREGNANCY OUTCOMES: MATERNAL
PREGNANCY OUTCOMES: NEONATAL

POST–BARIATRIC SURGERY PREGNANCY
CARE

INTRODUCTION

Obesity, defined as a body mass index (BMI) of 30 kg/m^2 or greater, is a growing epidemic. In the United States, 35% of adults and 17% of children are obese.[1] Obesity is associated with multiple medical morbidities, including type 2 diabetes mellitus, hypertension, heart disease, stroke, cancers, and obstructive sleep apnea. Obese women are at higher risk of adverse pregnancy outcomes when compared to women with a normal BMI.[2] Complications in pregnancy include gestational diabetes, gestational hypertension, preeclampsia, macrosomia, fetal anomalies, and need for cesarean section.

Weight loss can reduce the risks and complications of these medical conditions. Unfortunately, behavioral modifications and medical management prove to be unsuccessful in many individuals. Surgical therapy performed to manage obesity is the only effective and proven therapy for patients with severe obesity (BMI ≥ 35 kg/m^2).[3]

Bariatric operations are some of the most commonly performed surgeries. In 2011, over 340,000 bariatric procedures were performed worldwide, with more than 120,000 procedures performed in North America.[4] The majority of these surgeries are performed in reproductive-aged women.[5] In addition, the use of bariatric surgery in the adolescent population is rising.[6] This poses significant implications for women prior to and during pregnancy. Clinicians caring for reproductive-aged women need to be familiar with the various types of bariatric surgeries, the recommendations for management in pregnancy, and the associated complications and risks to both the patient and her fetus.

Current indications for bariatric surgery include a BMI of 40 kg/m^2 or greater or a BMI of 35 kg/m^2 or greater with comorbid medical conditions.[7] Individuals meeting criteria should also have attempted and failed other weight loss treatments. In addition, patients are expected to be psychologically stable.

Weight loss from bariatric surgery occurs through two general mechanisms: restriction of intake or malabsorption of ingested food. Procedures may have a combination of both malabsorptive and restrictive components. The Roux-en-Y gastric bypass, which is a mixed malabsorptive-restrictive surgery, is the most commonly performed surgery for weight loss in the United States. It involves creation of a small gastric pouch that is directly connected to a portion of the jejunum known as the "Roux limb," thereby bypassing the rest of the stomach and duodenum. The Roux limb is then linked to the remaining segment of intestine in a Y-shaped enteroenterostomy. The adjustable gastric band is another common procedure that is entirely restrictive in nature. It involves placement of a fluid-filled band around the fundus of the stomach, reducing its functional volume. Depending on the type of procedure performed, patients may be at risk for micronutrient deficiencies, decreased absorption of medications, dumping syndrome, and gastric ulcers. It is important for medical providers to consider these potential complications in pregnant women with a history of bariatric surgery.

Weight loss after bariatric surgery can restore the normal hormonal milieu, thereby improving ovulatory dysfunction and infertility.[8-11] It is important to counsel women on the improvement in fertility and to discuss options for contraception. Due to the malabsorptive nature of some of the surgical procedures, there is an increased risk of oral contraceptive failure.[12] Alternative nonoral forms of hormonal contraception should therefore be considered.[10] Despite improved fertility rates after weight loss, bariatric surgery should not be used as a primary treatment for infertility.

The current recommendation is for women to wait 12–18 months after bariatric surgery prior to pursuing pregnancy. This is due to the potential concern that rapid postoperative weight loss and subsequent nutrient deficiencies may result in adverse effects on the pregnancy.[13] Although the recommendation is to delay conception for at least 12 months following bariatric surgery, data suggest that pregnancy outcomes tend to be favorable among patients who conceive within 1 year. Observational studies did not note any significant differences in obstetric and neonatal complications, including fetal growth restriction, preterm delivery, preterm premature rupture of membranes, preeclampsia, gestational diabetes, cesarean delivery, or congenital anomalies, among postsurgical patients conceiving prior to or after the 12- to 18-month window.[14] Limited data also suggest that the length of time to conception following surgery does not affect total postoperative weight loss.[15]

Weight loss in obese women prior to pregnancy generally results in more favorable outcomes for both the mother and the neonate.[16] Despite bariatric surgery, most women remain obese at the start of pregnancy.[17] Interpreting pregnancy outcomes in women after bariatric surgery can be challenging due to the different control groups, which include obese women without bariatric surgery, the same women prior to their bariatric surgery, or the general obstetric population. In general, pregnancy outcomes in women following bariatric surgery are more favorable than when compared to obese women who have not undergone a weight loss procedure.

PREGNANCY OUTCOMES: MATERNAL

Bariatric surgery leads to higher rates of diabetes remission when compared to other weight loss methods.[18] The return to normal blood glucose levels and discontinuation of diabetes-related medications occurs soon after surgery.[19,20] Pregnancy outcomes are improved as these women enter pregnancy in a euglycemic state and avoid the pregnancy complications associated with pregestational diabetes.[21] Observational studies have also demonstrated a reduction in the incidence of gestational diabetes mellitus among pregnant women who have undergone bariatric surgery.[22-24] Although the risk of gestational diabetes in these women is lower than in obese women who have not had surgery, the risk is still higher than the baseline risk.[25-27] Studies comparing pre– and post–bariatric procedure pregnancy outcomes also demonstrated a significant reduction in the risk of gestational diabetes.[28,29] Outside pregnancy, the most common procedures, including gastric bypass, sleeve gastrectomy, and gastric banding, all lead to an improvement in diabetes.[30] It is not certain if the type of surgical procedure affects the rate and outcome of gestational diabetes in pregnancy.

In addition to diabetes, bariatric surgery improves other cardiovascular risk factors, such as hypertension and dyslipidemia.[31] These women are at lower risk for developing hypertensive complications in a future pregnancy. Observational studies have demonstrated that the incidence of preeclampsia is reduced in women after weight loss surgery when compared to both obese women and pregnancies in the same women prior to bariatric surgery.[23,26,32]

Obesity is a definite risk factor for cesarean section, with the magnitude of risk correlated to the degree of obesity.[33] The risk of cesarean section persists in patients post–bariatric surgery, the majority of whom remain obese after surgery, when compared to nonobese pregnant patients.[25,34] Cesarean section rates are not higher in pregnant women after bariatric surgery than in their obese nonsurgical counterparts.[34,35]

PREGNANCY OUTCOMES: NEONATAL

Medically indicated preterm deliveries are more common among obese women due to obesity-related comorbidities, such as hypertension and diabetes.[36] Pregnancy after bariatric surgery is associated with a reduction in these iatrogenic preterm births.[23] The association between obesity and spontaneous preterm deliveries is less clear. Earlier studies demonstrated that obesity is not associated with an increased risk of spontaneous preterm birth,[36] but more recent, larger studies suggested that the risk is increased, particularly for preterm deliveries prior to 28 weeks.[37] The data regarding preterm delivery after bariatric surgery are also mixed. Prior studies did not show an increased risk of postsurgical preterm birth,[17,25] although a more recent, larger study found that women after bariatric surgery are at higher risk of both indicated and spontaneous preterm deliveries.[38]

Maternal obesity is a significant risk factor for macrosomia, infants who are large for gestational age, and later offspring obesity.[39] The risk is greatest for women with class III obesity (BMI $\geq$ 40 kg/m^2).[40] Pregnancies following bariatric surgery result in lower mean birth weights and a reduction in the incidence of macrosomia.[22,23,26] Meanwhile, postsurgical infants have also been shown to have an increased risk of being born small for gestational age (SGA) when compared to babies born to both nonobese and obese women.[22,24,27,38,41] The risk for SGA may be highest with malabsorptive procedures, including gastric bypass.[35]

Perinatal complications, including the risk of stillbirth and neonatal mortality, do not seem to be increased in pregnancies following weight loss surgery, although the data are limited due to the rarity of these outcomes.[25,38] There is theoretical concern regarding an increase in congenital anomalies, particularly neural tube defects, due to potential postsurgical nutrient deficiencies. However, large population-based studies have found no significant difference in the rate of congenital malformations in post–bariatric surgery pregnancies when compared to the general pregnant population.[22,25] In fact, data have shown that the rate of anomalies is higher with increasing maternal BMI regardless of preconception bariatric surgery.[42]

POST–BARIATRIC SURGERY PREGNANCY CARE

Although preconception weight loss surgery generally results in better pregnancy outcomes, maternal and neonatal risks still exist and should be considered when caring for a pregnancy after bariatric surgery. Care should be multidisciplinary, involving an obstetrician, bariatric surgeon, and nutritionist.

Due to the anatomic and physiologic changes involved with bariatric surgery, micronutrient deficiencies are common, particularly after malabsorptive procedures.[43] Most frequently, serum iron, folate, B_{12}, calcium, and vitamin D levels are affected.[44] Bypass operations eliminate the primary absorption sites—the duodenum and proximal jejunum—for iron, folate, vitamin D, and calcium. Vitamin B_{12} deficiency occurs as a result of the reduced gastric acid content and intrinsic factor available in the smaller gastric pouch of surgeries with a restrictive component. Gastric bands may need to be adjusted by a bariatric surgeon so that oral intake can be increased in pregnancy.[45] Preoperative deficiencies, reduced oral intake, malabsorption, inadequate supplementation, and increased nutritional requirements of pregnancy make pregnant women especially prone to clinically significant deficiencies. Studies have demonstrated that post–bariatric surgery pregnant patients are at higher risk of anemia (hemoglobin < 10 mg/dL) when compared to other obese parturients.[46]

Micronutrient supplementation during pregnancy should be optimized to reduce the risk of potential adverse pregnancy outcomes related to nutritional deficiencies. Potential adverse outcomes include fetal anomalies (e.g., neural tube defects due to folic acid deficiency, microphthalmia due to vitamin A deficiency, and fetal intracranial hemorrhage due to vitamin K deficiency) as well as maternal complications, such as Wernicke's encephalopathy, caused by nausea and vomiting of pregnancy.

Currently, there are no established guidelines on nutritional supplementation in pregnant patients after bariatric surgery. Most experts agree that supplementation should be tailored to the type of bariatric procedure and to any existing deficiencies.[47] A comprehensive assessment of micronutrient levels, including iron, ferritin, vitamin B_{12}, folate, calcium, and vitamin D levels, and a complete blood cell count should be obtained early in pregnancy. If abnormal values are noted, the appropriate supplementation should be initiated. Levels should be assessed at least every trimester and more frequently in the case of documented deficiencies.

Generally, patients should be instructed to continue with their prepregnancy regimen. Prenatal vitamins should either include or be supplemented with at least 50–100 µg of elemental iron, 400–800 μg of folate, and 1000–1500 μg of calcium, in addition to 60 g of dietary protein.[13] Parenteral forms of certain micronutrients should be considered if oral intake does not correct existing laboratory abnormalities. Vitamin A supplementation should not exceed 5000 IU daily due to risks of congenital malformations. Consultation with a nutritionist should be considered to ensure that patients are following the appropriate dietary regimens and recommended supplementation.

Early screening for gestational diabetes is recommended for women at high risk of unrecognized type 2 diabetes (women with obesity, history of gestational diabetes, or known impaired glucose metabolism).[48] Patients with a history of gastric bypass may be unable to tolerate the 50-g glucose load used to screen for gestational diabetes due to the dumping syndrome. Patients with the dumping syndrome experience abdominal discomfort, nausea, vomiting, and diarrhea after ingesting a high glycemic load. The sugar load rapidly enters the small intestine from the stomach, causing fluid shifts into the lumen of the bowel, resulting in small bowel distention. Hyperinsulinemia followed by hypoglycemia results in tachycardia, palpitations, and diaphoresis. These women should forego the traditional testing for gestational diabetes. Instead, home glucose monitoring for at least 1 week between 24 and 28 weeks of pregnancy should serve as gestational diabetes screening.[48] Sugars should be assessed fasting and 1 or 2 hours after meals. Women with restrictive procedures or those who do not report symptoms of the dumping syndrome can undergo the routine screening for gestational diabetes.

Absorption of medications and subsequent bioavailability may be reduced in patients with malabsorptive components to their bariatric surgery as these procedures reduce the functional surface area of the intestine. Drug dosages and administration of medications may therefore need to be adjusted when prescribing medications to this group of patients.[49] An additional consideration is the reduced postoperative size of the stomach and the effect of certain medications. For example, the use of nonsteroidal anti-inflammatory drugs poses an increased risk of gastric ulceration.[50]

A high index of suspicion must be maintained for bariatric-related operative complications in pregnancy. Complications include bowel obstructions, hernias, band erosion or migration, and anastomotic leaks.[51-54] Pregnant women with a history of bariatric surgery, particularly gastric bypass, who present with abdominal pain or other unusual gastrointestinal symptoms should be evaluated for complications, such as intestinal obstruction, volvulus, or intussusception. Increased abdominal pressure and upward displacement of the bowel due to the enlarging pregnant uterus increase the risk of intestinal complications.[55] Consultation with a bariatric surgeon and radiologist is strongly advised as imaging with abdominal computed tomography (CT) or magnetic resonance imaging (MRI) should be performed if indicated.[56] Keeping a high index of suspicion and a strong sense of urgency to rule out serious complications of bariatric surgery will reduce both maternal and fetal/neonatal morbidity.[55]

A history of bariatric surgery should not affect management of labor and delivery. Women post–bariatric surgery may deliver vaginally, with cesarean delivery reserved for the standard obstetrical indications.[47] Because obesity often persists despite weight loss surgery, providers should appreciate the obesity-related concerns of labor and delivery, including longer labor patterns, more failed inductions, and increased need for cesarean section.[17,57,58]

In terms of the fetus and neonate, serial ultrasounds for fetal growth should be performed in the third trimester due to the risk of SGA in pregnancies following bariatric surgery. There are also case reports of infants of women with previous weight loss surgery presenting with nutritional deficiencies.[59] Therefore, micronutrient supplementation and screening for deficiencies should continue in the postpartum period for breastfeeding women.

CONCLUSION

As the frequency of bariatric surgery is on the rise, particularly among reproductive-aged women, providers need to be familiar with its implications in pregnancy. Overall, both maternal and fetal/neonatal outcomes are improved in pregnancies following bariatric procedures. Pregnancy management of the postsurgical patient includes appropriate micronutrient supplementation, alternative methods for gestational diabetes screening, and serial ultrasounds for fetal growth, in addition to an awareness of the potential surgical complications of these procedures. The risk of adverse outcomes can be reduced with multidisciplinary care involving the obstetrician, bariatric surgeon, nutritionist, and radiologist.

REFERENCES

1. Ogden CL, Carroll MD, Kit BK, Flegal KM. Prevalence of childhood and adult obesity in the United States, 2011–2012. *JAMA*. 2014;311(8):806.
2. Cnattingius S, Bergstrom R, Lipworth L. Prepregnancy weight and the risk of adverse pregnancy outcomes. *N Engl J Med*. 1998:338(3):147.
3. Scirmer B, Schauer P. The surgical management of obesity. In: Brunicardi C, Andersen DK, Billiar TR, et al., eds. *Schwartz's Principles of Surgery*. 9th ed. New York: McGraw-Hill; 2009:997.
4. Buchwald H, Olen DM. Metabolic/bariatric surgery worldwide 2011. *Obes Surg*. 2013;23(4):427.
5. Santry HP, Gillen DL, Lauderdale DS. Trends in bariatric surgical procedures. *JAMA*. 2005;294(15):1909.
6. Tsai WS, Inge TH, Burd RS. Bariatric surgery in adolescents: recent national trends in use and in-hospital outcome. *Arch Pediatr Adolesc Med*. 2007;161(3):217.
7. NIH Conference. Gastrointestinal surgery for severe obesity. Consensus Development Conference Panel. *Ann Intern Med*. 1991;115(12):956.
8. Teitelman M, Grotegut CA, Williams NN, Lewis JD. The impact of bariatric surgery on menstrual patterns. *Obes Surg*. 2006;16(11):1457.
9. Eid GM, Cottam DR, Velcu LM, et al. Effective treatmnet of polycystic ovarian syndrome with Roux-en-Y gastric bypass. *Surg Obes Relat Dis*. 2005;1(2):77.
10. Merhi ZO. Weight loss by bariatric surgery and subsequent fertility. *Fertil Steril*, 2007;87(2):430.
11. Shekelle PG, Newberry S, Maglione M. Bariatric surgery in women of reproductive age: special concerns for pregnancy. Evid Rep Technol Assess (Full Rep). 2008;(169):1–51.
12. Paulen ME, Zapata LB, Cansino C, Curtis KM, Jamieson DJ. Contraceptive use among women with a history of bariatric surgery: a systematic review. *Contraception*. 2010;82(1):86.
13. Beard JH, Bell RL, Duffy AJ. Reproductive considerations and pregnancy after bariatric surgery: current evidence and recommendations. *Obes Surg*. 2008;18(8):1023.
14. Wax JR, Cartin A, Wolff R, Lepich S, Pinette MG, Blackstone J. Pregnancy following gastric bypass for morbid obesity: effect of surgery-to-conception interval on maternal and neonatal outcomes. *Obes Surg*. 2008;18(12):1517.
15. Dao T, Kuhn J, Ehmer D, Fisher T, McCarty T. Pregnancy outcomes after gastric-bypass surgery. *Am J Surg*. 2006;192(6):762.
16. Schummers L, Hutcheon JA, Bodnar LM, Lieberman E, Himes KP. Risk of adverse pregnancy outcomes by prepregnancy body mass index: a population-based study to inform prepregnancy weight loss counseling. *Obstet Gynecol*. 2015;125(1):133.
17. Wax JR, Cartin A, Wolff R, Lepich S, Pinette MG, Blackstone J. Pregnancy following gastric bypass surgery: maternal and neonatal outcomes. *Obes Surg*. 2008;18(5):540.
18. Sjostrom L, Peltonen M, Jacobson P, et al. Association of bariatric surgery with long-term remission of type 2 diabetes and with microvascular and macrovascular complications. *JAMA*. 2014;311(22):2297.
19. Rubino F. Is type 2 diabetes an operable intestinal disease? A provocative yet reasonable hypothesis. Diabetes Care. 2008;31:S290.

20. Courcoulas AP, Goodpaster BH, Eagleton JK, et al. Surgical vs. medical treatments for type 2 diabetes mellitus: a randomized clinical trial. *JAMA.* 2014: 149(7):707.

21. Spanakis E, Gragnoli C. Bariatric surgery, safety and type 2 diabetes. *Obes Surg.* 2009;19(3):363.

22. Kjaer MM, Nilas L. Pregnancy after bariatric surgery—a review of benefits and risks. *Acta Obstet Gynecol Scand.* 2013;92(3):264.

23. Maggard MA, Yermilov I, Li Z, et al. Pregnancy and fertility following bariatric surgery: a systematic review. *JAMA.* 2008;300(19):2286.

24. Lesko J, Peaceman A. Pregnancy outcomes in women after bariatric surgery compared with obese and morbidly obese controls. *Obstet Gynecol.* 2012;119(3):547.

25. Sheiner E, Levy A, Silverberg D, et al. Pregnancy after bariatric surgery is not associated with adverse perinatal outcome. *Am J Obstet Gynecol.* 2004;190(5):1335.

26. Berlac JF, Skovlund CW, Lidegaard O. Obstetrical and neonatal outcomes in women following gastric bypass: a Danish national cohort study. *Acta Obstet Gynecol Scand.* 2014;93(5):447.

27. Johansson K, Cnattingius S, Naslund I, et al. Outcomes of pregnancy after bariatric surgery. *N Engl J Med,* 2015;372(23):814.

28. Aricha-Tamir B, Weintraub AY, Levi I, Sheiner E. Downsizing pregnancy complications: a study of paired pregnancy outcomes before and after bariatric surgery. *Surg Obes Relat Dis.* 2012;8(4):434.

29. Burke AE, Bennett WL, Jamshidi RM, et al. Reduced incidence of gestational diabetes with bariatric surgery. *J Am Coll Surg.* 2010;211(2):169.

30. Hutter MM, Schirmer BD, Jones DB, et al. First report from the American College of Surgeons Bariatric Surgery Center Network: laparoscopic sleeve gastrectomy has morbidity and effectiveness positioned between the band and the bypass. *Ann Surg.* 2011;254(3).420.

31. Ricci C, Gaeta M, Rausa E, Macchitella Y, Bonavina L. Early impact of bariatric surgery on type II diabetes, hypertension, and hyperlipidemia: a systematic review, meta-analysis and meta-regression on 6,587 patients. *Obes Surg.* 2014;24(4):522.

32. Galazis N, Docheva N, Similis C, Nicolaides K. Maternal and neonatal outcomes in women undergoing bariatric surgery: a systematic review and meta-analysis. *Eur JObstet Gynecol Reprod Biol.* 2014;181:45.

33. Weiss JL, Malone FD, Emig D, et al. Obesity, obstetric complications and cesarean delivery rate—a population-based screening study. *Am J Obstet Gynecol.* 2004;190(4):1091.

34. Patel JA, Patel NA, Thomas RL, Nelms JK, Colella JJ. Pregnancy outcomes after laparoscopic Roux-en-Y gastric bypass. *Surg Obes Relat Dis.* 2008;4(1):39.

35. Kjaer MM, Lauenborg J, Breum BM, Nilas L. The risk of adverse pregnancy outcome after bariatric surgery: a nationwide register-based matched cohort study. *Am J Obstet Gynecol.* 2013;208(6):464.

36. McDonald SD, Han Z, Mulla S, Beyene J, Knowledge Synthesis Group. Overweight and obesity in mothers and risk of preterm birth and low birth weight infants: systematic review and meta-analyses. *BMJ.* 2010;341:3428.

37. Cnattingius S, Villamor E, Johansson S, et al. Maternal obesity and risk of preterm delivery. *JAMA.* 2013:309(22):2362.

38. Roos N, Neovius M, Cnattingius S, et al. Perinatal outcomes after bariatric surgery: nationwide population based matched cohort study. BMJ. 2013;347:6460.

39. Yu Z, Han S, Zhu J, Sun X, Ji C, Guo X. Pre-pregnancy body mass index in relation to infant birth weight and offspring overweight/obesity: a systematic review and meta-analysis. *PLoS One.* 2013;8(4):e61627.

40. Lusiv O, Mah J, Beyene J, McDonald SD. The effects of morbid obesity on maternal and neonatal health outcomes: a systematic review and meta-analyses. *Obes Rev.* 2015;16(7):531.

41. Belogolobkin V, Salihu HM, Weldesalasse H, et al. Impact of prior bariatric surgery on maternal and fetal outcomes among obese and non-obese mothers. *Arch Gynecol Obstet.* 2012;285(5):1211.

42. Josefsson A, Bladh M, Wirehn AB, Sydsjo G. Risk for congenital malformations in offspring of women who have undergone bariatric surgery. A national cohort. *Br J Obstet Gynecol.* 2013;120(12):1477.

43. Ledoux S, Msika S, Moussa F, et al. Comparison of nutritional consequences of conventional therapy of obesity, adjustable gastric banding, and gastric bypass. *Obes Surg.* 2006;16(8):1041.

44. Devlieger R, Guelinckx I, Jans G, Voets W, Vanholsbeke C, Vansant G. Micronutrient levels and supplement intake in pregnancy after bariatric surgery: a prospective cohort study. *PLoS One.* 2014;9(12):e114192.

45. Martin LF, Finigan, KM, Nolan TE. Pregnancy after adjustable gastric banding. *J Obstet Gynecol.* 2000;95(6):927.

46. Shai D, Shoham-Vardi I, Amsalem D, Silverberg D, Levi I, Sheiner E. Pregnancy outcome of patients following bariatric surgery as compared with obese women: a population-based study. *J Matern Fetal Neonatal Med.* 2014;27(3):275.

47. American College of Obstetrics and Gynecology. Practice Bulletin 105: bariatric surgery and pregnancy. *Obstet Gynecol.* 2009;113(6):1405.

48. American College of Obstetrics and Gynecology. Practice Bulletin 137: gestational diabetes mellitus. *Obstet Gynecol.* 2013;122(2):406.

49. Stein J, Stier C, Raab H, Weiner, R. Review article: the nutritional and pharmacological consequences of obesity surgery. *Aliment Pharmacol Ther.* 2014; 40(6):582.

50. Miller AD, Smith KM. Medication and nutrient administration considerations after bariatric surgery. *Am J Health Syst Pharm*. 2006;87(2):1852.

51. Andreasen LA, Nilas L, Kjaer MM. Operative complications during pregnancy after gastric bypass—a register-based cohort study. *Obes Surg*. 2014:24(10):1634.

52. Caranta DG, Lee Am, Pennington D, Zelig CM. Complications from Roux-en-Y gastric bypass mistaken for medical complications in gravid patients. *Obstet Gynecol*. 2014:124(2):464.

53. Wax JR, Wolff R, Cobean R, Pinette MG, Blackstone J, Cartin A. Intussusception complicating pregnancy following laparoscopic Roux-en-Y gastric bypass. *Obes Surg*. 2007;17(7):977.

54. Suffee MT, Poncelet C, Barrat C. Gastric band slippage at 30 weeks' gestation: diagnosis and laparoscopic management. *Surg Obes Relat Dis*. 2012;8(3):366.

55. Moore KA, Ouyang DW, Whang EE. Maternal and fetal deaths after gastric bypass surgery for morbid obesity. *N Engl J Med*. 2004:351(7):721.

56. Altieri MS, Telem DA, Kim P, Gracia G, Pryor AD. Case review and consideration for imaging and work evaluation of the pregnant bariatric patient. *Surg Obes Relat Dis*. 2015;11(3):667.

57. Vahratian A, Zhang J, Troendle JF, Savitz DA, Siega-Riz AM. Maternal prepregnancy overweight and obesity and the pattern of labor progression in term nulliparous women. *Obstet Gynecol*. 2004;104(5):943.

58. Poobalan AS, Aucott LS, Gurung T, Smith WC, Bhattacharya S. Obesity as an independent risk factor for elective and emergency caesarean delivery in nulliparous women—systematic review and meta-analysis of cohort studies. *Obes Rev*. 2009;10(1):28.

59. Celiker MY, Chawla A. Congenital B_{12} deficiency following maternal gastric bypass. *J Perinatol*. 2009;29(9):640.

Contraceptive Management

CHAPTER 27

Renee E. Mestad, MD, MSCI

Zevidah Vickery, MD, MSCI

INTRODUCTION

More than half the female population of the United States is overweight or obese. Thirty-two percent of women aged 20–39 and 40% of women aged 40–59 are obese.[1] One-third of adolescent females aged 12–19 are overweight and obese, with 20% qualifying as obese.[1] Overweight and obese women are no less likely to be sexually active and therefore at risk of pregnancy than normal-weight women.[2] Adolescent females in the higher-weight categories have a higher risk of unintended pregnancy than their normal-weight peers due to lower self-esteem and less confidence negotiating condom and contraception use.[2]

Obesity increases several maternal and fetal risks associated with pregnancy, including gestational diabetes, preeclampsia, fetal macrosomia, emergency cesarean section, and stillbirth. In addition, pregnancy can exacerbate pregestational

TABLE 27-1 World Health Organization BMI Classification[a]

Weight Classification	*BMI (kg/m^2)*
Underweight	<18.5
Normal weight	18.5–24.99
Overweight	25–29.99
Obese	≥30
Class I obese	30–34.99
Class II obese	35–39.99
Class III obese	≥40

[a]Adapted from World Health Organization. BMI classification 2015. http://apps.who.int/bmi/index.jsp?introPage=intro_3.html. Accessed May 22, 2015.

comorbidities such as hypertension, diabetes, and obesity. Obese women should plan their pregnancies to optimize their health and minimize maternal and fetal complications.

Until recently, however, obese women have been excluded from contraception trials, in which participants are generally limited to within 130% of their ideal body weight.[2] Therefore, health care providers experience difficulty counseling their obese patients about the safety and efficacy of contraception methods available in the United States.

For the purposes of this chapter, the World Health Organization (WHO) body mass index (BMI) classification system is used.[3] A BMI of 30 kg/m^2 is considered obese (Table 27-1).

CONTRACEPTION OPTIONS

The contraception options available in the United States are listed in Table 27-2 along with their pregnancy rates with perfect use (efficacy), typical use (effectiveness), and continuation at 1 year. All methods are more effective than no method. However, as sterilization, intrauterine devices (IUDs), and the subdermal contraceptive implant do not require patient compliance to work properly, their pregnancy rates with typical use approach perfect use pregnancy rates. Both the American Congress of Obstetricians and Gynecologists (ACOG) and the American Academy of Pediatrics recommend intrauterine devices and the subdermal contraceptive implant as first-line contraceptives for women of all ages as they are long-acting, reversible contraceptive (LARC) methods.[4,5] Their effectiveness is as high as that of sterilization without being permanent. The Medical Eligibility Criteria tables produced by the Centers for Disease Control and Prevention (CDC) provide assistance in determining which methods are appropriate for obese patients (Table 27-3). Methods in category 1 do not have any restrictions. Current evidence indicates the benefits of methods in category 2 outweigh the risks. The methods in categories 1 and 2 can be considered safe for otherwise-healthy obese women.[6]

TABLE 27-2 Contraceptive Method Options Available in the United States[a]

Method	Typical Use	Perfect Use	Women Continuing at 1 Year, %
Male sterilization	0.15	0.1	
Female sterilization	0.5	0.5	100
Subdermal contraceptive implant	0.05	0.05	84
Intrauterine devices			
Copper	0.8	0.6	78
Levonorgestrel	0.2	0.2	80
Depo-Provera	6	0.2	56
Oral contraceptives	9	0.3	67
Contraceptive patch	9	0.3	67
Contraceptive ring	9	0.3	67
Diaphragm	12	6	57
Condom			
Male	18	2	43
Female	21	5	41
Sponge			36
Nulliparous	12	9	
Parous	24	20	
Withdrawal	22	4	46
Spermicides	28	18	47
None	85	85	42

[a]Adapted from Cunningham G. Contraception and sterilization. In Hoffman B, Schorge J, Schaffer J, Halvorson L, Bradshaw K, Cunningham G, eds. *Williams Gynecology.* 2nd ed. New York: McGraw-Hill; 2012.

EMERGENCY CONTRACEPTION

There are three methods of emergency contraception available in the United States: levonorgestrel (LNG), 150 mg orally; ulipristal acetate (UPA), 30 mg orally; and the copper intrauterine device (IUD). LNG is available over the counter in branded and generic forms (Plan B One Step, Next Choice One Dose, Take Action, My Way) and is recommended by the manufacturer to be taken within 72 hours after unprotected intercourse to decrease risk of pregnancy by 88%.[7] UPA (Ella) requires a prescription. Both can be used up to 150 hours after unprotected intercourse, although UPA has a

TABLE 27-3 Centers for Disease Control and Prevention Medical Eligibility Criteria[a]

	CHC	POP	DMPA	Implant	LNG IUD	Cu IUD
Obesity	2[b]	1	1	1	1	1
	COC P, R					
Malabsorptive bariatric surgery	3	1	3	1	1	1

Abbreviations: CHC, combined hormonal contraceptives (pill, patch, ring); COC, combined oral contraceptive; Cu IUD, copper IUD; DMPA, depo medroxyprogesterone acetate; Implant, progestin-only subdermal contraceptive implant; LNG IUD, levonorgestrel intrauterine device; P, patch; POP, progestin-only pill; R, ring.
[a]Adapted from http://www.cdc.gov/reproductivehealth/UnintendedPregnancy/PDF/Legal_Summary%20Chart_English_Final_TAG508.pdf. Accessed April 26, 2015.
[b]1, no restrictions; 2, benefits outweigh proven or theoretical risks; 3, proven or theoretical risks generally outweigh benefits; 4, unacceptable health risk.

higher success rate (65% fewer pregnancies at 24 hours to 42% fewer pregnancies at 72 hours) when compared to LNG.

Randomized trials of both LNG and UPA indicated obesity increases the risk of failure for both oral methods. For women using LNG, risk of pregnancy quadrupled in obese (BMI > 30) women when compared to normal-weight or underweight women (odds ratio [OR] 4.41, 95% confidence interval [CI] 2.05, 9.44). Obese women using UPA demonstrated a nonstatistically significant doubled risk of pregnancy (OR 2.62, 95% CI 0.89, 7.00). With regard to weight, these methods ceased to be beneficial at 70 kg for LNG and 88 kg for UPA.[8] Analysis of phase 3 trials of UPA indicated twice the pregnancy rate of women weighing over 85 kg when compared to women weighing less than 85 kg (3.4% vs. 1.6%).[9] Of note, few participants in these trials had a BMI above 35 kg/m^2.

Women in these weight categories should consider a copper IUD (Paragard). The copper IUD is recommended for up to 5 days after unprotected intercourse. Thirty years of data from around the world gives the copper IUD pregnancy rate of 0.09% when used as emergency contraception.[10] Its effectiveness is not affected by weight and has the advantage of providing continued contraception for up to 10 years.

MOST EFFECTIVE METHODS

The most effective methods prevent pregnancy over 99% of the time and do not require participation by the user for their high effectiveness.

Sterilization

Permanent sterilization is a highly reliable method of contraception for women confident they have completed childbearing. In the United States, female sterilization is one of the most popular methods of contraception, following oral contraceptives.[11] About 10% of women had partners who had undergone vasectomy.[11] Vasectomy is highly effective, with an estimated failure rate of 0.15%.[12] This method should be considered as the health and weight of the female patient are not affected. The couple needs to be counseled that vasectomy is not immediately effective, and another method of contraception should be used until semen analysis verifies azospermia. In addition, if the relationship ends, the woman will need another method of contraception.

Female sterilization involves occlusion of the fallopian tubes, whether by laparotomy, minilaparotomy, laparoscopy, or hysteroscopy. Because the mechanism of action involves mechanical occlusion of the fallopian tubes, efficacy should not be affected by weight or obesity. There is no data to support or refute this idea.

Approximately half of female sterilizations occur in the immediate postpartum period with partial salpingectomy.[11] After a vaginal delivery, access to the peritoneal cavity through a small umbilical incision may be difficult depending on the patient's abdominal adipose distribution. Other authors have found the Alexis (Applied Medical, Rancho Santa Margarita, CA) can facilitate visualization of the anatomy.[13] Distribution of abdominal adipose tissue may impede access to the fallopian tubes during cesarean section regardless of the larger incision. In the event fallopian tubes can be visualized but not safely brought to the incision, Filshie clips are an option. While found to be acceptably effective for interval sterilization, Filshie clips had a statistically significantly higher pregnancy rate after 24 months than partial salpingectomy in a multicenter trial.[11,14] Cumulative pregnancy probability for the clip was 0.017 versus 0.004 in the partial salpingectomy group.

Currently, most abdominal interval female sterilizations are performed laparoscopically. Initial analysis of the Collaborative Review of Sterilization (CREST), a large, multicenter, cohort study from 1978 to 1987, did not factor in BMI or weight in their evaluation of efficacy for each method.[15] A secondary analysis of the data looked at risk factors resulting in increased complications. Obesity was found to be an independent risk factor for complications, OR 1.7 (95% CI 1.2, 2.6). Of the 21 women in whom entrance or pneumoperitoneum could not be achieved, 15 (71%) were obese. Other independent risk factors included diabetes mellitus and previous abdominal or pelvic surgery.[16] However, most of these data were collected in the early years of laparoscopic surgery; technique and instruments have improved, especially due to laparoscopic bariatric surgery, since the mid-1980s when data collection concluded.[11] Also, more current data comparing laparoscopic abdominal surgery to laparotomy indicated a 70%–80% reduced risk of infection when using a laparoscopic approach instead of the open approach for obese patients. For this reason, laparoscopic sterilization should be considered over minilaparotomy.[17]

Hysteroscopic sterilization offers a means of female sterilization that avoids entering the abdominal cavity, general anesthesia, and their accompanying risks. Essure® (Bayer Health Pharmaceuticals) is the method of hysteroscopic sterilization available in the United States. Approved in 2002 by the US Food and Drug Administration (FDA), Essure is a nickel-titanium coil microinsert introduced into the fallopian tube ostia hysteroscopically.[18] This stimulates a local tissue reaction, resulting in fallopian tube occlusion within 90 days. The manufacturer recommends occlusion be confirmed by hysterosalpingogram at the end of the 90 days. In the interim, women should use a second method of contraception or abstain from sexual intercourse. About 5% of patients will not experience tubal occlusion at 90 days.[19] While surgeons may have more difficulty accessing the cervix in the office and prefer to perform the procedure in the operating room, data indicate equal sterilization success regardless of BMI or location of procedure.[18]

TABLE 27-4 Levonorgestrel Intrauterine Devices and Amenorrhea[a]

	1 Year	2 Year	3 Years
Skyla®	6%		12%
Liletta®	19%	26%	38%

[a]Adapted from Bayer Healthcare Pharmaceuticals Inc. Skyla (LNG IUS). Package insert 2013. http://labeling.bayer-healthcare.com/html/products/pi/Skyla_PI.pdf. Accessed May 17, 2015; and from Actavis: Liletta (LNG IUS). Package insert 2015. http://pi.actavis.com/data_stream.asp?product_group=1960&p=pi&language=E. Accessed May 17, 2015.

Intrauterine Devices

In the United States, one nonhormonal and three hormonal devices (IUDs) are available. They are all T shaped. The three hormonal IUDs all contain the progestin hormone LNG and include Mirena®, Skyla®, and Liletta™. The mechanism of action of the LNG IUD includes thickening of cervical mucus to prevent sperm entrance into the uterus, inhibition of capacitation or survival of sperm, and possible prevention of implantation. Mirena contains 52 mg of LNG, releasing 20 µg/d. It is approved for 5 years of use and is FDA approved to manage menorrhagia.[20] Skyla is slightly smaller than Mirena and contains 13.5 mg of LNG, releasing 14 µg/d. It is approved for 3 years of use.[21] Liletta contains 52 mg of LNG, releasing 18.6 µg/d. It is approved for 3 years of use and is the same size as Mirena.[22] While neither Skyla nor Liletta has FDA approval to manage menorrhagia, both devices decrease bleeding and can result in amenorrhea (Table 27-4).

The nonhormonal IUD available in the United States is the Paragard®. It has an exposed surface area of 380 m² of thin copper wire wrapped around a polyethylene frame with barium.[23] It is approved for 10 years of use and does not have any effect on menstrual bleeding after the first few months.

Serum LNG levels have been noted to be lower in obese women using an LNG IUD.[24] However, as the mechanisms of action for both the LNG IUD and the copper IUD are local, these methods maintain their efficacy regardless of the patient's weight. An analysis of Contraceptive CHOICE data demonstrated no difference in failure rate of 1/100 woman-years (WY) between normal-weight, overweight, and obese women.[25] In addition, the IUDs do not affect weight, lipid, or glucose metabolism.

Inserting the IUDs may be difficult for obese patients. Ultrasound guidance can be helpful when bimanual exam cannot provide information about uterine size or position. Also, an IUD can be inserted at the time of diagnostic or therapeutic dilation and curettage for patients with abnormal uterine bleeding.

Contraindications to IUD use no longer include nulliparity or adolescence as they did in the past (Table 27-5).

Subdermal Contraceptive Implant

The subdermal contraceptive implant currently available in the United States is Nexplanon®. It is a progestin-only contraceptive containing etonogestrel (ENG) 68 mg in a single implant that is inserted subdermally in the medial aspect of the nondominant upper arm.[26] Prior to Nexplanon, Implanon® was the subdermal contraceptive

TABLE 27-5 Contraindications to IUD Use

Pregnancy or suspicion of pregnancy
Abnormalities of the uterus resulting in distortion of the uterine cavity
Acute pelvic inflammatory disease or current behavior suggesting a high risk for pelvic inflammatory disease
Postpartum endometritis or postabortal endometritis in the past 3 months
Known or suspected uterine or cervical malignancy
Genital bleeding of unknown etiology
Mucopurulent cervicitis
Allergy to any component of IUD
A previously placed IUD that has not been removed
Copper IUD–specific contraindication
   Wilson's disease
LNG IUD specific contraindications
   Cannot be used for postcoital contraception
   Known or suspected breast cancer or other progestin-sensitive cancer
   Acute liver disease or liver tumor (benign or malignant)
   Hypersensitivity to any component of Mirena

implant available in the United States. Both were manufactured by the same pharmaceutical company, the only differences being the applicator and that Nexplanon contains barium sulfate to facilitate radiologic identification. Implanon was discontinued in 2012.

The mechanisms of action include ovulation suppression and thickening of cervical mucus. The progestin also affects the endometrium, resulting in altered uterine bleeding patterns, ranging from amenorrhea to almost-daily bleeding. In clinical trials, 11% of women discontinued use of the ENG implant because of bleeding irregularities.[26]

The clinical trials did not include women greater than 130% their ideal body weight, creating questions about the effectiveness of this method for obese women. One small pharmacokinetic study compared 13 obese women to 4 normal weighted women. The study found plasma ENG concentrations to be 47% lower in obese women than in normal weighted women.[27] Projected ENG concentrations were 133 pg/mL, 102 pg/mL, and 98 pg/mL. Ovulation suppression is noted when plasma ENG concentrations are greater than 90 pg/mL.[28] As plasma concentrations approach this lower limit, there is concern about this method's effectiveness in the third year.[27]

This theoretical increased failure has not been demonstrated clinically. The Contraceptive CHOICE Project evaluated the failure rate of 1168 participants who chose the ENG implant.[25] Twenty-eight percent were overweight, and 35% were obese. One pregnancy was reported among 1377 WY of use. The participant had a BMI of 31. The pregnancy occurred 4 days after insertion and was likely an undiagnosed pregnancy rather than a method failure. The cumulative failure rate for all participants was 0/100 WY, and it was 0.23/100 WY for obese participants.

Studies of the 6-rod LNG contraceptive implant (Norplant®) indicated an increased risk of weight gain.[29] However, analysis of Contraceptive CHOICE Project data indicated race was the predictor for weight gain among users of the ENG implant.[30] Prior to adjustment, mean weight change over 12 months was 2.1 kg (range –16.3 to 32.7 kg). After adjusting for race, no difference in weight change was noted, except for African

American women. Weight and BMI at initiation of method did not influence weight change.

Currently, the CDC Medical Eligibility Criteria gives the ENG implant a category 1 rating for obese patients and a 1 or 2 rating for most of the other comorbidities associated with obesity, including hypertension, thromboembolism, and diabetes.[6]

VERY EFFECTIVE METHODS

The very effective methods are 90%–99% effective at preventing pregnancy.

Combined Hormonal Contraceptives

Combined hormonal contraceptives (CHCs) contain both an estrogen and a progestin. The methods considered CHCs are the combined oral contraceptive (COC) pill, contraceptive patch, and contraceptive ring. The primary mechanism of action of CHCs is via the negative-feedback inhibition of the hypothalamic-pituitary-ovarian (HPO) axis, resulting in ovulation suppression. In addition, the progestin thickens cervical mucus, preventing sperm penetration of the cervix.

Pharmacokinetics of Hormonal Contraception in Obese Women

Data concerning efficacy of hormonal contraceptives are conflicting. Some indicate no difference in efficacy between normal-weight women and obese women, while others find an increased contraceptive failure rate in obese women.[2] Obesity can affect hormonal pharmacokinetics in several possible ways: bioavailability, hepatic clearance, and volume of distribution of drugs, depending on lipophilic properties or binding globulins.

Using a COC with ethinyl estradiol (EE) 30 µg and LNG 150 µg with a 21-/7-day hormone to hormone-free cycle, pharmacokinetics were compared between normal-weight women (BMI 19–24.9 kg/m^2) and obese women (BMI 30–39 kg/m^2).[31] Serum levels of EE, LNG, E2 (estradiol), and progesterone were drawn at various time points in a 28-day pill pack cycle, as well as administration of twice-weekly pelvic ultrasounds to evaluate ovarian follicular development. While peak serum concentrations of EE and LNG were lower in the obese group, trough concentrations did not differ. Prior research has demonstrated that peak serum LNG concentrations do not contribute to contraceptive efficacy, but trough concentrations do contribute.[32] In addition, there was no statistically significant difference in follicular development between the two groups.[31] There were 2 ovulations, 1 in each group. The normal-weight participant demonstrated compliant use; the obese patient had missed several pills.

Edelman et al. examined the effect of obesity on the HPO axis and ovulation suppression.[33] Nonobese (BMI < 25) and obese (BMI > 30) women received two cycles of an oral contraceptive pill containing EE 20 µg and LNG 100 µg using the 21-/7-day hormone regimen. During 2 inpatient stays, the first admission at the end of the hormone pills of the first cycle (around day 21) and the second admission at the end of the hormone-free pills, at the beginning of the next pack, serum levels of estrogen, progesterone, follicle-stimulating hormone (FSH), luteinizing hormone (LH), inhibin B, and sex hormone–binding globulin (SHBG) were drawn, some multiple times during the inpatient stays, to assess HPO activity. They found the LNG half-life was twice as long in obese women as in nonobese women (52 vs. 26 hours). This resulted in a lower maximum concentration of LNG on day 1 of cycle 2 and a longer time to reach steady state in obese women (10 vs. 5 days). Distribution volume did not differ. Twice as many obese women than nonobese women demonstrated E2 levels indicating development of a dominant follicle and progesterone levels demonstrating ovulation. While these findings provide credibility to the idea that obesity affects hormonal contraceptive pharmacokinetics resulting in higher HPO activity and possible ovulation, the study only used indirect measures of ovulation and did not address all possible mechanisms of action of hormonal contraceptives. The authors recommended against making any practice changes based on their findings for this reason and other limitations of the study.

Subsequent research investigated ways to address the prolonged time to LNG steady-state concentration as this in combination with imperfect compliance could result in clinical COC failure. They investigated using either a higher-dose COC (30 µg EE/150 µg LNG) in the 21-/7-day cyclic regimen and using the lower-dose pill (EE 20 µg/100 µg LNG) without the hormone-free period.[34] Several serum pharmacokinetic parameters were measured as well as ovarian follicle size and cervical mucus. All participants had a BMI of at least 30 kg/m². Participants were randomized to one of the two groups after 2 cycles of the low-dose COC with hormone-free weeks. Prior to randomization, both groups demonstrated the extended time to steady state, and almost half demonstrated follicular development. After randomization, the increased-dose participants continued to have a longer time to steady state (12 days), while those in the low-dose continuous regimen maintained the steady-state LNG concentration. Both groups saw a significant decline in developed follicles, from 45% to 9%. The mean BMI in the continuous participants was 38 kg/m², while that of the higher-dose participants was 41 kg/m². As follicular development is necessary for ovulation and fertility, this study offered two ways to counter the possible adverse effects of altered pharmacokinetics on contraceptive efficacy for obese women: The provider can either prescribe an increased-dose COC or prescribe a continuous regimen if a low-dose COC is desired.

Clinical Efficacy of Combined Hormonal Contraceptives In Obese Women

There is concern about the efficacy of CHCs in obese women. One Cochrane review of 5 studies between 2002 and 2012 found results for 2 COCs, 1 for the transdermal patch and 1 each for an implant and vaginal ring not available in the United States.[35] One COC study found an increased risk (relative risk [RR] 2.49) for women with a BMI of 25 or greater. The other did not find any difference. The patch study analyzed results according to weight deciles. There were 15 pregnancies, 9 in women greater than 73 kg, 7 in women greater than 80 kg, and 5 in women greater than 90 kg. The other 6 were in women weighing between 52 and 74 kg. The overall conclusion was that these methods remain effective when used properly given limited data.

McNicholas et al., evaluated unintended pregnancy rates among 1523 participants in the Contraceptive CHOICE Project who opted for a CHC method.[36] They did not find a statistically significant difference in cumulative 3-year unintended pregnancy rates when comparing participants with a BMI less than 25 (8.44%), 25–30 (11.03%), 30–40 (8.61), and greater than 40 (10.84%). Secondary analysis of the European Active Surveillance Study on Oral Contraceptives did not find a correlation between BMI and oral contraceptive failure.[37]

TABLE 27-6 Contraindications to Combined Hormonal Contraceptive Use

Pregnancy
Uncontrolled hypertension
Smokers older than 35 years
Diabetes with vascular involvement
Thrombogenic heart arrhythmias
Thrombogenic cardiac valvulopathies
Cerebrovascular or coronary artery disease
Migraine headaches with aura
Thrombophlebitis or thromboembolic disorders
History of deep vein thrombophlebitis or thrombotic disorders
Undiagnosed abnormal genital bleeding
Known or suspected breast carcinoma
Cholestatic jaundice of pregnancy or jaundice with oral contraceptive pill use
Hepatic adenomas or carcinomas or active liver disease with abnormal liver function
Carcinoma of the endometrium or other known or suspected estrogen-dependent neoplasia

Contraindications and Considerations

While CHC methods are very effective, there are several contraindications, particularly to the estrogen component, including uncontrolled hypertension, diabetes with vascular involvement, coronary artery disease, and thromboembolic disorders (Table 27-6).

Another significant concern is weight gain due to use of CHCs. Perceived weight gain frequently contributes to discontinuation. Women already struggling with obesity are unlikely to initiate use of these methods due to this misconception. A Cochrane review evaluating effects of CHCs on weight found little-to-no weight changes.[38] Five studies compared COCs to a placebo or no intervention, and 1 compared a skin patch to a placebo. None found any change in weight. Four studies in the Cochrane review comparing different hormonal formulations found mean weight changes ranging from a loss of 0.67 kg in one study to a gain of 0.70 kg in another. A longitudinal Swedish study from 1981 to 2006 found the use of COCs was not associated with weight increase, only age.[39]

Thromboembolism is another concern for CHC use by obese women. The background rate of venous thromboembolism (VTE) for women of reproductive age not using CHCs ranges from 0.7 to 3.8 per 10,000 WY in database studies to 3.8 to 12.2 per 10,000 WY in cohort studies.[40] Pregnancy increases this risk 6 times in the third trimester and 20 times in the first 6 weeks postpartum.[41] Canadian data indicated obesity doubles the risk of deep vein thrombosis and triples the risk of pulmonary embolus in pregnancy. While European data demonstrated a 3-fold increase in VTE for obese women (BMI > 30) using CHCs, the risk during CHC use is still lower than that of pregnancy.[40] However, there are few safety data for women with a BMI greater than 40.[2] Otherwise-healthy obese women at risk of pregnancy can be considered candidates for the CHC methods, although progestin-only methods should be encouraged for patients with other comorbidities. Of note, and relevant to women of any BMI, new use of a CHC method whether by stopping and restarting, switching methods, or being a first-time user, temporarily increases the VTE risk. Therefore, if a patient is satisfied with her current CHC method, consider continuing it regardless of new formulations.

Benefits

In addition to preventing unplanned pregnancy, CHCs help manage menstrual difficulties suffered by many obese women, chiefly irregular bleeding, heavy bleeding, and endometrial hyperplasia.[42] In addition, COCs can decrease the risk of ovarian cancer by up to 50% in women taking them for at least 10 years.[43] This is not insignificant given pelvic masses are more difficult to detect via pelvic exam and ultrasound in obese women.

Combined Oral Contraceptive Pill

Popularly known as *the pill, birth control pill*, and *birth control*, COCs available in the United States all contain EE as the estrogen and a variety of progestins. There is 1 pill containing ethinyl valerate, Natazia® (Bayer), currently available. Estrogen doses commonly range from 20 to 50 µg, although a 50-µg dose is not frequently prescribed. In 2011, Lo Loestrin Fe (Warner Chilcot) became available, containing 10 µg of EE. COC formulations can be monophasic, where hormonal dosing is the same throughout the pack, or multiphasic, where dosing varies throughout the pack. Packaging can consist of the 21-day regimen (21 days of hormones, 7 days of placebo pills); 24-day regimen (24 days of hormones, 4 days of placebo pills); or the continuous regimen, which does not have any placebo pills. As most studies indicating increased failure rates used the 21-day regimen, the 24-day and continuous regimens likely decrease the risk of escape ovulation noted previously as a possible mechanism of action for contraceptive failure.[42]

If a pill is missed, that pill should be taken on realization and the current days pill also taken. Some nausea may be experienced. If several pills are missed or a lower dose is being used (10–20 µg), then escape ovulation is possible, and a barrier method or abstinence should be used for the next 7 days.

Traditionally, initiation waited until the first Sunday after the first day of the next menstrual cycle. The *quick start* method improves short-term compliance and decreases risk of pregnancy prior to the next menstrual cycle.[44] Another method of contraception or abstinence should be used if not initiating within the first 5 days of bleeding.

Contraceptive Patch

Currently, Ortho Evra® is the only transdermal contraceptive patch available in the United States. A new patch is applied weekly for 3 weeks, followed by a patch-free week for a withdrawal bleed.[45] The patch contains EE 35 µg/d and norelgestromin 150 µg/d. It is applied to the shoulder, back hip, or buttocks; adhesion improves if rubbing alcohol is applied to clean the skin of oils and allowed to dry prior to patch administration. The patch should not be applied to the breast as direct estrogen administration to the area can cause significant tenderness.

As noted previously, efficacy appears to be decreased for women weighing more than 90 kg (198 lb).[34] Also, there is concern for increased risk of VTE due to reports of increased hepatic synthesis of estrogen-sensitive procoagulants when compared to COCs and the vaginal ring.[46] However, data indicating an increased clinical risk have been conflicting, demonstrating no risk (OR 0.9, 95% CI 0.5–1.6) to a small increased risk (OR 2.4, 95% CI 1.1–5.5),[2] which is lower than the VTE risk of pregnancy.

Contraceptive Ring

There is only 1 contraceptive ring available in the United States, Nuvaring®. It is a polymeric vaginal ring containing 11.7 mg ENG and 2.7 mg EE, which releases on average 0.12 mg/d of ENG and 0.015 mg/d of EE.[47] The ring is placed inside the vagina behind the symphysis pubis for 3 weeks and then removed for 1 week for a withdrawal bleed. It does not need to fit around the cervix.

Reanalysis of phase 3 clinical trials demonstrated weight did not affect the efficacy of the contraceptive ring.[2] As well, estrogen-sensitive procoagulants that increased with the patch actually decreased with the ring.[46] However, there are few data demonstrating a clinical relevance in VTE risk with the ring.

Off-label use of both the patch and the ring for continuous use is common. The ring can remain in the vagina up to 4 full weeks (removing the old ring the same time as replacing it with the new one) with consistent efficacy. Continuous use with the patch is more difficult as many insurance companies will not pay for more than 3 patches per month. Women may experience breakthrough bleeding in the second month of continuous use.

Progestin-Only Contraceptives

The very effective category of progestin-only contraceptives includes delivery by injection and pills.

Progestin-Only Injection

There are two available preparations of the progestin-only contraceptive injection, depo medroprogesterone acetate (DMPA; Depo-Provera®) intramuscular (IM) and subcutaneous (SC). Both consist of medroxyprogesterone acetate and are administered every 13 weeks. Depo-Provera intramuscular injection is available in vials and prefilled syringes, each containing 1 mL of medroxyprogesterone acetate sterile aqueous suspension 150 mg/mL.[48] Depo-Provera subcutaneous injection is also available in vials and prefilled syringes containing a dose of 104 mg/0.65 mL. It is able to use a lower dose of progestin as it is absorbed more slowly than the intramuscular dose.[49] Both methods suppress ovulation, increase cervical mucus viscosity, and create an endometrium unfavorable for implantation.

The manufacturer's package insert lists several contraindications, including known or suspected pregnancy, active thrombophlebitis or a history of thromboembolic disorders or cerebrovascular disease, current or suspected breast malignancy, allergy to the medication components, significant liver disease, or undiagnosed vaginal bleeding.[48] The CDC Medical Eligibility Criteria, however, list DMPA in category 2, finding the benefits of the method outweigh the risks.[6]

The efficacy of either administration route is not affected by obesity.[42,48] Almost half the women in the American clinical trials and a quarter of those in the European trials qualified as overweight or obese. There were no pregnancies in the overweight/obese women in either trial.

Weight gain is a concern of both patients and health care providers as overweight and obese women rarely want to gain more weight. In a Cochrane review, one study comparing adolescents using DMPA to those using nonhormonal contraception found weight changes of 10.3% and 2.8%, respectively.[29] The DMPA-using participants also had a larger increase of body fat and decrease of lean body mass. Little difference was found when comparing them to COC users, however. Two retrospective studies compared weight gain of users of DMPA to those using a nonhormonal IUD. One study found little difference in weight change, while the other study found a mean difference of 2.28, 2.71, and 3.71 at years 1, 2, and 3, respectively. These weight differences were found in women in the normal and overweight groups, but not in the obese group (BMI > 30).[29] Counseling women about these data may help avoid discontinuation due to misinformation or concerns.

Bone mineral density (BMD) loss, particularly among adolescent women, is another concern. In 2004, the FDA issued a black box warning against the use of DMPA for more than 2 years due to studies indicating longer return to normal BMD with prolonged use of DMPA.[48] Quality studies have yet to demonstrate that this translates into a clinically relevant increased risk of fracture. One study that found an increased fracture risk also found the DMPA users had an increased fracture risk prior to DMPA initiation (incidence rate ratio [IRR] 1.28 before and IRR 1.23 after initiation).[50] In a committee opinion, the ACOG stated DMPA can be used for a duration of more than 2 years; bone loss appears to return to normal after discontinuation. Adolescent patients should not be followed with dual-energy x-ray absorptiometry (DXA) scans as they have not been validated in nonmenopausal populations.[51] As with any method of contraception, the benefits and risks must be weighed against those of pregnancy in patients at risk of pregnancy.

Bleeding irregularities are common, ranging from daily spotting to amenorrhea. The amenorrhea that develops after more than a year's use makes DMPA a common management for women with heavy periods that result in iron deficiency anemia. However, ovulation suppression can continue up to a year after discontinuation, making this method less than ideal for women planning pregnancy within a few years.[52]

Progestin-Only Contraceptive Pills

Oral progestin-only pills (POPs) for contraception are taken daily. They do not reliably suppress ovulation, but thicken cervical mucus and induce endometrial atrophy as the mechanism of action. As mucus changes are not sustainable more than 24 hours, the POP must be taken every 24 hours with very little grace period. Women more than 3 hours late taking this medication need to abstain or use a second method of contraception for 48 hours. This is a continuous method, without any hormone-free intervals.

The contraindications are similar to those for DMPA. As these pills do not contain estrogen, they are an option for patients in whom combined hormonal methods are contraindicated.

Only 1 study of POP effect on weight was recognized in a Cochrane review of progestin-only contraceptives and their effects on weight. It compared 2 POPs and did not find a difference in weight changes.[29] No studies comparing POPs to nonhormonal contraceptive methods were recognized.

MODERATELY EFFECTIVE AND EFFECTIVE METHODS

The moderately effective and effective methods are less than 90% effective and require use with every act of vaginal intercourse. This group includes the various natural family-planning methods, barrier methods, and spermicides. There are no data concerning the effect weight and BMI have on their effectiveness. Many obese women experience irregular menstrual cycles, making the natural family-planning methods difficult to follow as they often require menstrual regularity. Diaphragms require refitting with weight gain or loss of more than 10 pounds. In addition, diaphragms, sponges, caps, and the female condom may be difficult to insert or remove for the morbidly obese woman. These methods will not affect the woman's health or weight status.

CONCLUSION

Obese and overweight women of reproductive age suffer from lack of adequate education regarding contraception. They are as sexually active as their thinner contemporaries yet risk unintended pregnancies at greater rates than other women. As mentioned, the risks of those unplanned pregnancies for overweight and obese women may be greater than for thinner women, whose pregnancies, at every gestational milestone, are less complicated. It behooves providers of women's health care to address the contraceptive needs of their overweight and obese patients at each and every visit.

Contraception has not been adequately studied in overweight and obese women. With a majority of reproductive aged women now having a BMI above 25, researchers must include, and perhaps focus on, heavier women in studies on the use, risks, and benefits of contraceptive methods. Data have been limited and inconsistent thus far. This creates an information gap, limiting providers' ability to counsel patients comprehensively. While available data confirm little apparent differences in failure rates, particularly among the highly effective methods such as IUDs and the implant, further research is needed to elucidate any health risks that may be higher in the obese population. Additional benefits to obese women, such as endometrial protection to this group at high risk of cancer, need further study as well.

REFERENCES

1. Ogden C, Carroll M, Kit B, Flegal K. Prevalence of childhood and adult obesity in the United States, 2011–2013. *JAMA*. 2014;311(8):806–814.

2. Higginbotham S. Contraceptive considerations in obese women: SFP guidelines. *Contraception*. 2009; 80(6):583–590.

3. World Health Organization. BMI classification 2015. http://apps.who.int/bmi/index.jsp?introPage=intro_3.html. Accessed November 30, 2016.

4. ACOG Committee Opinion Number 539. Adolescents and long acting reversible contraception: implants and intrauterine devices. *Obstet Gynecol*. 2012;120(4):983–988.

5. Policy Statement American Academy of Pediatrics. Contraception for adolescents. Pediatrics 2014;134(4): e1244-e1256.

6. Curtis K, Jatlaoui T, Tepper N, Zapata L, Horton L, Jamieson D, Whiteman M. US selected practice recommendations for contraceptive use, 2016. MMWR 2016. http://www.cdc.gov/mmwr/volumes/65/rr/rr6504a1.htm?s_cid=rr6504a1_w#B-1-1_down, Accessed November 28, 2016.

7. Teva. Plan B One Step package insert. 2009. http://www.accessdata.fda.gov/drugsatfda_docs/label/2009/021998lbl.pdf. Accessed May 17, 2015.

8. Glasier A, Cameron S, Blithe D, et al. Can we identify women at risk of pregnancy despite using emergency contraception? Data from randomized trials of ulipristal acetate and levonorgestrel. *Contraception*. 2011;84:363–368.

9. Moreau C, Trussell J. Results from pooled phase III studies of ulipristal acetate for emergency contraception. *Contraception*. 2012;86:673–680.

10. Cleland K, Zhu H, Gosdstuck N, Cheng L, Trussell J. The efficacy of intrauterine devices for emergency contraception: a systematic review of 35 years of experience. *Hum Reprod*. 2012;27(7):1994–2000.

11. Peterson HB. Sterilization. *Obstet Gynecol*. 2008; 111(1):189–203.

12. Pollack A, Thomas L, Barone M. Female and male sterilization. In: Hatcher RA, Trussell J, Nelson AL, Cates W Jr, Stewart FH, Kowal D, eds. *Contraceptive Technology*. 19th rev. ed. New York: Ardent Media; 2007:531–573.

13. Simmons K, Edelman A. Contraception in the setting of obesity and bariatric surgery. In: Allen R, Cwiak C, eds. *Contraception for the Medically Challenging Patient*. New York: Springer; 2014:157–180.

14. Rodriguez M, Seuc A, Sokal D. Comparative efficacy of postpartum sterilisation with titanium clip versus partial salpingectomy: a randomised controlled trial. *BJOG*. 2013;120:108–112.

15. Peterson H, Trussell J, Hughes E, Taylor L. The risk of pregnancy after tubal sterilization: findings from the US Collaborative Review of Steriliation (CREST). *Am J Obstet Gynecol*. 1996;174(4):1161–1170.

16. Jamieson D, Hillis S, Duerr A, Marchbanks P, Costello C, Peterson H. Complications of interval laparoscopic tubal sterilization: findings from the United Stated

Collaborative Review of Sterilization. *Obstet Gynecol.* 2000;96(6):997–1102.

17. Shabanzadeh DM, Sørensen LT. Laparoscopic surgery compared with open surgery decreases surgical site infection in obese patients. *Ann Surg.* 2012;256(6):934–945.

18. Anderson T, Yunker A, Scheib S, Callahan T. Hysteroscopic sterilization success in outpatient versus office setting is not affected by patient or procedural characteristics. *J Minim Invasive Gynecol.* 2013;20(6):858–863.

19. Connor V. Essure: a review six years later. *J Minim Invasive Gynecol.* 2009;16(3):282–290.

20. Bayer Healthcare Pharmaceuticals Inc. Mirena (LNG IUS). Package insert 2014. http://labeling. bayerhealthcare.com/html/products/pi/Mirena_PI.pdf. Accessed May 17, 2015.

21. Bayer Healthcare Pharmaceuticals Inc. Skyla (LNG IUS). Package insert 2013. http://labeling.bayer-healthcare.com/html/products/pi/Skyla_PI.pdf. Accessed May 17, 2015.

22. Actavis. Liletta (LNG IUS). Package insert 2015. http://pi.actavis.com/data_stream.asp?product_group=1960&p=pi&language=E. Accessed May 17, 2015.

23. Teva. Paragard (copper IUD). Package insert 2013. http://www.paragard.com/Pdf/ParaGard-PI.pdf. Accessed May 17, 2015.

24. Pocius K, Dutton C. Update on hormonal contraception and obesity. *Curr Obstet Gynecol Rep.* 2015;4:61–68.

25. Xu H, Wade J, Peipert J, Zhao Q, Madden T, Secura G. Contraceptive failure rates of etonogestrel subdermal implants in overweight ad obese women. *Obstet Gynecol.* 2012;120(1):21.

26. Merck and Company Inc. Nexplanon. Package insert 2014. http://www.merck.com/product/usa/pi_circulars/n/nexplanon/nexplanon_pi.pdf. Accessed May 20, 2015.

27. Mornar S, Chandra A, Mistretta S, Neustadt A, Martinez G, Gilliam M. Pharmacokinetics of the etonogestrel contraceptive implant in obese women. *Am J Obstet Gynecol.* 2012;207(2):110.e1–6.

28. Diaz S, Pavez M, Moo-Young C, Bardin CW, Croxatto HB. Clinical trial with 3-keto-desogestrel subdermal implants. *Contraception.* 1991;44(4):393–408.

29. Lopez L, Edelman A, Chen M, Otterness C, Trussell J, Helmerhorst F. Progestin-only contraceptives: effects on weight. *Cochrane Database Syst Rev.* 2013;(7):CD008815. doi:10.1002/14651858.CD008815. pub3.

30. Vickery Z, Madden T, Zhao Q, Secura GM, Allsworth JE, Peipert JF. Weight change at 12 months in users of three progestin-only contraceptive methods. *Contraception.* 2013;88(4):503–508.

31. Westhoff C, Torgal A, Mayeda E, Pike M, Stanczyk F. Pharmakokinetics of a combined oral contraceptive in obese and normal-weight women. *Contraception.* 2010;81:474–480.

32. Rahimy M, Cromie M, Hopkins M, Tong D. Lunelle™ monthly contraceptive injection (medroxyprogesterone acetate and estradiol cypionate injectable suspension): effects of body weight and injection sites on pharmacokinetics. *Contraception.* 1999;60:201–208.

33. Edelman A, Carlson N, Cherala G, Munar M, Stouffer L, Cameron J, Stanczyk F, Jensen J. Impact of obesity on oral contraceptive pharmacokinetics and hypothalamic-pituitary-ovarian activity. *Contraception* 2009;80(2):119.

34. Edelman A, Cherala G, Munar M, McInnis M, Stanczyk F, Jensen J. Correcting oral contraceptive pharmacokinetic alterations due to obesity: a randomized controlled trial. *Contraception* 2014;90:550.

35. Lopez LM, Grimes DA, Chen M, et al. Hormonal contraceptives for contraception in overweight or obese women. *Cochrane Database Syst Rev.* 2013;(4):CD008452. doi:10.1002/14651858.CD008452. pub3.

36. McNicholas C, Zhao Q, Secura G, Allsworth J, Madden T, Peipert J. Contraceptive failures in overweight and obese combined hormonal contraceptive users. *Obstet Gynecol.* 2013;121(3):585–592.

37. Dinger JC, Cronin M, Möhner S, Schellschmidt I, Minh T, Westhoff C. Oral contraceptive effectiveness according to body mass index, weight, age and other factors. *Am J Obstet Gynecol.* 2009;201:263.e1–9.

38. Gallo MF, Lopez LM, Grimes DA, Carayon F, Schulz KF, Helmerhorst FM. Combination contraceptives: effects on weight. *Cochrane Database Syst Rev.* 2014:(1):CD003987. doi:10.1002/14651858.CD003987.pub5.

39. Lindh I, Ellström A, Milsom I. The long-term influence of combined oral contraceptives on body weight *Hum Reprod.* 2011;26(7):1917–1924.

40. Edelman A, Jensen J. Obesity and hormonal contraception: safety and efficacy. *Semin Reprod Med.* 2012;30:479–485.

41. Sultan A, West J, Tata L, Fleming K, Nelson-Piercy C, Grainge M. Risk of first venous thromboembolism in and around pregnancy: a population-based cohort study. *Br J Haematol.* 2011;156:366–373.

42. Rodriguez M, Edelman A. Safety and efficacy of contraception, why should the obese woman be any different? *Rev Endocrinol Metab Disorders.* 2011;12:85–91.

43. Havrilesky L, Moorman P, Lowery W, et al. Oral contraceptive pills as primary prevention for ovarian cancer. *Obst Gynecol.* 2013;122(1):139–147.

44. Westoff C, Heartwell S, Edwards S, et al. Initiation of oral contraceptives using a quick start compared with

a conventional start, a randomized controlled trial. *Obstet Gynecol.* 2007;109(6):1270-1276.

45. Janssen Pharmaceuticals. Ortho Evra (transdermal contraceptive patch). Package insert. 2014. http://www.orthoevra.com/sites/default/files/assets/OrthoEvraPI.pdf. Accessed April 19, 2015.

46. Jensen J, Burke A, Barnhart K, Tillotson C, Messerle-Forbes M, Peters D. Effects of switching from oral to transdermal or transvaginal contraception on markers of thrombosis. *Contraception.* 2008;78(6):451-458.

47. Merck and Company Inc. Nuvaring (transvaginal contraceptive patch). Package insert. 2014. http://www.merck.com/product/usa/pi_circulars/n/nuvaring/nuvaring_pi.pdf. Accessed April 19, 2015.

48. Pfizer. Depo-Provera (depo medroxyprogesterone acetate IM). Package insert. 2015. http://labeling.pfizer.com/ShowLabeling.aspx?id=522. Accessed April 19, 2015.

49. Jaina J, Jakimiukb A, Bodec F, Rossd D, Kaunitze A. Contraceptive efficacy and safety of DMPA-SC. *Contraception.* 2004;70:269-275.

50. Lanza L, McQuay L, Rothman K, et al. Use of depot medroxyprogesterone acetate contraception and incidence of bone fracture. *Obstet Gynecol.* 2013;121:593-600.

51. ACOG Committee Opinion No. 602. Depot medroxyprogesterone acetate and bone effects. *Obstet Gynecol.* 2014;123:1398-1402.

52. Gardner J, Mishell D. Analysis of bleeding patterns and resumption of fertility following discontinuation of a long-acting injectable contraceptive. *Fertil Steril.* 1970;21:286-291.

Infertility Issues and Polycystic Ovary Syndrome

Shawky Z. A. Badawy, MD

INTRODUCTION

Polycystic ovary syndrome is one of the most common endocrinopathies in women during reproductive years. It is a complex disease process that leads to ovulatory dysfunction, infertility, irregular uterine bleeding, and various skin manifestations. The skin manifestations include hirsutism, oily skin, acneiform eruptions, and skin pigmentation known as achanthosis nigricans.[1]

There are certain manifestations of the polycystic ovary syndrome that also affect the health of women; one of these is obesity, which is present in about 30%–50% of patients with polycystic ovary syndrome. This will predispose women to what is known as metabolic syndrome. This metabolic syndrome includes prediabetes, diabetes, and hypertension.[2] Furthermore, there is the possibility for these patients to develop endometrial cancer if they are not treated properly.

The etiology of polycystic ovary syndrome is not known, but it may be due to some genetic predisposition. Polycystic ovary syndrome is reported to be present in 50% of sisters and 40% of mothers of patients with this disease process. The mode of inheritance is suggested to be autosomal or X-linked process. Aneuploides and polyploides of the X chromosome have been described. Deletion of the long arm of chromosome 11 was seen in some cases of polycystic ovary syndrome. The genes related to steroidogenesis and carbohydrate metabolism are suggested to be factors in the development of this syndrome.[3,4]

HISTORICAL ASPECTS AND DIAGNOSTIC CHARACTERISTICS

Polycystic ovary syndrome was first described in 1935 by Irving Stein and Michael Leventhal.[5] These two gynecologists from Chicago described a category of women with enlarged ovaries, irregular cycles, and infertility. The ovaries contained multiple cysts, which are follicles that have not ovulated. They treated these women with wedge resection of the ovaries; the women resumed ovulatory cycles, and some of them achieved pregnancy.[6] Stein-Leventhal syndrome remained the characteristic identification of this disease because of these two scientists and their contribution. Wedge resection was the main line of treatment in these patients until the late 1970s. At that time, endocrine science was not advanced, and hormonal assays, as we know today, were not present or available. Therefore, the Stein-Leventhal syndrome was a purely clinical and morphological diagnosis. In the mid-1970s, it became possible, due to the development of proper hormonal assays, to evaluate patients' gonadal hormones. Several societies developed criteria based on endocrine testing to rule out other diseases.

Diagnostic criteria were put forward by several societies and institutions. In the early 1990s, the National Institutes of Health (NIH) had a consensus meeting; afterward, certain criteria were published as diagnostic for patients with polycystic ovary syndrome[7]:

1. Anovulation, manifested by oligomenorrhea or amenorrhea
2. Excess androgen activity, manifested by hyperandogenemia or hypoandrogenism

Patients who fulfilled these two criteria would be diagnosed as having polycystic ovary syndrome.

In 2003, representatives of the American Society of Reproductive Medicine and the European Society of Human Reproduction and Embryology met in Rotterdam, the Netherlands, and developed the Rotterdam criteria for the diagnosis of polycystic ovary syndrome[8,9]:

1. Amenorrhea/oligomenorrhea
2. Hyperandrogenism/hyperandrogenemia
3. Polycystic appearance of the ovary on ultrasound

Two of the 3 criteria *must be present* for the diagnosis of polycystic ovary syndrome.
In 2006, the Androgen Excess Society met and published their criteria, which are similar to the Rotterdam criteria for the diagnosis of polycystic ovary syndrome.[10]

ENDOCRINOLOGY OF POLYCYSTIC OVARY SYNDROME

The hypothalamic-pituitary-ovarian axis and gonadotropin production are affected in the polycystic ovary syndrome, resulting in elevation of luteinizing hormone (LH) levels in relation to follicle-stimulating hormone (FSH) levels. As a result of that change, the ovary increases its production of androstenedione from the thecal cells under the affect of increased LH secretion. Androstenedione is metabolized to testosterone by 17-β-hydoxysteroid dehydrogenase. In addition, estrogen production is increased from two sources: the aromatization of testosterone to estradiol and the conversion of androstenedione to estrone in the fatty tissue. The end result of the excess estrogen production in these patients is the suppression of FSH and stimulation of LH levels. Therefore, the ratio of FSH to LH is in favor of excess LH, which leads to the activation of the thecal cells and increased production of androgens.[11]

The excess androgen production will inhibit the formation of steroid-binding globulins in the liver, and the free testosterone level will be elevated. This might be the case even if the total testosterone level is normal. With the elevation of the free testosterone level, accessibility to the tissues will be high; therefore, peripheral manifestations are developed in the skin in the form of acne eruptions, hirsutism, and oily skin.[12]

The excess estrogen production in these patients, without progesterone effect, will lead to stimulation of the endometrium to undergo proliferation. This process may proceed to hyperplasia; carcinoma of the endometrium could also develop in some of these patients.[13]

Hyperinsulinemia in patients with polycystic ovary syndrome will lead to increased androgen production from thecal cells in the ovaries. Furthermore, hyperinsulinemia inhibits the synthesis of steroid-binding globulins from the liver and adds to the finding of increased free androgens. This will lead to the androgenic properties in polycystic ovary syndrome.[14]

In some patients with polycystic ovary syndrome, it has been noticed that they also have some degree of hyperprolactinemia. This is due to the excess estrogen stimulation of the lactotropes.[15,16] Also, in about 30%–50% of patients with polycystic ovary syndrome, there is a slight elevation of dehydroepiandrosterone sulfate from the adrenal glands. This may be due to the excess estrogen level, which causes some blockage in the process of hydroxylation in the adrenal gland.[17]

The easy accessibility of testosterone to the skin associated with the increased activity of 5α-reductase leads to the high production of dihydrotestosterone, which leads to all the skin manifestations of patients with polycystic ovary syndrome.[18]

MANAGEMENT OF PATIENTS WITH POLYCYSTIC OVARY SYNDROME

Treatment of Infertility and Increased Weight

About 50% of patients with polycystic ovary syndrome are either overweight or obese. This leads to an increase in insulin levels due to an increase in insulin resistance. The end result will be the development of prediabetes or the full picture of diabetes. To help these patients achieve their goal, which includes management of the irregular cycles, skin manifestations, and infertility, they have to be counseled properly for weight loss. This is usually not an easy line of treatment; however, it should be discussed thoroughly with the patient and include referral to a weight loss program. Patients who lost weight have regained normal ovulatory cycles. If the cycles remain irregular, then the management will be more successful compared to management of overweight and obese patients.[19] The use of fertility medications in such patients will not be successful in induction of ovulation even with the use of high medication doses.

This failure is due to an increase in leptin in the serum and follicular fluid. Leptin acts through receptors in granulosa and thecal cells with inhibition of steroidogenesis.

Furthermore, in obese patients, there is a decrease in serum adiponectin, which leads to an increase in insulin levels that will stimulate more androgen secretion by the ovary. The end result of thecal cell change is failure of ovulation.[20]

Management of Hirsutism

Hirsutism is due to an increase in total testosterone production and an increase in free testosterone levels. The increase in the free testosterone levels is due to the decrease in steroid-binding globulins secreted by the liver. Also, increased activity of 5α-reductase in the skin converts the available testosterone to dihydrotestosterone. This conversion will lead to hirsutism, acne, and increased secretion of sebaceous glands, leading to oily skin.

One of the most effective lines of treatment for this condition is the use of steroidal oral contraceptives (combination birth control pill).[21] These pills contain ethinyl estradiol and a progestin. They suppress gonadotropins and decrease the secretion of androstenedione from the ovaries and will decrease the levels of testosterone. Usually, when these patients are put on the birth control pills, they will have normalized androgen levels within 6–8 weeks. They have to continue on the medication as long as they do not want to achieve a pregnancy. In addition to the reduction of testosterone production, the use of the birth control pill inhibits 5α-reductase activity in the skin; therefore, this will decrease the synthesis of dihydrotestosterone, and the end result will be marked improvement in the hirsutism and the oily skin. Note that the treatment will not abolish hirsutism; however, it will decrease the rate of hair growth and will prevent further stimulation of hair follicles. After a 6-month period of time when the rate of hair growth is stabilized, the patients could then use other cosmetic treatments to remove these stimulated hair follicles by either hydrolysis or laser treatment.

Patients who are on birth control pills should have no contraindications to their use, mainly smoking, uncontrolled hypertension, and poorly controlled diabetes. We also have to be certain there is no history of thromboembolic disease. If the patient has a family history of thromboembolic disease, then that could be explored by studying all the various thrombotic factors, including gene mutations.

Patients often ask about the type of birth control pill that is more effective. Note that the third generation of birth control pills containing desogestrel are better in these conditions than the first- and second-generation pills. This is due to the mechanism of action: Desogestrel binds totally to progesterone receptors and has no binding to androgen receptors. In contrast, norethindrone (first generation) and levonorgestrel (second generation) have affinity to androgen receptors, thus leading to some androgen effect. Also, another type of oral contraceptive pill is the variety that contains drospirenone as a progestin. It is an agonist of spironolactone that has been shown to be effective lowering the testosterone level and inhibiting 5α-reductase.[22]

Patients also ask questions related to the effect of birth control pills on future fertility. The available data suggest there is no negative effect of birth control pill use on future fertility. These data suggest that the fertility rate is the same as for patients who have not used a birth control pill.[23]

The Use of Metformin in Management of Polycystic Ovary Syndrome

Metformin, or Glucophage, suppresses hepatic gluconeogenesis and increases insulin sensitivity in peripheral tissues, thus increasing glucose utilization by muscles and fatty tissue. Metformin has been used in polycystic ovary syndrome to increase sensitivity to the insulin secreted by the pancreas in these patients and, as such, will prevent the development of diabetes. In addition, it has been found from clinical trials that the use of metformin helped those patients to lose weight. Furthermore, with this result, patients developed regular cycles; some of these patients showed evidence of ovulation and successful pregnancy.[24]

It has been shown that metformin will decrease insulin levels, and as such, it will decrease the stimulation of androstenedione production by the ovaries. The end result will be a decrease in testosterone production and testosterone levels in these patients. A side effect of metformin is the gastrointestinal problem of diarrhea, which usually occurs with high doses of the drug. This is why we usually recommend starting with a low dose of 500 mg daily, which might be increased to twice per day or higher according to the needs of the patient.

Management of Infertility

The workup for infertility in patients with polycystic ovary syndrome includes endocrine studies to rule out any other endocrinopathy. In addition, we test the male factor, especially if the partner is also obese. This will need proper attention as there might be a problem with the sperm picture in these patients. For the female patient, induction of ovulation is the standard of treatment provided that the patient has lost some weight if obesity has been seen since the beginning of the treatment regimen. The following have been used for induction of ovulation: clomiphene citrate, letrozole (aromatase inhibitor), gonadotropins in induction of ovulation, and surgery for treatment of polycystic ovary syndrome.

Clomiphene Citrate

Clomiphene citrate is a specific estrogen receptor modulator and acts as an estrogen agonist on the hypothalamic-pituitary axis and estrogen antagonist on the endometrium. This last effect is usually evident with high doses. For this reason, if these patients ovulate with this medication, they will need progesterone support of the luteal phase and the pregnancy for up to 12 weeks.

Clomiphene citrate acts by attaching itself to estrogen receptors in the hypothalamic area; this will facilitate the secretion of gonadotropin-releasing hormones, which will act on the pituitary gonadotropes, facilitating the secretion of FSH and LH. The ovary will respond by proper folliculogenesis with a rise in the estrogen level, which will stimulate the LH peak to trigger ovulation.

Usually, clomiphene citrate is successful in inducing ovulation in about 80% of patients who are anovulatory. The pregnancy rate is 50%, and the multiple-birth rate is 10%–15%. The clinician must begin with a small dose, 50 mg on days 3–7 of the cycle. If that does not produce a successful response, then the dose should be increased to either 100 or 150 mg for 5 days. The reason for gradually using higher doses is to avoid the antiestrogenic effect on the endometrium and cervical mucus.[25,26]

One of the main problems in induction of ovulation is the high testosterone level in these patients. This usually interferes with the actions of the fertility medications. For this reason, it would be helpful for the patients to use a combination of metformin and clomiphene citrate. This has been shown to facilitate the induction of ovulation because metformin lowers testosterone levels.

Some patients with polycystic ovary syndrome have slight elevation of the adrenal dehydroepiandrosterone sulfate. Again, this will interfere with the action of clomiphene citrate in facilitating the ovary response to gonadotropins. For this reason, in these patients we recommend a small dose (0.5 mg daily) of dexamethasone to be given at bedtime on days 3–7 of the cycle in addition to the fertility medication clomiphene citrate. This has been beneficial in facilitating induction of ovulation and successful pregnancy. Dexamethasone would then be discontinued once pregnancy is achieved.

Some of the patients with polycystic ovary syndrome have a slight elevation in serum prolactin level due to the stimulation of the lactotropes by the high estrogen levels present. To help these patients and to facilitate the response to clomiphene citrate, a small dose of dopamine agonist can be given to lower the prolactin level and thus facilitate ovulation.

Letrozole

The use of the aromatase inhibitor letrozole was approved by the Food and Drug Administration (FDA) for chemotherapeutic treatment of breast cancer. In 2000, several studies for the use of letrozole in induction of ovulation were presented at the American Society of Reproductive Medicine meeting. Letrozole inhibits aromatase enzyme and therefore inhibits the conversion of testosterone to estrogen. The end result will be the release of hypothalamic gonadotropin-releasing hormones and stimulation of gonadotropin secretion, which will lead to folliculogenesis and ovulation. It is effective, and some pregnancies have been reported. It is also suggested that it might be used as a first-line treatment to induce ovulation rather than reserving it for failure of clomiphene citrate in some patients.[27,28]

Gonadotropins in Induction of Ovulation

Usually, gonadotropin treatment is reserved for those cases that fail to respond to clomiphene citrate, metformin, and letrozole. The reason for that is the expense and the need for testing in the form of estradiol levels and sonograms to check follicle growth during the course of induction of ovulation. The incidence of multiple births is also higher at 35% or so compared to the use of clomiphene citrate. In addition, ovarian hyperstimulation syndrome is higher in patients who are treated with gonadotropins as compared to clomiphene citrate. There are two types of gonadotropins: recombinant and purified urinary. Both have the same effect on the ovary, and the pregnancy rate is nearly the same.[29]

Surgery for Treatment of Polycystic Ovary Syndrome

Stein and Leventhal in 1935 described polycystic ovary syndrome, and they treated affected patients with wedge resection of the ovaries. Some patients ovulated and achieved a pregnancy. However, the mode of action was not known. Recently, Judd et al. completed a study in which they evaluated androgen levels at baseline and followed them after the wedge resection of the ovaries.[30] It was found that the wedge resection of the ovaries reduced the concentration of androgens. However, that effect did not last for a long period of time because these androgen levels increased to the preoperative levels in a few months. Wedge resection has been discontinued as a preferred line of treatment of polycystic ovary syndrome. This surgery was replaced by the various fertility medications that have a good success rate without subjecting the patient to an operative procedure.

During the past three decades, the surgical treatment of polycystic ovary syndrome has been revived by what is known as laparoscopic drilling of the ovaries. In these cases, the patients are given general anesthesia, and laparoscopy is performed; using a unipolar needle cautery, several punctures are made in the tunica of the ovaries. Some of these studies have also documented a pregnancy rate after ovarian drilling that is equal to that using ovulation-inducing medications. Furthermore, some of the experimental studies in animals have shown that following ovarian drilling, some periovarian and peritubal adhesions formed which could delay or prevent fertility.[31–33] In a prospective clinical study to evaluate ovarian adhesions following ovarian drilling for polycystic ovary syndrome, it was found that adhesion formation developed in 60% of patients in the study.[34] In addition, some studies have documented a decrease in ovarian reserve following ovarian drilling.[35] The treatment of patients with polycystic ovary syndrome who desire pregnancy must take all these effects and side effects into consideration when ovarian drilling is considered for management.

CONCLUSION

In conclusion, polycystic ovary syndrome diagnosis and management have come a long way since the era of Stein and Leventhal. Today, we have facilities for endocrine evaluation, medications for successful induction of ovulation, and medication for treatment of cutaneous manifestations. Polycystic ovary syndrome is a common endocrinopathy in reproductive-age women. With modern developments we are able to help these patients overcome the manifestations of the disease and achieve successful pregnancies.

Future research may focus on new methods of induction of ovulation that are reasonable, easy to use, less expensive, and with a good pregnancy rate compared to clomiphene citrate and gonadotropins. The use of aromatase inhibitors in these patients is promising. More data will be useful for their application in our daily treatment of both obese and normal-weight women.

REFERENCES

1. Sheehan M. Polycystic ovarian syndrome: diagnosis and management. *Clin Med Res*. 2004;2(1):13–27.
2. Gambineri A, Pelusi C, Vicenmati V, et al. Obesity and the polycystic ovary syndrome. *Int J Obes Relat Metab Disord*. 2002;26:883–896.
3. Legro RS, Driscoll D, Strouss JF III, Dunaif A. Evidence for a genetic basis for hyperandrogenemia in polycystic ovary syndrome. *Proc Natl Acad Sci U S A*. 1998;95:14956–14960.
4. Meyer MF, Gerreshein F, Pfeiffer A, Epplen JT, Schatz H. Association of polycystic ovary syndrome with an interstitial deletion of the long arm of chromosome 11. *Exp Clin Endocrinol Diabetes*. 2000;108:519–523.
5. Stein IF, Leventhal ML. Amenorrhea associated with bilateral polycystic ovaries. *Am J Obstet Gynecol*. 1935;29:181–191.
6. Stein IF. Duration of infertility following ovarian wedge resection. *West J Surg*. 1964;72:237.
7. Zawadski JK, Dunaif A. Diagnostic criteria for polycystic ovary syndrome towards a rational approach. In: Dunaif A, Givens JR, Haseltine FP, Merriam GR, eds. *Polycystic Ovary Syndrome*. Boston: Blackwell Scientific; 1992:377–384.
8. The Rotterdam ESHRE/ASRM-Sponsored PCOS Consensus Workshop Group. Revised 2003 consensus on diagnostic criteria and long-term health risks related to polycystic ovarian syndrome. *Hum Reprod*. 2004; 19:41–47.
9. The Rotterdam ESHRE/ASRM-Sponsored PCOS Consensus Workshop Group. Revised 2003 consensus on diagnostic criteria and long-term health risks related to polycystic ovarian syndrome. *Fertil Steril*. 2004;81 (1):19–25.
10. Ricardo A, Eurico C, Didier D, et al. The Androgen Excess and PCOS Society criteria for the polycystic ovary syndrome: the complete task force report. *Fertil Steril*. 2009;91:456–488.

11. Rebar R, Judd HL, Yen SSC, et al. Characterization of the inappropriate gonadotropin secretion in polycystic ovary syndrome. *J Clin Invest*. 1976;57:1320.

12. Hatch R, Rosenfield RL, Kim MH, et al. Hirsutism: implications, etiology and management. *Am J Obstet Gynecol*. 1981;140:815–830.

13. Guidic LC. Endometrium in PCOS: implantation and predisposition to endocrine CA. *Best Pract Res Clin Endocrinol Metab*. 2006;20(2):235–244.

14. Dunaif A. Insulin resistance and the polycystic ovary syndrome: mechanism and implications for pathogenesis. *Endocr Rev*. 1997;18(6):774–800.

15. Bracero N, Zacur HA. Polycystic ovary syndrome and hyperprolactinemia. *Obstet Gynecol Clin North Am*. 2000;28(1):77–84.

16. Robin G, Catteau-Jonard S, Young J, et al. Physiopathological link between polycystic ovary syndrome and hyperprolactinemia: myth or reality? *Gynecol Obstet Fertil*. 2011;39(3):141–145.

17. Mei-Jau Chen, Chin-Der Chin, Jehn-Hsiahn Yang, et al. High serum dehydroepiandrosterone sulphate is associated with phenotypic acne, and a reduced risk of abdominal of abdominal obesity in women with polycystic ovary syndrome. *Hum Reprod*. 2010;26(1):227–234.

18. Kirshiner MA, Samojlik E, Silber D. A comparison of androgen production and clearance in hirsute and obese women. *J Steroid Biochem*. 1983;19(1B):607–614.

19. Clark AM, Thornley B, Tomlinson L, et al. Weight loss in obese infertile women results in improvement in reproductive outcome for all forms of fertility treatment. *Hum Reprod*. 1998;13(6):1502–1505.

20. Pandey SH, Pandy SU, Maheshwari A, Bhattacharya S. The impact of female obesity on the outcome of fertility treatment. *J Hum Reprod Sci*. 2010;3(2):62–67.

21. Yildiz BO. Oral contraceptives in polycystic ovary syndrome: risk benefit assessment. *Semin Reprod Med*. 2008;26(1):111–120.

22. Mathur R, Levin O, Aziz R. Use of eithinylestradiol/drospirenone combination in patients with the polycystic ovarian syndrome. *Ther Clin Risk Manag*. 2008;4(2):487–492.

23. Farrow A, Hull MG, Northstone K. Prolonged use of oral contraception before a planned pregnancy is associated with decreased risk of delayed conception. *Hum Reprod*. 2002;17(10):2754–2761.

24. Lord JM, Flight IHK, Norman RJ. Metformin in polycystic ovary syndrome: systematic review and meta-analysis. *BMJ*. 2003;327(7421):951–953.

25. Gysler M, March CM, Mishell DR Jr, et al. A decade's experience with an individualized clomiphene treatment regimen including its effect on the post coital test. *Fertil Steril*. 1982;37:161–167.

26. Roy S, Greenblatt RB, Mahesh VB, et al. Clomiphene citrate: further observations on its use in induction of ovulation in the human and on its mode of action. *Fertil Steril*. 1963;14:575.

27. Bayar U, Basaran M, Kiran S, et al. Use of an aromatase inhibitor in patients with polycystic ovarian syndrome: a perspective randomized trial. *Fertil Steril*. 2006;86:1447–1451.

28. Mitwally MFM, Casper RF. Use of aromatase inhibitor for induction of ovulation in patients with an inadequate response to clomiphene citrate. *Fertil Steril*. 2001;75:305–309.

29. Bayram N, van Wely M, van Der Veen F. Recombinant FSH versus urinary gonadotropins or recombinant FSH for ovulation induction in subfertility associated with polycystic ovary syndrome. *Cochrane Database Syst Rev*. 2001;(2):CD002121.

30. Judd HL, Rigg LA, Anderson DC, Yen SS. The effects of ovarian wedge resection on circulating gonadotropin and ovarian steroid levels in patients with polycystic ovary syndrome. *J Clin Endocrinol Metab*. 1976;43(2):347–355.

31. Amer SA, Li TC, Ledger WL. Ovulation induction using laparoscopic ovarian drilling in women with polycystic ovarian syndrome: predictors of success. *Hum Reprod*. 2004;19:1719–1724.

32. Mercorio F, Mercorio A, DiSpiezio Sardo A, et al. Evaluation of ovarian adhesion formation after laparoscopic ovarian drilling by second look mini-laparoscopy. *Fertil Steril*. 2008;89:1229–1233.

33. Kong GWS, Cheung LP, Lok IH. Effects of laparoscopic ovarian drilling in treating infertile anovulatory polycystic ovarian syndrome patients with and without metabolic syndrome. *Hong Kong Med J*. 2011;17:5–10.

34. Mercorio F, Mercorio A, DiSpiezio Sardo A, Barba GV, Pellicano M, Nappi C. Evaluation of ovarian adhesion formation after laparoscopic ovarian drilling by second look mini laparoscopy. *Fertil Steril*. 2008;89(5):1229–1233.

35. Kandil M, Selim M. Hormonal and sonographic assessment of ovarian reserve before and after laparoscopic ovarian drilling in PCOS. *BJOG Int Obstet Gynecol*. 205;112:1427–1430.

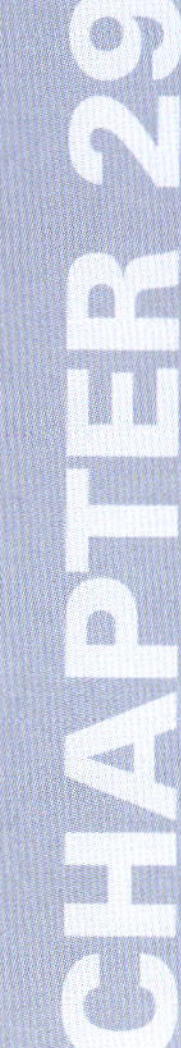

CHAPTER 29

Metabolic Syndrome

Maida Taylor, MD, MPH, FACOG

METABOLIC SYNDROME: HOW TO DEFINE HEALTH RISKS

In 1988, at the Banting Lecture at the annual meeting of the American Diabetes Association,[1] Dr. Gerald Reaven of Stanford University described a constellation of metabolic abnormalities associated with an increased risk for diabetes and atherosclerotic cardiovascular disease (CVD). This cluster of risk factors was designated "syndrome X," or insulin resistance syndrome. Dr. Reaven stated that persons with syndrome X[2] manifest glucose intolerance, dyslipidemia, abnormal uric acid metabolism, renal salt retention, increased sympathetic tone, and hypercoagulability due to increases in plasminogen activator inhibitor 1 (PAI-1).

As the defining features of syndrome X have evolved, researchers coined the term *metabolic syndrome* (metS) to describe the abnormalities that identify the segment of the population at risk for diabetes and atherosclerotic disease. But, there has been a lack of consensus on a precise definition of metS.

The World Health Organization, National Cholesterol Education Project, American Academy of Clinical Endocrinology, and International Diabetes Federation have published somewhat different diagnostic criteria (Table 29-1). Consequently, the National Heart, Lung, and Blood Institute and the American Heart Association in 2004 convened a conference to develop a meaningful definition of metabolic syndrome.[3] Clinical features they agreed on include the following:

TABLE 29-1 Metabolic Syndrome: Varying Definitions

	Blood Pressure	Lipids	Central Obesity	Glucose	Other	Diagnostic Requirements
WHO	On antihypertensive therapy or BP ≥ 140/90 mm Hg	Plasma triglycerides over 150 dL/mL and/or HDL-C < 35 mg/dL (men), < 39 mg/dL for women	BMI > 30 and/or waist-hip ratio > 0.9 (men), > 0.85 (women)	IGT or as in type 2 diabetes	Microalbuminuria (UAE ≥ 20 µg/min or albumin-creatinine ratio ≥ 30 mg/g)	Type 2 diabetes or IGT and 2 additional abnormalities; if GT normal, 3 required
NCEP ATP III	BP ≥ 130/85 mm Hg	Plasma triglycerides over 150 dL/mL and/or HDL-C < 40 mg/dL (men), < 50 mg/dL for women	Waist circumference > 102 cm (40 in.) (men), > 88 cm (35 in.) (women)	FBG ≥ 110 mg/dL		3 or more of criteria listed
AACE	Hypertension	Plasma triglycerides over 150 dL/mL and/or HDL-C <35 mg/dL (men), <45 mg/dL for women	Waist circumference > 102 cm (40 in.) (men), >88 cm (35 in.) (women)	IFG or as in type 2 diabetes	Insulin resistance, acanthosis nigricans, hyperuricemia. Minor criteria: hypercoagulability, coronary heart disease, polycystic ovarian disease, vascular endothelial dysfunction, microalbumenuria	Not specified

Abbreviations: IGT, Impaired Glucose Tolerance; UAE, Urinary Albumin Excretion; IFG, Impaired Fasting Glucose; AACE, American Association of Clinical Endocrinologists; NCEP ATP III, National Cholesterol Education Program, Adult Treatment Panel III; WHO, World Health Organization.

1. Abdominal obesity is the form of obesity most strongly associated with metS. It presents clinically as increased waist circumference.
2. Atherogenic dyslipidemia manifests in routine lipoprotein analysis by raised triglycerides and low concentrations of high-density lipoprotein (HDL) cholesterol and many times other lipoprotein abnormalities (e.g., increased remnant lipoproteins, elevated apolipoprotein B, small low-density lipoprotein [LDL] particles, and small HDL particles). All of these abnormalities have been implicated as independent atherogenic factors.
3. Elevated blood pressure strongly associates with obesity, and 50% of persons with hypertension also evidence insulin resistance.
4. Insulin resistance is present in the majority of people with metS. It strongly associates with other metabolic risk factors and correlates univariately with CVD risk. When glucose intolerance evolves into clinical diabetes, an elevated glucose level constitutes a major independent risk factor for CVD.

Revised ATP III metabolic syndrome* Oct 2005

Risk factor	Defining level
Abdominal obesity[†] (Waist circumference[‡])	
Men	≥102 cm (>40 in)
Women	≥88 cm (>35 in)
TG	≥150 mg/dL or Rx for ↑ TG
HDL-C	
Men	<40 mg/dL
Women	<50 mg/dL or Rx for ↓ HDL
Blood pressure	≥130/≥85 mm Hg or on HTN Rx
Fasting glucose	≥100 mg/dL or Rx for ↑ glucose

*Diagnosis is established when ≥3 of these risk factors are present.
[†]Abdominal obesity is more highly correlated with metabolic risk factors than is ↑ BMI.
[‡]Some men develop metabolic risk factors when circumference is only marginally increased.

FIGURE 29-1. Current revised diagnostic criteria for metabolic syndrome, National Cholesterol Education Program's Adult Treatment Panel III (ATP III). BMI, body mass index; HDL-C, high-density lipoprotein cholesterol; HTN, hypertension; Rx, prescription; TG, triglycerides.

5. A pro-inflammatory state, recognized clinically by elevations of C-reactive protein (CRP), is commonly present in persons with metS. Multiple mechanisms are involved, but obesity and excess adipose tissue cause the release of inflammatory cytokines such as CRP.
6. A prothrombotic state, characterized by increased plasma PAI-1 and fibrinogen, also is associated with metS, and the prothrombotic and pro-inflammatory states seem to be metabolically interconnected.

The National Heart, Lung, and Blood Institute/American Heart Association Conference set the criteria in Figure 29-1 for a diagnosis of metS. A person must have 3 or more of the following:

- Waist circumference greater than 102 cm in men or greater than 88 cm in women
- Serum triglycerides 150 mg/dL or greater
- HDL cholesterol less than 40 mg/dL in men or less than 50 mg/dL in women
- Systolic/diastolic blood pressure of 130/85 mm Hg or greater or taking hypertension medications
- Fasting plasma glucose level of 100 mg/dL or greater or taking diabetes mellitus medications

Malik and colleagues[4] quantified the impact of metS on CVD mortality. Relative to an individual with no metS risk factors, having 1 to 2 risk factors increased a patient's hazard ratio by more than 70%, to 1.73. Having 3 or more of the 5 risk factors associated with metS imposes a CVD mortality hazard ratio of 2.71 (Figure 29-2). The highest risks are associated with type 2 diabetes and CVD and with those with coincident CVD and type 2 diabetes mellitus.

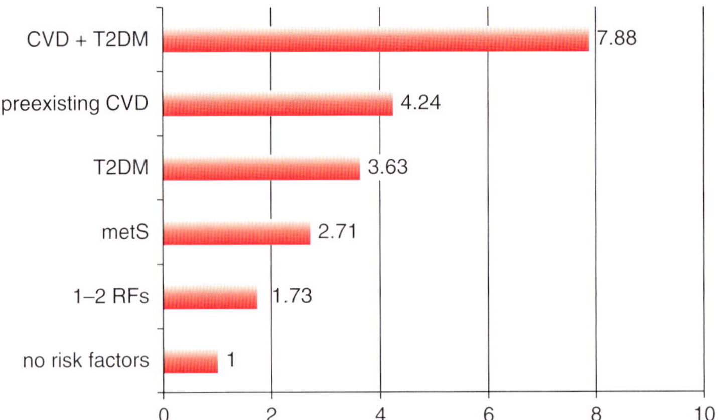

FIGURE 29-2. Hazard ratios for cardiovascular mortality with metabolic syndrome, diabetes, and cardiovascular disease (based on USA data adjusted for gender, age, smoking, physical activity, and total cholesterol). RF, risk factor; T2DM, type 2 diabetes mellitus. (From Malik S, Wong ND, Franklin SS, et al. Impact of the metabolic syndrome on mortality from coronary heart disease, cardiovascular disease, and all causes in United States adults. *Circulation.* 2004;110:1245–1250.)

Complexities Within the metS Parameters

Our understanding of the physiological disturbances associated with metS continues to evolve. A vast array of complexities and subtleties exist within the pathophysiology of insulin resistance, obesity, atherogenic dyslipidemia and hypertension, and metS, while defining a cluster of findings suffers from being too restrained.

The keystone in metS is central obesity, defined by waist circumference. Waist circumference is measured at the high point of the iliac crest at minimal respiration to the nearest 0.1 cm. There has been some research and discussion if waist or waist-hip ratio is a better measure for assessing risk. It is clear that while waist measurement offers some small challenges, hip measurement is difficult to do owing to poor placement of measuring tape and poor reproducibility. The default has become waist circumference.

In the Nurses' Health Study, with data generated over 8 years on 43,581 subjects, there was a strong positive association between waist circumference and the incidence of diabetes. Those women with a waist circumference greater than 38 inches had a diabetes relative risk (RR) of 22.4, relative to women in the normal waist circumference range of less than 28 inches. While the study also looked at body mass index (BMI) and waist-hip ratio, both of which were validated and predicted the same trend, waist circumference showed the sharpest gradient and was judged to be the best predictor of risk.[5]

Waist measurement is simple for patients to understand. Are your pants, belts, or dresses tight? You have gained weight. Are they loose? You have lost weight. Moreover, you have lost weight where it counts, from your abdomen. Some weight loss clinics suggested replacing regular weighing at home on a scale with a tape measure. And, when working with patients from economically disadvantaged communities, a retractable cloth tape measure is considerably cheaper than a scale and can be carried in a suitcase, briefcase, or purse.

TABLE 29-2 Country/Ethnic Group–Specific Waist Circumference Cut Points[a]

Country/Ethnic Group		*Waist Circumference*
United States	Male	102 cm (40 in.)
	Female	88 cm (35 in.)
Europids	Male	94 cm (37 in.)
	Female	80 cm (31 in.)
South Asian and Chinese	Male	90 cm (35 in.)
	Female	80 cm (31 in.)
Japanese	Male	85 cm (33 in.)
	Female	90 cm (35 in.)
Ethnic South and Central American	Use South Asian until more data are available	
Sub-Saharan Africans	Use European until more data available	
Eastern Mediterranean and Middle Eastern (Arab)	Use European until more data available	

[a]Tan CE, Ma S, Wai D, Chew SK, Tai ES. Can we apply the National Cholesterol Education Program Adult Treatment Panel definition of the metabolic syndrome to Asians? *Diabetes Care.* 2004;27(5):1182–1186. PMID:15111542.

Waist circumference cut points for CVD risk vary by race and ethnicity. The International Diabetes Foundation (IDF) suggested ethnic-specific values for waist circumference for different populations, although the normative values are not as well validated as the normative values in American and Europid groups (Table 29-2).

Due to a number of factors, the clinical correlates for the lower waist circumference cut points owe to the higher risk of diabetes and CVD, particularly in South Asians and Chinese populations and expatriate groups residing in Westernized societies. The thresholds for risk are lower for acquired traits, including age, obesity, abdominal obesity, and a high percentage of body fat. The risk for diabetes escalates in males from India at a BMI of 23 and waist circumference of 85 cm in men and 80 cm in women. At any given BMI, South Asians have a higher degree of central adiposity and a higher degree of insulin resistance.[6]

This body type, with thin arms and legs but a cylindrical trunk with chest, waist, and hip circumference being similar, has been termed *TOFI*, thin on the outside, fat on the inside. Moreover, South Asians, Asians, and Pacific Islanders evidence earlier onset of diabetes and CVD and have a significantly higher number of risk factors when diagnosed.[7] They manifest a higher prevalence of retinopathy; higher rates of hypertension; and higher levels of hemoglobin A_{1c} and total cholesterol, despite being younger at the time of diagnosis than Europids.

Inflammatory Markers and Prothrombotic Markers

In addition to high-sensitivity CRP (hsCRP), other cytokines (also called adipokines) are upregulated in obesity and are adipocyte-derived bioactive substances.

Adiponectin, a protective adipokine, is downregulated by intra-abdominal obesity. Adiponectin protects the endothelial vasculature by inhibiting foam cell formation and vascular remodeling, processes that promote the formation of atherosclerotic plaque. Adiponectin also improves insulin sensitivity, keeping blood sugar in check. Conversely, interleukin 6 (IL-6) is upregulated by intra-abdominal obesity. IL-6 is a pro-atherogenic hormone; it worsens insulin resistance and is therefore both pro-atherogenic and diabetogenic. Tumor necrosis factor alpha (TNF-α) is also upregulated in obesity, lowers insulin sensitivity in adipocytes, and increases free fatty acid production and triglycerides. TNF-α induces a procoagulant state, and when coupled with increased secretion of PAI-1, proatherogenic, pro-inflammatory, and procoagulant changes are further enhanced.

Consensus on Metabolic Syndrome Still Lacking

While much energy has been devoted to developing a definition for metS, it must be mentioned that many experts in the field do not believe that the term is a valuable and viable clinical construct. Coincident with the publication of the report of the National Heart, Lung, and Blood Institute/American Heart Association Conference on Scientific Issues Related to the Definition of metS, another consensus group comprising members of the Professional Practice Committee of the American Diabetes Association and an ad hoc committee of the European Association for the Study of Diabetes issued their own statement, arguing that the current definition of metS was still poorly characterized, did not sufficient identify persons at risk, and might lead patients and clinicians to neglect significant markers of disease that are not part of the cluster of risk factor delineated by metS. The committee stated the following:

> While there is no question that certain CVD risk factors are prone to cluster, we found that the metabolic syndrome has been imprecisely defined, there is a lack of certainty regarding its pathogenesis, and there is considerable doubt regarding its value as a CVD risk marker. Our analysis indicates that too much critically important information is missing to warrant its designation as a "syndrome." Until much needed research is completed, clinicians should evaluate and treat all CVD risk factors without regard to whether a patient meets the criteria for diagnosis of the "metabolic syndrome (p. 2289)."[8]

Nonetheless, the term *metabolic syndrome* has become embedded within our lexicon, in research protocols, and in clinical practice. Paul Huang has perhaps written the most cogent review of the topic, providing a working definition of metS and an excellent review of its clinical utility:

> The metabolic syndrome is a clustering of hyperglycemia/insulin resistance, obesity and dyslipidemia. It is important for several reasons. First, it identifies patients who are at high risk of developing atherosclerotic CVD and type 2 diabetes (T2D). Second, by considering the relationships between the components of metabolic syndrome, we may be able to better understand the pathophysiology that links them with each other and with the increased risk of CVD. Third, it facilitates epidemiological and clinical studies of pharmacological, lifestyle and preventive treatment approaches (p. 231).[9]

Metabolic syndrome should be regarded as one more algorithm for defining persons at risk. But, it is not sufficient. Consider the following three patient profiles:

Patient 1: Marcia
- 54-year-old white female
- Waist 93 cm (38 inches)
- Glucose 120 mg/dL
- Triglycerides 260 mg/dL
- Low-density lipoprotein 180 mg/dL

Patient 2: Mary
- 54-year-old white female
- Waist 93 cm (38 inches)
- Glucose 99 mg/dL
- Triglycerides 190 mg/dL
- High-density lipoprotein 55 mg/dL

Patient 3: Maria
- 54-year-old white female
- Waist 85 cm (33.5 inches)
- Glucose 145 mg/dL
- Triglycerides 120 mg/dL
- High-density lipoprotein 30 mg/dL

Only the first patient (with high waist circumference, elevated glucose, and elevated triglycerides) meets the current criteria for metS, but all 3 women have substantially elevated risk of CVD mortality.

So, a diagnosis of metS is in no way a comprehensive method for identifying high-risk individuals. But, the term constitutes a useful rubric that may help the clinician explain metabolic aberrations and risks to the patient. Using the term *metabolic syndrome* simplifies care by helping patients to understand the complexities of managing multiple interrelated metabolic aberrations; it helps conceptually when formulating a comprehensive approach to the manifold problems seen in these individuals. But, to truly address risk, each of the abnormalities subsumed by the term *metS* requires focus and attention, illumination, and intervention.

As illustrated by the case profiles, the predictive value of screening using the criteria for metS is not superior to tools like the Framingham Risk Score in defining 10-year risk of atherosclerotic vascular disease, but it does not assess risk for stroke, which has been correlated with metS criteria. Other screening tools, such as the Reynolds Risk Score,[10] are calibrated to predict stroke. Screening tools are useful adjuncts in patients with metS and actually may be easier to use and provide more accurate risk assessments than metS criteria.

The Framingham Risk Score offers 2 methods for calculating risk.[11] The first, the "General CVD Risk Prediction Using Lipids," includes gender, age, systolic blood pressure, current treatment for hypertension, current smoking, diabetes, and HDL and total cholesterol values for assessing risk. The second Framingham method, "General CVD Risk Prediction Using BMI," includes gender, age, systolic blood pressure, current treatment for hypertension, current smoking, diabetes, and BMI. Both of these methodologies yield a 10-year risk for coronary disease. The Reynolds Risk Score includes[12] gender, total cholesterol, HDL, systolic blood pressure, hsCRP, and parental history of heart attack or stroke under age 60.

The Continuum of Insulin Resistance, Prediabetes, and Diabetes

Insulin resistance is clearly a precursor to frank diabetes. There is a continuum, from insulin resistance to prediabetes to overt type 2 diabetes. Unfortunately, most people are not identified until they experience a sentinel cardiovascular event. And, while persons with type 2 diabetes have a 3-fold increased risk for coronary events, even those with prediabetes are at significant risk, a 2-fold increase, a level that demands our attention.

Current diagnostic criteria for frank diabetes are as follows[13]:

- Hemoglobin A_{1c} value greater than or equal to 6.5%
- Fasting plasma glucose greater than or equal to 126 mg/dL (7.0 mmol/L), with fasting defined as no caloric intake for at least 8 hours
- Two-hour plasma glucose greater than or equal to 200 mg/dL (11.1 mmol/L) during oral glucose tolerance test (75-mg glucose load)
- Patient with classic symptoms of hyperglycemia or hyperglycemic crisis, with random glucose greater than or equal to 200 mg/dL (11.1 mmol/L)

Current diagnostic criteria for prediabetes are as follows:

- Hemoglobin A_{1c} equal to 5.7%–6.4%
- Fasting plasma 100 (5.6 mmol/L) to 125 mg/dL (7.0 mmol/L), with fasting defined as no caloric intake for at least 8 hours
- Two-hour plasma glucose greater than or equal to 200 mg/dL (11.1 mmol/L) during oral glucose tolerance test (75-mg glucose load)
- Patient with classic symptoms of hyperglycemia or hyperglycemic crisis, with random glucose greater than or equal to 200 mg/dL (11.1 mmol/L)

According to the National Diabetes Education Program, 18–19 million US adults have type 2 diabetes, and another 86 million Americans have prediabetes and are at high risk of developing type 2 diabetes.[14]

METABOLIC SYNDROME AND WOMEN

According to the National Health and Nutrition Examination Survey (NHANES), the prevalence of metS has risen steadily over time, from 32.9% in 2003–2004, to 36.1% in 2007–2008, and to 34.7% in 2011–2012. While the prevalence in women dropped from 39.4% in 2007–2008 to 36.6% in 2011–2012 ($p = .03$), women continue to have significantly higher prevalence compared with men (36.6% vs. 30.3%, $p < .001$).

The prevalence of metS is highest in Hispanics, 35.4%, followed by non-Hispanic whites (33.4%) and blacks (32.7%). Fifty percent of people aged 60 years and older are thought to have metS.[15]

Given the ambiguities inherent in labeling a patient with a diagnosis of metS, obesity offers a simplified surrogate for risk. The 2015 report from NHANES[16] found that women were more likely to be obese than overweight, at 37% and 30%, respectively. Fewer than 30% of women over age 55 are normal weight or underweight. So, two-thirds of American women are over a normal weight. While menopausal women continue to blame their postmenopausal hormonal status on their weight problems, note that 3 of 4 men over age 55 are overweight or obese.

African Americans have the highest rates of obesity, with 39% of men and 57% of women affected. Of black women, 17% are now extremely obese. Obesity rates are high in all racial groups: for Mexican Americans, 38% of men and 43% of women; and for whites, 35% of men and 34% of women. Asian Americans were not accounted due to lack of adequate sampling.

Metabolic Syndrome and Reproductive Milestones

It cannot be emphasized enough that midlife signals the start of a marked escalation in the risk of metS and related disorders. Many reproductive milestones are associated with significant weight gain, specifically puberty, childbirth, and menopause. At puberty, girls stop exercising regularly, with a decline from more than 8 hours of vigorous activity to less than 2 hours per week. During pregnancy in the United States, 42% of women gain more than the recommended number of pounds, and for many, "baby weight" becomes permanent. Women who retain their pregnancy weight at 6 months postpartum are then 8.3 kg heavier 10 years later. This retained weight after each pregnancy contributes to increased risk of metS, diabetes, and CVD.

Gestational diabetes is a strong predictor of metS and type 2 diabetes mellitus, with the predictive risk approaching 70%. A history of preeclampsia predisposes to insulin resistance and hypertension. Obesity contributes to preeclampsia, and conversely, obesity-associated metabolic abnormalities, including elevated glucose, insulin and triglycerides, are associated with an increased risk of preeclampsia. Women with polycystic ovary syndrome, at any given BMI, are twice as likely to develop metS later in life and also are at risk for hypertension and type 2 diabetes mellitus.[17]

Metabolic Syndrome and Menopause

Menopause per se does not appear to increase the risk of metS and diabetes mellitus, but rather, menopause-related changes in body composition and fat distribution do confer added risks, probably mediated by a marked increase central obesity seen at midlife. The Study of Women Across the Nation (SWAN) more clearly delineated the timing of risk, specifically pinpointing the rise in risk to the perimenopause. SWAN followed 949 participants over 9 years. During the course of the study, 13.7% of women developed new-onset metS. The odds ratio specific for metS during the perimenopause was 1.45, while during the postmenopausal stage, the odds ratio dropped to 1.24, a statistically significant differential.[18]

The strongest associations between the development of metS were seen with increased levels of bioavailable testosterone and decreased sex hormone–binding globulin. Menopause provokes a relative hyperandrogenemia because estradiol decreases by 80%, while testosterone drops only 50%,[19] an altered hormonal milieu that hypothetically might lead to increased risk of CVD. This relative hyperandrogenemia is thought to provoke not only metabolic changes but also body conformational changes that enhance risk. Ley et al. measured sex-related and menopause-related differences in body composition and regional fat distribution; they used dual-energy x-ray absorptiometry (DEXA) in nonobese healthy volunteers. Postmenopausal women ($n = 70$) had a 20% greater fat mass ($p < .001$) than premenopausal women ($n = 61$). Body configuration and fat distribution shifted in postmenopausal women toward a more android fat distribution. While an android (upper body) fat distribution was most often seen in men (48.6%, $p < .001$), fat distribution in women shifted over time, with an android pattern seen in 38.3% of premenopausal women to 42.1% in postmenopausal women ($p < .001$). Conversely, the gynecoid body fat distribution declined, becoming less common in the postmenopausal women.

Not only do postmenopausal women possess more body fat, but also that fat is deposited in a pattern associated with negative metabolic effects and elevated risk of disease. It has been hypothesized that gluteal subcutaneous adipose tissue (GSAT) and abdominal subcutaneous adipose tissue (ASAT) exert opposing metabolic effects on fasting insulin, insulin resistance, and dyslipidemia. The operant mechanism is thought to be differential depot-specific gene expression in preadipocytes from different depot sites. Gluteal fat is resistant to upregulation of gene expression that enhances inflammatory responses, while abdominal adipocytes are less resistant to this effect. Measurements of arteriovenous blood from fat confirm that abdominal fat stores secrete 4 times the amount of pro-inflammatory IL-6 as gluteal fat stores. Visceral adipose tissue (VAT) has been less well studied owing to difficulty in obtaining serial intra-abdominal biopsies in human subjects. Animal models have confirmed that visceral fats store produce greater amounts of inflammatory cytokines.[20]

It is worth mentioning that many of the drugs often prescribed for common problems related to midlife are associated with weight gain. Progestins, antihypertensives, and antidepressants often cause weight gain. See Table 29-3 for a list of drugs implicated in weight gain and suggested alternative options.

TABLE 29-3 Drugs Associated With Weight Gain[a]

Category	Drug Class	Weight Gain	Alternatives—Weight Reducing in Parentheses
Psychiatric agents	Antipsychotic	Clozapine Risperidone Olanzapine Quetiapine Haloperidol Perphenazine Quetiapine	Ziprasidone Aripiprazole
	Antidepressants/mood stabilizers: tricyclic antidepressants	Amytriptyline Doxepin Imipramine Nortriptyline Trimipramine Mirtazapine	(Bupropion) Nefazodone Fluoxetine (short term) Sertraline (<1 year)
	Antidepressants/mood stabilizers: SSRIs	Fluoxetine? Sertraline? Paroxetine Fluvoxamine	Same as above
	Antidepressants/mood stabilizers: MAO inhibitors	Phenylzine Tranylcypromine	Same as above
	Lithium		Same as above

(Continued)

TABLE 29-3 Drugs Associated With Weight Gain[a] (*Continued*)

Category	Drug Class	Weight Gain	Alternatives—Weight Reducing in Parentheses
Neurologic agents	Anticonvulsants	Carbamazepine Gabapentin Valproate	Lamotrigine? (Topiramate) (Zonisamide)
Endocrinologic agents	Diabetes drugs	Insulin (weight gain differs with type and regimen used) Sulfonylureas Thiazolidinediones Sitagliptin? Metiglinide	(Metformin) (Acarbose) (Miglitol) (Pramlintide) (Exenatide) (Liraglutide)
Gynecologic agents	Oral contraceptives	Progestational steroids Hormonal contraceptives containing progestational steroids	Barrier methods IUDs
	Endometriosis treatment	Depot leuprolide acetate	Surgical methods
Cardiologic agents	Antihypertensives	α-Blocker? β-Blocker?	ACE inhibitors? Calcium channelblockers Aangiotensin-2 receptor antagonists
Infectious disease agents	Antiretroviral therapy	Protease inhibitors	None
General	Steroidal hormones	Corticosteroids Progestational steroids	NSAIDs
	Antihistamines/anticholinergics	Diphenhydramine? Doxepin? Cyproheptadine?	Decongestants Steroid inhalers

Abbreviations: ACE, angiotensin-converting enzyme; MAO, monoamine oxidase; NSAIDs, nonsteroidal anti-inflammatory drugs; SSRI, selective serotonin reuptake inhibitor.
[a]From Cheskin L. Prescription drugs that can cause weight gain. John Hopkins Health Alert. Accessed November 18, 2012. Can prescription drugs cause weight gain? http://www.drugs.com/article/weight-gain.html. Accessed May 20, 2015.

Metabolic Syndrome and Hormone Therapy

One might hypothesize that if menopause is associated with changes in habitus and fat mass that predispose to metS, perhaps hormone supplementation might avert or reverse these changes and lessen the risk of developing the abnormalities seen in metS. The 3-year Postmenopausal Estrogen/Progestin Intervention Study (PEPI) offered some early insights into the effects of hormone therapy (HT) on regulation of blood glucose and insulin. It must be noted that all women in PEPI had preexistent CVD, and the results may not be generalizable to a more normative population. Nonetheless, in PEPI, treatment with 0.625 mg CEs with or without medroxyprogestereone decreased fasting insulin by 16.1% and fasting blood glucose (FBG) declined 2.2 mg/dL, rather modest declines. The 2-hour postchallenge glucose increased 6.4 mg/dL, leading the authors to speculate that this might indicate a delay in glucose clearance.[21] The maximum improvements were seen in those patients who were the most hyperglycemic and hyperinsulinemic at the start of study.

The literature evaluating the effects of HT on glucose metabolism is confusing, given that most studies are small and that the types of estrogen, routes of delivery, and use of progestins are all highly variable. Results also appear to differ when hormones are taken by women without metS or type 2 diabetes mellitus.

Saltpeter et al.[22] did an extensive review and meta-analysis in 2006. The authors identified 107 randomized controlled trials encompassing a total of 33,315 subjects. In those studies measuring abdominal obesity (9 studies), HT benefited nondiabetic women compared with controls, increasing lean body mass (weighted mean difference [WMD] 3.3%; 95% CI 0.02, 6.6). When pooled, 5 studies showed reduced waist circumference in the HT group (WMD –0.8%; 95% CI –1.2, –0.4; $p < .05$), and 4 studies showed reductions in abdominal fat (–6.8%; 95% CI –11.8, –1.9). Eighteen studies included measures of insulin resistance and diabetes. Insulin resistance (homcostasis model assessment, HOMA-IR) was lowered in nondiabetic women on HT compared with controls (WMD 12.9%; 95% CI 8.6, 17.1; $p < .05$). Fasting glucose and fasting insulin also improved (WMD 2.5%; 95% CI 1.5, 3.5; and WMD 9.3%; 95% CI 4.9, 13.7, respectively). The risk of developing type 2 diabetes mellitus dropped by 30% (RR 0.7; 95% CI 0.6, 0.9). A greater reduction in HOMA-IR was observed for women with diabetes compared with those without diabetes ($p = .07$). Subgroup analysis suggested that the type of HT was not important, but the confidence intervals for this segment of the study were wide.

Two randomized trials, the Heart and Estrogen/Progestin Replacement Study (HERS) and the Women's Health Initiative (WHI) trial, reported the effect of 0.625 mg conjugated equine estrogen alone or combined with 2.5 mg medroxyprogesterone acetate (MPA) on new-onset diabetes. In HERS, the incidence of diabetes was 6.2% in the HT group and 9.5% in the placebo group (relative hazard 0.65 [95% CI 0.48–0.89]; $p = .006$). Diabetes risk was not mediated by weight or waist circumference.[23] In the WHI estrogen-only arm, the cumulative incidence of treated diabetes was 8.3% in the CE arm and 9.3% in the placebo arm (hazard ratio 0.88; 95% CI 0.77–1.01; $p = .072$). During the first year, insulin resistance declined in the estrogen group, but this differential disappeared at the 3- and 6-year follow-up visits. For the CE/progestin arm (CE/MPA) of the WHI, the cumulative incidence of treated diabetes was 3.5% in the CE/MPA group and 4.2% in the placebo group (hazard ratio 0.79; 95% CI 0.67–0.93; $p = .004$). Adjusting for waist circumference and BMI did not lessen the effect. This suggests that any effect of HT on the risk of diabetes is not mediated through alterations in body configuration or fat distribution.

The E3N (Etude Epidemiologique de Femmes de la Mutuelle Générale de l'Education Nationale) cohort study from France evaluated similar findings on the effect of oral and transdermal HT on the risk of new-onset diabetes in a cohort of postmenopausal French women. New-onset diabetes was reduced in ever users of HT (hazard ratio = 0.82 [0.72–0.93]), compared to never users. Adjustment for BMI during follow-up rather than baseline BMI did not substantially modify this association. Oral estrogen was associated with a greater decrease in diabetes risk than transdermal HT (hazard ratio = 0.68 [0.55–0.85] vs. 0.87 [0.75–1.00]).[24]

FUTURE RESEARCH

Continuing research is needed to enhance our understanding of the factors predisposing to insulin resistance. Clearer biometric criteria are needed, and better algorithms for delineating long-term risks may help clinicians identify when to initiate critically needed interventions.

Studies are needed to define the pathways of insulin resistance and obesity and when dysfunction begins. More work is needed on the genetic basis for the disorder, the genetics of obesity and insulin regulation, and how obesity during pregnancy might induce epigenetic changes that induce an increased risk of metabolic dysregulation in offspring. The role of adipokine signaling and modulating appetite and satiety needs further illumination. It remains to be seen whether therapeutics are able to regulate adipokines, such as leptin, which suppresses hunger, and if so, whether obesity and insulin functionality will be altered.

We need better understanding of how reproductive events and hormonal therapies affect the risk of developing diabetes and heart disease, especially the effects of hormonal contraception during reproductive years and menopausal HT in younger and older menopausal women. Studies are presently under way to look at the effects of oral contraceptives, vaginal rings, and implants on women with metS or diabetes mellitus and later incidence of metS or diabetes mellitus. Genistein and other phytoestrogens are being studied to see if they will lessen the risk of metS or diabetes mellitus in menopausal women. Strength training and aerobic exercise, including Zumba, are being tested as methods to limit the long-term progression of disease.

The National Institutes of Health conducted a trial that closed in 2009, examining the impact of CE or raloxifene on total-body fat mass, total abdominal fat area, and visceral abdominal fat area. Results have yet to be reported. Dehydroepiandrosterone (DHEA) and testosterone have also been studied to explore whether anabolic activity of these steroids might improve body composition and energy balance.

More information and education are needed about the ethnic differences in insulin resistance and rapid rate of progression of disease in these groups. Studies are under way to explore possible difference in the development of type 2 diabetes in Asian versus White populations. Last, the lessons learned from the American Diabetes Prevention Program are being translated and implemented in other countries to determine if metformin, lifestyle, and other measures will mitigate adverse outcomes in diverse populations.

CONCLUSION

With two-thirds of the US population now falling into the class of overweight or obese, the risk factors associated with type 2 diabetes mellitus and CVD are ubiquitous. Women accrue excess pounds during puberty and pregnancy and at menopause. The close association between reproductive landmarks and weight gain gives credence to the myth that obesity is a hormone-related disorder. But, behavior undeniably contributes far more to obesity than changes in estrogen across the reproductive life span. In adolescence, physical activity decreases at least 7% per year, with the declines more marked in girls.[25] McMurray reported that moderate physical activity and vigorous physical activity declined by 65%–70% during adolescence, with the most significant declines seen in girls who progress from normal weight to obesity.[26]

Women who gain excess weight during pregnancy, when evaluated 21 years later, were twice as likely to be overweight and 4 times as likely to be obese (OR 2.15 and 4.49, respectively).[27] Indeed, menopause and loss of endogenous estrogens may be associated with a decline in basal metabolic rate of 200 calories per day. Also important are the decrease in physical activity at midlife and the increased incidence of disability after age 50. Few, if any women, compensate for declining physical activity by reducing calorie intake.

The "metabolic syndrome," while by no means an all-encompassing formula for identifying women at risk for diabetes and CVD, is a useful construct when trying to explain to patients the physiological aberrations of insulin resistance. The linkage between intra-abdominal fat mass, central obesity, and upregulation of inflammatory cytokines provides an elegantly simple explanation of the dysfunctions associated with insulin dysregulation.

While there is ongoing debate about which method is best for assessing cardiovascular risk (waist circumference, waist-hip ratio, BMI, skinfold thickness, water weighing, computed tomographic scan, or magnetic resonance imaging), measurement of waist circumference is quick, simple, and cheap. Patients can assess their progress during treatment either by using a tape measure or by putting on an old, tight pair of jeans that once fit but are now too tight. While calorie restriction is the best approach to weight loss, aerobic exercise selectively targets abdominal fat mass, improves insulin sensitivity, and is a necessary adjuvant in the treatment of metS.

Ryan found that weight loss and exercise markedly improved CVD risk factors in older sedentary women (mean age 59) with a history of gestational diabetes mellitus and with type 2 diabetes. While body fat declined 11%–12% and subcutaneous abdominal fat dropped by 10%, visceral fat mass decreased by 27% during this 6-month interventional trial.[28] While reproductive medicine has focused intensely on obesity during pregnancy, these lifestyle interventions are highly effective in modifying risk factors in older women.

REFERENCES

1. Reaven GM. Banting lecture 1988: role of insulin resistance in human disease. *Diabetes*. 1988;37:1595–1607.
2. Canadian Association of Cardiovascular Prevention and Rehabilitation. An interview with Gerald Reaven: syndrome X: the risks of insulin resistance. http://www.cacpr.ca/information_for_public/archived_issues/2000s/0009Reaven.pdf. September 2000. Accessed November 11, 2016.
3. Grundy SM, Brewer HB Jr, Cleeman JI, Smith SC Jr, Lenfant C; American Heart Association; National Heart, Lung, and Blood Institute. Definition of metabolic syndrome: report of the National Heart, Lung, and Blood Institute/American Heart Association conference on scientific issues related to definition. *Circulation*. 2004;109(3):433–438. PMID: 14744958.
4. Malik S, Wong ND, Franklin SS, et al. Impact of the metabolic syndrome on mortality from coronary heart disease, cardiovascular disease, and all causes in United States adults. *Circulation*. 2004;110:1245–1250.
5. Carey VJ, Walters EE, Colditz GA, et al. Body fat distribution and risk of non-insulin-dependent diabetes mellitus in women: the Nurses' Health Study. *Am J Epidemiol*. 1997;145:614–619.
6. Tan CE, Ma S, Wai D, et al. Can we apply the National Cholesterol Education Program Adult Treatment Panel definition of the metabolic syndrome to Asians? *Diabetes Care*. 2004;27:1182–1186.
7. Raymond NT, Varadhan L, Reynold DR, et al. Higher prevalence of retinopathy in diabetic patients of South Asian ethnicity compared with white Europeans in the community: a cross-sectional study. *Diabetes Care*. 2009;32(3):410–415.
8. Kahn R, Buse J, Ferrannini E, Stern M. American Diabetes Association; European Association for the Study of Diabetes. The metabolic syndrome: time for

a critical appraisal: joint statement from the American Diabetes Association and the European Association for the Study of Diabetes. *Diabetes Care.* 2005;28(9):2289–2304. PMID: 16123508.

9. Huang PL. A comprehensive definition for metabolic syndrome. *Dis Model Mech.* 2009;2(5–6):231–237. doi:10.1242/dmm.001180.

10. Ridker PM, Buring JE, Rifai N, Cook NR. Development and validation of improved algorithms for the assessment of global cardiovascular risk in women: the Reynolds Risk Score. *JAMA.* 2007;297:611–619.

11. Framingham Heart Study. Cardiovascular disease (10-year risk). https://www.framinghamheartstudy.org/risk-functions/cardiovascular-disease/10-year-risk.php. Accessed June 15, 2015.

12. Reynolds Risk Score calculation. http://www.reynoldsriskscore.org/Default.aspx. Accessed June 15, 2015.

13. American Diabetes Association. Standards of medical care in diabetes—2014. *Diabetes Care.* 2014;37(Suppl 1): S14–S80. doi:10.2337/dc14-S014. PMID: 24357209.

14. National Diabetes Education Program. National Institutes of Health. Guiding principles for the care of people with or at the risk for diabetes. http://ndep.nih.gov/hcp-businesses-and-schools/guiding-principles/principle-01-identify-undiagnosed-diabetes-and-prediabetes.aspx. Accessed April 1, 2015.

15. Aguilar M, Bhuket T, Torres S, Liu B, Wong RJ. Prevalence of the metabolic syndrome in the United States, 2003–2012. *JAMA.* 2015;313(19):1973–1974. doi:10.1001/jama.2015.4260.

16. Yang L, Colditz GA. Prevalence of overweight and obesity in the United States, 2007–2012. *JAMA Intern Med.* 2015 Jun 22. doi:10.1001/jamainternmed.2015.2405. [Epub ahead of print] PMID: 26098405.

17. Bentley Lewis R, Koruda K, Seely EW. The metabolic syndrome in women. *Nature Clin Pract Endocrinol Metab.* 2007;3(10):696–704. doi:10.1038/ncpendmet0616.

18. Janssen I, Powell LH, Crawford S, Lasley B, Sutton-Tyrrell K. Menopause and the metabolic syndrome: the Study of Women's Health Across the Nation. *Arch Intern Med.* 2008;168(14):1568–1575. doi:10.1001/archinte.168.14.1568. PMID: 18663170. PMCID: PMC2894539.

19. Yongmei L, Jingzhong D, Bush TL, et al. Relative androgen excess and increased cardiovascular risk after menopause: a hypothesized relation. *Am J Epidemiol.* 2001;154(6):489–494. doi:10.1093/aje/154.6.489.

20. Pinnick KE, Nicholson G, Manolopoulos KN, et al. MolPAGE Consortium. Distinct developmental profile of lower-body adipose tissue defines resistance against obesity-associated metabolic complications. *Diabetes.* 2014;63:3785–3797.

21. Espeland MA, Hogan PE, Fineberg SE, et al. Effect of postmenopausal hormone therapy on glucose and insulin concentrations. PEPI Investigators. Postmenopausal Estrogen/Progestin Interventions. *Diabetes Care.* 1998;21(10):1589–1595. PMID: 9773716.

22. Salpeter SR, Walsh JM, Ormiston TM, Greyber E, Buckley NS, Salpeter EE. Meta-analysis: effect of hormone replacement therapy on components of the metabolic syndrome in postmenopausal women. *Diabetes Obes Metab.* 2006;8(5):538–554.

23. Vittinghoff E, Shlipak MG, Varosy PD, et al. Heart and Estrogen/Progestin Replacement Study Research Group. Risk factors and secondary prevention in women with heart disease: the Heart and Estrogen/Progestin Replacement Study. *Ann Intern Med.* 2003;138(2):81–89. PMID: 12529088.

24. De Lauzon-Guillain B, Fournier A, Fabre A, et al. Menopausal hormone therapy and new-onset diabetes in the French Etude Epidemiologique de Femmes de la Mutuelle Générale de l'Education Nationale (E3N) cohort. *Diabetologia.* 2009;52(10):2092–2100. doi:10.1007/s00125-009-1456-y.

25. Dumith SC, Gigante DP, Domingues MR, Kohl HW 3rd. Physical activity change during adolescence: a systematic review and a pooled analysis. *Int J Epidemiol.* 2011;40(3):685–698. doi:10.1093/ije/dyq272. Epub 2011 Jan 18. PMID: 21245072.

26. McMurray RG, Harrell JS, Creighton D, Wang Z, Bangdiwala SI. Influence of physical activity on change in weight status as children become adolescents. *Int J Pediatr Obes.* 2008;3(2):69–77. doi:10.1080/17477160701789794. PMID: 18465433.

27. Mamun AA, Kinarivala M, O'Callaghan MJ, Williams GM, Najman JM, Callaway LK. Associations of excess weight gain during pregnancy with long-term maternal overweight and obesity: evidence from 21 y postpartum follow-up. *Am J Clin Nutr.* 2010;91(5):1336–1341. doi:10.3945/ajcn.2009.28950. Epub 2010 Mar 17. PMID: 20237138.

28. Ryan AS. Improvements in insulin sensitivity after aerobic exercise and weight loss in older women with a history of gestational diabetes and type 2 diabetes mellitus. *Endocr Res.* 2016:1–7. [Epub ahead of print] PMID: 26925596.

Botanicals and Other Supplements

CHAPTER 30

Maida Taylor, MD, MPH, FACOG

COMPLEMENTARY AND ALTERNATIVE MEDICINE FOR WEIGHT LOSS AND GLYCEMIC CONTROL

Defining Complementary and Alternative Medicine

Complementary and alternative medicine (CAM) can be used for weight loss and glycemic control. Alternative medicine comprises several systematic medical practices based on models of health and disease that differ from the medical physiology that underpins Western allopathic medicine (Table 30-1). One of the oldest practices

489

TABLE 30-1 Complementary and Alternative Medicine (CAM) Headings in MEDLINE

Acupuncture
Anthroposophy
Biofeedback
Chiropractic
Color therapy
Diet fads
Eclecticism
Electric stimulation
Homeopathy
Kinesiology
Massage
Medicine, traditional
Mental healing
Moxibustion
Music therapy
Naturopathy
Organotherapy
Radiesthesia
Rejuvenation
Relaxation techniques
Therapeutic touch

within this rubric is traditional Chinese medicine (TCM), a system that defines health as a harmonious balance of the essential life force known as *Qi* (pronounced "Chee"). TCM also includes acupuncture and is used to promote wellness and to treat disease by regulating the flow of Qi along meridians that course through the body.

Mind-body medical systems view health as a balance of conscious and unconscious influences of mind on bodily functions. Mind-body medicine include manipulative and body-based systems like chiropractic, osteopathy, and massage, which are said to rebalance or realign the body through manipulation. Meditation, hypnosis, music, and prayer fall under this aegis. Mind-body medicine also includes energy-modulating modalities, such as therapeutic touch, Qi Gong, and magnets, which supposedly reorder bioelectric fields in or around the body to promote wellness and healing.

The most commonly used CAM practices are biologic-based therapies, such as botanical medicine, dietary supplements, vitamins, minerals, and orthomolecular medicine. Use of botanicals has been increasing steadily over the past 40 years. The reasons are manifold. Botanicals, despite a lack of evidence, are perceived as safer than conventional pharmaceuticals. They are promoted and perceived as supporting wellness, rather than treating disease. Any person can walk into any health food store, purchase whatever products they like without consulting a health care provider, thereby exercising a high degree of control and autonomy over their health care. CAM treatments harmonize with the philosophical and ethical values of many people. They offer natural alternatives that are unprocessed and unrefined. Many consumers are impressed by the seemingly vast traditional and historical record supporting the use of CAM products, despite the fact that the record is limited to observation, anecdote, and testimonials.

Nonetheless, the rate of use of CAM continues to escalate. In the data collected during the first National Health and Nutrition Examination Survey (NHANES) in 1971–1974, 22% of adults under 50 and 27% of those over 27 used dietary supplements. By NHANES 2003–2006, rates reached 45% and 67%, respectively.

Reasons for Using Botanicals and Supplements

Weight loss is reportedly one of the top 20 reasons people take dietary supplements.[1] Research suggests that 15% of US adults have used a weight loss dietary supplement at some point in their lives, with higher rates of use in women reporting (20.6%) than in men (9.7%).[2] In the weight loss marketplace, 85% of clients for products, programs, and services are women.

Women (and men) with metabolic syndrome (metS) and other obesity-related health issues are likely to use botanicals and supplements promoted for appetite suppression, weight loss, glycemic control, metabolic stimulation, and cholesterol lowering. The offerings are vast. The products discussed next are arranged alphabetically; this list is by no means exhaustive. It is merely an attempt to highlight products, and some representative clinical trials when available, that may help clinicians, who are likely to be asked about them in the course of counseling patients with metS. A detailed review of many products can be found in an Internet textbook by Evans and Bahng.[3] While it focuses on botanicals and supplements for diabetes, many of the products promoted for weight loss are covered in detail. Also, see the National Institutes of Health provides a Fact Sheet for Health Professionals reviewing weight loss supplementswebsite.[4] Excellent patient educational materials are also available at the institute's website. Also see a 2015 article by Ríos et al. on natural products for the treatment of type 2 diabetes mellitus (T2DM).[5]

BOTANICALS AND SUPPLEMENTS FOR WEIGHT LOSS AND GLYCEMIC CONTROL

α-Lipoic Acid

α-Lipoic acid, also called thioctic acid (not to be confused with α-linolinic acid, also designated as ALA) is marketed primarily as a "weight loss" and "energy" supplement and as an antioxidant. It is reported to improve insulin sensitivity after both intravenous and oral therapy. One recent study included 12 patients with T2DM (mean ± SD; age 52.9 ± 9.9 years; body mass index 33.9 ± 7.4 kg/m^2) for treatment with oral α-lipoic acid, 600 mg twice daily for 4 weeks. Twelve subjects with normal glucose tolerance served as a control. Using a euglycemic clamp technique, both glucose disposal rate (M) and insulin sensitivity index increased. In fact, the insulin sensitivity index in patients with T2DM did not differ statistically from the index in normal controls at the end of the treatment period. CAM practitioners typically recommend α-lipoic acid 600–1200 mg/d in tablet form. Food sources for α-lipoic acid include liver, spinach, broccoli, brussels sprouts, peas, potatoes, and yeast.

Agaricus blazei Murill

Agaricus blazei Murill (ABM) is a mushroom native to Brazil, also known as the royal sun mushroom or *cogumelo do sol* in Brazil or *himematsutake* in Japan. Extracts are marketed seemingly as a panacea for everything: cancer, T2DM, high cholesterol, arteriosclerosis, liver disease, and hematologic and gastrointestinal disorders. It is said to boost immunity and act as an adaptogen, an agent that helps with physical and psychological stress. In Japan, extracts are approved and sold as food additives. The mushroom is eaten and brewed as a tea. It is supposed to enhance insulin secretion from islets.

It does in fact improve the viability and proliferation of islets in diabetic and normal rats. A clinical randomized, double-blind, placebo-controlled trial enrolled 72 subjects with T2DM taking gliclazide and metformin for more than 6 months. The enrolled patients were randomly assigned to receive either a supplement of ABM extract or a placebo (cellulose) 1500 mg daily for 12 weeks. The homeostasis model assessment for insulin resistance (HOMA-IR) was the principle outcome measurement. At the end of the study, subjects who received the supplement of ABM extract ($n = 29$) showed a significantly lower HOMA-IR index (3.6 [SD 2.5] vs. 6.6 [SD 7.4], $p = .04$) than the control group ($n = 31$). The plasma adiponectin concentration increased 20% in the ABM group, while decreasing 12% in the placebo arm ($p < .001$).[6]

Allium sativum (Garlic)

Kitchen or garden variety garlic (*Allium sativum*) is promoted for dyslipidemia. In clinical trials, garlic supplementation yielded modest reduction in total cholesterol with no significant changes in low-density lipoprotein (LDL) or high-density lipoprotein (HDL) cholesterol levels. A meta-analysis of 13 trials found that garlic reduced the total cholesterol level significantly more than a placebo, with a weighted mean decline of –15.7 mg/dL (confidence interval [CI] –25.6 to –5. 7 mg/dL). While these data suggest that garlic is superior to placebo, the effect size was modest and far from robust. The authors concluded that garlic is probably of questionable value.[7] There is limited evidence that garlic lowers blood sugar in patients with T2DM.

Aloe vera

Aloe vera is a cactus-like desert plant and is the source of a gel used for a number of dermatological conditions. In the Arabian peninsula, parts of the aloe plant are used in traditional folk medicine for diabetes, said to stimulation β-cell function.

A recent study tested aloe vera gel complex (Aloe QDM complex) in people with prediabetes or early diabetes mellitus. Participants ($n = 136$) were randomly assigned to interventional or control groups and evaluated at baseline and at 4 and 8 weeks. While trending down, body fat and weight, blood sugar, insulin level ($p = .04$), and HOMA-IR ($p = .047$) were not statistically significant at 8 weeks. As is common in such studies, these marginal outcomes were reported as positive findings, reminding readers to go back to the primary sources when evaluating the literature.[8] *Aloe vera* has been linked to severe diarrhea, electrolyte abnormalities, and hepatotoxicity.

Bitter Orange (Synephrine)

Bitter orange is the common name for *Citrus aurantium*. This plant is a source of synephrine alkaloids, which mimic the action of epinephrine and norepinephrine. Whether bitter orange and synephrine impose cardiovascular and central nervous system risks like those seen with epinephrine and norepinephrine is unknown. Bitter orange is supposed to exert two effects: increased energy expenditure and appetite suppression.

When ephedra was banned in 2004 by the Food and Drug Administration (FDA),[9] botanical manufacturers substituted bitter orange in their weight loss formulations.

According to a review by Stohs et al.,[10] 23 small clinical trials used bitter orange, with a total enrollment of 360 subjects. In most, bitter orange was used in combination with caffeine and other supplements. Of the subjects, 44% consumed a bitter orange/p-synephrine-only product. The published literature noted small or no increase in heart rate or blood pressure, and there was no alteration in electrocardiograms, serum chemistry, blood cell counts, or urinalysis. p-Synephrine alone as well as in combination appeared to increase resting metabolic rate and energy expenditure and provided modest increases in weight loss at 6 to 12 weeks. The authors concluded that the evidence of efficacy and safety is far from robust.

Caffeine

Caffeine is almost in its own dietary class, which would include caffeine-containing herbs such as guarana (*Paullinia cupana*), kola or cola nut (*Cola nitida*), yerba mate (*Ilex paraguariensis*) and green tea (*Camellia sinensis*). Most often consumed in coffee and teas, caffeine is also added to weight loss supplements, frequently without being listed on the product label.

Caffeine is a methylxanthine and stimulates the central nervous system, heart, and skeletal muscles. It is estimated 100 mg of caffeine increases energy expenditure by approximately 9.2 kcal/h. Most clinical trials of caffeine have employed combination agents. In long-term observational studies, caffeine consumption was associated with a slight restriction in weight gain over time. Of the 18,417 men and 39,740 women enrolled in either the Health Professionals Follow-Up Study or Nurses' Health Study, men who increased their caffeine intake during the 12 years of observation gained 0.43 kg less than those who decreased their consumption, and women gained 0.35 kg less.

In 2014, Gurley et al.[11] published a detailed review of caffeine-containing supplements. They identified only 5 placebo-controlled studies that lasted more than 8 weeks using ephedra-free formulations. All the trials used multibotanicals with bitter orange and an ephedra substitute. Compared to placebo, these products led to 0 to 3.1 kg greater weight loss than that seen with placebo.

The FDA has advised limiting caffeine intake to 400 mg/d to avoid significant adverse effects.[12]

Caffeine Levels	
Coffee, 8 oz (237 mL)	95–200 mg[a]
Coffee, 8 oz decaffeinated	2–12 mg
Espresso, 1 oz (30 mL)	47–75 mg
Espresso, decaffeinated, 1 oz.	0–15 mg
Black tea, 8 oz (237 mL)	14–70 mg
Black tea, decaffeinated, 8 oz	0–12 mg
Green tea, 8 oz (237 mL)	24–45 mg

[a]Darker roast coffees generally have less caffeine.

Cinnamon

Cinnamon is used as a spice and is made from the inner bark of trees in the genus *Cinnamomum*. Cinnamon has an extensive history in folk medicine regarding its use for gastrointestinal disorders, respiratory problems, and diabetes. More recently, it has been promoted for glucose control, weight loss, and lipid disorders.

There is a distinct species difference between types of cinnamon sold. True cinnamon includes Ceylon cinnamon, *Cinnamomum zeylanicum*, and *Cinnamomum verum*. Of commercial cinnamon, 90% is a closely related species, *Cinnamomum burmannii*, also known as Indonesian cinnamon, Indonesian cassia, or Java cinnamon, and is designated as cassia in common labeling. This distinction between true cinnamon and cassia is not trivial. One teaspoon of cassia-type cinnamon contains 5–12 mg coumarin. The European Food Safety Authority has recommended no more than 0.1 mg coumarin intake from food daily per 2.2 pounds (1 kg) of body weight. For the generic 70-kg man, the upper limit of intake is 7 mg of coumarin. Therefore, dietary intake of cassia should be limited to 1 teaspoon per day for the average person. Ceylon cinnamon, true cinnamon, contains only traces of coumarin.[13] But, it is the high-coumarin cassia that is said to improve glucose tolerance.

The Cochrane Collaborative reviewed cinnamon in 2012 and identified 10 prospective, randomized controlled trials (RCTs), with 577 participants with types 1 and 2 diabetes mellitus. Eight studies were judged to be at high or unclear risk of bias, and the remaining 2 at moderate risk. Most studies used cinnamon cassia with a mean dose of 2 g daily for 4 to 16 weeks. The impact on glucose was inconclusive. There was no discernible effect on glycosylated hemoglobin A_{1c} (HbA_{1c}), serum insulin, or postprandial glucose. None of the trials reported health-related quality of life, morbidity, mortality, or costs.[14]

A more recent review and meta-analysis of cinnamon, glucose, and lipid levels was published in 2013. In patients with T2DM, 10 RCTs with 543 patients were included. Cinnamon doses between 120 mg/d and 6 g/d for 4 to 18 weeks lowered fasting plasma glucose by –24.59 mg/dL (95% CI –40.52 to –8.67 mg/dL); total cholesterol –15.60 mg/dL (95% CI, –29.76 to –1.44 mg/dL); LDL cholesterol (LDL-C) –9.42 mg/dL (95% CI –17.21 to –1.63 mg/dL); and triglycerides –29.59 mg/dL (95% CI –48.27 to –10.91 mg/dL); they also raised HDL cholesterol (HDL-C) 1.66 mg/dL (95% CI 1.09 to 2.24 mg/dL). No significant change in HbA_{1c} was noted.[15]

Due to a lack of sufficient evidence, neither the National Center for Complementary and Alternative Medicine (NCCAM) nor the American Diabetes Association recommends the use of cinnamon supplementation. Nonetheless, owing to minimal safety concerns around cinnamon, CAM practitioners continue to recommend its use, often in large doses.

Chitosan

Chitosan is a polysaccharide extracted from the exoskeletons of crustaceans. It supposedly absorbs fat, reducing its nutritional and caloric impact. The fat trapped, however, appears to be clinically insignificant.[16] In a Cochrane Collaborative review of 13 trials, chitosan (when taken for 4 weeks to 6 months) reduced body weight by a mean of 1.7 kg compared with placebo. The authors noted that the trials were poor quality, and that in the well-designed studies, chitosan was minimally effective.[17]

Chromium Picolinate

Chromium, after calcium, is the most commonly purchased mineral supplement in the United States. The most commonly sold form is chromium picolinate, although CAM dietary experts assert that trivalent chromium is the most effective form for glucose intolerance. It is promoted for diabetes, obesity, metS, and T2DM.

The mechanism of action suggested is enhanced insulin binding, insulin receptor number, insulin internalization, and β-cell sensitivity. In reviewing chromium intake and effects on glucose intolerance, the FDA has said that the relationship between chromium picolinate intake and insulin resistance is highly uncertain.[18] Three reviews have been published to date, the first concluding that there may be some clinical efficacy but there is insufficient documentation of long-term benefit and safety.[19] In 2013, a Cochrane review analyzed 9 RCTs of chromium picolinate for weight loss; the trials included 622 overweight or obese participants. Subjects received 200–1000 µg per day for 8 weeks to 6 months. Six of the trials included resistance or weight training. Overall, chromium picolinate supplementation reduced body weight by 1.1 kg more than placebo, but weight loss had no correlation to the dose of chromium picolinate administered.[20] Another review was published that same year with 11 RCTs that included 866 overweight or obese individuals. The studies used chromium picolinate 137 to 1000 µg for 8 to 26 weeks. Chromium appeared to reduce body weight by 0.5 kg and percentage body fat by 0.46% more than placebo. Similar findings were reported in an earlier meta-analysis of 12 trials.[21]

Coenzyme Q10

Coenzyme Q10 is a cofactor used in oxidative metabolism. Supplements are often recommended as an adjunct for patients taking HMG CoA (3-hydroxy-3-methylglutaryl coenzyme A) reductase inhibitors to lessen side effects thought to be due to depletion of naturally occurring coenzyme Q10 by the action of statins. The most often posited benefit of coenzyme Q10 is mitigation of statin-induced myopathy, although the available studies to date have failed to document significant benefit.[22]

Small studies have suggested that coenzyme Q10 might affect both T2DM and metS. In a 2015 meta-analysis, 7 trials were identified that included 356 patients. Neither coenzyme Q10 alone nor coenzyme Q10 plus fenofibrate improved glycemic control, LDL-C, HDL-C, and blood pressure, but triglycerides and total cholesterol did improve significantly. The authors noted that the studies were small, underpowered, and often poorly designed.[23] In a recent trial, 64 patients with T2DM were randomly assigned to receive either 200 mg coenzyme Q10 or placebo daily for 12 weeks. Serum HbA_{1c} concentration decreased in the group treated with coenzyme Q10.[24]

Coccinia indica (Ivy Gourd)

Coccinia indica (ivy gourd) is a creeping vine that has been used in traditional Indian Ayurvedic medicine to treat diabetes and is postulated to have insulinlike activity. In a small trial, 60 patients (aged 35–60 years) with T2DM were randomly assigned to placebo or treatment using 1 g extract of coccinia for 90 days. Fasting and postprandial blood glucose levels decreased by 16% and 18%, respectively ($p < .05$), and HbA_{1c} declined 0.6%.[25] Further study is needed to confirm and validate these findings.

Coconut Oil

Coconut oil is being touted as a healthy fat, said to improve the lipid profile and lower the risk for cardiovascular disease, stroke, and Alzheimer disease. It is said to also promote weight loss and lower the risk of diabetes. None of these claims have been substantiated. Coconut oil is a saturated fat containing predominantly medium-chain triglycerides, which are metabolized differently from the long-chain triglycerides found in most other oils. In a small trial, 40 obese women were told to cook with 2 tablespoons coconut oil or soybean oil each day. After 3 months, in the women given coconut oil, waist circumference dropped from 39 inches to 38.5 inches ($p = .005$). While reported as significant, the change is not clinically meaningful. HDL increased and LDL decreased in the coconut group.[26]

Coleus forskohlii (Forskolin)

Forskolin is extracted from the root of the *Coleus forskohlii* plant, which is grown in India and Thailand. Studies are limited; in 1 small RCT, 19 overweight or obese females aged 18–40 years were given either forskolin (250 mg twice daily) or placebo while maintaining their usual diet for 12 weeks. There was no effect on weight.[27] A similar study in men also found no effect.

Fiber

Increased intake of fiber is one of the mainstays of dietary recommendations for weight loss and glycemic control.[28] A wide variety of fiber sources have been prompted as weight loss aids, including oat bran, psyllium, glucomannan, and guar gum.

There are two types of dietary fiber: soluble and insoluble.

- Soluble fiber absorbs water and forms a gelatinous, viscous gel that slows gastric emptying, thus providing an increased sensation of satiety. Soluble fiber is provided by oatmeal, oat cereal, lentils, apples, oranges, pears, oat bran, strawberries, nuts, flaxseeds, beans, dried peas, blueberries, psyllium, cucumbers, celery, and carrots.
- Insoluble fiber also adds bulk to stool and improves gastrointestinal motility. Insoluble fiber is found in whole wheat, whole grains, wheat bran, corn bran, seeds, nuts, barley, couscous, brown rice, bulgur, zucchini, celery, broccoli, cabbage, onions, tomatoes, carrots, cucumbers, green beans, dark leafy vegetables, raisins, grapes, fruit, and root vegetable skin.
- Both types of fiber have been associated with lowered risk of cardiovascular disease, diabetes, constipation, diverticulitis, and obesity.

As a nutritional intervention, advising patients to increase fiber intake is far simpler than almost any other diet construct and has been proven to be an effective approach that is easy for patients to follow. In 1 study, 240 adults with metS were randomized to 1 of 2 diets. One-half of the group were told to follow the American Heart Association's (AHA's) diet, which includes recommendations to eat more fruits, vegetables, high-fiber foods, fish, and lean protein and to reduce salt, sugar, fat, and alcohol intake. The other half were counseled to increase their fiber intake to 30 g or more each day. At 12 months, mean change in weight was –2.1 kg (95% CI –2.9 to –1.3 kg) in the high-fiber diet group versus –2.7 kg (CI –3.5 to –2.0 kg) in the AHA diet group. Dropout rates were 9.9% and 12.6% in the high-fiber and AHA diet groups, respectively ($p = .55$). Seven subjects in the high-fiber diet group and 1 in the AHA diet group ($p = .066$) developed diabetes. The more complex AHA diet led to 1.7 kg more weight loss, but the simplified recommendation to increase fiber intake appeared to be a reasonable recommendation for individuals who find complex recommendations hard to follow.[29]

β-Glucan, the soluble fiber in oat bran and barley, has been shown to lower insulin resistance, dyslipidemia, hypertension, and obesity. Similar claims for other types of fiber are less well documented.[30] Studies of other fiber have been less convincing. Glucomannan is a soluble dietary fiber derived from konjac root (*Amorphophallus konjac*). Like other fibers, glucomannan absorbs water, increasing feelings of satiety and slowing gastric emptying. In a review of glucomannan, encompassing 6 RCTs with 293 subjects, the authors concluded that glucomannan had little effect on weight loss.[31]

Guar gum is a soluble fiber from the Indian cluster bean, *Cyamopsis tetragonolobus*. Pittler et al. found 20 RCTs of guar gum and pooled data from 11 trials, which included 203 adults with metabolic risk factors. Guar gum did not produce any substantive weight loss.[32] The same authors reviewed 1 RCT of psyllium, a water-soluble fiber from the husks of seeds from the *Plantago ovate* plant. No significant weight loss was observed.

Other popular diet fiber supplements include α-cyclodextrin, which is a soluble fiber derived from corn; African mango seed; and inulin-type fructans, a naturally occurring polysaccharide that is added to many foods to increase the fiber content. Inulin had no impact on weight in overweight and obese children.[33]

For simple tables with the fiber content of common foodstuffs, see the Harvard Health blog[34] or the Mayo Clinic website.[35]

Fish Oil

Omega-3 polyunsaturated fatty acids (n-3 PUFAs) include eicosapentaenoic acid (EPA, 20:5n-3) and docosahexaenoic acid (DHA, 22:6n-3) from seafood and α-linolenic acid from plants. Generally thought to improve cardiovascular risk, including blood pressure, arrhythmias, and triglycerides, PUFAs have also been suggested to improve glycemic control. The benefits, however, are far from clear.

In a systematic review, researchers identified 16 studies for inclusion in their analysis, with 18 separate cohorts comprising 540,184 individuals and 25,670 cases of incident diabetes mellitus. Overall, consumption of fish or seafood was not associated with lower risk of diabetes. Fish oil supplements also failed to provide risk reduction.[36] A review by Hruby (2015) found no effect of fish oil on insulin sensitivity, insulin secretion, β-cell function, or glucose tolerance.[37]

Garcinia

Garcinia cambogia (hydroxycitric acid, HCA) is marketed under the brand name Citramax, which is made from the pulp and rind of the fruit of this tree. The active compound is said to be HCA, and it supposedly has effects on lipogenesis, glycogen synthesis, appetite, and weight loss. In 89 overweight women, those taking *Garcinia cambogia* (800 mg, 30–60 minutes before meals for a total daily dose of 2.4 g/d [1.2 g HCA]) and given a 1200-kcal diet for 12 weeks lost significantly more weight (3.7 kg) than those receiving placebo (2.4 kg).[38]

A meta-analysis of 12 RCTs with 706 participants examined the effects of HCA on weight loss; 9 of the trials were judged adequate for inclusion. HCA appeared to reduce body weight by approximately 0.88 kg more compared to placebo. When only well-designed studies were included in the analysis, no effect was seen. The authors concluded that *Garcinia cambogia*/HCA lacked sufficient proof of efficacy as a weight loss supplement.[39]

Ginseng (*Panax ginseng, Panax quiquefolius*)

Ginseng is made from root of the ginseng plant and is eaten whole, powdered, or brewed as a tea or decoction. It is said to be an adaptogen, an agent that enhances the body's ability to tolerate illness and to adapt to environmental, physical, and emotional stresses. Three types of ginseng are commonly recommended: (1) *Panax ginseng* (Asian Ginseng); (2) *Panax quinquefolis* (American red ginseng, ARG); and (3) *Eleutherococcus senticosus* (Siberian ginseng, which is not a true ginseng). Both Asian and American ginseng contain ginsenosides, thought to be the active ingredient, although in differing amounts. *Eleutherococcus* was employed by Soviet military and Olympic trainers to enhance athletic performance and endurance.[40]

Ginseng is mixed into energy drinks with other stimulants, and as might be expected, reported side effects include agitation, diarrhea, headache, nervousness, and insomnia. These are not necessarily attributable to ginseng itself. Anaphylaxis and drug-herb interactions have also been reported.

Shishtar et al.[41] published a systemic review of ginseng and glucose intolerance in 2014. The group identified 16 relevant studies of fasting blood glucose ($n = 770$), 10 of fasting plasma insulin ($n = 349$), 9 for glycated hemoglobin ($n = 264$), and 7 that employed the HOMA-IR ($n = 305$). Ginseng significantly reduced fasting blood glucose compared to the control (MD = –0.31 mmol/L [95% CI –0.59 to –0.03], $p = 0.03$), but no significant effects were seen on fasting plasma insulin, glycated hemoglobin, or the HOMA-IR. Most trials were short and included subjects with only modest glycemic impairments. Needless to say, the authors concluded that further studies are needed. To that end, 11 trials are listed on the ClinicalTrials.gov registry (https://ClinicalTrials.gov).

Gymnema sylvestre

Gymnema sylvestre is a herb native to India and Sri Lanka. Chewing the leaves suppresses the perception of sweet taste. In both humans and animals, it has hypoglycemic effects, possibly acting as an insulin secretagogue. An extract, GS4, has been used as a treatment in 2 nonrandomized clinical trials, showing improvement in fasting glucose and HbA_{1c}. No well-designed trials have been conducted.

Hoodia (*Hoodia gordonii*)

Hoodia gordonii is a succulent plant used by the San people of the Kalahari Desert as an appetite suppressant on long hunting excursions. *Hoodia* was widely marketed in the United States as a weight loss product starting in 2002. In an RCT, 49 healthy overweight women aged 18–50 years were randomized to receive *Hoodia gordonii* purified extract (2220 mg/d) or placebo twice daily while on an ad libitum diet for 15 days.[42] Subjects reported more nausea, emesis, and abnormal skin sensation than controls, and researchers found significant increases in blood pressure, heart rate, bilirubin, and alkaline phosphatase ($p < 0.05$) in the *Hoodia* group. There were no differences in food intake or weight during the course of the trial.

Inositol

The inositol is a phosphoglycan sugar that has 9 isomeric forms and is involved in the synthesis of lipids, cell membranes, and cell growth and acts as a second messenger in insulin signaling. When insulin binds its receptor, mediators of phosphoglycans are generated by hydrolysis of glycosylphosphatidylinositol lipids in cell membranes. These mediators then enter cells and alter insulin signaling mechanisms. D-Chiro-inositolphosphoglycan mediator activates pyruvate dehydrogenase phosphatase, while myoinositolphosphoglycan mediator inhibits cyclic adenosine monophosphate–dependent protein kinase A.[43]

In hyperglycemic states, production of myoinositol increases to support insulin activity and to promote glucose uptake. Excretion of myoinositol also increases in hyperglycemia, and ultimately the combination of increased utilization and excretion leads to stores becoming depleted. Myoinositol depletion decreases insulin sensitivity and impairs glucose uptake.

Both D-chiro- and myoinositol have been used to treat polycystic ovary syndrome and infertility, with improvements in glucose tolerance, decreased serum androgens, and ovulation in this syndrome. It has not been extensively studied for other indications. Of note is a recent study examining the efficacy of myoinositol in the prevention of gestational diabetes. At 12–13 weeks of gestation, 220 pregnant women were randomized to myoinositol or placebo. The gestational diabetes mellitus rate was significantly reduced in the myoinositol group compared with controls, 14.0% versus 33.6%, respectively ($p = .001$; odds ratio 0.34; 95% confidence interval 0.17–0.68). This effect was confirmed by the fact that the HOMA-IR was also better in the inositol group.[44]

Linoleic Acid

Conjugated linoleic acid (CLA) is derived from linoleic acid and is present as both a *trans* fatty acid and a *cis* fatty acid. Research has suggested that CLA enhances weight loss by promoting adipose cellular apoptosis. While animal studies suggested that CLA decreases weight and fat mass, studies in humans have not been able to show a significant effect on body weight, body composition, or weight regain related to either of the CLA isomers.

A systematic review of CLA was done in 2012. The authors found 15 RCTs of CLA, but only 7 were included in the review. A meta-analysis revealed a statistically significant difference in weight loss favoring CLA over placebo (mean difference –0.70 kg; 95% CI –1.09, –0.32) and a small significant difference in fat loss favoring CLA (MD –1.33 kg; 95% CI –1.79, –0.86; $I(2) = 54\%$). The magnitude of these effects is small and less than convincing.[45]

Magnesium

Based on observational data, magnesium deficiency suggests low levels are associated with poor glucose control in people with overt diabetes. However, in clinical trials, supplementation of magnesium has not yielded clear evidence of any positive benefits in T2DM. Hruby et al., reporting from Framingham group, studied 2582 community-dwelling participants 26–81 years old with impaired fasting glucose

(≥ 5.6 to < 7.0 mmol/L) or impaired glucose tolerance (2-h postload glucose ≥ 7.8 to < 11.1 mmol/L), insulin resistance, or hyperinsulinemia. Over 7 years, those in the highest quintile for magnesium intake had a 47% reduction in the likelihood of progressive metabolic impairment or of developing frank diabetes compared to those in the lowest quintile.[46] The correlation was weakened when corrected for fiber intake, but persisted in those with metabolic abnormalities at baseline, lowering the risk of progressing to overt diabetes.

Momordica charantia (Bitter Melon)

The *Momordica charantia* (bitter melon) plant, grown in Africa, Asia, and South America, is known as "vegetable insulin." Efird et al.[47] published a review of the available trials on bitter melon and diabetes. The authors identified 21 clinical studies, but only 4 randomized studies were found, and just 1 trial was of high quality. In that single study, fructosamine decreased significantly after 4 weeks of intake of 2000 mg/d of bitter melon, compared with baseline levels. No change was seen in fasting glucose or 2-hour glucose tolerance measurements.[48] The Cochrane Collaborative also published a review. Three RCTs of up to 3 months were found with a total enrollment of 350 subjects. Only 1 study was peer reviewed. Two RCTs using 2 different preparations both showed no statistically significant differences in outcome measures compared to placebo.[49] Thus, the efficacy of *Momordica* is unproven.

Opuntia streptacantha (Nopal)

The prickly pear cactus or nopal cactus (*Opuntia streptacantha*) grows in desert regions of North America. It is commonly used in Mexican cooking and is used as a folk remedy by Mexican American individuals with diabetes. A study by Lopez Romero measured glucose tolerance in 7 normal persons and 15 with T2DM. Subjects were fed a high-carbohydrate breakfast or a breakfast high in soy protein, with both breakfasts given with and without nopal. Individuals with T2DM who consumed the high-carbohydrate breakfast plus nopal evidenced lower area under the curve for glucose (287 ± 30) than for those who consumed the breakfast with high-carbohydrate only (443 ± 49).[50]

Raspberry Ketone

Raspberry ketone is an aromatic compound derived from red raspberries (*Rubus idaeus*) and has some similarities to capsaicins and synephrines (see the discussion of bitter melon). One RCT has been reported in the literature; it used a proprietary product, Prograde Metabolism™ (METABO), containing 2000 mg of raspberry ketone, caffeine, bitter orange, ginger, garlic, cayenne, L-theanine, and pepper extract along with B vitamins and chromium.[51] Subjects were calorie restricted to 500 calories less than estimated needs and also exercised 60 minutes 3 times a week. During the 8-week study, the METABO group lost significantly more body weight than subjects taking the placebo, 1.9 kg versus 0.4 kg, and lost more fat mass. Results were reported for only 45 completers of 70 who enrolled in the study. No intent-to-treat analysis was done.

Trigonella foenum-graecum (Fenugreek)

Fenugreek (*Trigonella foenum-graecum*) is a member of the family Fabaceae, which includes beans, peas, and other legumes. Fenugreek is used in small amounts as a food flavoring and in traditional medicine in Asia to treat diabetes. The active compound in fenugreek is called *trigonelline* and supposedly lowers blood sugar. Recently, a glucagon-like peptide 1 receptor compound was isolated in fenugreek seeds.[52]

Neelakantan et al., in a recent review, identified 10 trials of fenugreek. Overall, fenugreek significantly lowered fasting blood glucose by –0.96 mmol/L (95% CI –1.52, –0.40; I^2 = 80%; 10 trials); 2-hour postload glucose by –2.19 mmol/L (95% CI –3.19, –1.19; I^2 = 71%; 7 trials); and HbA_{1c} by –0.85% (95% CI –1.49%, –0.22%; I^2 = 0%; 3 trials) as compared with controls.[53]

White Kidney Bean/Bean Pod (*Phaseolus vulgaris*)

White kidney bean or bean pod (*Phaseolus vulgaris*) is a legume from Latin America and is supposed to act as a fat blocker, like chitosan. In a RCT from Italy,[54] 60 overweight women aged 20–45 were given a 2000- to 2200-calorie meal plan and a pill with 445 mg dried aqueous extract of *Phaseolus vulgaris* (Phase 2 Starch Neutralizer IV) or a placebo once daily before eating a carbohydrate-rich meal. After 1 month, women in the interventional arm lost significantly more weight (mean weight loss 2.93 kg) than those receiving the placebo (mean weight loss 0.35 kg), lost more fat mass and adipose tissue thickness, and decreased their waist-hip-thigh circumference. Another small trail in the United States found no differences in outcome between treatment versus placebo. A third trial enrolled 124 subjects, with 117 completers, and used 1000 mg *Phaseolus vulgaris* 3 times per day before meals plus calorie restriction (500 kcal/d less than basal). The study found that those receiving *Phaseolus vulgaris* lost significantly more body weight (2.91 vs. 0.92 kg) and body fat (2.23 vs. 0.65 kg).[55] Open-label follow-up showed fairly good maintenance of weight loss.

Yohimbe (*Pausinystalia yohimbe*, Yohimbine)

Yohimbe (*Pausinystalia yohimbe, Pausinystalia johimbe*) is derived from the bark of an evergreen tree. Yohimbine is an adrenergic exerting agonist effects on α_2 receptor. It is promoted to enhance libido, in body building, and as a weight loss supplement. Yohimbine hydrochloride is sold as a prescription drug for erectile dysfunction. Pittler and Ernst[53] identified 3 trials of yohimbe, 2 negative and 1 positive. Yohimbe is considered potentially toxic, causing hypertension, headaches, anxiety, agitation, tachycardia, myocardial infarction, cardiac failure, and death. The toxic threshold has not been established. Yohimbe should not be recommended for weight loss. It should only be used under close medical supervision for the approved indication.

REGULATORY ISSUES AND BOTANICAL MEDICINES

The majority of Americans believe that over-the-counter drugs, vitamins, botanical products, and dietary supplements are subject to testing by the FDA, much like prescription drugs. In actuality, these alternatives are marketed without documentation of efficacy or safety because botanical medicines are not subject to the regulatory statutes that apply to pharmaceutical products. Potential defects in manufacturing include lack of standardization of active ingredients (if known); adulteration; contamination with heavy metals, dirt, and pesticides; and wide variation in constituents due to growing conditions and extraction techniques.

On March 29, 2015, Consumer Lab, an independent health and nutritional testing service, under the Freedom of Information Act obtained results from the FDA on inspections of 483 dietary supplement manufacturing facilities.[56] In 2014, of these sites, 62% received letters of noncompliance with "current good manufacturing practices" (cGMPs). Frequent infractions included failure to verify the identity of a dietary supplement ingredient and failure to establish specifications for identity, purity, strength, or composition of the finished product. In 2015, the Office of the Attorney General of New York State bought herbal products from 4 national retailers: GNC, Target, Walmart, and Walgreens. Four of 5 products tested using DNA bar coding, a genetic DNA fingerprint for plant type, contained traces of the herbs listed on the label.[57] Many products contained only filler agents, including rice powder, radish powder, legume powder, asparagus, and house plant material. In other states, attorneys general are stepping around the FDA and initiating their own fraud investigations. These states include Connecticut, the District of Columbia, Hawaii, Idaho, Indiana, Iowa, Kentucky, Massachusetts, Mississippi, New Hampshire, Pennsylvania, and Rhode Island.[58]

Private agencies have established testing programs to document and verify that supplements contain material specified on the label and that they are free of contaminants and adulterants. The US Pharmacopeia (USP) certifies products for quality, standardization, and purity. Verified products are listed on the USP website.[59] Consumer Lab also tests products at the request of manufacturers. Access to their list of verified products requires a nominal subscription fee.[60] Note that botanical medicines manufactured in Europe are subjected to more stringent regulation and testing than US products; therefore, brands from Germany, Switzerland, and the United Kingdom offer more consistent, higher-quality products.

ADVISING ON THE USE OF CAM

When a health care provider advises, recommends, or supports the use of a specific CAM remedy, even an over-the-counter product, that provider is judged to be a "learned expert" and legally is judged to hold responsibility and liability for poor outcomes. Selling and distributing supplements in one's office heightens the risk of liability. Because botanical medicines are exempt from the statutes that govern drug safety, the health care professional who recommends botanical medicine assumes most of the burden of liability should adverse outcomes occur. Practicing defensively may help to mitigate exposure to liability.

One should document the reason the patient wants to incorporate botanicals and supplements in a therapeutic regimen and research any possible drug-herb interactions before making recommendations. Patients should be given handouts about supplements. WebMD, Medline Plus, and other sites have well-researched monographs available online for patients. Patients must be duly warned about potential adverse events. Copies of handouts should be added to the patient's chart to document informed consent. Provide listings of quality products from reputable manufacturers or provide links to the US Pharmacopeia or Consumer Lab websites for lists of verified products. At follow-up visits, query and then document compliance, satisfaction, and any adverse events. Adverse events should be reported through MedWatch[61] or poison control.

Supplements should be stopped before any planned surgeries because many herbal/botanical medicines affect coagulation. Discontinue all supplements at least 4–6 weeks before any scheduled major surgical procedures. See Table 30-2 for a list of supplements known to affect clotting.

TABLE 30-2 Botanicals and Coagulation[a]

Salicylate-containing supplements
Black cohosh
Meadowsweet flower
Poplar bark or buds
Sweet birch bark
Willow bark
Wintergreen leave
Supplements inhibiting platelet function
Angelica
Bromelain
Cayenne fruit
Chinese skullcap root
Danshen
Dong quai
Feverfew
Fish oil
Garlic
Ginger
Ginkgo
Ginseng
Licorice
Papain
Policosanol
Pycnogenol (in smokers)
Red clover
Reishi and relshi fruit bodies
Resveratrol
Saw palmetto
Turmeric root
Tocopherols, mixed
Tocotrienols
Vitamin E

For a more definitive listing, please see Cordier W, Steenkamp V. Herbal remedies affecting coagulation: a review [review]. *Pharm Biol.* 2012;50(4):443–452. doi:10.3109/13880209.2011.611145. Epub 2011 Dec 2. PMID: 22136282.
[a]Botanicals that interfere with clotting and should be discontinued prior to surgery.

CONCLUSION

While some CAM therapies may affect weight and glycemic control, for most products convincing evidence of efficacy is lacking. The public also holds to the false belief that everything on the shelf in a health food store is subject to FDA scrutiny, testing, and approval. If information on efficacy is scant, information on safety is even more illusive. Products may carry substantial risks that are not easily identified. Due to a lack of regulatory oversight and inadequate reporting, it may take years for a dangerous supplement to be taken off the market. Ephedra, a popular weight loss product, was banned in 2004. The ban was initiated only after 155 deaths and 15,000 adverse events were recognized. These counts are probably underenumerated, given that fewer than 1 in 10 adverse reactions are reported, even for pharmaceuticals.[62] After the ban of ephedra, sales of products like green coffee bean extract or raspberry ketones surged, indicating the insatiable appetite people have for something, anything, to control overeating and obesity.

There is no magic bullet, no quick fix to this problem. Food is available everywhere, and we are constantly bombarded by advertisements inducing us to eat. This impels our patients to wander the aisles of the health food store on a quest for some illusory Holy Grail that promises weight loss without diet or exercise.

Calorie restriction, moderate exercise, and the judicious use of pharmaceuticals to treat metabolic disorders are parts of the only reasonable, reliable course for both providers and patients hoping to stave off the consequences of metS and obesity. The Diabetes Prevention Program[63] clearly demonstrated that lifestyle is as effective as or more effective than drug therapy in preventing the progression of metS. Lifestyle is also more cost effective.[64] Compared to the placebo, the cost per additional quality-adjusted life-year (QALY) totaled $1100 for the lifestyle intervention, versus $31,300 for treatment with metformin. All clinicians know the great inertia and resistance encountered when trying to motivate patients to eat less and move more. But, even small changes, like eliminating sugary beverages or walking 10 minutes 3 times a day, yield improvements in body mass and glycemic control.

In reviewing the clinical utility of supplements, a small number are safe, and a few may be effective. Advising patients to increase fiber intake—a simple, easy dietary change—may lead to modest weight loss and may also improve glycemic control and lipid profile. Fish oil and linoleic acid are probably safe, but whether they are effective for weight loss or glucose homeostasis is questionable. Magnesium is safe, but again its role in weight loss and glycemic control is unproven. More studies are needed to define the role of inositol in disorders of glucose and insulin metabolism. At least 20 trials are currently in progress[65] assessing the impact of inositol in women with gestational diabetes, infertility, and polycystic ovary syndrome. A large body of literature exists on the health benefits and relative safety of ginseng. More definitive research on glucose metabolism is pending, with 14 studies presently in progress looking at effects on insulin, glucose, and metS.[66]

REFERENCES

1. Bailey RL, Gahche JJ, Miller PE, Thomas PR, Dwyer JT. Why US adults use dietary supplements. *JAMA Intern Med.* 2013;173:355–361.

2. Blanck HM, Serdula MK, Gillespie C, et al. Use of nonprescription dietary supplements for weight loss is common among Americans. *J Am Diet Assoc.* 2007;107:441–447.

3. Evans JL, Bahng M. Non-pharmaceutical intervention options for type 2 diabetes: diets and dietary supplements (botanicals, antioxidants, and minerals). In: De Groot LJ, Beck-Peccoz P, Chrousos G, et al., eds. *Endotext.* South Dartmouth, MA: MDText.com; 2000– (updated March 4, 2014). http://www.ncbi.nlm.nih.gov/books/NBK279062/.

4. National Institutes of Health, Office of Dietary Supplements. Dietary supplements for weight loss: fact sheet for health professionals. https://ods.od.nih.gov/factsheets/WeightLoss-HealthProfessional/#en96.

5. Ríos JL, Francini F, Schinella GR. Natural products for the treatment of type 2 diabetes mellitus. *Planta Med.* 2015;81(12–13):975–994. doi:10.1055/s-0035-1546131. Epub 2015 Jul 1. PMID: 26132858.

6. Hsu CH, Liao YL, Lin SC, Hwang KC, Chou P. The mushroom *Agaricus blazei* Murill in combination with metformin and gliclazide improves insulin resistance in type 2 diabetes: a randomized, double-blinded, and placebo-controlled clinical trial. *J Altern Complement Med.* 2007;13(1):97–102. PMID: 17309383.

7. Stevinson C, MH, Ernst E. Garlic for treating hypercholesterolemia. A meta-analysis of randomized clinical trials. *Ann Intern Med.* 2000;133(6):420–429. PMID: 10975959.

8. Choi HC, Kim SJ, Son KY, Oh BJ, Cho BL. Metabolic effects of aloe vera gel complex in obese prediabetes and early non-treated diabetic patients: randomized controlled trial. *Nutrition.* 2013;29(9):1110–1114. doi:10.1016/j.nut.2013.02.015. Epub 2013 Jun 2. PMID: 23735317.

9. Food and Drug Administration. FDA issues regulation prohibiting sale of dietary supplements containing

ephedrine alkaloids and reiterates its advice that consumers stop using these products. http://www.fda.gov/NewsEvents/Newsroom/PressAnnouncements/2004/ucm108242.htm. Released February 6, 2004. Last updated March 29, 2013. Accesses November 3, 2016.

10. Stohs SJ, Preuss HG, Shara M. A review of the human clinical studies involving *Citrus aurantium* (bitter orange) extract and its primary protoalkaloid p-synephrine. *Int J Med Sci.* 2012;9(7):527–538. Epub 2012 Aug 29. PMID: 22991491. PMCID: PMC3444973.

11. Gurley BJ, Steelman SC, Thomas SL. Multi-ingredient, caffeine-containing dietary supplements: history, safety, and efficacy. *Clin Ther.* 2015;37(2):275–301. doi:10.1016/j.clinthera.2014.08.012. Epub 2014 Sep 26. PMID: 25262198.

12. USDA National Nutrient Database for Standard Reference, Release 26; Journal of Analytical Toxicology, 2006; Starbucks, 2014; Food and Chemical Toxicology, 2014; Keurig, 2014. Modified from http://www.mayoclinic.org/healthy-lifestyle/nutrition-and-healthy-eating/in-depth/caffeine/art-20049372. Accessed November 3, 2016.

13. Wang YH, Avula B, Nanayakkara NP, Zhao J, Khan IA. Cassia cinnamon as a source of coumarin in cinnamon-flavored food and food supplements in the United States. *J Agric Food Chem.* 2013;61(18): 4470–4476. doi:10.1021/jf4005862. Epub 2013 Apr 29. PMID: 23627682.

14. Leach MJ, Kumar S. Cinnamon for diabetes mellitus. *Cochrane Database Syst Rev.* 2012;(9):CD007170. doi:10.1002/14651858.CD007170.pub2. PMID: 22972104.

15. Allen RW, Schwartzman E, Baker WL, Coleman CI, Phung OJ. Cinnamon use in type 2 diabetes: an updated systematic review and meta-analysis. *Ann Family Med.* 2013;11(5):452–459. doi:10.1370/afm.1517.

16. Gades MD, Stern JS. Chitosan supplementation and fat absorption in men and women. *J Am Diet Assoc.* 2005;105(1):72–77. PMID: 15635349.

17. Jull AB, Ni Mhurchu C, Bennett DA, Dunshea-Mooij CA, Rodgers A. Chitosan for overweight or obesity. *Cochrane Database Syst Rev.* 2008;(3):CD003892.

18. Trumbo PR, Ellwood KC. Chromium picolinate intake and risk of type 2 diabetes: an evidence-based review by the United States Food and Drug Administration. *Nutr Rev.* 2006;64(8):357–363. PMID: 16958312.

19. Suksomboon N, Poolsup N, Yuwanakorn A. Systematic review and meta-analysis of the efficacy and safety of chromium supplementation in diabetes. *J Clin Pharm Ther.* 2014;39(3):292–306. doi:10.1111/jcpt.12147. Epub 2014 Mar 17. PMID: 24635480.

20. Tian H, Guo X, Wang X, et al. Chromium picolinate supplementation for overweight or obese adults. *Cochrane Database Syst Rev.* 2013;11:CD010063. doi:10.1002/14651858.CD010063.pub2. PMID: 24293292.

21. Onakpoya I, Posadzki P, Ernst E. Chromium supplementation in overweight and obesity: a systematic review and meta-analysis of randomized clinical trials. *Obes Rev.* 2013;14(6):496–507. doi:10.1111/obr.12026. Epub 2013 Mar 18. PMID: 23495911.

22. Banach M, Serban C, Sahebkar A, et al.; Lipid and Blood Pressure Meta-analysis Collaboration Group. Effects of coenzyme Q10 on statin-induced myopathy: a meta-analysis of randomized controlled trials. *Mayo Clin Proc.* 2015;90(1):24–34. doi:10.1016/j.mayocp.2014.08.021. Epub 2014 Nov 14. PMID: 25440725.

23. Suksomboon N, Poolsup N, Juanak N. Effects of coenzyme Q(10) supplementation on metabolic profile in diabetes: a systematic review and meta-analysis. *J Clin Pharm Ther.* 2015. doi:10.1111/jcpt.12280. [Epub ahead of print] PMID: 25913756.

24. Kolahdouz MR, Hosseinzadeh-Attar MJ, Eshraghian MR, Nakhjavani M, Khorami E, Esteghamati A. The effect of coenzyme Q10 supplementation on metabolic status of type 2 diabetic patients. *Minerva Gastroenterol Dietol.* 2013;59(2):231–236. PMID: 23831913.

25. Kuriyan R, Rajendran R, Bantwal G, Kurpad AV. Effect of supplementation of *Coccinia cordifolia* extract on newly detected diabetic patients. *Diabetes Care.* 2008;31:216–220.

26. Assunção ML, Ferreira HS, dos Santos AF, Cabral CR Jr, Florêncio TM. Effects of dietary coconut oil on the biochemical and anthropometric profiles of women presenting abdominal obesity. *Lipids.* 2009;44(7): 593–601. doi:10.1007/s11745-009-3306-6. Epub 2009 May 13. PMID: 19437058.

27. Henderson S, Magu B, Rasmussen C, et al. Effects of *Coleus forskohlii* supplementation on body composition and hematological profiles in mildly overweight women. *J Int Soc Sports Nutr.* 2005;2:54–62. doi:10.1186/1550-2783-2-2-54. PMID: 18500958. PMCID: PMC2129145.

28. Ma Y, Olendzki BC, Wang J, et al. Single-component versus multicomponent dietary goals for the metabolic syndrome: a randomized trial. *Ann Intern Med.* 2015;162:248–257. doi:10.7326/M14-0611.

29. Ma Y, Olendzki BC, Wang J, Persuitte GM, et al. Single-component versus multicomponent dietary goals for the metabolic syndrome: a randomized trial. *Ann Intern Med.* 2015;162(4):248–257. doi:10.7326/M14-0611. PMID: 25686165. PMCID: PMC4456033.

30. El Khoury D, Cuda C, Luhovyy BL, Anderson GH. Beta glucan: health benefits in obesity and metabolic syndrome. *J Nutr Metab.* 2012;2012:851362. doi:10.1155/2012/851362.

31. Onakpoya I, Posadzki P, Ernst E. The efficacy of glucomannan supplementation in overweight and obesity: a systematic review and meta-analysis of randomized

clinical trials. *J Am Coll Nutr.* 2014;33(1):70–78. doi:10.1080/07315724.2014.870013. PMID: 24533610.

32. Pittler MH, Ernst E. Dietary supplements for body-weight reduction: a systematic *Am J Clin Nutr.* 2004;79(4):529–536. PMID: 15051593.

33. Liber A, Szajewska H. Effect of oligofructose supplementation on body weight in overweight and obese children: a randomised, double-blind, placebo-controlled trial. *Br J Nutr.* 2014;112(12):2068–2074. doi:10.1017/S0007114514003110. Epub 2014 Oct 20. PMID: 25327394

34. Ferrari N. Making one change—getting more fiber—can help with weight loss. http://www.health.harvard.edu/blog/making-one-change-getting-fiber-can-help-weight-loss-201502177721. Posted February 17, 2015. Updated April 9, 2015.

35. Mayo Clinic. Nutrition and healthy eating. Chart of high-fiber foods. http://www.mayoclinic.org/healthy-lifestyle/nutrition-and-healthy-eating/in-depth/high-fiber-foods/art-20050948. Posted October 8, 2015.

36. Wu JH, Micha R, Imamura F, et al. Omega-3 fatty acids and incident type 2 diabetes: a systematic review and meta-analysis. *Br J Nutr.* 2012;107(Suppl 2): S214–S227. doi:10.1017/S0007114512001602. PMID: 22591895. PMCID: PMC3744862.

37. Hruby A, Yanai H, Hamasaki H, et al. Effects of intake of fish or fish oils on the development of diabetes. *J Clin Med Res.* 2015;7(1):8–12. doi:10.14740/jocmr1964w. Epub 2014 Oct 16. PMID: 25368695. PMCID: PMC4217746.

38. Mattes RD, Bormann L. Effects of (–)-hydroxycitric acid on appetitive variables. *Physiol Behav.* 2000; 71:87–94.

39. Onakpoya I, Hung SK, Perry R, Wider B, Ernst E. The use of garcinia extract (hydroxycitric acid) as a weight loss supplement: a systematic review and meta-analysis of randomised clinical trials. *J Obes.* 2011;2011:509038.

40. Baranov AI. Medicinal uses of ginseng and related plants in the Soviet Union: recent trends in the Soviet literature. *J Ethnopharmacol.* 1982;6(3):339–353.

41. Shishtar E, Sievenpiper JL, Djedovic V, et al. The effect of ginseng (the genus *Panax*) on glycemic control: a systematic review and meta-analysis of randomized controlled clinical trials. *PLoS One.* 2014;9(9):e107391. doi:10.1371/journal.pone.0107391. eCollection 2014. PMID: 25265315. PMCID: PMC4180277.

42. Blom WA, Abrahamse SL, Bradford R, et al. Effects of 15-d repeated consumption of *Hoodia gordonii* purified extract on safety, ad libitum energy intake, and body weight in healthy, overweight women: a randomized controlled trial. *Am J Clin Nutr.* 2011;94(5): 1171–1181. doi:10.3945/ajcn.111.020321. Epub 2011 Oct 12. PMID: 21993434.

43. Cheang KI, Essah P, Nestler JE. A paradox: the roles of inositolphosphoglycans in mediating insulin sensitivity and hyperandrogenism in the polycystic ovary syndrome. *Hormones.* 2004, 3(4):244–251.

44. D'Anna R, Di Benedetto A, Scilipoti A, et al. Myo-inositol supplementation for prevention of gestational diabetes in obese pregnant women: a randomized controlled trial. *Obstet Gynecol.* 2015;126(2): 310–315. doi:10.1097/AOG.0000000000000958. PMID: 26241420.

45. Onakpoya IJ, Posadzki PP, Watson LK, Davies LA, Ernst E. The efficacy of long-term conjugated linoleic acid (CLA) supplementation on body composition in overweight and obese individuals: a systematic review and meta-analysis of randomized clinical trials. *Eur J Nutr.* 2012;51(2):127–134. doi:10.1007/s00394-011-0253-9. Epub 2011 Oct 12. PMID: 21990002.

46. Hruby A, Meigs JB, O'Donnell CJ, Jacques PF, McKeown NM. Higher magnesium intake reduces risk of impaired glucose and insulin metabolism and progression from prediabetes to diabetes in middle-aged americans. *Diabetes Care.* 2014;37(2):419–427. doi:10.2337/dc13-1397. Epub 2013 Oct 2. PMID: 24089547. PMCID: PMC3898748.

47. Efird JT, Choi YM, Davies SW, Mehra S, Anderson EJ, Katunga LA Potential for improved glycemic control with dietary *Momordica charantia* in patients with insulin resistance and pre-diabetes. *Int J Environ Res Public Health.* 2014;11(2):2328–2345. doi:10.3390/ijerph110202328.

48. Tongia A, Tongia SK, Dave M. Phytochemical determination and extraction of *Momordica charantia* fruit and its hypoglycemic potentiation of oral hypoglycemic drugs in diabetes mellitus (NIDDM). *Indian J Physiol Pharmacol.* 2004;48:241–244.

49. Ooi CP, Yassin Z, Hamid TA. *Momordica charantia* for type 2 diabetes mellitus. *Cochrane Database Syst Rev.* 2010;(2):CD007845. doi:10.1002/14651858. CD007845.pub2. Update in: *Cochrane Database Syst Rev.* 2012;8:CD007845. PMID: 20166099.

50. López-Romero P, Pichardo-Ontiveros E, Avila-Nava A, et al. The effect of nopal (*Opuntia ficus indica*) on postprandial blood glucose, incretins, and antioxidant activity in Mexican patients with type 2 diabetes after consumption of two different composition breakfasts. *J Acad Nutr Diet.* 2014;114(11):1811–1818. doi:10.1016/j.jand.2014.06.352. Epub 2014 Aug 12. PMID: 25132122.

51. Lopez HL, Ziegenfuss TN, Hofheins JE, et al. Eight weeks of supplementation with a multi-ingredient weight loss product enhances body composition, reduces hip and waist girth, and increases energy levels in overweight men and women. *J Int Soc Sports Nutr.* 2013;10(1):22. doi:10.1186/1550-2783-10-22. PMID: 23601452. PMCID: PMC3639826.

52. King K, Lin NP, Cheng YH, Chen GH, Chein RJ. Isolation of positive modulator of glucagon-like peptide-1 signaling from *Trigonella foenum-graecum* (fenugreek) seed. *J Biol Chem*. 2015. pii: jbc.M115.672097. [Epub ahead of print] PMID: 26336108.

53. Neelakantan N, Narayanan M, de Souza RJ, van Dam RM. Effect of fenugreek (*Trigonella foenum-graecum* L.) intake on glycemia: a meta-analysis of clinical trials. *Nutr J*. 2014;13:7. doi:10.1186/1475–2891–13–7. PMID: 24438170. PMCID: PMC3901758.

54. Celleno L, Tolaini MV, D'Amore A, Perricone NV, Preuss HG. A dietary supplement containing standardized *Phaseolus vulgaris* extract influences body composition of overweight men and women. *Int J Med Sci*. 2007;4(1):45–52. PMID: 17299581. PMCID: PMC1796956.

55. Grube B, Chong WF, Chong PW, Riede L. Weight reduction and maintenance with IQP-PV-101: a 12-week randomized controlled study with a 24-week open label period. *Obesity (Silver Spring)*. 2014;22(3): 645–651. doi:10.1002/oby.20577. Epub 2013 Sep 5. Erratum in: *Obesity (Silver Spring)*. 2014;22(10):2274–2275. PMID: 24006357.

56. ConsumerLab.com. Recalls and warnings. https://www.consumerlab.com/recall_detail.asp?recallid=10799. Posted March 30, 2015.

57. O'Connor A. New York attorney general targets supplements at major retailers. *New York Times, Well* blog. http://well.blogs.nytimes.com/2015/02/03/new-york-attorney-general-targets-supplements-at-major-retailers/?_r=1. Posted February 3, 2015.

58. O'Connor A. Safety of herbal supplements pulls prosecutors together. *New York Times, Well* blog. http://well.blogs.nytimes.com/2015/03/09/safety-of-herbal-supplements-pulls-prosecutors-together/. Posted March 9, 2015.

59. US Pharmacopeial Convention. Find USP verified dietary supplements. http://www.usp.org/usp-verification-services/usp-verified-dietary-supplements/verified-supplements.

60. ConsumerLab.com. Where to buy products. https://www.consumerlab.com/products.asp.

61. Food and Drug Administration. MedWatch: The FDA safety information and adverse event reporting program. http://www.fda.gov/Safety/MedWatch/. Last update August 19, 2016.

62. Hazell L, Shakir SA. Under-reporting of adverse drug reactions: a systematic review. *Drug Saf*. 2006;29(5):385–396. PMID: 16689555.

63. National Institutes of Health, National Institute of Diabetes and Digestive and Kidney Diseases. Diabetes Prevention Program. http://www.niddk.nih.gov/about-niddk/research-areas/diabetes/diabetes-prevention-program-dpp/Pages/default.aspx.

64. Herman WH, Hoerger TJ, Brandle M, et al. The cost-effectiveness of lifestyle modification or metformin in preventing type 2 diabetes in adults with impaired glucose tolerance. *Ann Intern Med*. 2005;142(5):323–332.

65. ClinicalTrials.gov. Search results: "inositol." https://clinicaltrials.gov/ct2/results?term=inositol&pg=5. Accessed March 30, 2016.

66. ClinicalTrials.gov. Search results: "inositol + glucose." https://clinicaltrials.gov/ct2/results?term=ginseng+glucose&Search=Search. Accessed March 30, 2016.

Menopause and Perimenopausal Issues

CHAPTER 31

Leah Kaufman, MD, FACOG

SCOPE OF THE ISSUE OF OBESITY IN THE MENOPAUSAL TRANSITION

Menopause is defined as the natural end to a woman's menstrual cycle at the average age of 51 years and ranging between 45 and 55 years.[1] This period of time may also be associated with physiologic symptoms, such as vasomotor symptoms or "hot flashes," mood lability, anxiety, depression, weight gain, insomnia, and fatigue. Many of these symptoms have been attributed to the menopausal transition secondary to a decline in ovarian function.[1] The percentage of obese individuals in our population can be assessed through the National Health and Nutrition Examination Survey (NHANES). The 2011–2012 survey data were assessed for body mass index (BMI) stratification[2]; they revealed that 33.9% of US adults aged 20 years and older were overweight, 35.1% were obese, and 6.4% were extremely obese, with a BMI greater than or equal to 40. These numbers jump significantly in the perimenopausal period. When assessed in the NHANES data set last so stratified in 2007 (showing no change in trends since 2003–2004), 41.1% of women aged 40–59 were obese compared to 30.5% aged 20–39 years. When evaluated by ethnicity, 53% of non-Hispanic black women, 51% of Mexican women, and 39% of non-Hispanic white women aged 40–59 were obese. Over age 60, these numbers increased to 61% for non-Hispanic black women but decreased to 37% for both non-Hispanic white and Mexican women.[3] Baseline obesity can affect many of the symptoms described as well as potentially affect the perimenopausal-to-menopausal transition.[1]

TIMING OF ONSET OF OBESITY

The physiology of menopause in all women surrounds the cessation of ovulation due to a loss of ovarian follicles, which in turn reduces ovarian production of estradiol, the most biologically active form of estrogen. This process then will cause an increase in circulating follicle-stimulating hormone (FSH) and a decrease in inhibin, which inhibits the release of FSH. The elevated FSH also increases the rate of follicular loss.[4] Menopause is reached when the follicular number reaches approximately 1000.[5]

There has been some debate regarding the impact of obesity on the timing of menopause. There are studies that discussed an increase in BMI as positively associated with a later onset of menopause, using elevation of hormonal levels as a marker for timing.[6,7] There are also as many studies that showed no association between BMI and age of menopause onset. One study showed a modest prolongation of the age of menopause from 50.1 years to 50.4 years but using a BMI of 21.9 and 26.2, respectively.[8] It is clear in these studies that current smoking was associated with an earlier age of menopause, and increasing parity delayed onset of menopause, but these are additional confounding factors in many of the studies in assessing obesity.[9,10] As the current existing data stand, obesity independent of smoking, parity, and exercise history cannot be associated with an early or late onset for timing of menopause. Newer studies looking at insulin resistance in conjunction with the metabolic syndrome rather than purely BMI cutoffs alone in comparison to age of final period or time of menopause seemed to show more of an association and may be the direction for further investigation.[11]

PERIMENOPAUSE, OBESITY, AND THE METABOLIC SYNDROME

Addressing perimenopausal and postmenopausal women with respect to their metabolic syndrome comorbidities rather than categorization purely by obesity class is clearly prudent given the fact that menopausal status alone is associated with a 60% increased risk of the metabolic syndrome even after adjusting for confounding factors, including age, BMI, household income, and activity. These factors include those listed in Table 31-1.

Postmenopausal women have an increase in total cholesterol, low-density lipoprotein (LDL), triglycerides, and lower high-density lipoprotein (HDL), with the greatest change in LDL during the perimenopausal-to-menopausal transition. Triglycerides also increase in the early postmenopausal period and are highly associated

TABLE 31-1 Features of the Metabolic Syndrome

1. Central obesity
2. Insulin resistance
3. Dyslipidemia
    a. Elevated triglycerides
    b. Small, dense LDL particles
    c. Reduced HDL
4. High blood pressure
5. Hypercoagulable state
6. Pro-inflammatory state

with increasing abdominal fat content and insulin resistance. Abdominal obesity is associated with hyperinsulinemia and type 2 diabetes risk.[12] During menopause, central obesity is greater as lipase activity is greater and response to lipolysis is lower. These changes result in decreasing estrogens, with the relative hyperandrogenism resulting in central obesity. Studies have shown such changes result in increased appetite, decreased exercise and lipolysis, as well as mood disorders, which are discussed further in this chapter.[13] The menopausal transition will increase the risk for all women for central obesity, relative insulin insensitivity, and dyslipidemia.

A high waist circumference, reflective of central obesity and low sex hormone-binding globulin (SHBG) level are independent risk factors for metabolic disease in the perimenopausal transition.[14] Cutoffs for morbidity of elevated risk for waist circumference is generally seen above 35 inches in women when compared with women with waist sizes of 28 inches or less. This risk translates to an increase in cardiovascular and cancer risk in these patients. Waist circumference has also been observed to increase in the perimenopause.[15] The woman who enters menopause with preexisting central obesity and underlying baseline comorbidities will have a greater risk that will be further exacerbated with further weight gain.

PERIMENOPAUSE AND ASSESSMENT FOR ENDOMETRIAL CANCER

In the obese as well as nonobese woman, the perimenopausal variation in hormonal function may cause irregular vaginal bleeding. In the obese perimenopausal patient, a decrease in progesterone in addition to an increase in androstendione conversion to estrone and decreased SHBG further exacerbate this pattern.[16] While the average woman has a lifetime risk of endometrial cancer of 3%, the risk is doubled in overweight women (BMI > 25 to <29.5) and redoubled in obese women (BMI > 30). The same study that showed this increase also found a dose response to obesity exposure with increased risk of endometrial cancer in patients with persistence of obesity or magnitude of increase, with 35% weight gain in the 20s associated with a 10-year earlier diagnosis of endometrial cancer.[17] This enhanced risk is in part secondary to the increase in circulating estrone and estradiol levels from adipose tissue,[18] which is elevated by 40% in postmenopausal women with a BMI greater than 30.

The clinician must thus have a heightened awareness in this patient population and perform endometrial sampling as clinically indicated. Given the potential risk of anesthesia associated with patient habitus or comorbidities, including cardiovascular disease and sleep apnea, an office sample is preferred if technically possible. With an irregular bleeding pattern, an endometrial biopsy should be performed to rule out hyperplasia or cancer. For the perimenopausal patient with irregular bleeding and particularly in the obese patient, the first priority must be to rule out endometrial cancer. Some authors have suggested saline infusion sonography or transvaginal ultrasound on all such patients with irregular bleeding, but there are no endometrial thicknesses that consistently are predictive of hyperplasia or cancer in these patients. While intracavitary assessment is helpful in the diagnosis of other pathology, such as polyps or fibroids, sampling must be considered if the bleeding pattern is irregular in the perimenopausal patient, with risk further increased for the obese patient as outlined previously.[19]

When these patients are postmenopausal, sonographic assessment can be more useful. In a meta-analysis published by Timmermans et al. in 2010, studies evaluating various cutoffs for endometrial thickness in postmenopausal patients with vaginal bleeding were evaluated, revealing that it was a highly sensitive predictor for cancer of the uterus. At 4 mm, sensitivity was 94.8% with a specificity of 46.7%; at 5 mm, the sensitivity was 90.3% and the specificity was 54%; at 3 mm, sensitivity was increased to 97.9% but at a specificity of 35.4%.[20]

A joint practice bulletin released by the American College of Obstetricians and Gynecologists and the Society of Gynecologic Oncology recommended premenopausal patients be evaluated clinically outside of their sonographic findings and sampled as clinically appropriate. This is because of the lack of correlation between thickness and hyperplasia or cancer in patients in the perimenopause or premenopausal period. With postmenopausal patients, it is appropriate to start evaluation directly with endometrial biopsy or sonography.[21]

Treatment of the irregular bleeding with progesterone either continuous or cyclic oral or through a progesterone intrauterine device (IUD) should be considered.[22] For control of symptoms and treatment of the endometrium, the delivery system has been debated. In cases of endometrial hyperplasia in particular, a levonorgestrel-releasing intrauterine system (LNG-IUS) is more efficacious than oral treatment in the rate of regression of the lesion and is not dependent on regular patient administration.[23] Control of symptoms in the perimenopause can be achieved through the LNG-IUS through the menopausal transition, with cyclic progestins, or with low-dose oral contraceptive pills. For the obese patient with medical contraindications to oral contraceptives, a LNG-IUS may be the ideal choice. Depending on the severity of symptoms and the irregularity of cycles, with potentially very heavy flow and severe anemia associated with the hemorrhage when it does occur, treatment can improve patient quality of life, decrease risk of emergent hospitalization, and combat the risk of endometrial cancer.

INCIDENCE AND TREATMENT OF VASOMOTOR SYMPTOMS

Vasomotor symptoms are also encountered by approximately 65% of women transitioning through the menopause.[16] Women report vasomotor symptoms related to hypoestrogenism mainly in the first 5 years of menopause. As they progress through menopause, these symptoms become less pronounced, although symptoms unrelated to hormonal levels (e.g., arthralgias, myalgias, and insomnia) remain unchanged. There has been debate regarding whether obese women have more or less vasomotor symptoms during their transition. Several studies have shown that symptoms in obese women are both more frequent and increased over their counterparts with BMI less than 30.[24]

There appear to be multiple reasons why obese women have more symptoms that are tied to the changes in hormonal levels in the perimenopause and menopausal transition. Estradiol levels are higher in obese postmenopausal women, but the inhibin and estradiol levels are inversely related to BMI in the premenopausal years for the obese woman. As the inhibin levels are lower in obese patients, the FSH levels are more elevated in obese women during the perimenopause. These relative associations in the obese and normal-weight patient pre-, peri-, and postmenopause are demonstrated in Figure 31-1. Postmenopause, when the ovarian contribution of

FIGURE 31-1.
(A) Estradiol by menopausal stage
(*P* < .001). (B) FSH by menopausal stage
(*P* = .008). (C) Inhibin by menopausal stage
(*P* = .004). (From Freeman E, Sammel M, Lin H, Gracia CR. Obesity and reproductive hormone levels in the transition to menopause. *Menopause*. 2010;17:718–726.)

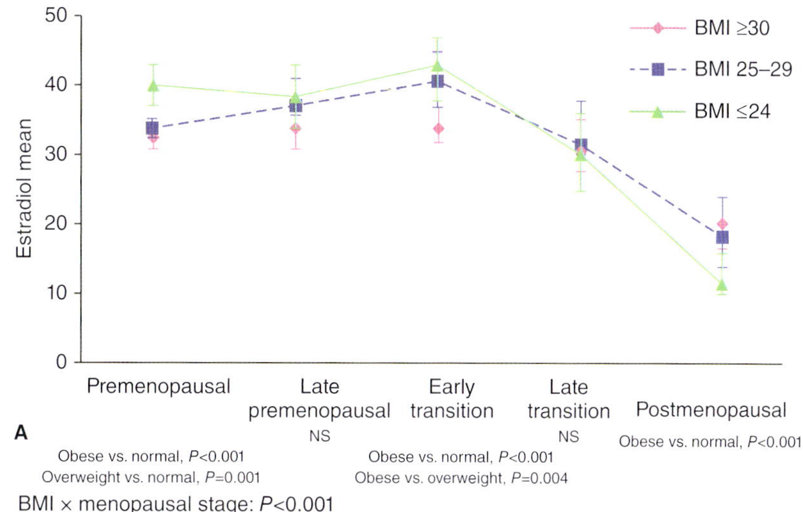

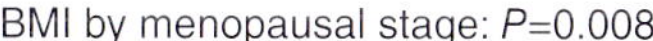

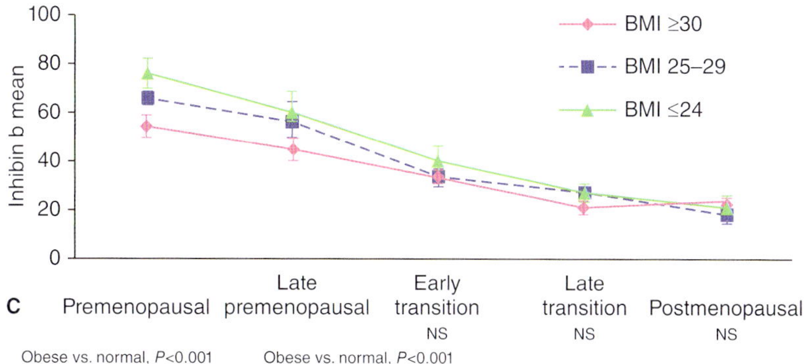

estrogen is greatly reduced, the peripheral conversion in adipose tissue accounts for the increase in levels in the obese over normal-weight woman.[25]

Huang et al. studied women who were overweight and obese at the transition to menopause, with BMI between 25 and 50. Approximately 50% of these patients described significant symptoms. A decrease in weight (on average 5.5 kg), decrease in BMI, and decrease in abdominal circumference over a 6-month period resulted in a significant reduction in vasomotor symptoms. This reduction of symptoms persisted when the authors controlled for use of oral or transdermal estrogens or selective serotonin reuptake inhibitors (SSRIs), thus suggesting that intensive patient counseling and even modest weight loss can have an impact on quality of life for these patients.[26]

If weight loss is not practical for these patients, hormone replacement therapy has been proven to be 75% efficacious relative to placebo for the treatment of vasomotor symptoms.[27] Many studies, however, excluded obese patients because of concern with respect to medical comorbidities; these success rates are thus not confined to our patient population of the peri- to postmenopausal female with a BMI greater than 30. Al-Safi and Santoro[28] published a list of contraindications to hormonal therapy. Although obese women may have endometrial cancer, venous thromboembolism (VTE), history of stroke or coronary artery disease, unexplained vaginal bleeding, or other problems outlined in Table 31-2, obesity itself was not a contraindication to the treatment of symptoms with hormones. An additional important consideration is that immobility is a contraindication to hormone therapy in these patients, and the obese patient may have limited mobility. A comprehensive review of the patient's history and status is essential to tailoring treatment to her symptoms and needs. In their review, Al-Safi and Santoro also outlined that, given the likely comorbid conditions in these patients, the avoidance of smoking, reduction of alcohol intake, and dressing in layers may all provide an improvement in symptomatic relief.

Serotonin overloading the receptor site at the hypothalamus, affecting thermoregulation, is one of the proposed mechanisms for vasomotor symptoms in the peri- and postmenopausal patient. Targeting treatment at this site may be an effective means of symptomatic relief. SSRIs such as paroxetine and fluoxetine and SNRIs (selective serotonin-norepinephrine reuptake inhibitors) such as venlafaxine have been shown

TABLE 31-2 Contraindications to Hormonal Therapy[a]

- History of breast or endometrial cancer
- Atypical ductal hyperplasia of the breast
- History of venous thromboembolic disease
- History of coronary artery disease or stroke
- Unexplained vaginal bleeding
- Uncontrolled hypertension
- Migraine headaches (may increase risk of stroke)
- Active liver disease (decreases estrogen metabolism)
- Immobilization
- Active gallbladder disease
- Porphyria (may be exacerbated)
- Hypertriglyceridemia (may increase venous thromboembolic disease)

[a]Data from Al-Safi ZA, Santoro N. Menopausal hormone therapy and menopausal symptoms. *Fertil Steril.* 2014;101:905–915.

to provide approximately 62% and 61% reduction, respectively, in vasomotor symptoms when compared with placebo. Efficacious dosing for venlafaxine ranges from 37.5 to 75 to 150 mg per day.[28] Specifically, there was a reduction in symptoms by 62.2% and 64.4% in the patients taking 12.5 or 25 mg of paroxetine, respectively, when taken over 6 weeks when compared to a 37.8% reduction in patients on placebo. This study focused on patients who were postmenopausal and did not select for BMI. The relative efficacy and range of included BMIs was not reported. The main side effects cited were a dose-dependent headache, nausea, and sleep disturbance.[29] The side effect of decreased libido that concerns many of our peri- and postmenopausal patients does not appear to be an issue with treatment at doses for vasomotor symptoms but rather of concern in the range for depressive symptoms.

Clonidine, by reducing hypothalamic norepinephrine levels and peripheral vascular reactivity, is another nonhormonal option for the treatment of vasomotor symptoms. Doses range from 0.025 to 0.075 mg twice daily for the oral treatment to 0.1 mg per day for the transdermal treatment, with results showing a 34% reduction in symptoms compared to 24% for placebo.[29] One benefit in this selection for the obese patient is the potential for improvement of any comorbid mild hypertension while improving symptoms. In selection of delivery systems, while no studies of efficacy in these patients with either oral and transdermal clonidine exist, newer randomized studies of oral contraceptives looked at relative efficacy in obese patients. Kaunitz et al. randomized 1500 patients to the transdermal patch versus an oral contraceptive pill in a patient population that was 30% obese, and the BMI range went to 60. The study showed equal efficacy for these obese patients with the transdermal delivery system.[30] A trial of transdermal delivery, if preferable to the patient, is thus reasonable for these patients.

Gabapentin is another nonhormonal treatment for vasomotor symptoms, with a 45% reduction in symptoms compared to 29% reduction in symptoms for use of placebo. The main side effects seen were dizziness and drowsiness. Central action in the hypothalamus is also hypothesized as the mechanism of action for gabapentin. For patients with an issue of sleep disturbance associated with restless leg syndrome, gabapentin may be an ideal nonhormonal selection as it appears to improve these symptoms.[29] With respect to safety in the obese patient, gabapentin has been used in patients undergoing weight reduction surgery to control perioperative pain, with safety and efficacy in studies where the minimal BMI cutoff was 40.[31]

DEPRESSION IN OBESITY AND MENOPAUSE

Perimenopausal and menopausal women also have a higher risk of symptoms of depression and anxiety, which has been linked to obesity. As with many of the studies on obesity, eliminating level of physical activity as a confounding factor is difficult, but this is clearly an issue that needs to be addressed with the obese perimenopausal patient.[1] An approach to this issue through counseling, activity modification, and exercise should be considered. Many of the pharmacologic treatments used here (as well as for vasomotor symptoms), such as SSRIs or NSRIs, may exacerbate the weight gain seen in the perimenopausal period.[32] As outlined previously, such an increase in weight gain could further worsen symptoms of depression and anxiety, and proper monitoring of a patient's weight in addition to symptomatology with follow-up is essential.

DIRECTIONS FOR FUTURE RESEARCH

There appear to be modest direct associations between elevated BMI and age to last menses, but these are based on studies where the comparisons are in patients with a BMI of 21.9 versus 26.2. When looking at multiple studies, the associations are inconsistent, seeming to be more likely associated with insulin resistance and the metabolic syndrome. One potential area for future research would be to evaluate the age at last period in women of normal, obese, and morbidly obese BMIs with and without impaired glucose tolerance. This would further assist in counseling patients with respect to expectations for menopause and cancer risk in this already high-risk population.

An additional area of needed research is that of expansion of evaluation of efficacy and safety of the medications used for vasomotor symptoms in the obese patient population. Most of what is found with respect to safety is extrapolated from the anesthesia and bariatric patient data and transposed with efficacy from normal-weight counterparts. Relative efficacy and dosing trials done for vasomotor symptoms with patients who have morbid obesity (BMI > 40) are needed to most effectively care for these women.

SUMMARY

There are thus many clear physiologic reasons for an increase in symptomatology for the perimenopausal obese patient, the treatments for which can make a tremendous difference in quality of life. Continued monitoring for further weight gain and depressive symptoms is essential in these patients, as is full understanding of their comorbid conditions. Obesity alone should not be considered a contraindication for the medical treatment of perimenopausal symptoms. The practitioner caring for the peri- and postmenopausal obese woman must also have heightened awareness of their increased risk of endometrial cancer and have a low threshold for testing when symptomatology arises. Simple interventions in all of these areas can have a tremendous impact on these patients.

REFERENCES

1. Keller C, Larkey L, Distefano JK, et al. Perimenopausal obesity. *J Womens Health.* 2009;19(5):987–996.
2. Fryar C, Carroll M, Ogden C. Prevalence of overweight, obesity and extreme obesity among adults: United States, 1960–1962 through 2011–2012. National Cancer Center for Health Statistics. http://www.cdc.gov/nchs/data/hestat/obesity_adult_11_12/obesity_adult_11_12.htm. Accessed October 6, 2016.
3. Ogden CL, Carroll MD, McDowell MA, Flegal KM. *Obesity Among Adults in the United States—No Statistically Significant Change Since 2003–2004.* Hyattsville, MD: National Center for Health Statistics; 2007. NCHS data brief no. 1. http://www.cdc.gov/nchs/data/databriefs/db01.pdf. Accessed September 30, 2015.
4. Takahashi T, Johnson K. Menopause. *Med Clin North Am.* 2015;99:521–534.
5. Gold E. The timing of the age at which natural menopause occurs. *Obstet Gynecol Clin North Am.* 2011;38:425–440.
6. Reynolds RF, Obermeyer CM. Age at natural menopause in Spain and the United States: results from the DAMES project. *Am J Hum Biol.* 2005;17:331–340.
7. Greendale G, Hogan P, Kritz-Silverstein D, et al. Age at menopause in women participating in the postmenopausal estrogen/progestins interventions (PEPI) trial: an example of bias introduced by selection criteria. *Menopause.* 1995;2:27–34.
8. Akahoshi M, Soda M, Nakashima E, et al. The effects of body mass index on age at menopause. *Int J Obes.* 2002;26:961–968.
9. Bromberger JT, Matthews KA, Kuller LH, et al. Prospective study of the determinants of age at menopause. *Am J Epidemiol.* 1997;145:124–133.

10. Den Tonkelaar I, Seidell J. Fat distribution in relation to age, degree of obesity, smoking habits, parity and estrogen use: a cross-sectional study of 11,825 Dutch women participating in the DOM project. *Int J Obes.* 1990;14:753–761.

11. Sowers M, McConnell D, Yosef M, et al. Relating smoking, obesity, insulin resistance, and ovarian biomarker changes to the final menstrual period. *Ann N Y Acad Sci.* 2010;1204:95–103.

12. Carr M. The emergence of the metabolic syndrome with menopause. *J Clin Endocrinol Metab.* 2003;88:2404–2411.

13. Teede H, Lombard C, Deeks A. Obesity, metabolic complications and the menopause: an opportunity for prevention. *Climacteric.* 2010;13:203–209.

14. Janssen I, Powell LH, Crawford S, et al. Menopause and the metabolic syndrome: the study of women's health across the nation. *Arch Intern Med.* 2008;168:1568–1575.

15. Zhang C, Rexrode KM, van Dam RM, et al. Abdominal obesity and the risk of all-cause, cardiovascular, and cancer mortality: 16 years of follow up in US women. *Circulation.* 2008;117:1658–1667.

16. Zhang Y, Lui H, Yang S, et al. Overweight, obesity and endometrial cancer risk: results from a systematic review and meta-analysis. *Int J Biol Markers.* 2014;29:e21–e29.

17. Lingeng L, Risch H, Irwin M, et al. Long-term overweight and weight gain in early adulthood in association with risk of endometrial cancer. *Int J Cancer.* 2011;129:1237–1243.

18. Cauley JA, Gutai JP, Kuller LH, Ledonne D, Powell JG. The epidemiology of serum sex hormones in postmenopausal women. *Am J Epidemiol.* 1989;129:1120–1131.

19. Diagnosis of abnormal uterine bleeding in reproductive aged women. Practice bulletin no. 128. American College of Obstetricians and Gynecologists. *Obstet Gynecol.* 2012;120:197–206.

20. Timmermans A, Opmeer B, Khan K, et al. Endometrial thickness measurement for detecting endometrial cancer in women with postmenopausal bleeding: a systematic review and meta-analysis. *Obstet Gynecol.* 2010;116:160–167.

21. Endometrial cancer. Practice bulletin no. 149. American College of Obstetricians and Gynecologists and Society of Gynecologic Oncologists. *Obstet Gynecol.* 2015;125:1006–1026.

22. Yoo H, Lee M, Ko Y, et al. The efficacy of the levonorgestrel-releasing intrauterine system in perimenopausal women with menorrhagia or dysmenorrhea. *Arch Gynecol Obstet.* 2012;285:161–166.

23. Hashim H, Zayed A, Ghayaty E, et al. LNG-IUS treatment of non-atypical endometrial hyperplasia in perimenopausal women: a randomized controlled trial. *J Gynecol Oncol.* 2013;24:128–134.

24. Da Fonsca A, Bagnoli V, Souza M. Impact of age and body mass on the intensity of menopausal symptoms in 5968 Brazilian women. *Gynecol Endocrinol.* 2013;29:116–118.

25. Freeman E, Sammel M, Hui Lin, et al. Obesity and reproductive hormone levels in the transition to menopause. *Menopause.* 2010;17:718–726.

26. Huang A, Subak L, Wing R, et al. An intensive behavioral weight loss intervention and hot flushes in women. *Arch Intern Med.* 2010;170:1161–1167.

27. Maclennen A, Broadbent J, Lester S, et al. Oral oestrogen and combined oestrogen/progestin therapy versus placebo for hot flushes. *Cochrane Database Syst Rev.* 2004;(4);CD002978.

28. Al-Safi Z, Santoro N. Menopausal hormone therapy and menopausal symptoms. *Fertil Steril.* 2014;101:905–915.

29. Stearns V, Beebe K, Iyengar M, et al. Paroxetine: controlled release in the treatment of menopausal hot flashes. A randomized controlled trial. *JAMA.* 2003;289:2827–2834.

30. Kaunitz A, Portman D, Westhoff C, et al. Low-dose levonorgestrel and ethinyl estradiol patch and pill: a randomized controlled trial. *Obstet Gynecol.* 2014;123:295–303.

31. Hassani V, Abdolreza P, Nasim N, et al. The effect of gabapentin on reducing pain after laparoscopic gastric bypass surgery in patients with morbid obesity: a randomized clinical trial. *Anesth Pain Med.* 2015;5:e22372.

32. Davis SR, Castelo-Branco C, Chedraui P, et al. Understanding weight gain at menopause. *Climacteric.* 2012;15:419–429.

Perioperative Management of Obese Patients

Brian Thompson, MD

Dennis Brown, MD

INTRODUCTION

The Obesity Epidemic

The most widely used classification of obesity is the body mass index (BMI).[1] Between 1986 and 2000, the number of individuals with BMIs greater than 30, 40, and 50 kg/m^2 were reported to have doubled, quadrupled, and quintupled, respectively, in the United States.[2]

The Obesity Paradox

Obesity has long been considered to be a risk factor for poor outcomes from a variety of surgical procedures, yet recent studies of critically and chronically ill patients suggested that overweight and obese patients may paradoxically have better outcomes than "normal"-weight patients.[3] Mullen et al.[3] demonstrated, in a prospective multi-institutional risk-adjusted study of 118,707 patients undergoing nonbariatric surgery, that the highest rates of death occurred in the underweight and morbidly obese, and the lowest rates were found in the overweight and moderately obese patients. This study revealed that there was a progressive increase in the likelihood of a complication with increasing BMI that was almost entirely due to increasing rates of infection. They hypothesized that metabolic regulation and immune response are highly integrated. Malnourished patients have protein calorie malnutrition, which impairs immunologic response mechanisms; obese patients are known to have a low-grade inflammatory response, which primes their immune system.[3]

PREOPERATIVE EVALUATION AND PREPARATION

Despite emerging evidence of the "obesity paradox," there are recommendations for the preoperative evaluation and preparation of obese patients. The extent of the preoperative evaluation depends on the assessment of their surgical risk and the degree of surgery-specific risk.

Major surgery is accompanied by an increased demand for oxygen consumption. This places increased demands on the cardiorespiratory system.[4] If patients are unable to increase their oxygen delivery to meet these requirements, they have increased mortality.[5]

Patient Preoperative Surgical Risk

Preoperative risk assessment always starts with an in-depth history and comprehensive physical examination. Will the patient be able to tolerate the physiological stresses of the planned surgery? The American College of Cardiology and American Heart Association (ACC/AHA) have established clinical predictors of cardiac risk. Patients can be categorized as having minor, intermediate, and major risks. However, a more important predictor of risk is the patient's functional capacity. This assessment helps us understand how combined cardiopulmonary function will tolerate the stress of surgery. This can be readily ascertained using a simple set of questions adopted from the Duke Activity Status Index. This concept measures a patient's physiologic response by determining the metabolic equivalent tasks (METs). One MET is 3.5 mL/min/kg average resting oxygen consumption in a 70-kg, 40-year-old man.[4] The ACC/AHA guidelines state the patients with exercise tolerance of greater than 4 METs may proceed to major surgery without further investigation.[4] Patients with poor exercise tolerance (<4 METs) have significantly greater cardiovascular and neurological complication (20.4% vs. 10.4%, $p < 0.001$).[6]

Surgical Procedure Risk

In addition to risk assessing the patient, one must risk adjust the surgical procedure. The ACC/AHA has classified procedures into high, intermediate, and low.[4] In this algorithm, risk is defined as the combined risk of cardiac death and nonfatal myocardial infection. Perhaps the most utilized predictor of postoperative death is the American Society of Anesthesiologists (ASA) scoring system.[4,7]

Preoperative Investigations

Ramaswamy et al.[8] investigated the efficiency of extensive preoperative testing in morbidly obese patients undergoing gastric bypass. They analyzed 193 patients who routinely had chest x-rays, arterial blood gas (ABG) tests, spirometry, electrocardiograms (ECGs), stress echoes, basic metabolic panel (BMP), complete blood cell counts (CBCs), coagulation profiles, thyroid function tests, and B_{12} and serum iron studies. Only 4% of chest x-rays showed abnormalities, none of which required preoperative intervention. Of the ECGs, 15% were abnormal, but none required preoperative intervention. Spirometry evaluations found 21% of patients had abnormalities. Preexisting asthma was predictive of obstructive physiology. BMI was predictive of restrictive physiology. ABGs identified 1 case of severe hypoxemia requiring intervention. Echo cardiography showed 2% abnormalities, and previous history of cardiac disease was the only risk factor. Routine CBCs did not identify 84% and 50% of the patients with iron and vitamin B_{12} deficiencies.

The authors[8] concluded that routine preoperative testing in these morbidly obese patients should include CBC, electrolyte, ECG, and anemia studies. Coagulation profiles, chest x-rays, cardiac stress tests, and pulmonary function tests should be performed based on patient history of bleeding tendencies and cardiopulmonary disease. Patients with major clinical predictors of risk (e.g., poor functional capacity and high surgical-specific risk) should be considered for more in depth preoperative testing.

POTENTIAL IN-DEPTH PREOPERATIVE TESTS FOR SUSPECTED HIGH-RISK PATIENTS

Echo Cardiography

Echo cardiography provides information concerning wall motility, valvular disease, and systolic and diastolic function. The ACC/AHA, however, has found that there is a poor correlation between ECG and a patient's functional capacity. Thus, it is not felt to be a consistent predictor of perioperative ischemic events.[9]

Exercise Electrocardiography

Exercise electrocardiography has been shown to have a sensitivity of 81% for multivessel coronary disease but a specificity of only 66%.[10] Patients with an estimated 7 METS or a heart rate greater than 130 without demonstrable ischemia are at low risk.[11]

Cardiopulmonary Exercise Testing (the Gold Standard)

Presently, most preoperative surgical patients have evaluation of either their cardiac or their pulmonary system in isolation. Inherently, it would seem that concurrent exercise testing of both systems would provide a more accurate assessment of the patient's ability to withstand the stress of surgery. Exercise testing requires that oxygen consumption and carbon dioxide production be measured while the patient exercises on a bicycle. The anaerobic threshold is determined, which is the point at which oxygen delivery is insufficient and anaerobic metabolism begins. A 12-lead ECG is simultaneously obtained to evaluate for ischemia and arrhythmia.[4] In major abdominal surgery, patients with aerobic thresholds less than 11 mL/kg/min have significantly higher mortality rates than those with higher aerobic thresholds (18% vs. 0.8%).[12]

PULMONARY RISK FACTORS REQUIRING IN-DEPTH PREOPERATIVE EVALUATIONS

Obstructive sleep apnea (OSA), obesity hypoventilation syndrome (OHS), and pulmonary hypertension (PH) are gaining increasing recognition as pulmonary risk factors for patients undergoing noncardiac surgery.[13]

Obstructive Sleep Apnea

Young et al. estimated the prevalence of OSA with an apnea-hypopnea index (AHI). The apnea-hypopnea index is defined as the number of apneic and hypopnea events that occur per hour of sleep. The prevalence of OSA with an AHI of 15 or higher in patients aged 30–69 with a BMI greater than 40 is noted to be 42%–55% for men and 16%–24% for women.[14]

Screening for OSA should start with questions about daytime sleepiness, heavy snoring and sudden awakening with the need to catch a breath, and apnea witnessed by a partner.[13] Hypertension; short, thick neck; BMI greater than 30; narrow oropharynx; and retrognathia may be found by physical exam.[13] Patients with a high suspicion for OSA should have polysomnography (PSG) to confirm or rule out the diagnosis.

Gupta et al., using PSG and pulse oximetry data for OSA diagnosis in 101 patients undergoing orthopedic surgery, found a statistically significant higher incidence of postoperative serious complications which include intensive care unit [ICU] days, reintubations, and cardiac events (24 vs. 9 complications, $p = .004$) and hospital length of stay (6.8 vs. 5.1 days, $p < .007$).[15] Other studies involving patients undergoing noncardiac surgery have confirmed that patients with OSA have a higher incidence of postoperative hypoxemia ($p = .009$), overall complications ($p = .003$), unplanned ICU transfer ($p = .069$), and longer hospital length of stay ($p = .049$) compared to controls.[13]

When using general anesthesia, the possibility of difficult intubation and induction should be considered. Use of ASA guidelines for management of the difficult airway may be necessary.[16] Extubation should be considered only after full reversal of neuromuscular blockade. Because patients with OSA are more prone to perioperative oxygen desaturation, opioids should be minimized. Intravenous acetaminophen, tramadol, pregabalin, and cyclooxygenase 2 (COX-2) inhibitors have been useful in postoperative opioid-sparing protocols. The patients' continuous positive airway pressure (CPAP) apparatus and settings should be instituted as soon as possible postoperatively to avoid airway obstruction and desaturation. A 16% absolute risk reduction in the rate of respiratory failure was reported in a bariatric surgery population with the use of noninvasive ventilation during the first 48 hours after extubation.[17]

Obesity Hypoventilation Syndrome

Obesity hypoventilation syndrome is characterized by the triad of chronic daytime hypercapnia ($PaCO_2 > 45$ mm Hg), sleep disordered breathing, and obesity with a BMI greater than 30 kg/m^2.[18] To compensate for chronic respiratory acidosis, patients with

OHS have high serum bicarbonate levels. Patients with known OSA and high serum bicarbonate levels should be considered for the diagnosis of OHS.

Mortality as high as 23% has been reported in untreated patients with OHS compared to 9% in matched obese cohorts.[19] Because of the chronic hypercapnia, these patients have blunting of their respiratory drive and have a high risk of respiratory failure after elective surgery (44.4% vs. 2.6% in controls).[20]

The perioperative management of these patients is similar to patients with OSA. Preparation for a possible difficult intubation, full reversal of neuromuscular blockage, opioid sparing, and early use of CPAP should be considered. In patients for whom the positive airway pressure settings are not known, an empiric inspiratory positive airway pressure of 16–18 cm H_2O and expiratory airway pressure of 9–10 cm H_2O can be initiated.[21]

Pulmonary Hypertension

Symptoms and signs of PH evolve slowly over time. Initially, patients experience subtle exertional dyspnea and fatigue. Eventually, exertional chest pain, syncope, peripheral edema, ascites, and pleural effusion may be present.[22]

Chest x-ray may reveal enlargement of central pulmonary arteries with attenuation of peripheral vessels. The ECG may have evidence of right ventricular hypertrophy, an R wave/S wave ratio that is greater than 1 in lead V, and right bundle branch block. Echocardiography can estimate the pulmonary artery pressure and assess right ventricular size, thickness, and function. However, the definitive diagnosis of PH requires right heart catheterization. PH is confirmed when the mean pulmonary artery pressure is greater than 25 mm Hg at rest or greater than 30 mm Hg during exercise.[14] PH is classified by the World Health Organization into groups based on etiologies of left heart disease, chronic lung disease, chronic thromboembolic disease, and unclear multifactorial mechanisms.[22]

PERIOPERATIVE RISK IN PATIENTS WITH PULMONARY HYPERTENSION

Kaw et al. confirmed that patients with PH undergoing elective noncardiac surgery were more likely than non-PH patients to develop congestive heart failure ($\#p < .001$), hemodynamic instability ($p < .002$), sepsis ($p < .005$), and respiratory failure ($p < .004$).[23] These patients also had longer ICU stays ($p < .04$), a higher 30-day readmission rate ($p < .008$), and longer mechanical ventilation ($p < .002$).

Risk Reduction Strategies in Patients with Pulmonary Hypertension

Perioperative pulmonary artery catheter monitoring allows for accurate measurement of pulmonary artery pressure, mixed venous oxygen saturation, cardiac output, central venous pressure (CVP), and pulmonary capillary wedge pressure. This information can be used to guide administration of fluids and vasopressors.[13] General anesthesia is most commonly used in patients with PH. Spinal anesthesia is usually avoided due to its profound sympatholytic effect.[13] Key factors in the intraoperative management of these patients is to avoid hypertension, hypothermia, and acidosis.[13] Refraction hypotension can be managed by prompt intra-aortic balloon counterpulsation, left ventricular assist device, or extracorporeal membrane oxygenation.[24]

SURGICAL SITE INFECTION REDUCTION STRATEGIES

Perioperative plans to reduce surgical site infections (SSIs) should be utilized for all weight classes. Surgical infections result from a complex set of factors, and addressing just one issue will not result in the desired reductions. Developing a process of care across the preoperative, intraoperative, and postoperative spectra of care will yield the best results. Standardized SSI protocols that reduce variations in the process of care have been utilized to reduce superficial, deep, and organ space infections.

Surgical Site Infection Bundle

Surgical infections result from an interplay of bacterial dose, bacterial virulence, and host resistance.

$$SSI = \frac{Bacterial\ dose \times Bacterial\ virulence}{Host\ Resistance}$$

Other than antimicrobial stewardship, there is little one can do to affect bacterial virulence. For this reason, most SSI bundles have concentrated on reducing bacterial bioburden and increasing host resistance.

Preoperative Measures to Reduce SSI

Preoperative patient education should be a cornerstone of any SSI bundle. Patients should be made to understand that they have responsibilities to stop smoking and if diabetic to optimize their glycemic control. Preoperative skin hygiene with chlorhexidine gluconate showers or wipes will reduce skin bioburden and may be a part of a colony reduction program for methicillin-resistant *Staphylococcus aureus* (MRSA). If a complex gynecologic tumor reduction procedure is planned, consideration of a preoperative oral antibiotic, mechanical bowel prep should be considered. If the patient is protein calorie malnourished, it may be possible to improve the patient's nutrition with dietary supplements. In severely malnourished patients, should preoperative hyperalimentation be employed until the patient's serum albumin has improved? If the patient is immune suppressed, for example, is receiving high doses of steroids, is it possible to taper or discontinue the patient's steroids? These questions have not been answered fully and will require further studies to determine what a best practice is.

PERIOPERATIVE GLYCEMIC CONTROL

Diabetes mellitus affects 8.3% of the US population.[25]) Abdelmolak et al. retrospectively reviewed records of 35,000 patients who received noncardiac surgery and found that 21% of those without a diagnosis of diabetes were hyperglycemic, and approximately half of those had undiagnosed diabetes.[26]

In 2012, the Endocrine Society published clinical practice guidelines. They recommended blood glucose testing in all patients on admission to the hospital (including admissions for surgery), regardless of diabetic status, and further monitoring of nondiabetics with blood glucose levels greater than 140 mg/dL. These patients and all diabetics (who have not had hemoglobin A_{1c} [HbA_{1c}] testing in the previous 2–3 months) should have HbA_{1c} determination.[27]

It is postulated that hyperglycemia is associated with increased production and impaired scavenging of reactive oxygen species,[28] polymorphonuclear neutrophil dysfunction,[29] and decreased intracellular killing.[30,31]

Many studies have been published linking preoperative and intraoperative hyperglycemia to poor outcomes. Noordzij et al.[32] found that preoperative blood glucose levels greater than 200 mg/d were associated with a 2.1-fold increased risk of overall mortality and 4-fold increased cardiovascular mortality risk.

Current data offer no concrete guidance on whether an elective procedure should be cancelled in light of a given level of hyperglycemia.[33] It would seem reasonable not to cancel surgery if the patient has mild-to-moderate hyperglycemia. Cancelling surgery may be considered if the serum glucose is above 350 mg/dL or the patient displays ketoacidosis.[34,35] The triad of hyperglycemia (blood glucose > 250 mg/dL), acidosis (arterial pH < 7.3, serum bicarbonate < 18 mg/L, anion gap > 10), and ketonemia (urine and serum ketone positive) strongly support the diagnosis of ketoacidosis.[36]

Collectively, both diabetics and hyperglycemic nondiabetics should be treated, perhaps with different blood glucose targets; there is evidence that treating hyperglycemia may be more beneficial for nondiabetics compared with diabetics.[33] Currently, at our institution, preoperative surgery patients receive a blood glucose test, and known diabetics receive blood sugar and HbA_{1c} (if not determined within previous 2–3 months) tests on arrival to the preoperative testing area. If the fasting blood sugar is above 100 our diabetes management team is notified. A team member communicates with the patient, primary care physician, anesthesiologist, and surgeon in an effort to develop a plan for preoperative and intraoperative glycemic control. Our goal is to keep the intraoperative and postoperative blood sugars less than 180 mg/dL. Tight glucose control (80–110 mg/dL) has not been shown to improve outcomes.[35] We encourage intravenous insulin drips and discourage sliding scale insulin protocols. Basal/bolus insulin protocols are then developed in the postanesthesia care unit by a collaboration of our clinical diabetic educators (glycemia "swat team") with the anesthesiologist and surgeon.

Our institution has adopted the Cleveland Clinic protocol for perioperative glucose control.[33]

INTRAOPERATIVE MANAGEMENT

Patient Safety Checklist

Intraoperative management of the patient begins prior to the surgery itself with the initiation of the patient safety checklist or "time-out." There are various patient safety checklists from different organizations. One example is the World Health Organization's Surgical Safety Checklist.[34] Use of this checklist begins prior to the induction of anesthesia, continues with a time-out prior to the skin incision, and then a final check occurs prior to the patient leaving the operating room. The WHO checklist is conveniently located on one placard. Institution of the WHO Surgical Safety Checklist was noted to decrease in-hospital complication rates. The decrease was noted to be significant, resulting in a reduction of complications from 19.9% prior to institution of the WHO checklist to 11.5% thereafter. In addition, a reduction in inpatient admission length of stay was noted.[35]

Antibiotic Prophylaxis

It is well known that the perioperative use of prophylactic antibiotics results in a decrease in SSI rates for cesarean sections. Recommended regimens include the use of a first-generation cephalosporin such as cefazolin given within 60 minutes of the start of surgery. For patients who have a significant allergy to cefazolin, then the use of clindamycin with an aminoglycoside would be appropriate.[36]

The timing of prophylactic antibiotics has also been reviewed. In a study involving 29 hospitals, for antibiotics requiring a short duration of infusion (e.g., with cefazolin), a decreased risk of SSI was noted if the prophylactic antibiotics were given within 30 minutes of the start of the surgery as compared to antibiotics given between 31 and 60 minutes prior to the start of surgery. They found a decrease, although not statistically significant, in SSIs from 2.4% to 1.6%.[37] Therefore, with antibiotics of shorter duration to administration, including cefazolin, there may be additional benefit of administration within 30 minutes of the start of surgery as compared to within 60 minutes.

The dosage of antibiotics in obese patients has also been evaluated. Secondary to the pharmacokinetics of obese patients, higher dosing of antibiotics for prevention of SSIs is indicated.[38] Recommendations for dosing of patients with cefazolin for those patients with a weight less than 120 kg is cefazolin 2 g IV given within 60 minutes of incision time. However, for patients who weigh greater than or equal to 120 kg, a higher dose is indicated. In these patients, cefazolin 3 g IV is given within 60 minutes of incision time.[38]

The redosing intervals of antibiotics for prevention of SSIs for lengthy surgical cases has also been reviewed. For cefazolin, a common antibiotic for obstetrical and gynecologic procedures, the half-life of cefazolin is noted to be 1.2 to 2.2 hours in adults who have normal renal function. Therefore, redosing of cefazolin is recommended, if surgery is still occurring, 4 hours from the start of the preoperative dose. The 4 hours is equivalent to approximately 2 half-lives of cefazolin. In patients who have a significant allergy to cefazolin, if clindamycin and gentamycin are utilized, dosing recommendations include clindamycin 900 mg IV with a redosing interval of 6 hours, if surgery is still occurring, based on a half-life of 2 to 4 hours in adults with normal renal function. For gentamicin, recommended dosing is 5 mg/kg given as a single dose. In addition, if a large amount of blood is lost at surgery, redosing is also recommended.[38]

Skin Preparation

Various solutions exist for disinfection of the skin to decrease the bacterial load and surface contamination at the site of the incision. These solutions include povidone-iodine, chlorhexidine gluconate, and alcohol-based solutions. A review of the literature provided differing results. A Cochrane review of 6 trials involving skin preparation at the time of cesarean section noted no statistical difference in wound infection or endometritis rates involving the various methods of skin preparation. In this review, there was no clear difference regarding which skin preparation was most effective in reducing infection rates.[39] However, in an evaluation of a skin preparation of chlorhexidine-alcohol versus povidone-iodine, chlorhexidine-alcohol was noted to have reduced rates of SSI in clean contaminated surgery. When 849 subjects were evaluated, the overall infection rate in the chlorhexidine-alcohol group was 9.5% compared to 16.1% in the povidone-iodine group.[40]

Preoperative Hair Removal

Preoperative hair removal has been evaluated for reduction of postoperative infection rates. A Cochrane review of 14 trials noted no difference statistically in the incidence of SSIs if preoperative hair removal was performed, although the number of participants in the studies were not sufficient for definitive conclusions.[41] In addition, it was noted that if hair removal is needed, clipping of the hair appears to result in fewer surgical infections when compared to hair removal via shaving of the skin.

Venous Thromboembolism Prophylaxis

Both obesity and surgery, as well as pregnancy, are risk factors for venous thromboembolism (VTE). Patients having surgery that is longer than 45 minutes in surgical length time should receive VTE prophylaxis.[42,43] For patients who are at moderate risk for a thrombotic event and are not at a high risk of bleeding, Gould et al.,[43] as well as the American College of Obstetrics and Gynecology, recommended a variety of methods, including the use of low molecular weight heparin, low-dose unfractionated heparin, as well as mechanical methods through the use of intermittent pneumatic compression.

Intraoperative Patient Warming

The avoidance of perioperative and intraoperative hypothermia cannot be overstated. Complications of perioperative hypothermia are many and include wound infection, reduced drug metabolism, and increased blood loss.[44] Clinical guidelines have been established for the management of perioperative hypothermia.[45] Intraoperative recommendations for assessment of perioperative hypothermia include the identification of risk factors for perioperative hypothermia, monitoring of the patient's temperature throughout the surgery, evaluation for any evidence of hypothermia during the surgical case, and communication with the surgical team of any findings.[45]

During the course of the surgery, Hooper et al.[45] recommended actions that include decreasing exposure of skin to lower temperatures as well as patient warming measures, which can include cotton blankets and surgical drapes. These would be considered passive warming procedures. In addition, the surrounding operating room temperature is recommended to be between 20°C and 25°C. It is also recommended that patient warming be instituted through forced-air warming if any or a combination of the following factors occur, for example: the surgery is longer than 30 minutes in duration, if the patient is at increased risk for hypothermia, or if the patient is hypothermic at the time of surgery. Alternatives may also be used. These would include warming of the intravenous fluids, warming of the irrigation fluids, as well as circulating water garments or mattresses.[45] Hooper et al.[45] have developed clinical care algorithms not only for intraoperative recommendations and interventions but also for the preadmission and preoperative time periods as well as the postoperative phase of patient care.

Retained Foreign Bodies at the Time of Surgery

The incidence of retained foreign bodies at the time of surgery has been estimated at 1 in 5500 surgeries based on a review at a tertiary care center.[1] Of these, the most common retained foreign body was a surgical sponge. This occurred for 68% of the incidents. In addition, the most common location of a retained sponge was the abdomen or pelvis. Other retained bodies included needles as well as a surgical instrument. Of note, 62% of the time the surgical count was correct. In addition, imaging intraoperatively for evaluation of a foreign body only detected a foreign body 67% of the time. Finally, it should be noted that the incidence of retained surgical needles was only 9% in their study.[46]

Obesity, defined as a BMI greater than or equal to 30, has also been noted to be a risk factor for retained foreign bodies at the time of surgery.[47] Al-Qurayshi et al.[47] noted that the highest frequency of retained foreign bodies was with gastrointestinal surgeries. Gynecologic procedures, cardiovascular surgeries, and musculoskeletal surgeries also had an increased frequency of retained foreign bodies. Of the patients with retained foreign bodies who were obese, obesity was only a risk factor for a retained foreign body if the patient had undergone abdominopelvic surgery.

SURGICAL MANAGEMENT

The surgical management of various hysterectomy techniques is important to consider in regard to the obese patient. Various methods for hysterectomy include abdominal, vaginal, and laparoscopic routes. Harmanli et al.[48] evaluated the effects of obesity on the abdominal hysterectomy route. Their study evaluated 357 women; of these, 172 were considered obese. The obese patients had a higher occurrence of hypertension and were more commonly of African American descent. In the obese patients, on average, operative time was 22 minutes longer; however, the duration of hospitalization was the same, at approximately 3 days, when compared to nonobese patients. The difference in the incidence of urinary tract injury, bowel injury, postoperative bleeding, as well as blood product transfusion rates between obese and nonobese patients was similar and not statistically significant. Interestingly, of statistical significance was a lower incidence of postoperative ileus in obese patients. The nonobese group had a higher incidence of postoperative ileus. Overall, there was no significant difference in outcomes of obese versus nonobese patients when performing a total abdominal hysterectomy.

Harmanli et al.[49] also reviewed vaginal hysterectomy and any obesity effects. They studied 324 patients who underwent vaginal hysterectomy. Of these, 149 were considered obese. The surgical indications for hysterectomy were similar for both obese and nonobese patients. For vaginal hysterectomies, the duration of surgery was not statistically different between obese and nonobese patients. Also, the duration of hospitalization was similar. In addition, the incidence of complications was similar for both obese and nonobese patients; complication incidence included the rate of urinary tract and bowel injury as well as conversion to laparotomy to complete the hysterectomy. Their conclusion was that there was no statistical difference in the outcomes, over the short term, when comparing obese and nonobese patients who underwent vaginal hysterectomy.

Isik-Akbay et al.[50] compared the effects of obesity on abdominal and vaginal hysterectomies. They studied 369 obese patients. As would be expected, there was a shorter hospitalization and shorter length of surgery for the hysterectomies performed via a vaginal approach. When complications were evaluated, there was a statistically increased incidence of postoperative fevers, wound complications, urinary tract infections, and ileus in the patients who underwent an abdominal approach as compared to a vaginal approach for hysterectomy. Their conclusion was to suggest a vaginal approach for hysterectomy.

The obesity effect has also been evaluated for the laparoscopic hysterectomy approach.[51,52] Morgan-Ortiz et al.[51] evaluated 209 patients who underwent a total laparoscopic hysterectomy; of these individuals, 50 patients were considered to be obese with a BMI greater than or equal to 30.[51] When comparing obese and nonobese patients, Morgan-Ortiz et al.[51] noted that the length of surgery for the obese patient subgroup undergoing laparoscopic hysterectomy was statistically longer as compared to patients with a normal BMI. However, the incidence of conversion to laparotomy to complete the surgery was similar among obese and nonobese patients, as was the duration of hospitalization. Surgical blood loss was greater for obese patients undergoing laparoscopic hysterectomy as compared to patients with a normal BMI of less than 25, although the difference in the amount of blood loss was not statistically significant between the two groups.

Harmanli et al.[52] also evaluated supracervical and total laparoscopic hysterectomies performed on obese patients. Harmanli et al.[52] noted a higher incidence of blood transfusion in the obese patient group undergoing laparoscopic hysterectomy. In addition, in their study, they noted a higher incidence of laparotomy conversion for hysterectomy completion in the obese patient subgroup. The incidence of urinary tract complications was similar in both obese and nonobese subgroups, and there were no bowel injuries noted in any group. However, when analysis was performed of subgroups of obese and nonobese patients undergoing total versus supracervical hysterectomy, differences were identified among the subgroups. The lowest incidence of urinary tract injuries was noted in the nonobese patient subgroup who underwent a supracervical hysterectomy as compared to an obese patient who underwent a total laparoscopic hysterectomy. The risk of urinary tract injury was 0.3% in the nonobese laparoscopic supracervical hysterectomy subgroup compared to 3.2% in the obese total laparoscopic hysterectomy subgroup.[53] In addition, the risk of serious complications, which included urinary tract injury, VTE, and vaginal cuff dehiscence, was the least (1.7%) in the nonobese laparoscopic supracervical hysterectomy group as compared to the subgroup of obese patients who underwent a laparoscopic total hysterectomy, where the incidence was noted to be 7.9%.[52]

POSTOPERATIVE MANAGEMENT

The postoperative management of the obese patient continues with the same guidelines and principles as intraoperative management. This includes postoperative patient warming in the recovery suite, continued glycemic control, and VTE prophylaxis. Early ambulation, aggressive pulmonary toilet, and early oral feeding are also encouraged. Finally, the care of the obese patient continues with appropriate discharge planning and follow-up.

SUMMARY

Obesity is considered a risk factor during surgical procedures. However, we do need to consider the obesity paradox, by which obese and overweight patients may have improved outcomes when compared to patients considered to have a normal weight.

The surgical management of obese patients begins in the office setting, when consideration begins for surgical management of the patients. This includes appropriate preoperative evaluation and preparation as well as the identification of surgical risk for the patient. Preoperative testing may include not only blood work but also testing specific to the surgical risk of the patient. This testing may include not only chest x-ray, cardiac stress testing, or pulmonary function tests, but also, if indicated, echo cardiography and exercise testing.

As practitioners, we must also recognize the importance of pulmonary risk factors, including OSA, OHS, and PH. As with all patients, reduction strategies for SSI, perioperative glucose control, as well as prophylactic antibiotics, VTE prevention, and choice of surgical route remain of great importance.

As the rates of obesity continue to increase, the perioperative management of the obese patient cannot be overstated.

REFERENCES

1. Poirier P, Giles TD, Bray GA, et al. Obesity and cardiovascular disease: pathophysiology, evaluation and effect of weight loss: an update of the 1997 American Heart Association scientific statement on obesity and heart disease from the Obesity Committee of the Council on Nutrition, Physical Activity and Metabolism. *Circulation*. 2006;113:898–918.
2. Sturm R. Increases in clinically severe obesity in the United States, 1986–2000. *Arch Intern Med*. 2003;163:2146–2148.
3. Mullen JT, Moorman DW, Davenport DL. The obesity paradox, body mass index and outcomes in patients undergoing non-bariatric general surgery. *Ann Surg*. 2009;250(1):166–172.
4. Jones C, Sritharon K, Abu Habsa M. Identification and management of perioperative cardiovascular risk. *Br J Hospital Med*. 2010;71(1):M12–M15.
5. Shoemaker WC. Cardio-respiratory patterns of surviving and non-surviving postoperative patients. *Surg Gynecol Obstet*. 1972;134:810–814.
6. Reitty DF, McNealy MJ, Doerner D, et al. Self-reported exercise tolerance and the risk of serious perioperative complications. *Arch Intern Med*. 1999;159:2185–2192.
7. Mangano DT. Perioperative cardio morbidity. *Anesthesiology*. 1990;72:153–184.
8. Ramaswamy A, Gonzalez R, Smith CD. Extensive preoperative testing is not necessary in morbidly obese patients undergoing gastric bypass. *J Gastrointest Surg*. 2004;8159–8165. doi:10.1016/j.gassur.2003.11.001.
9. Fleisher IA, Beckman JA, Brown KA, et al. ACC/AHA 2007 guidelines on perioperative cardiovascular evaluation and care for non-cardio surgery: a report of the American College of Cardiology/American Heart Association Task Force on Practice Guidelines. *Circulation*. 2007;116:c418–c500.
10. Detrano R, Giantressi R, Mulvihill D, et al. Exercise-induced ST segment depression in the diagnosis of multi-vessel coronary disease; a meta analysis. *J Am Coll Cardiol*. 1989;14:1501–1508.
11. Hollenberg SM. Pre-operative cardiac risk assessment. *Chest*. 1999;115:51S–75S.
12. Older P, Hall A, Hader R. Cardio pulmonary exercise testing as a screening test for perioperative management of major surgery in the elderly. *Chest*. 1999;116:355–362.
13. Bhatejice P, Kaw R. Emerging risk factors and prevention of perioperative pulmonary complications. *Sci World J*. 2014;2014:546758.
14. Young T, Peppard PE, Taheri S. Excess weight and sleep disordered breathing. *J Appl Physiol*. 2005;99(4):1592–1599.
15. Gupta RM, Parvizi J, Hanssen AD, Gay PC. Post-operative complications in patients with obstructive sleep apnea syndrome undergoing hip or knee replacement: a case-control study. *Mayo Clin Proc*. 2001;76(9):897–905.
16. Rosenblatt WH, Whipple J. The difficult airway algorithm of the American Society of Anesthesiologists. *Anesth Analg*. 2003;96(4):1233.
17. El Solh AA, Aqualina A, Pineda L, Dhanvantri V, Erant B, Bouquin P. Non invasive ventilation for presentation of post-extubation respiratory failure in obese patients. *Eur Respir J*. 2006;28(3):588–595.
18. Kaw R, Chung F, Pasupuleti V, Mehta J, Gay PC, Hernandez AV. Meta-analysis of the association between obstructive sleep apnea and post-operative outcome. *Br J Anesth*. 2012;109(6):897–906.
19. Nowbar S, Burkart KM, Gonzales R, et al. Obesity-associated hypoventilation in hospitalized patients: prevalence, effects and outcome. *Am J Med*. 2004;116(1):1–7.
20. Kaw R, Pasupuleti V, Walker E, et al. Obesity hypoventilation syndrome: an emergency and unrecognized risk factors among surgical patients. In: Proceedings

of the American Thoracis Society Annual Meeting; May 2001; Denver, CO.

21. Chan EH, Lam D, Wong J, Mokhlesi B, Chung F. Obesity hypoventilation syndrome: a review of epidemiology, pathophysiology and perioperative considerations. *Anesthesiology*. 2012;117:188–205.

22. Rubin L, Hopkins W, Mandel J, Finlay G. Clinical Features and Diagnosis of Pulmonary Hypertension in Adults. *UptoDate*. Accessed November 27, 2016.

23. Kaw R, Pasupuleti V, Deshpande A, Hamich T, Walker E, Minai OA. Pulmonary hypertension: an important prediction of outcomes in patients undergoing non-cardio surgery. *Respir Med*. 2011;105(4):619–624.

24. Keogh AM, Mayer E, Benza RL, et al. Interventional and surgical modalities of treatment in pulmonary hypertension. *J Am Coll Cardiol*. 2009;54(1):567–577.

25. Centers for Disease Control and Prevention. National Diabetes Fact Sheet, 2011. https://www.cdc.gov/diabetes/pubs/pdf/ndfs_2011.pdf. Accessed November 27, 2016.

26. Abdelmolak B, Abdelmolak JB, Knittel J, et al. The prevalence of undiagnosed diabetes in non-cardiac surgery patients, an observational study. *Can J Anesthes*. 2010;57:1058–1064.

27. Umpeirrez GE, Hellmon R, Korytkowski MT, et al. Management of hyperglycemia in hospitalized patients in non-critical core setting: an Endocrine Society Clinical practice guideline. *J Clin Endocrinol Metab*. 2012;97:16–38.

28. Van den Berghe G. How does blood glucose control with insulin save lives in intensive care? *J Chin Invest*. 2004;114:1187–1195.

29. Rassids AJ, Marrin CA, Arrnda J, et al. Insulin infusion improves neutrophil function in diabetic cardiac surgery patients. *Anesth Analg*. 1999;88:1011–1016.

30. Neilson CP, Hindson DA. Inhibition of polymorphonuclear leukocyte respiratory burst by elevated glucose concentrations in vitro. *Diabetes*. 1989;38:1031–1035.

31. Kwon S, Thompson R, Dellinger P, et al. Importance of perioperative glycemia control in general surgery: a report from the Surgical Care and Outcomes Assessment Program. *Ann Surg*. 2013;257:8–14.

32. Noordzij PG, Buersma E, Schreiner F, et al. Increased preoperative glucose levels are associated with perioperative mortality in patients undergoing non-cardiac, nonvascular surgery. *Eur J Endocrinol*. 2007;156:137–142.

33. Abdelmolak B. Anesthesiologist's guide to perioperative glycemic management. *Refresh Courses Anesthesiol*. 2014;42(1):1–11.

34. Weiser TG, Haynes AB, Lashoher A, et al. Perspectives in quality: designing the WHO surgical safety checklist. *Int J Qual Health Care*. 2010;22(5):365–370. doi:10.1093/intqhc/mzq039.

35. Haugen AS, Softeland E, Almeland SK, et al. Effect of the world health organization checklist on patient outcomes: a stepped wedge cluster randomized controlled trial. *Ann Surg*. 2015;261(5):821–828. doi:10.1097/SLA.0000000000000716.

36. American College of Obstetricians and Gynecologists. ACOG practice bulletin no. 120: use of prophylactic antibiotics in labor and delivery. *Obstet Gynecol*. 2011;117(6):1472–1483. doi:10.1097/AOG.0b013e3182238c31.

37. Steinberg JP, Braun BI, Hellinger WC, et al. Trial to Reduce Antimicrobial Prophylaxis Errors (TRAPE) Study Group. Timing of antimicrobial prophylaxis and the risk of surgical site infections: results from the trial to reduce antimicrobial prophylaxis errors. *Ann Surg*. 2009;250(1):10–16. doi:10.1097/SLA.0b013e3181ad5fca.

38. Bratzler DW, Dellinger EP, Olsen KM, et al. Society for Healthcare Epidemiology of America. Clinical practice guidelines for antimicrobial prophylaxis in surgery. *Am J Health Syst Pharm*. 2013;70(3):195–283. doi:10.2146/ajhp120568.

39. Hadiati DR, Hakimi M, Nurdiati DS, Ota E. Skin preparation for preventing infection following caesarean section. *Cochrane Database Syst Rev*. 2014;(9):CD007462. doi:10.1002/14651858.CD007462.pub3.

40. Darouiche RO, Wall MJ Jr, Itani KM, et al. Chlorhexidine-alcohol versus povidone-iodine for surgical-site antisepsis. *N Engl J Med*. 2010;362(1):18–26. doi:10.1056/NEJMoa0810988.

41. Tanner J, Norrie P, Melen K. Preoperative hair removal to reduce surgical site infection. *Cochrane Database Syst Rev*. 2011;(11):CD004122. doi:10.1002/14651858.CD004122.pub4.

42. Committee on Gynecologic Practice. Committee opinion no. 619: gynecologic surgery in the obese woman. *Obstet Gynecol*. 2015;125(1):274–278. doi:10.1097/01.AOG.0000459870.06491.71.

43. Gould MK, Garcia DA, Wren SM, et al. American College of Chest Physicians. Prevention of VTE in nonorthopedic surgical patients: antithrombotic therapy and prevention of thrombosis, 9th ed: American College of Chest Physicians evidence-based clinical practice guidelines. *Chest*. 2012;141(2 Suppl): e227S–e277S. doi:10.1378/chest.11-2297.

44. Carpenter L, Baysinger CL. Maintaining perioperative normothermia in the patient undergoing cesarean delivery. *ObstetGynecological Surv*. 2012;67(7): 436–446. doi:10.1097/OGX.0b013e3182605ccd.

45. Hooper VD, Chard R, Clifford T, et al. ASPAN. ASPAN's evidence-based clinical practice guideline for the promotion of perioperative normothermia: second edition. *J Perianesth Nurs*. 2010;25(6):346–365. doi:10.1016/j.jopan.2010.10.006.

46. Cima RR, Kollengode A, Garnatz J, et al. Incidence and characteristics of potential and actual retained foreign object events in surgical patients. *J Am Coll Surg.* 2008;207(1):80–87. doi:10.1016/j.jamcollsurg.2007.12.047.

47. Al-Qurayshi ZH, Hauch AT, Slakey DP, Kandil E. Retained foreign bodies: risk and outcomes at the national level. *J Am Coll Surg.* 2015;220(4):749–759. doi:10.1016/j.jamcollsurg.2014.12.015.

48. Harmanli O, Dandolu V, Lidicker J, Ayaz R, Panganamamula UR, Isik EF. The effect of obesity on total abdominal hysterectomy. *J Womens Health.* 2010;19(10):1915–1918. doi:10.1089/jwh.2010.2032.

49. Harmanli OH, Dandolu V, Isik EF, Panganamamula UR, Lidicker J. Does obesity affect the vaginal hysterectomy outcomes? *Arch Gynecol Obstet.* 2011;283(4):795–798. doi:10.1007/s00404-010-1422-4.

50. Isik-Akbay EF, Harmanli OH, Panganamamula UR, Akbay M, Gaughan J, Chatwani AJ. Hysterectomy in obese women: a comparison of abdominal and vaginal routes. *Obstet Gynecol.* 2004;104(4):710–714. doi:10.1097/01.AOG.0000140685.30899.24.

51. Morgan-Ortiz F, Soto-Pineda JM, Lopez-Zepeda MA, Peraza-Garay Fde J. Effect of body mass index on clinical outcomes of patients undergoing total laparoscopic hysterectomy. *Int J Gynaecol Obstet.* 2013;120(1):61–64. doi:10.1016/j.ijgo.2012.08.012.

52. Harmanli O, Esin S, Knee A, Jones K, Ayaz R, Tunitsky E. Effect of obesity on perioperative outcomes of laparoscopic hysterectomy. *J Reprod Med.* 2013;58(11–12):497–503.

CHAPTER 33

Minimally Invasive Surgery and Surgical Approach

Norman F. Angell, MD, PhD, MBA

INTRODUCTION

Obesity is a major surgical obstacle. Obesity not only decreases access to the surgical field but also alters the anatomical relationships between the abdominal wall and the abdomen. The surgeon must understand not only anatomy in normal-weight women but also how obesity alters normal anatomy. Obesity affects the choice of incisions, size of incisions, closure of incisions, and choice of instruments (retractors, long instruments, etc.). Obesity affects these decisions about open surgery and minimally invasive surgery (MIS).

Before booking a case surgeons, must evaluate their own surgical skills, their hospital's operating room, and the other specialists needed to care for the patient

TABLE 33-1 Optimizing Outcome

Resources	1. Skill/experience of surgeon 2. Equipment 3. Anesthesiologist 4. Assistants
Plan the operation	1. Route (vaginal, abdominal, minimally invasive) 2. Antibiotics, blood, VTE prophylaxis 3. Incision 4. Closure
Postoperative care	1. VTE prophylaxis 2. Intensive care 3. Glycemic control 4. Nursing care

(Table 33-1). The skill and experience of the surgeon are paramount. If experienced in the needed operation, it may only be necessary to ask a more experienced surgeon who has dealt with obesity in the operation to assist. If the surgeon is relatively inexperienced, it may be prudent to refer the patient to a more experienced surgeon and serve as assistant at the operation if possible. The surgeon must be certain that the equipment needed is available, which may mean a wide operating table designed for obese patients, long instruments, proper retractors, and so on. Obesity is a significant problem for the anesthesiologist, and the surgeon must be certain that the anesthesiologist is comfortable with the anesthetic challenges posed by obese patients (see Chapter 25). Experienced assistants are important in an operation in which obesity is a significant problem. A preoperative conference with the operating room personnel, the anesthesiologist, and the assistants can be helpful in performing the operation safely.

GENERAL NEEDS OF OBESE PATIENTS REQUIRING SURGERY

Preoperative Care

Obese women may have important comorbidities. Primary care physicians and other subspecialists need to be aware of the upcoming surgery to advise the appropriate preoperative evaluation and treatment of medical problems. Routine preoperative clearance by the patient's medical physician will identify problems and allow optimization of care for these diseases prior to surgery. This is especially true in patients with diabetes, hypertension, vascular disease, heart disease, and asthma. Nutritional assessment and recommendations should be addressed as many obese patients may have significant nutritional deficiencies.

Preoperative anesthesia evaluation is crucial. The anesthesiologist will evaluate the airway, plan for a difficult intubation, and evaluate medical problems of special importance to safe anesthetic care and identify any further preoperative workup that will be needed. Also, during this preoperative visit the anesthesiologist will have the opportunity to discuss these issues with the patient.

Intraoperative Care

Deep Vein Thrombosis Prophylaxis

Obese patients are at high risk for deep vein thrombosis (DVT) and possible life-threatening sequelae, including pulmonary emboli (PE). Prophylaxis with sequential compression devices and heparin is advised. Shorter-action unfractionated heparin should be employed during surgery, but if there is a low probability of continued blood loss, patients can be switched to long-acting, low molecular weight heparin postoperatively so that only 1 injection per 24 hours is needed rather than administering unfractionated heparin more frequently. Ambulation may be difficult but is perhaps the most important aspect of DVT prophylaxis. You should consider continuing prophylaxis for 4 weeks after surgery.[1] While this will decrease the risks for the development of DVT/PE, it will not eliminate the possibility of a thrombotic event. The patient should be counseled concerning the signs and symptoms of thrombosis that require evaluation.

Prophylactic Antibiotics

Obese women are at increased risk for wound infection and should be given prophylactic antibiotics. Antibiotics should be appropriately dosed based on weight and need to be administered far enough prior to the incision to ensure that adequate tissue levels are present. Fat has decreased blood supply, and extra time may be needed for absorption. The precise time required for tissue levels is unclear, but 15–60 minutes prior to the incision should be sufficient.[2] If surgery is prolonged or there a large amount of blood is lost, then antibiotics should be redosed. Postoperative antibiotics should not be given in the absence of an established infection.

Postoperative Care

Intensive care admission may need to be scheduled in advance of the operation or intraoperative events may require emergent admission to the intensive care unit; the surgeon must be certain that such intensive care is available. Prolonged intubation of obese patients may be required, and intensive care unit admission in many hospitals is necessary for ventilator support and management.

Medical colleagues may be needed for help in postoperative care. Glycemic control has been shown to be important in reducing the risk of infection both preoperatively and postoperatively. Many of the comorbidities present in obese patients may be exacerbated postoperatively and require expert management. If medical specialists were involved in the preoperative care of the patient, they will be aware of the patient's needs and familiar with the patient's care.

Nursing care for obese patients is challenging but important. There must be enough nursing staff available to assist patients in promptly getting out of bed and to assist in walking. The proper equipment must be at hand, such as hoists, to allow the staff members to help the patient out of bed and avoid injury to themselves. Unfortunately, injuries to the staff in assisting obese patients are common.[3] There is evidence that recommended DVT prophylaxis with sequential compression devices (SCDs) is routinely ignored by patients and nursing staff.[4] It is important for everyone involved in the care of obese patients to be aware of the importance of postoperative compliance with recommendations.

ANATOMY CONSIDERATIONS

There are three aspects of anatomy that must be considered: the bony pelvis; abdominal wall anatomy (muscles, fascias, vasculature, nerves); and the shape and relationship of the overlying fat. A review of normal anatomy may be found in any basic anatomy text.

Bony Pelvis

The diameters of the bony pelvis are important but often ignored. There is a significant difference in the diameter 3 cm above the pubic symphysis (location of a Pfannenstiel incision) and the diameter between the anterior superior spines, resulting in greater access to the pelvis if the incision is made between the anterior superior spines (Figure 33-1). While a Pfannenstiel incision for a cesarean section places the surgeon directly above the lower uterine segment, this incision limits the surgeon access in any other type of surgery. This is rarely the incision of choice in obese patients undergoing gynecologic surgery.

Relationship of Fat to the Abdominal Wall

Obesity does not alter the underlying abdominal wall but can markedly alter the surface relationships to the abdominal wall (Figure 33-2). To judge the relationship of surface markers and the abdominal wall, the surgeon must take into account the thickness of the overlying fat and the shape of the fat. An "apple" body shape affects the distance between the surface and the abdominal wall but may not greatly affect the relationship to the abdominal wall. However, a large panniculus (pear body shape) can dramatically alter these relationships. With a large panniculus, the umbilicus no longer marks the bifurcation of the aorta but instead places the umbilicus over the lower pelvis. Because of this relationship, a transverse incision at or above the

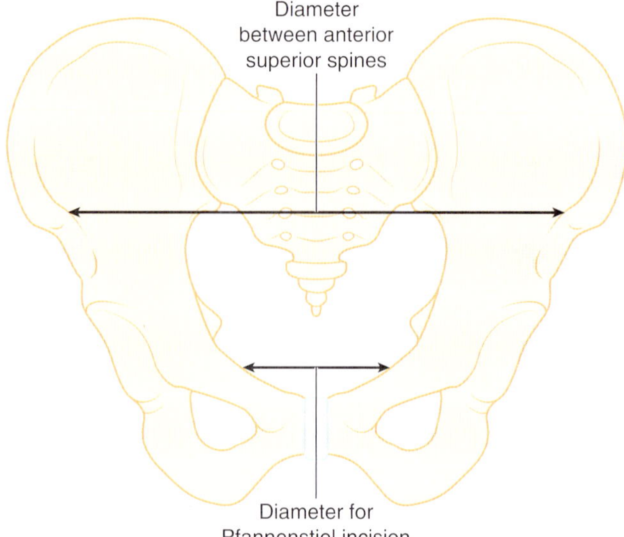

FIGURE 33-1. An incision between the anterior superior spines results in greater access to the pelvis.

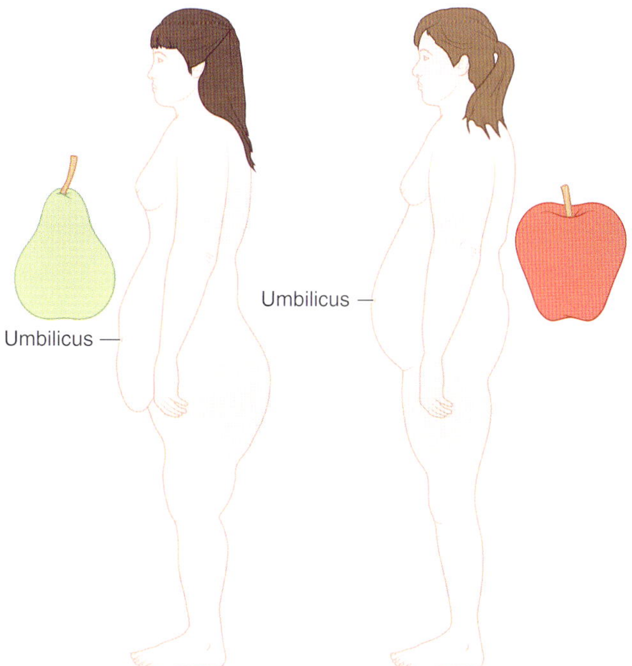

FIGURE 33-2. Body shape must be taken into account concerning incisions in both open and minimally invasive operations.

umbilicus (often with splitting of the rectus muscles) may provide excellent exposure for gynecologic surgery. While the final decision may need to be made after induction of anesthesia, the surgeon must discuss the incision possibilities in depth with the patient preoperatively.

OPEN SURGERY

Incisions

The choice of incision and the size of the incision are crucial decisions made by the surgeon. The wrong decision or limiting the size of the incision may markedly increase the difficulty of the operation or at times prevent safe surgery in the pelvis. The importance of the choice of incision is amplified by the presence of obesity, and obesity often requires altering the choice of incision. The choice must always be made primarily on maximizing the safety of the operation, but the decision has several other considerations that are also important (time of performance, healing, cosmesis) (Table 33-2).

Midline Incision

The midline incision is the incision of choice for any operation that may require access to the upper abdomen, particularly in operations for gynecological cancers. The incision is relatively quick to perform, can be readily extended if necessary, and avoids blood vessels and nerves. The midline incision may result in more pain, longer healing, and an increased risk of wound separation. In the setting of a large panniculus, the midline incision may not reach the pelvis without dealing with the fold of the panniculus.

TABLE 33-2 Incision

Type of Incision	Positive Aspects	Negative Aspects
Midline	1. Quickest 2. Avoids vessels, nerves 3. Can be extended 4. Upper abdomen can be accessed	1. Wound healing 2. Cosmesis 3. Problem in lower limit of incision with panniculus
Transverse	1. Good healing 2. Pain	1. Increase in operative time 2. Size limited 3. Limitation of access of upper abdomen
Muscle splitting	1. Increase in access 2. Decision intraoperatively	1. Increase in operative time 2. Slight increase in risk (bleeding, pain)
Minimally invasive	1. Small incisions 2. Quicker recovery 3. Less blood loss 4. Less pain	1. Difficulty in manipulation of fat layer 2. Need for long instruments 3. Anesthesia issues (deep Trendelenburg)

Transverse Incisions

Many gynecologic surgeons prefer transverse incisions. Transverse incisions heal well, decrease problems with wound separation, and are cosmetically superior. However, obesity may limit the use of transverse incisions. Transverse incisions limit the size of the incision and limit access to the upper abdomen (of particular importance in operations for cancer). Transverse incisions may increase difficulty in retracting the fat layer. These incisions increase operative time, and damage to the epigastric vessels can result in significant bleeding or a hematoma.

Location of a Transverse Incision: The decision concerning location of a transverse incision often must be made after the patient is under anesthesia. The surgeon must determine the relationship between the panniculus and the pelvis. An overhanging panniculus often places the area around the umbilicus directly over the pelvis, and a transverse incision below or above the umbilicus can provide good exposure of the pelvis. Some surgeons may choose to elevate the panniculus to allow the incision under the panniculus where there is less overlying fat. The panniculus can be taped to the skin and then secured to the operating table, or penetrating clamps can be placed in the panniculus so tape or cords can be attached to secure them to the operating table. Newer self-retaining adhesive retractors can be useful (Retentus Panniculus Retractor™, GSuared Medical; Traxi Panniculus Retractor™, Clinical Innovations). The surgeon must consider postoperative healing of the incision, which is then under the overlying panniculus.[5] The location of this incision may severely limit access because of the anatomy of the bony pelvis (see previous discussion).

Extension of Transverse Incision via Muscle Splitting: Muscle splitting procedures can significantly improve visualization and access though a transverse incision and should be considered if necessary.

Maylard Incision: Partial or full division of the rectus muscles is easily and quickly performed to obtain increased access to the pelvis. To perform the Maylard incision procedure, the anterior rectus fascia is opened transversely. The rectus muscle is then undermined, and a moist, open 4 by 4 is used to elevate the muscle, which is then divided via electrocautery. If the muscle is divided more than 50% of its width, it is recommended that the inferior epigastric vessels be divided and sutured. After the muscles are divided, the peritoneum is opened transversely. In closure, there is no need to suture the muscles as they heal by forming a new aponeurosis. Risks of this incision include bleeding from the cut edges or from the cut inferior epigastric vessels if they are not completely sutured.

Cherney Incision: If the incision has been made close to the pubic symphysis and more exposure is needed, the Cherney incision technique can be employed. The rectus muscles are mobilized by cutting the tendons 1–2 cm from the insertion of the tendons into the pubic bone. During closure, the tendons must be sutured. This technique can give good exposure to the space of Retzius and the pelvic sidewall.

Panniculectomy

In massively obese women, the usual incisions may not allow adequate exposure of the operating field. Consideration should be given to panniculectomy to allow easier access to the pelvis. While panniculectomy is a relatively simple procedure, many gynecologists would prefer to ask for help from a general surgeon or plastic surgeon to perform this procedure. Recent studies have shown that combined panniculectomy and pelvic surgery is safe and effective.[6,7]

Retractors

Use of the appropriate retractor can improve access to the field in obese women.

Balfour Retractor

The Balfour retractor is commonly utilized by gynecologic surgeons. The use of the upper arm and appropriate size blades can help in exposure in obese women. The Balfour fourth blade attachment is crucial to retract the upper pole of the incision. Long malleable retractors must be available to retract the thick fat layer.

O'Sullivan-O'Connor Retractor

While the O'Sullivan-O'Connor retractor is not as flexible as the Balfour, long blades are available for this instrument. It is expected that it has limited use in very obese women.

Bookwalter Retractor

The Bookwalter retractor provides a great deal of flexibility in providing access to the field and often may be the instrument of choice. Deep blades are available and can be placed in the most advantageous locations. Attaching the instrument to the operating table provides great stability and strength in retraction. The surgeon must be willing to move the retractor blades as the operation evolves.

Mobius Elastic Retractor™

The Mobius elastic retractor can be useful in obese patients. The retractor is available in a range of sizes. The working area ranges from 3.2 to 28 cm³ to 113 to 227 cm³. The largest size can be used in incisions that range from 12 to 17 cm and thus is the most likely size to be useful in obese patients.

Vaginal Retractors

The usual vaginal retractors (Deavor, right angle) may be difficult to use in obese patients because the thighs may interfere with the handles. Breisky-Navratil retractors avoid this problem because of the axial design of the handle. This retractor is available in 3 sizes, but the largest is most likely to be used, so that at least 3 of the largest size should be available. The smaller sizes may also be useful, particularly anteriorly.

Wound Closure

Wound complications in obese women are higher. Wound complications include wound infection, wound separation, and wound dehiscence. Good decisions concerning closing the wound can minimize these complications. These decisions include choice of suture and technique.

Choice of Suture

In general, the choice of suture for closure of the abdominal wall should be delayed absorbable products. A suture that minimizes inflammation should be considered. In patients for whom poor healing would be predicted because of comorbidities (such as chronic steroid use), the surgeon should consider permanent suture in closure because of the tensile strength. However, permanent sutures can cause inflammation (silk) or can stretch with load (polypropylene, nylon). Rather than a permanent suture, the use of a higher-gauge, long-acting suture may be a better choice (double-strand polydioxanone 0 or 1 gauge).

Closure Technique

Closure of the Abdomen: A mass closure (including peritoneum and fascia in the stitch) of the abdomen with a running stitch is usually adequate, but many surgeons use a Smead-Jones closure in high-risk wounds. The Smead-Jones closure has a low incidence of complications, and in high-risk wounds has been found superior in decreasing wound infection and the incidence of incisional hernia,[8] but the Smead-Jones closure increases operative time. One should consider placing stay sutures in massively obese women or in women who have comorbidities that increase loss of wound integrity.

Dead Space Closure: The question of closure of subcutaneous fat to close potential dead space is uncertain. A Cochrane review of noncesarean surgery showed inadequate data to support or refute subcutaneous closure.[9] Of importance was a study included in this review that showed no difference in closure versus nonclosure of midline incisions with at least 3 cm in fat thickness.[10] Such midline incisions place the maximum stress on the incision. A meta-analysis of trials related to subcutaneous versus no subcutaneous closure after cesarean section showed a small decrease in the risk of wound disruption in women with more than 2 cm in fat thickness (largely because of a decrease in wound seroma).[11] More recently, a study failed to show any difference in wound complications in closure versus no closure in cesarean section with Pfannenstiel incisions.[12] Subcutaneous closure remains a surgeon choice, with no clear guidance from data. The surgeon must take into account the danger of increasing the risk of infection by increasing the amount of foreign material in the wound, particularly because of the limited blood supply in fat. If closure is chosen, then it is recommended that small-gauge and minimally reactive suture be used (such as 3-0 polyglactin).

Use of Drains: The use of drains in the wound is discouraged. Data have shown that drains do not improve outcomes in terms of wound disruption or wound infection and may be detrimental.[13]

Skin Closure: The use of staples to close the skin decreases operating time; this is accentuated in the large incisions needed for surgery in obese women. To account for the increased load on the wound that fat produces, the staples are often left in place longer (a week or more) and replaced with adhesive strips.[14] However, despite these maneuvers, the risk of wound separation is increased in obese women in whom staples were used.[15] Because of these limitations with staples, the surgeon should consider the use of subcuticular closure in a stable patient despite the extra operative time required. A small-gauge, absorbable suture is adequate (0000 polyglactin or poliglecaprone). Studies have shown a subcuticular closure decreases the chances of wound separation. Subcuticular closure may improve patient satisfaction as many patients are upset by the idea of staples, and there is discomfort associated with removal (travel to have the staples removed and the removal itself).

MINIMALLY INVASIVE SURGERY

The advantages of MIS are well documented, and despite the challenges that obesity adds, the use of MIS may improve the care of obese women. The wide use of laparoscopy in bariatric surgery has provided experience in treating obese women and has also resulted in production of instruments that are suited for treatment of obese women. Experience has shown that laparoscopic gynecologic surgery can be performed safely and effectively in obese women.[16]

Robotic surgery has similar problems in the obese as traditional laparoscopy but adds the problem of interference of extreme obesity in docking the robot. Robotic surgery has been shown to perform similarly to traditional laparoscopy and can be used in obese patients.[17]

Vaginal hysterectomy is the ultimate in MIS but may be very difficult in obese women. Obese women are more likely to be nulligravid because of the problems in conception posed by obesity. As a result, uterine decensis is less likely. Massive thighs and a redundant vagina in obese women can cause great difficulty in vaginal surgery. Even with proper leg placement and the use of special retractors, access through the vagina can be challenging to the surgeon and the surgical assistants.

Closed Versus Open Technique for Laparoscopy

While the use of the closed technique for laparoscopy by gynecologists is more common, obesity presents problems with this technique. Long Verres needles are available for use in obese patients, but difficulty in elevating the abdominal wall is usual in obese women and may make placement of the Verres needle difficult. The open (Hasson) technique may be a better choice in obese patients to decrease the chances of a failed entry.[18] Because of the underlying fat, the skin incision may need to be bigger, but the fascial/peritoneal incision is unchanged by the fat. Taking advantage of the thinner area above the umbilicus can make entry easier. Closure of a fascial incision can be difficult under a deep layer of fat, but this task is made easier because of the placement of the fascial sutures used in securing the Hasson cannula.

Port Placement

Careful planning of the placement of the camera port and other ports is crucial to performance of the operation. While not unique to treating obese women, the history of previous surgery must be considered in the placement of ports, particularly the initial (camera) port. The previous discussion of the relation of a large panniculus and the abdominal wall and the abdomen is of particular importance. The traditional placement of the camera port beneath the umbilicus may place this port considerably caudal to the bifurcation of the aorta and may place the camera too close to the pelvis for effective visualization. Placement of the camera port often must be cephalad of the umbilicus in patients with a large panniculus but must also be considered in a patient with an apple body habitus. There is an additional advantage to this port placement as the fat layer is often thinner above the umbilicus.

Placement of the accessory ports can be planned under direct vision after the camera port is in place. Longer trocars are available and usually must be used. A perpendicular insertion will give the shortest distance to the peritoneal cavity, but an angular placement will place less stress on the port and aims the port into the pelvis, which will ease manipulation of instruments. A decision must be made at surgery concerning this angle. The surgeon must also judge the length of operative instruments needed in the case and must be certain that the proper size instruments are available. Take into account the distances to the pelvic organs in placement of the ports. The size of the patient's thighs is sometimes not taken into account, and interference of the thighs in manipulating instruments can cause major problems.

Additional Exposure Problems

The supracervical operation avoided problems with the vaginal portion of a total laparoscopic hysterectomy (TLH) or the laparoscopically assisted vaginal hysterectomy (LAVH). However, supracervical hysterectomy has been made more difficult now that many surgeons are hesitant to employ the power morcellator. A TLH avoids most vaginal surgery but may sacrifice optimal support of the vagina in a patient who has a high risk of dehiscence of the vagina because of the increased pressure placed on the cuff by obesity. In LAVH, more extensive vaginal surgery is required with exposure problems but may allow better support of the vagina. To perform the vaginal portions of the operations, the surgeon must have expert assistance in retraction via the assistants and must have a choice of retractors, including Breisky-Navratil retractors in a range of sizes.

Port Closure

It is recommended that port size great than 5 mm be closed. If the open (Hasson) technique is used, then closure of the camera port is simplified. If a 5-mm camera is used, then closure is not necessary. Closure of port incisions in the obese patient is difficult, but instruments are available to help in this crucial but awkward portion of the operation. The Carter-Tomson™ instrument is useful, but in the obese the Carter-Tomson II™ instrument simplifies that closure. The Carter-Tomson II provides greater length and adds traction to help in the placement of sutures.

SUMMARY

Obesity presents special challenges to the gynecologic surgeon. The choice of open surgery, vaginal surgery, or laparoscopic or robotic surgery depends on the surgery required, the resources of the operating room, and the experience of the surgeon and the surgical team. Careful consideration of the route chosen will optimize the outcome of the surgery for the patient.

The team approach to care is critical to optimize the care of obese patients. Careful and honest assessment of the surgeons' experience and available resources are needed prior to the operation. Referral to a regional hospital may be in the patient's best interest if all components needed for optimal care are not available locally.

REFERENCES

1. Clarke-Pearson DL, Abaid LN. Prevention of venous thromboembolic events after gynecologic surgery. *Obstet Gynecol.* 2012;119(1):155–167.
2. Sullivan SA, Smith T, Chang E, Hulsey T, Vandorsten JP, Soper D. Administration of cefazolin prior to skin incision is superior to cefazolin at cord clamping in preventing postcesarean infectious morbidity: a randomized, controlled trial. *Am J Obstet Gynecol.* 2007; 196(5):455 e1–e5.
3. Walden CM, Bankard SB, Cayer B, et al. Mobilization of the obese patient and prevention of injury. *Ann Surg.* 2013;258(4):646–650; discussion 650–651.
4. Brady MA, Carroll AW, Cheang KI, Straight C, Chelmow D. Sequential compression device compliance in postoperative obstetrics and gynecology patients. *Obstet Gynecol.* 2015;125(1):19–25.
5. Gallagher S, Gates JL. Obesity, panniculitis, panniculectomy, and wound care: understanding the challenges. *J Wound Ostomy Continence Nurs.* 2003;30(6):334–341.
6. Hardy JE, Salgado CJ, Matthews MS, Chamoun G, Fahey AL. The safety of pelvic surgery in the morbidly obese with and without combined panniculectomy: a comparison of results. *Ann Plast Surg.* 2008 Jan;60(1):10–13. doi:10.1097/SAP.0b013e318058ad7d.
7. Sinno S, Shah S, Kenton K, et al. Assessing the safety and efficacy of combined abdominoplasty and gynecologic surgery. *Ann Plast Surg.* 2011 Sep;67(3): 272–274. doi:10.1097/SAP.0b013e3181f9b245.
8. Sivam NS, Suresh S, Hadke MS, Kate V, Ananthakrishnan N. Results of the Smead-Jones technique of closure of vertical midline incisions for emergency laparotomies—a prospective study of 403 patients. *Trop Gastroenterol.* 1995;16(4):62–67.
9. Gurusamy KS, Toon CD, Davidson BR. Subcutaneous closure versus no subcutaneous closure after noncesarean surgical procedures. *Cochrane Database Syst Rev.* 2014;(1):CD010425.
10. Cardosi RJ, Drake J, Holmes S, et al. Subcutaneous management of vertical incisions with 3 or more centimeters of subcutaneous fat. *Am J Obstet Gynecol.* 2006 Aug;195(2):607–614; discussion 614–616. Epub 2006 Jun 21.
11. Chelmow D, Rodriguez EJ, Sabatini MM. Suture closure of subcutaneous fat and wound disruption after Cesarean delivery: a meta-analysis. *Obstet Gynecol.* 2004;103(5):974–980.
12. Esmer AC, Goksedef PC, Akca P, et al. Role of subcutaneous closure in preventing wound complications after cesarean delivery with Pfannenstiel incision: a randomized clinical trial. *J Obstet Gynaecol Res.* 2014;40:728–735. doi:10.1111/jog.12229.
13. Ramsey PS, White AM, Guinn DA, et al. Subcutaneous tissue reapproximation, alone or in combination with drain, in obese women undergoing cesarean delivery. *Obstet Gynecol.* 2005 May;105(5 Pt 1):967–973.
14. Mackeen AD, Berghella V, Larsen ML. Techniques and materials for skin closure in caesarean section. *Cochrane Database Syst Rev.* 2012 Nov 14;(11):CD003577. doi:10.1002/14651858.CD003577. pub3.
15. Tuuli MG1, Rampersad RM, Carbone JF, Stamilio D, Macones GA, Odibo AO. Staples compared with subcuticular suture for skin closure after cesarean delivery: a systematic review and meta-analysis. *Obstet Gynecol.* 2011 Mar;117(3):682–690.
16. McIlwaine K, Manwaring J, Ellett L, et al. The effect of patient body mass index on surgical difficulty in gynaecological laparoscopy. *Aust N Z J Obstet Gynaecol.* 2014 Dec;54(6):564–569.
17. Gallo T, Kashani S, Patel DA, Elsahwi K, Silasi DA, Azodi M. Robotic-assisted laparoscopic hysterectomy: outcomes in obese and morbidly obese patients. *JSLS.* 2012;16(3):421–427.
18. Ahmad G, O'Flynn H, Duffy JM, Phillips K, Watson A. Laparoscopic entry techniques. *Cochrane Database Syst Rev.* 2012 Feb 15;(2):CD006583. doi:10.1002/14651858.CD006583.pub3.

Endometrial Cancers

Rinki G. Agarwal, MD

INTRODUCTION

Endometrial cancer is the fourth-most-common cancer diagnosed in women in the United States, following breast, lung, and colorectal cancer in frequency. It accounts for 6% of all cancers in women, with an estimated 54,870 new cases in 2015. It is the most common gynecologic malignancy in the United States. One in 40 women will develop endometrial cancer in their lifetime, and the American Cancer Society estimated there would be 10,470 deaths from this disease in 2016. Endometrial cancer is typically a disease seen in perimenopausal and postmenopausal women. The likelihood of developing an endometrial cancer is rare before the age of 40 (<5%), and the risk increases thereafter, with median age at diagnosis of 63. Caucasian women are twice as likely to be affected.

Endometrial cancers can be divided into 2 categories: type 1 and type 2.[1] *Type 1* endometrial cancer includes endometrioid adenocarcinoma grades 1 and 2 and is more frequent. It is recognized to be estrogen related and hormonally dependent. It typically arises in patients with a hyperestrogenic state. Excess estrogen exposure can result from a variation of the normal reproductive physiology, as is seen in anovulatory cycles, polycystic ovary disease, prolonged perimenopause or late menopause with anovulatory bleeding pattern, or obesity. Alternatively, estrogen excess can be

""

the result of iatrogenic administration or estrogen-secreting ovarian tumors. The risk of endometrial neoplasia is greater for nulliparous women. It is hypothesized that this process may be related to prolonged periods of infertility, correlating with anovulatory menstrual cycles, excessive serum levels of androstenedione, and lack of monthly sloughing of the endometrial lining. These tumors are typically estrogen and progesterone receptor (PR) positive and have a high sensitivity to progestins. Patients have a favorable prognosis, and 5-year survival of approximately 85%. Obesity in particular increases the risk of type 1 endometrial cancers.

Type 2 endometrial cancers represent the opposite end of the spectrum. These tumors are typically more aggressive. They do not need a hyperestrogenic environment for development. These cancers are high grade, display high-risk cell types, and are not hormonally driven. Examples include grade 3 endometrioid adenocarcinomas and serous, clear cell, and undifferentiated cancers. Type 2 tumors have a higher incidence of deep myometrial invasion and, in comparison to type 1, a higher metastatic potential. Because these tumors are frequently estrogen receptor negative, they have low response rates to progestins. They have a relatively poor prognosis, with a 5-year survival of 58%. Patients with type 2 cancers are typically thinner and older and have no apparent stigmata or history to suggest a hyperestrogenic state. Type 2 tumors are not associated with obesity.

EPIDEMIOLOGIC EVIDENCE SUPPORTING ROLE OF OBESITY IN ENDOMETRIAL CANCER

Over 60% of adults in the United States have a body mass index (BMI) over 25, making them either overweight or obese. In a UK study, data from the Clinical Practice Research Datalink (CPRD) was utilized to examine associations between BMI and risk of individual cancers, adjusting for potential confounders. Each 5-kg/m^2 increase in BMI was linearly associated with cancers of the uterus, gallbladder, kidney, cervix, and thyroid and leukemia. Of endometrial cancers in this study, 41% could be attributable to excess weight.[2]

In the United States, the incidence of endometrial cancer increased every year from 1987 to 1998, and the disease-specific mortality has doubled, paralleling the rise in obesity during the same time frame.[3] From 1999 to 2011, the incidence of endometrial cancer has increased within African Americans, Latinos, and Asian Pacific Islanders, while it has stayed relatively stable in whites (Figure 34-1). Decreases in the use of unopposed estrogen for hormone replacement therapy in the United States should have resulted in a decrease in endometrial cancer. But, this anticipated decrease was not seen and has been attributed to the rising incidence of obesity. It is estimated that 70%–90% of patients with type 1 endometrial cancer are obese.[4] Obesity is a risk factor for neoplasia in both pre- and postmenopausal patients. Obesity and nulliparity are dominant risk factors for premenopausal endometrial cancer.[5]

Several studies have evaluated the relationship of obesity indices to the risk of endometrial cancer.[6,7] These studies showed that obesity increases the risk of endometrial neoplasia in a dose-dependent fashion; that is, women with a weight exceeding 78 kg (171 lb) are at a 2.3-fold increased risk over women with a weight of 58 kg (127 lb). A large meta-analysis of prospective studies that included 22,300 patients analyzed the association between anthropometric measures and endometrial cancers;

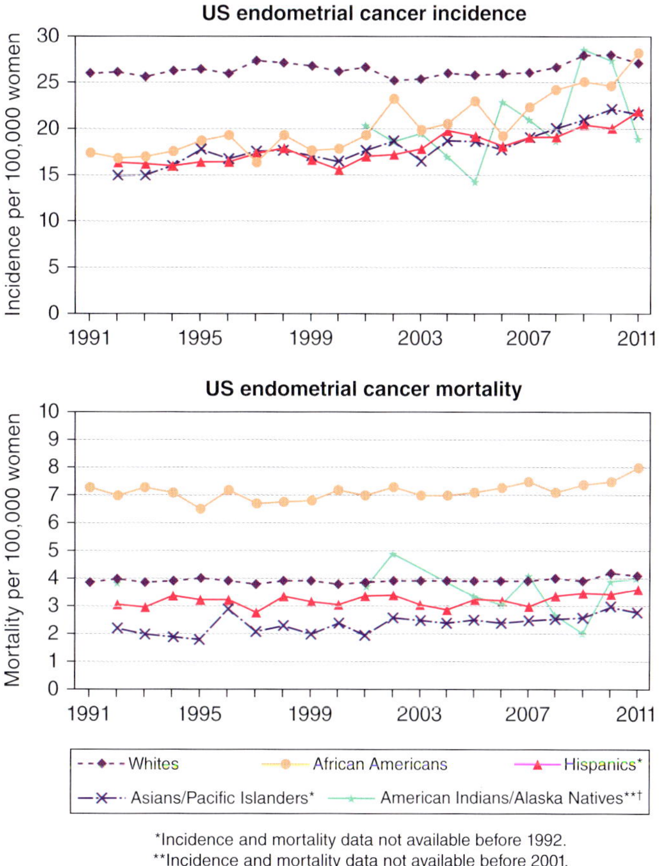

FIGURE 34-1. US endometrial cancer incidence and mortality from 1991 to 2011. (From Surveillance, Epidemiology, and End Results (SEER) Program and National Center for Health Statistics. Additional statistics and charts are available at the SEER website http://seer. cancer.gov.)

it found that the relative risk (RR) for a 5-unit increment in the BMI was 1.54. The risk curve was nonlinear, with a steeper increase in risk in the overweight and obese BMI ranges.[8]

Adult weight gain increases risk, and avoidance of weight gain may be protective. Baseline weight and weight gain in adulthood are associated with increased endometrial cancer risk.[9] A 20-kg (45-lb) weight gain has an RR of 2.75. In 2 large studies, current weight and adult weight gain conferred greater risk of endometrial cancer in never users of postmenopausal hormonal therapy (RR = 5.35) compared to ever users (RR = 2.53) or current users (RR = 1.44).[8,9]

Body fat distribution also appears to have an effect on the risk of endometrial cancer. Patients with a greater waist-to-hip circumference ratio, abdomen-to-thigh skin ratio, and suprailiac-to-thigh skin ratio have an increased risk of endometrial cancer. This suggests that increased upper body fat localization increases the risk for endometrial cancer.

The effect of diet and dietary interventions in the obese population and the risk of endometrial cancer have been evaluated. A higher rate of endometrial cancer in the West and lower rates in Eastern societies suggest a role for nutrition due to the presence of a higher amount of animal fat in the typical Western diet. Both total energy intake and diet components seem to have an effect on risk. Meats, sugar, and eggs increase risk. Fruits, vegetables, and whole grain breads are protective, especially if the foods are high in beta carotene or lutein. Exercise is inversely related to endometrial cancer risk, especially in the overweight and obese patient. The protection is dose dependent, with women who exercise 5 times/week at lower risk than women who never or occasionally exercise (hazard ratio = 0.77).[10]

MECHANISM

The biologic basis for the increased risk of endometrial neoplasia from obesity may be manifold—related to endocrine, metabolic, and inflammatory effects. These effects are felt to be dose dependent. The endocrine effects of obesity are related to estrogen excess. Adipose tissue expresses aromatase, an enzyme that converts adrenally secreted peripheral androstenedione to estrone. Estrone is then converted by 17-hydroxysteroid dehydrogenase into estradiol, the dominant postmenopausal estrogen. The excessive total aromatase levels found in the obese patient lead to excessive circulating estrogen. Estrogen stimulates proliferation in normal endometrium and consequently is considered mitogenic. In the Postmenopausal Estrogen/Progestin Interventions (PEPI) Trial, use of unopposed estrogen for 3 years led to the development of endometrial hyperplasia in 62% of study participants.[11] Chronic anovulation is common in obese premenopausal women, resulting in prolonged low progesterone levels. Coupled with unopposed estrogen from increased aromatase, an increased risk of neoplasia results. There is also increased androgen production, which negatively affects the circulating sex hormone–binding globulin (SHBG) levels by inhibiting synthesis in the liver. This leads to an increased level of unbound, and therefore bioavailable, estrogen. In the postmenopausal woman, high baseline follicle-stimulating hormone (FSH) levels stimulate aromatase, contributing further to higher levels and greater bioavailability of estradiol.

Obesity can lead to insulin resistance, diabetes, or metabolic syndrome. Insulin resistance is associated with elevated levels of insulinlike growth factor 1 (IGF-1). IGF-1 is a stimulus for proliferative activity in breast, colon, and endometrial tissue, leading to an increased risk of neoplasia. Progesterone deficiency can also affect IGF-1 activity due to lower levels of IGF-1–binding proteins (IGFBPs) and higher circulating free IGF-1 levels.[12] In the premenopausal female, hyperinsulinemia can cause stimulation of the hypothalamic-pituitary axis, leading to increased luteinizing hormone (LH) levels and hypersecretion of the ovarian androgens. This in turn causes anovulatory cycles and polycystic ovary disease. Hyperinsulinemia also decreases the amount of SHBG synthesis, which again leads to increased levels of bioavailable estrogen.

Inflammation has a key role in the normal menstrual cycle, and chronic inflammation has an indirect role in tumor initiation and progression, potentially by affecting insulin sensitivity.[12] Adiponectin, a cytokine, is an inverse marker for insulin resistance.[13] Levels of adiponectin are inversely proportional to the risk of endometrial cancer[14]; that is, lower levels indicate insulin resistance and a high risk of endometrial cancer.[15] Conversely, high levels of adiponectin have decreased endometrial cancer risk.[12]

Pro-inflammatory cytokines like tumor necrosis factor alpha (TNF-α), C-reactive protein, interleukin 6, and cytokine receptors like soluble TNF receptors 1 and 2 and interleukin 1 receptor antagonist have all been shown to have a positive correlation with the risk of endometrial cancer in postmenopausal women.[12]

Adipose-derived stem cells (ASCs) are cells within the adipose tissue vascular stroma that have plasticity and can differentiate into many different tissues, such as adipose tissue, heart muscle, cartilage, and so on. ASCs secrete growth factors, cytokines, and inflammatory cells and interact with cancer cells and may thereby have a role in tumor initiation, metastasis, and survival. Numerous studies have looked the role of ASCs in breast, ovarian, lung, pancreatic, and other cancers. There has been a study evaluating ASCs in endometrial cancer in a mouse model; it demonstrated that visceral adiposity increased the omental adipose stem cells and increased tumor vascularity.[13,16,17] The exact mechanism by which ASCs may contribute to tumor initiation or progression in endometrial cancer remains to be elucidated.

DIAGNOSTIC EVALUATION

Evaluation for endometrial neoplasms is prompted by abnormal uterine bleeding, typically postmenopausal bleeding. Routine screening for endometrial neoplasms is not currently recommended except in patients known to have Lynch syndrome, who have a 40%–60% lifetime risk of endometrial cancer. Lynch syndrome is an autosomal dominant genetic condition resulting from defects in DNA-mismatch repair genes (such as *MLH1*, *MSH2*, *MSH6*, *PMS2*, *EPCAM*) that results in an increased predisposition to cancers of colon, rectum, uterus, ovaries, stomach, small intestine, hepatobiliary tract, upper urinary tract, brain, and skin. To date, although it is recognized that overweight and obese women are at increased risk for endometrial cancer, there are no preventive or enhanced screening guidelines for this patient population. A high degree of suspicion should be maintained and diagnostic evaluation performed in patients with abnormal bleeding over 40 years. In addition, patients with an increased risk of endometrial neoplasms such as hyperestrogenic states (obesity, polycystic ovary syndrome [PCOS], chronic anovulation, tamoxifen exposure) with prolonged unexplained bleeding should be assessed. The typical diagnostic evaluation includes an ultrasound-based assessment of the endometrial thickness and an endometrial sampling.

Imaging

Ultrasound evaluation of endometrial thickness can be used in the assessment of abnormal uterine bleeding. In the postmenopausal woman, an endometrial thickness of 4 mm or greater is considered abnormal and may prompt further evaluation, such as endometrial sampling. An ultrasound is readily available in gynecology offices and is commonly used for this assessment. In the obese patient, the thickness of subcutaneous fat and resulting sound attenuation present diagnostic challenges. Transabdominal imaging using a standard 7-mHz ultrasound transducer can be 94%

attenuated in a patient with 8-cm subcutaneous tissue before it reaches the peritoneal cavity. Using "penetration mode" by lowering the frequency of the transducer to allow better penetration and using a technique called "tissue harmonic imaging," by which the presence of fat actually increases the beam frequency and image quality, may improve imaging. Also, placing the patient in a modified lateral decubitus position may help displace the fatty tissue and aid in transabdominal scanning.[18]

Transvaginal scanning is superior to transabdominal studies for evaluation of endometrial thickness, especially in the obese patient. The transvaginal route avoids the problem of adipose attenuation by the thickened abdominal wall. Visualization of the adnexa in obese women using a transvaginal ultrasound can be more difficult. In the United Kingdom Collaborative Trial of Ovarian Cancer Screening (UKCTOCS) study, visualization of the ovaries in postmenopausal women decreased with being overweight (odds ratio [OR] = 0.953) or obese (OR = 0.715).[19] Due to these considerations, a combination of both transabdominal and transvaginal ultrasound evaluation should be considered on a case-by-case basis for complete assessment of the pelvic structures.

A higher BMI is independently associated with thicker endometrium, and the degree of endometrial thickness correlates to the BMI.[20,21] This may affect interpretation using the standard criterion of 4 mm for endometrial thickness and lead to additional and potentially unnecessary procedures.

Although computerized tomographic (CT) imaging is not the initial study of choice to evaluate the endometrium, occasionally CT studies will be used for further evaluation. CT imaging is also used for assessment of metastatic endometrial cancer. In this scenario, the quality of CT imaging is affected by obesity and may require utilization of specialized obesity protocols. Most modern CT machinery has software algorithms designed to adjust for obesity that employ noise reduction techniques.[22] Obese patients receive a higher dose of radiation for CT scans and radiography compared to the nonobese patient. It is estimated that diagnostic CT scans increase exposure of target tissue to radiation by as much as 62% due to the higher-power settings required to obtain imaging.

Endometrial Sampling

Endometrial sampling with an office biopsy or with curettage is the standard for establishing the diagnosis of hyperplasia/cancer. An office endometrial biopsy has 91%–99% accuracy in diagnosis of cancer and correlates well with endometrial curettings.[23] A histologic evaluation allows confirmation of the diagnosis, assigns a grade for the cancer, and allows for evaluation for other sources for bleeding, such as polyps, atrophy, endometritis, and cervical cancer. As most endometrial cancers in obese patients are type 1, a simple office biopsy is typically sufficient to make the diagnosis. There are, however, challenges in obtaining an adequate endometrial sample, particularly with an office biopsy alone. In many cases, sampling will require a procedure in the operating room with additional staff and equipment that can meet the challenges that morbidly obese patients present. When an office biopsy is nondiagnostic or inadequate or if the patient symptoms are not congruent with the pathology, formal dilation and curettage are required. Hysteroscopy can provide confirmation that the endometrial cavity was accessed and can allow for a visually directed biopsy.

Complete assessment of cavities that are distorted by anatomical obstacles such as leiomyoma or scarring from previous endometrial ablations can be difficult. Stenosis of the cervix from atrophy or previous treatment for dysplasia can also contribute to difficulty in obtaining a sample.

TREATMENT OF ENDOMETRIAL CANCER

Surgery

Surgery is the mainstay of treatment for endometrial cancer. Patients undergoing standard treatment using surgery followed by adjuvant therapy based on risk factors have comparatively high disease-specific survival. Surgery has the advantage of immediate and effective palliation of bleeding and pain-related symptoms. Standard surgical treatment of endometrial cancer includes a hysterectomy, bilateral salpingo-oophorectomy, and staging with lymphadenectomy. The extent of surgical staging and the need for lymphadenectomy with endometrial cancer are major controversies in the field of gynecologic oncology. Although a thorough discussion of this issue is beyond the scope of this chapter, it should be noted that performing a formal retroperitoneal node dissection in obese patients can be challenging and may not be warranted.

A higher incidence of medical comorbidities, including hypertension, diabetes mellitus, obstructive sleep apnea, and venous stasis, requires preoperative optimization to improve outcomes. A consultation with an anesthesiologist, careful history, and airway assessment for difficult intubation should be considered in all obese patients. Special attention should be given to the possibility of obstructive sleep apnea. Obesity increases complications such as surgical site infection, venous thromboembolism, and wound complications. Informed consent for these increased risks should be part of preoperative counseling.[24] A detailed description of perioperative considerations in the obese patient is discussed in Chapters 25 and 32.

Surgical staging can be accomplished via a laparotomy or a minimally invasive surgical technique. Compared to laparotomy, minimally invasive surgery offers advantages in the obese patient. Minimally invasive techniques are considered to be feasible, safe, and comparable in staging with the added advantage of decreased postoperative complications, such as would healing and infection rates, and quicker return to baseline function.

In the Lap2 trial, 2616 patients were randomized to surgical staging of endometrial cancer by laparotomy (920 patients) or laparoscopy (1696 patients). The majority of patients were successfully staged laparoscopically, with an overall conversion rate of 26% from laparoscopy to laparotomy, demonstrating the feasibility of comprehensive surgical staging using laparoscopy. The conversion rates were associated with the BMI, with an increase from 17.5% in patients with a BMI of 25 to 57.1% in patients with a BMI greater than 40. The operative times were longer for the laparoscopy group. However, the laparoscopic group had a shorter hospital stay and fewer postoperative complications.

In several reported studies, and in my own experience, there is a lower conversion rate (6%) from robotic-assisted laparoscopic staging to laparotomy. In our study, the operating room times were longer, but surgical times were similar between laparoscopy and laparotomy, due to increased setup time prior to start of surgery.[25]

Rates of completion of the surgery laparoscopically, performance of lymphadenectomy, and lymph node counts were not affected by BMI. Similar findings have been reported in other large series.[26–28] In a retrospective study comparing survival after robotic surgery with standard laparoscopy, there was no significant difference in survival (3-year survival 93.3% and 93.6%), disease-free survival (DFS) (3-year DFS 83.3% and 88.4%, respectively), or tumor recurrence (14.8% and 12.1).[29] Outcomes from robotic surgery have also been shown to be comparable to those reported in the Surveillance, Epidemiology, and End Results database from the National Cancer Institute (NCI), with 88.7% overall survival at 5 years.[30] In conclusion, the oncologic outcome of robotic-assisted laparoscopic staging and feasibility of completion of surgery are equal to laparoscopy and the surgical parameters such as operative time, blood loss, conversion rates, and complications have been reported to be lower, making it the most used platform for endometrial cancer staging.

A Society of Gynecologic Oncology (SGO) task force white paper in 2012 reviewed use of the robotic platform for endometrial cancer in several large retrospective studies and accepted it as an alternative standard-of-care platform for minimally invasive surgery for staging of endometrial cancer.[31] Further, the task force consensus appears to be that a prospective trial evaluation of robotic surgery may not be feasible. Surgical staging in the obese patient is possible and should be considered the initial step in management in all patients unless there are specific contraindications. This is particularly relevant in this patient group as they are more likely to have disease with a good prognosis.

Chemotherapy for Endometrial Cancer

Chemotherapy is used in endometrial cancer in the presence of early-stage disease with adverse histology, advanced-stage disease, or with recurrent disease. Cancer outcomes are directly related to adequate dosage and frequency of chemotherapy. There is growing evidence of underdosing of chemotherapy in obese patients, with poorer outcomes noted posttreatment in breast, colon, and gynecologic malignancies.[32–36] With some exceptions, chemotherapy drug-dosing calculations are typically performed using the body surface area (BSA), which is calculated from patient weight and height. Numerous formulas are available for chemotherapy dosing and may have some variation in the calculation of BSA. The American Society of Clinical Oncology (ASCO) does not recommend any particular formula.

Chemotherapy drugs have a narrow therapeutic index, and dose intensity is directly related to efficacy, toxicity, and survival. In an increasingly obese population, there has been well-intentioned but misguided underdosing of chemotherapy due to concerns for toxicity. This is typically done by adjusting the dose on ideal body weight or adjusted body weight index instead of actual body weight. But, there is evidence that undertreatment with chemotherapy by adjustment of dosage or intensity led to poorer DFS and overall survival. Studies showed that close to 40% of obese patients were given treatment not based on actual body weight but on ideal/adjusted body weight or with a BSA capped at 2.0 m^2.

An expert panel was convened by ASCO to perform a systematic review of the available medical literature. The panel looked at 56 studies on cytotoxic chemotherapy dosing strategies for overweight and obese patients with cancer. The review excluded

TABLE 34-1 ASCO Clinical Practice Guideline on Appropriate Chemotherapy Dosing for Obese Adult Patients[a]

- Full weight-based chemotherapy doses should be used in the treatment of the obese patient, particularly when the goal of treatment is cure.
- Clinicians should respond to all treatment-related toxicities in the same way in obese patients as in nonobese patients.
- If a dose reduction is used in response to toxicity, consideration should be given to the resumption of full weight-based doses for subsequent cycles, especially if a possible cause for the toxicity (e.g., impaired renal, hepatic function) has been resolved. There is no evidence to support the need for greater dose reductions for obese patients compared with nonobese patients to manage toxicities.
- The use of a fixed dose is rarely justified (except for a few select agents).

[a]From Grigg JJ, et al. Appropriate Chemotherapy Dosing for Obese Adult Patients With Cancer: American Society of Clinical Oncology Clinical Practice Guideline. *J Clin Oncol* 2012;30(13):1553-1561.

leukemia studies and did not address dosing of novel targeted agents. The panel did an extensive review of all available literature to assess the use of BSA and fixed-dose chemotherapy calculations, clinical toxicities, and management of toxicities to determine the optimal chemotherapy dose in the obese patients. In 2012, ASCO released recommendations for dosing of chemotherapy in obese patients in a clinical practice guideline. The key recommendations are given in Table 34-1.

Radiation

Obesity presents challenges with radiation therapy as well. Radiotherapy planning is highly dependent on high-quality imaging; that is, the better the imaging, the more likely it allows for calculation of better planned target volumes (PTVs) and lead to better outcomes from radiotherapy. Because imaging quality is affected by adipose tissue in the obese patient,[37] this interferes with planning of radiation. Dosimetry calculations, adequate coverage of target areas, and consistency of positioning are all considerations in planning that need to be specifically addressed. This may require additional time spent planning for optimizing treatment and minimizing toxicities. Errors in radiation planning and delivery can be introduced by variability in positioning (setup error) and target organ motion. Skin mobility (motions of skin in relation to the internal anatomy) is higher in obese patients compared to those with a normal BMI, which can lead to systematic setup errors.

In patients undergoing radiation for endometrial cancer, the magnitude of setup errors using daily image guidance due to shifts of the target tissue have been noted to be greater in all dimensions (vertical, longitudinal, and lateral) with higher BMIs, introducing more systematic error.[38] Calculation of the mean systematic error using image-guided radiation therapy (IGRT) for the first 5 fractions of daily radiation and applying this mean to all subsequent fractions has been proposed to decrease setup error and resultant overall margin requirements for optimizing planning target volumes at reasonable cost. In patients undergoing daily image-guided intensity-modulated radiation therapy (IMRT) for abdominal tumors, the 3-dimensional (3-D) conformal imaging-based displacement of the target tissue was significantly greater in the overweight (BMI > 25) compared to the nonobese patient and required set corrections to reduce systematic error. The requisite planning target volumes were greater in the overweight group if daily image guidance was not employed.[39]

TABLE 34-2 Types of Brachytherapy and Applicators Available

Type of Brachytherapy	*Types of Applicators*
Low-dose brachytherapy	• Standard tandem and ovoid (Figure 34-2) • Simon Heyman capsules: intrauterine sources (Figure 34-3)
High-dose brachytherapy	• Rotte Y applicator: with customizable arms for maximizing uterine coverage (Figure 34-4)

These studies demonstrated the systematic error in the treatment planning and a need for image-guided radiation to optimize treatment.

In a Gynecologic Oncology Group (GOG) study of endometrial cancer in obese patients, there were more cutaneous toxicities and fewer gastrointestinal toxicities.[40] This was related to the higher doses of radiation exposure to the skin to have adequate treatment to the target organ. Also, due to increased visceral fat, there is more protection of the gastrointestinal tract and therefore lower gastrointestinal toxicity.

Morbid obesity may preclude patients from standard treatment for endometrial cancer using surgical staging followed by adjuvant therapy. In patients with inoperable cancer, a combination of external beam radiation and brachytherapy or brachytherapy alone has been used effectively as primary treatment. The types of brachytherapy applicators are listed in Table 34-2 and Figures 34-2 to 34-5. Patients treated with primary radiation therapy using pelvic radiation, brachytherapy, or a combination were found to have disease-specific survivals of 65%–88% in various series (Table 34-3). The severe complication rate from radiation ranged from 10% to 17%. A high likelihood of death from noncancer causes was noted, as would be expected of a high-risk patient population.

Hormonal Therapy

A high proportion of endometrial cancers related to obesity are well-differentiated endometrioid adenocarcinomas that have a high expressivity of hormonal receptors and have elevated unopposed estrogen levels. Hormonal therapy, which counteracts the proliferative stimulatory effect of estrogen, is an important modality to consider for prevention and primary treatment of endometrial hyperplasia/carcinoma. In young patients desirous of preserving the uterus for future fertility, and in a patient who is medically inoperable, hormonal therapy can be considered. For

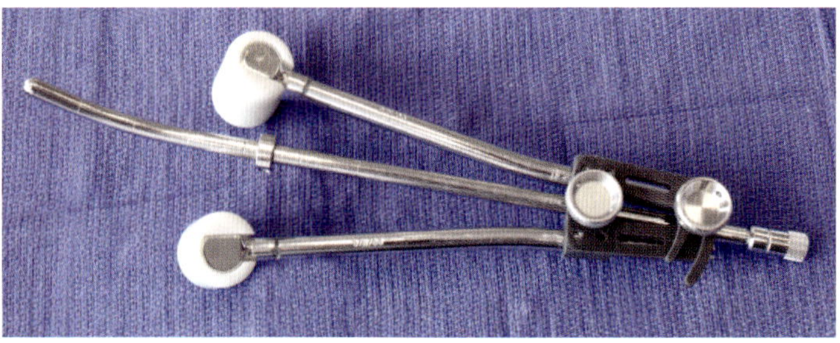

FIGURE 34-2. Tandem and ovoid applicator.

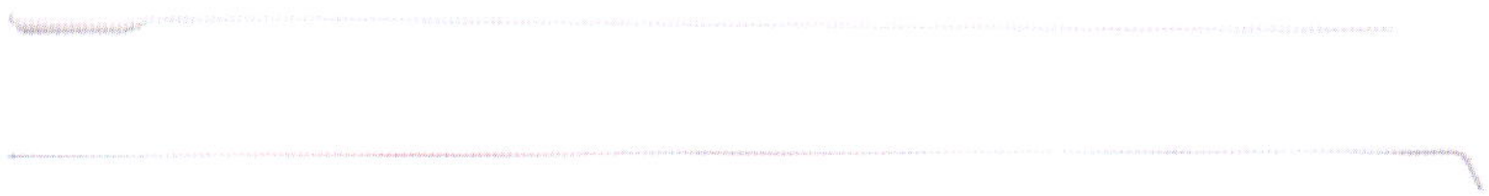

FIGURE 34-3. Heyman capsules.

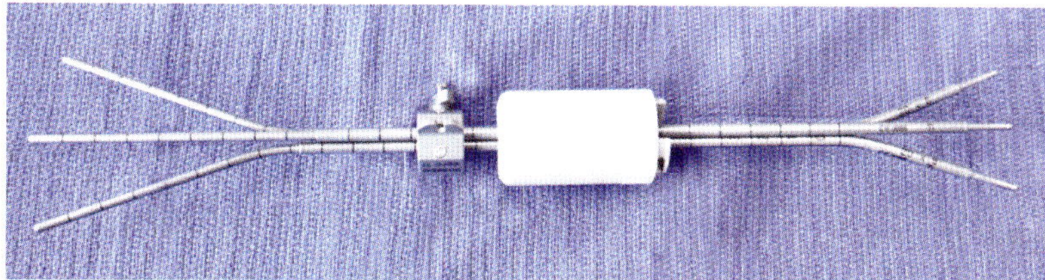

FIGURE 34-4. Rotte Y applicator.

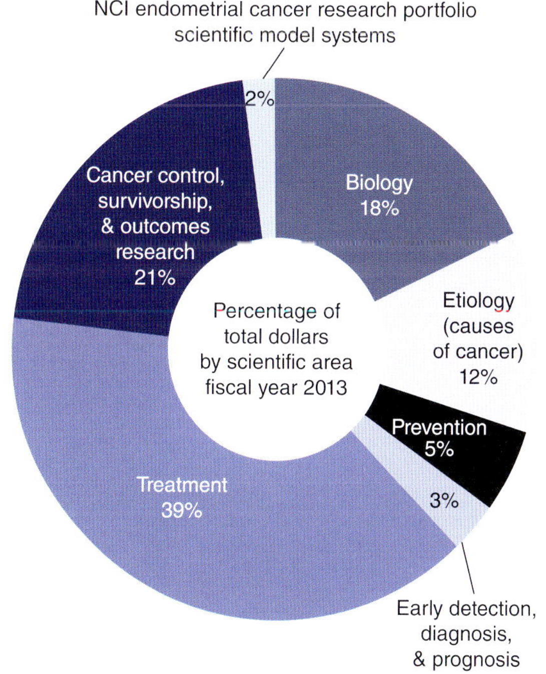

FIGURE 34-5. Endometrial cancer research portfolio for the National Cancer Institute (NCI) for the year 2013—distribution of funding into scientific outline area codes. (From National Cancer Institute [NCI] Funded Research Portfolio. Only projects with assigned common scientific outline area codes are included. A description of relevant research projects can be found on the NCI Funded Research Portfolio website.)

TABLE 34-3 Primary Radiation Therapy for Endometrial Cancer

Reference	Number of Patients	Stages	Age (Median)	Treatment	DSS	Pelvic Failures (%)	Complications
Grigsby et al.[57]	69	I	72	EBRT + BT: 49 Low-dose EBRT + BT: 9 BT-11	5 year: 76.8 10 year: 33.3	6.1 18.2	Severe complications = 16%: EBRT + BT
Taghian et al.[58]	104	I–IV	68.8	EBRT + BT: 52 BT: 52	5 year: 65.9 10 year: 58.6	8.3	Severe complications = 17.3%
Rose et al.[59]	64	I–II		EBRT + BT: 48 BT: 10	No difference in survival compared to surgically treated controls		Severe complications = 17% Noncancer death: 36%
Chao et al.[60]	101	I	71	EBRT + BT: 10 EBRT + midline shield + BT: 62 BT: 26	5 year: 84% (1A) and 80% (1B)	0	Noncancer death in older patients
Rouanet et al.[53]	250		68	EBRT + BT	DFS: 65.8 at 5 years, 66 at 10 years OS: 76.5 at 5 years and 68 at 10 years	24.1% (19.6% isolate and 4.5% with distant metastases)	
Fishman et al.[61]	54	I–II			80 (I) 85 (II)		Significantly shorter overall survival compared to operable patients
Chao et al.,[62] Niazi et al.[63]	38	I–II		EBRT + BT: 8 BT: 30	78%: all stages		Late toxicities: 10.5%
Kupelian et al.[64]	152			EBRT + BT: 36 BT = 116	5 year: 87% (I) 88% (II) 49% (III–IV)		

BT, brachytherapy; DFS, disease-free survival; DSS, disease-specific survival; EBRT, external beam radiation therapy; OS, overall survival.

years, hormonal therapy was, and in many cases still is, the preferable systemic treatment for metastatic or recurrent disease. Hormonal therapy has the potential of prolonging the progression-free survival in patients with recurrent disease, and in select patients can be as effective as chemotherapy with lower toxicity and cost. The literature includes numerous reports of uterine preservation with successful live births in younger patients with uterine preservation. Options for hormonal therapy include progestogenic agents and antiestrogenic agents.

Progestogens induce differentiation of the endometrial glandular epithelium and stroma in well-differentiated and receptor-positive cancers. Progesterone receptors (PRs) are present in 2 forms: PR-A and PR-B. PR-A is present in the nucleus, even in the absence of progesterone. PR-B is located in the cytosol but will translocate to the nucleus in the presence of progesterone. Progesterone can have a lasting response in a majority of endometrial cancers. The effect appears to be mediated through inhibition of the cell cycle, decreased cancer cell invasion, differentiation to a secretory phenotype, and downregulation of cellular adhesion molecules. It can inhibit cancer cell growth by enhancing activity of cell cycle checkpoint regulating genes p53 and p21. It may induce apoptosis by inhibiting the antiapoptotic activity of the nuclear factor kappa B[41], a primary transcription factor that can be activated in neoplastic transformation. Progestins have been used for treatment of endometrial cancer for over 50 years. Effective doses of medroxyprogesterone acetate for endometrial cancer range from 160 to 1000 mg/d. Higher doses have not been shown to be more effective. Side effects of progesterone include increased risk of thromboembolic events, peripheral edema, shortness of breath, anxiety, increased appetite, and weight gain.

Progesterone can also be used for prevention in patients at increased risk of cancer. Use of progesterone for at least 10 days each month concurrent with estrogen for hormone replacement was protective. Patients who received less than 10 days of progesterone therapy were at increased risk of endometrial cancer. Patients were at greatest risk of developing cancer if treated with estrogen alone. Estrogen with cyclic progesterone was associated with an increased risk if used for greater than 5 years.

In patients at high risk of endometrial cancer, such as Lynch syndrome, a prospective study of oral contraceptives or depot medroxyprogesterone acetate showed a decrease in the proliferative immune marker ki-67 in biopsies posttreatment when compared to pretreatment biopsies. A subset of patients had poor histologic response to exogenous progesterone. A possible explanation was that there was an increased expression of proteins that are inhibitors of apoptosis. These proteins included survivin, an inhibitor of the Wnt signaling pathway [sFRP1 (secreted frizzled-related protein) and sFRP2] that inhibits endometrial proliferation, and inhibitors of estrogen driven endometrial proliferation [retinaldehyde dehydrogenase 2 (RALDH2)].[42]

To date, data for empiric use of progesterone therapy for prevention of endometrial cancer in patients with obesity have not been directly studied. Given that about 25% of endometrial hyperplasia and cancer in the general population will respond to progesterone therapy, it is possible that improved understanding of the molecular pathways and an ability to predict response using tissue biomarkers may improve our ability to offer medically tailored therapy to this group of patients for prevention and treatment in the future.

Antiestrogenic therapy—such as tamoxifen and other selective estrogen receptor modulators (SERMs), GnRH (gonadotropin-releasing hormone) agonists, and aromatase inhibitors (AIs)—have been studied in endometrial cancer. Tamoxifen increases expression of PRs in the endometrium. It has shown a response rate of 10% in recurrent endometrial cancers, and the response was more favorable in patients with endometrioid histology and lower-grade tumors.[43] Because of the increase in PR expressivity by tamoxifen, the GOG studied use of tamoxifen with megestrol acetate in an alternating 3-week course and reported a 27% response rate.[44] GnRH agonists were studied due to the expression of GnRH receptors on endometrial cancer cells and did not show consistency in response rates.

Early studies have shown the effectiveness of AIs in the primary, adjuvant, and recurrent settings.[17,26,45] AIs suppress the conversion of androstenedione to estrone by 90%–98% in postmenopausal women. AIs have been used for treatment due to under-expression of PRs in some neoplastic endometrium, and they are of particular interest in the obese population due to higher expression of aromatase in the excessive adipose tissue. Patients treated with anastrozole have a significantly greater improvement in proliferative index as measured by ki-67 and a decrease in the estrogen and aromatase receptor expression, but no change in the PR expression.[46] AIs cannot be used in premenopausal women due to an upregulation of FSH, which counteracts the effect and can also lead to ovarian hyperstimulation.

OUTCOMES FOR THE MORBIDLY OBESE

Mortality rates for malignancies have been reported to be higher in obese patients. In the Cancer Prevention II study sponsored by the American Cancer Society, over 1 million participants were followed longitudinally for mortality. Mortality rates from all cancers combined in the overweight were 52% higher for men and 62% higher for women. For men, the RR of death was 1.52 (95% confidence interval, 1.13 to 2.05); for women, the RR was 1.62 (95% confidence interval, 1.40 to 1.87). This increase in mortality in both men and women with elevated BMIs was seen across a broad spectrum of malignancies, including those of the esophagus, colon and rectum, liver, gallbladder, pancreas, and kidney. This was also true for death due to non-Hodgkin lymphoma and multiple myeloma. Significant trends of increasing risk with higher BMI values were observed for death from cancers of the stomach and prostate in men and for death from cancers of the breast, uterus, cervix, and ovary in women.[47] The highest risk for women was for death from cancer of the corpus, not otherwise specified, with a RR of 6.25 for those with a BMI greater than 40 (Table 34-4).

Obesity may directly affect survival, as patients are more likely to die of comorbidities. In assessment of disease-specific mortality, obesity leads to a higher likelihood

TABLE 34-4 Mortality From Uterine Corpus Cancers According to BMI[a]

BMI Category	Number of Deaths	Death Rate	Relative Risk
18.8–24.9	333	10.68	1
25.0–29.9	225	15.68	1.50
30.0–34.9	105	26.05	2.53
35.0–39.9	25	30.16	2.77
>40.0	16	60.83	6.25

[a]Data reproduced from mortality from cancers of the uterine corpus according to BMI in US women in the Cancer Prevention Study II: 1982–1998. Calle EE, Thun MJ, Petrelli JM, Rodriguez C, Heath CW Jr. Body-mass index and mortality in a prospective cohort of US adults. *N Engl J Med.* 1999;341(15):1097–1105.

of receiving nonstandard care if patients are poor surgical candidates or are too ill to complete all recommended treatments, including chemotherapy and radiation. As previously discussed, dosing deficiencies in patients treated with chemotherapy and radiation therapy contribute to suboptimal care. There has been concern that obesity may also cause innate biologic changes, such as metabolic dysregulation due to increased circulation of insulin, IGF-1, adipokines, cytokines, and pro-angiogenic factors. These factors are important in cell cycle regulation, vascularization, tumor initiation, and cell proliferation and may lead to more aggressive behavior with worse outcomes.

Although some studies suggested poorer outcomes in endometrial carcinoma for obese patients, not all studies reached the same conclusion. Unlike breast cancer, for which the outcomes are related to BMI prediagnosis and during survivorship, there is unclear evidence that such an effect is present for the obese patient for endometrial cancer.[48] In a secondary analysis of the MRC-ASTEC (Medical Research Council–A study of treatment of endometrial cancer) trial, patients with early endometrial cancer were stratified by BMI, and there was no difference in survival.[49]

Since 2004, the annual incidence of endometrial cancers have been stable in Caucasians, but increasing in African American women by 1.9% per year. The mortality from endometrial cancer has remained stable in the Caucasian and African American population in the United States. In considering if obesity affects survival in patients with endometrial cancer, as it appears to in breast and prostate cancer, a retrospective review of outcomes relating to BMI was performed from patients enrolled in GOG 99 (a randomized trial of surgery with or without adjuvant radiation therapy).[40,50] The BMI was available for 380/392 patients enrolled in the study, which included stage IB–IIB (occult) disease. These patients were stratified by BMI into categories of underweight (<18.5), normal (18.5 to 24.9), overweight (25.0 to 29.9), obese (30.0 to 39.9), and morbidly obese (≥40.0) to study effect in recurrence-free interval, overall survival, and treatment-related toxicity. Of these patients, 41% were obese, and 12% were morbidly obese. Disease-specific survival was not adversely affected in the obese subgroup (hazard ratio [HR] = 1.48, 95% CI 0.82–2.70, p = .196) but was lower in the morbidly obese patients (HR = 2.77, 95% CI 1.21–6.36, p = .016), compared to patients with a BMI less than 30. A higher BMI was more frequently noted in the African American patients (73%) compared to non–African Americans (50%). The HR for overall survival was 2.24 for African American patients compared to non–African American patients. When BMI was controlled for, the HR decreased to 1.61. This suggests that BMI has a confounding effect on race as a prognostic factor for endometrial cancer. Morbidly obese patients had a higher rate of 66.7% of death from non–cancer-related deaths compared to 43% for patients with a BMI less than 40.

Quality of Life

Pretreatment assessment of the functional, emotional, and social well-being of patients using validated assessment tools have shown that patients who are obese have significantly worse baseline quality of life compared to nonobese patients.[51] A meta-analysis to assess the association of BMI with the quality of life for obese endometrial cancer survivors showed that the obese survivors had poor physical, social, and role functioning compared to nonobese survivors. Emotional and cognitive functioning did not show differences.[3,52] The quality of life is affected by limited mobility, decreased physical endurance, associated comorbidities, and social discrimination. There may also be decreased quality of life from increased treatment-related side effects or tolerance.[53]

Interventions suggested to improve the quality of life have been studied. In the Survivors of Uterine Cancer Empowered by Exercise and Healthy Diet (SUCCEED) trial, patients were randomized to either a 6-month period of exercise and lifestyle modification or standard care. For a unit decrease in the BMI, patients reported an improvement in their sense of well-being.[54] Furthermore, the central nervous system neural response to high-calorie foods changed in patients in the experimental arm, suggesting that behavior modification may have real benefits in these patients.[55] The REWARD (Revving-up Exercise for sustained Weight loss by Altering neurological Reward and Drive) study is also investigating the effect of activity and lifestyle modifications on weight and other metrics such as fitness, behavior, and eating habits.[56]

Bariatric Interventions

Weight loss has a direct protective impact on the risk of endometrial cancer. Weight loss also allows for improved physical conditioning (less cardiopulmonary load and an improvement in musculoskeletal disorders, fatigue) and avoidance of sedentary habits. Bariatric surgery for management of obesity is discussed in Chapter 9. Bariatric surgery is typically advised for patients with a BMI greater than 40 and for patients with BMI greater than 35 with at least 2 obesity-related comorbidities. Endometrial cancer is an obesity-related comorbidity and therefore should be considered an indication for aggressive management of obesity. After effective treatment of endometrial cancer, the obese patient with cancer continues to have significant risk for survival and quality of life related to obesity. Addressing this risk with lifestyle management interventions is of paramount importance. Referral for bariatric surgery and advocacy for coverage of bariatric surgery by insurance companies for this indication would seem beneficial and warrants future research. Lifestyle interventions with diet, exercise, and bariatric surgery should be considered when working to optimize all aspects of endometrial cancer care, including prevention, management, and survivorship.

FUTURE DIRECTIONS

A multimodal approach is required to tackle the profound growing problem of obesity and its impact on health. Education and training of all providers involved in the care of the growing US obese population regarding the risk for endometrial and other cancers and their management are important. Improving our knowledge at a genomic and cellular levels of the changes that lead to cancer development in the obese population is necessary. Research regarding appropriate screening and prevention mechanisms and a concerted effort in development of consensus guidelines for care of these patients is necessary. Improvement in the traditional therapeutic tools at our disposal, such as surgery, chemotherapy, radiation, and hormonal therapies, so that they can be used safely and more effectively in these medically complex situations is past due. Appropriate support for providers involved in the care of these patients in terms of research interest, funding, additional support staffing, and reimbursements have not kept up with the changing times.

Finally, development of programs that will focus on an overall improvement in health with diet, exercise, and other heretofore underdeveloped or unknown tools is

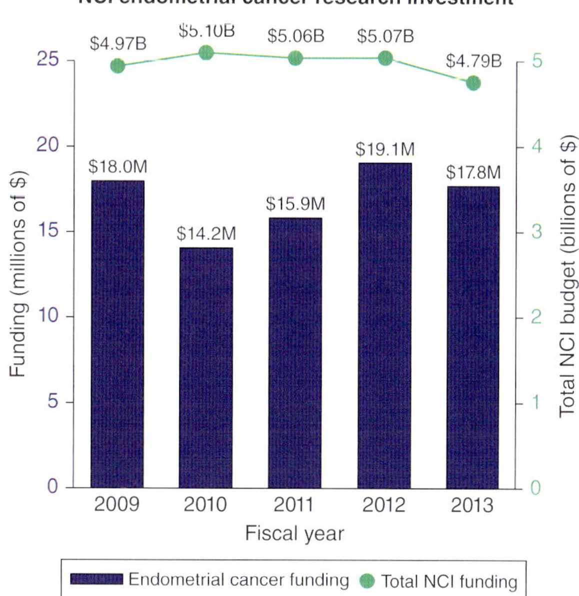

FIGURE 34-6. National Cancer Institute endometrial cancer research investment. (From NCI Office of Budget and Finance.)

necessary (Figure 34-5). Unfortunately, the current research programs are significantly underfunded (Figure 34-6). Although endometrial cancer is the fifth-most-common cancer among US women, the percentage of NCI dollars spent on endometrial cancer research in 2013 was a mere 0.3% of the total federal research budget. Meanwhile, it is estimated that $2.6 billion will be spent on the care for endometrial cancer patients in 2014. Efforts to bring the funding up to a level commensurate with the scope of the problem are imperative.

REFERENCES

1. Bokhman JV. Two pathogenetic types of endometrial carcinoma. *Gynecol Oncol*. 1983;15(1):10–17.

2. Bhaskaran K, Douglas I, Forbes H, dos-Santos-Silva I, Leon DA, Smeeth L. Body-mass index and risk of 22 specific cancers: a population-based cohort study of 5.24 million UK adults. *Lancet*. 2014;384(9945):755–765.

3. Fader AN, Arriba LN, Frasure HE, von Gruenigen VE. Endometrial cancer and obesity: epidemiology, biomarkers, prevention and survivorship. *Gynecol Oncol*. 2009;114(1):121–127.

4. von Gruenigen VE, Gil KM, Frasure HE, Jenison EL, Hopkins MP. The impact of obesity and age on quality of life in gynecologic surgery. *Am J Obstet Gynecol*. 2005;193(4):1369–1375.

5. Soliman PT, Oh JC, Schmeler KM, et al. Risk factors for young premenopausal women with endometrial cancer. *Obstet Gynecol*. 2005;105(3):575–580.

6. Goodman MT, Hankin JH, Wilkens LR, et al. Diet, body size, physical activity, and the risk of endometrial cancer. *Cancer Res*. 1997;57(22):5077–5085.

7. Swanson CA, Potischman N, Wilbanks GD, et al. Relation of endometrial cancer risk to past and contemporary body size and body fat distribution. *Cancer Epidemiol Biomarkers Prev*. 1993;2(4):321–327.

8. Aune D, Navarro Rosenblatt DA, Chan DS, et al. Anthropometric factors and endometrial cancer risk: a systematic review and dose-response meta-analysis of prospective studies. *Ann Oncol*. 2015; 26(8):1635–1648.

9. Chang SC, Lacey JV Jr, Brinton LA, et al. Lifetime weight history and endometrial cancer risk by type of menopausal hormone use in the NIH-AARP diet and health study. *Cancer Epidemiol Biomarkers Prev.* 2007;16(4):723–730.

10. Gierach GL, Chang SC, Brinton LA, et al. Physical activity, sedentary behavior, and endometrial cancer risk in the NIH-AARP diet and health study. *Int J Cancer.* 2009;124(9):2139–2147.

11. Effects of hormone replacement therapy on endometrial histology in postmenopausal women. The postmenopausal estrogen/progestin interventions (PEPI) trial. The writing group for the PEPI trial. *JAMA.* 1996;275(5):370–375.

12. Dossus L, Lukanova A, Rinaldi S, et al. Hormonal, metabolic, and inflammatory profiles and endometrial cancer risk within the EPIC cohort—a factor analysis. *Am J Epidemiol.* 2013;177(8):787–799.

13. Freese KE, Kokai L, Edwards RP, et al. Adipose-derived stems cells and their role in human cancer development, growth, progression, and metastasis: a systematic review. *Cancer Res.* 2015;75(7):1161–1168.

14. Linkov F, Kokai L, Edwards R, et al. The role of adipose-derived stem cells in endometrial cancer proliferation. *Scand J Clin Lab Invest Suppl.* 2014;244:5458; discussion 57–58.

15. Soliman PT, Wu D, Tortolero-Luna G, et al. Association between adiponectin, insulin resistance, and endometrial cancer. *Cancer.* 2006;106(11):2376–2381.

16. Klopp AH, Zhang Y, Solley T, et al. Omental adipose tissue-derived stromal cells promote vascularization and growth of endometrial tumors. *Clin Cancer Res.* 2012;18(3):771–782.

17. Ma BB, Oza A, Eisenhauer E, et al. The activity of letrozole in patients with advanced or recurrent endometrial cancer and correlation with biological markers—a study of the national cancer institute of canada clinical trials group. *Int J Gynecol Cancer.* 2004;14(4):650–658.

18. Modica MJ, Kanal KM, Gunn ML. The obese emergency patient: imaging challenges and solutions. *Radiographics.* 2011;31(3):811–823.

19. Sharma A, Burnell M, Gentry-Maharaj A, et al. Factors affecting visualization of postmenopausal ovaries: descriptive study from the multicenter United Kingdom Collaborative Trial of Ovarian Cancer Screening (UKCTOCS). *Ultrasound Obstet Gynecol.* 2013;42(4):472–477.

20. Andolf E, Dahlander K, Aspenberg P. Ultrasonic thickness of the endometrium correlated to body weight in asymptomatic postmenopausal women. *Obstet Gynecol.* 1993;82(6):936–940.

21. Sit AS, Modugno F, Hill LM, Martin J, Weissfeld JL. Transvaginal ultrasound measurement of endometrial thickness as a biomarker for estrogen exposure. *Cancer Epidemiol Biomarkers Prev.* 2004;13(9):1459–1465.

22. Schindera ST, Odedra D, Mercer D, et al. Hybrid iterative reconstruction technique for abdominal CT protocols in obese patients: assessment of image quality, radiation dose, and low-contrast detectability in a phantom. *AJR Am J Roentgenol.* 2014;202(2):W146–W152.

23. Clark TJ, Mann CH, Shah N, Khan KS, Song F, Gupta JK. Accuracy of outpatient endometrial biopsy in the diagnosis of endometrial cancer: a systematic quantitative review. *BJOG.* 2002;109(3):313–321.

24. Committee on Gynecologic Practice. Committee opinion no. 619: gynecologic surgery in the obese woman. *Obstet Gynecol.* 2015;125(1):274–278.

25. Dorzin E, Nguyen L, Anderson E, Bunn D, Cunningham M. Effect of body mass index on conversion rates and complications among patients undergoing robotic surgery for endometrial cancer. *Gynecol Oncol.* 2015;137(April):200–201.

26. Bellone S, Shah HR, McKenney JK, Stone PJ, Santin AD. Recurrent endometrial carcinoma regression with the use of the aromatase inhibitor anastrozole. *Am J Obstet Gynecol.* 2008;199(3):e7–e10.

27. Tang KY, Gardiner SK, Gould C, Osmundsen B, Collins M, Winter WE 3rd. Robotic surgical staging for obese patients with endometrial cancer. *Am J Obstet Gynecol.* 2012;206(6):513.e1–513.e6.

28. Subramaniam A, Kim KH, Bryant SA, et al. A cohort study evaluating robotic versus laparotomy surgical outcomes of obese women with endometrial carcinoma. *Gynecol Oncol.* 2011;122(3):604–607.

29. Cardenas-Goicoechea J, Adams S, Bhat SB, Randall TC. Surgical outcomes of robotic-assisted surgical staging for endometrial cancer are equivalent to traditional laparoscopic staging at a minimally invasive surgical center. *Gynecol Oncol.* 2010;117(2):224–228.

30. Kilgore JE, Jackson AL, Ko EM, et al. Recurrence-free and 5-year survival following robotic-assisted surgical staging for endometrial carcinoma. *Gynecol Oncol.* 2013;129(1):49–53.

31. Ramirez PT, Adams S, Boggess JF, et al. Robotic-assisted surgery in gynecologic oncology: a Society of Gynecologic Oncology consensus statement. Developed by the Society of Gynecologic Oncology's Clinical Practice Robotics Task Force. *Gynecol Oncol.* 2012;124(2):180–184.

32. Horowitz NS, Wright AA. Impact of obesity on chemotherapy management and outcomes in women with gynecologic malignancies. *Gynecol Oncol.* 2015;138(1):201–206.

33. Lee CS, Murphy DJ, McMahon C, et al. Visceral adiposity is a risk factor for poor prognosis in colorectal cancer patients receiving adjuvant chemotherapy. *J Gastrointest Cancer.* 2015;46(3):243–250.

34. Wu W, Liu X, Chaftari P, et al. Association of body composition with outcome of docetaxel chemotherapy in metastatic prostate cancer: a retrospective review. *PLoS One.* 2015;10(3):e0122047.

35. Chan DS, Vieira AR, Aune D, et al. Body mass index and survival in women with breast cancer-systematic literature review and meta-analysis of 82 follow-up studies. *Ann Oncol.* 2014;25(10):1901–1914.

36. Tran BH, Nguyen TJ, Hwang BH, et al. Risk factors associated with venous thromboembolism in 49,028 mastectomy patients. *Breast.* 2013;22(4):444–448.

37. Modica MJ, Kanal KM, Gunn ML. The obese emergency patient: Imaging challenges and solutions. *Radiographics.* 2011;31(3):811–823.

38. Lin LL, Hertan L, Rengan R, Teo BK. Effect of body mass index on magnitude of setup errors in patients treated with adjuvant radiotherapy for endometrial cancer with daily image guidance. *Int J Radiat Oncol Biol Phys.* 2012;83(2):670–675.

39. Choi M, Fuller CD, Wang SJ, et al. Effect of body mass index on shifts in ultrasound-based image-guided intensity-modulated radiation therapy for abdominal malignancies. *Radiother Oncol.* 2009;91(1):114–119.

40. von Gruenigen VE, Tian C, Frasure H, Waggoner S, Keys H, Barakat RR. Treatment effects, disease recurrence, and survival in obese women with early endometrial carcinoma: a Gynecologic Oncology Group study. *Cancer.* 2006;107(12):2786–2791.

41. Kim JJ, Sefton EC, Bulun SE. Progesterone receptor action in leiomyoma and endometrial cancer. *Prog Mol Biol Transl Sci.* 2009;87:53–85.

42. Lu KH, Loose DS, Yates MS, et al. Prospective multicenter randomized intermediate biomarker study of oral contraceptive versus depo-provera for prevention of endometrial cancer in women with lynch syndrome. *Cancer Prev Res (Phila).* 2013;6(8): 774–781.

43. Thigpen T, Brady MF, Homesley HD, Soper JT, Bell J. Tamoxifen in the treatment of advanced or recurrent endometrial carcinoma: a Gynecologic Oncology Group study. *J Clin Oncol.* 2001;19(2):364–367.

44. Fiorica JV, Brunetto VL, Hanjani P, et al. Phase II trial of alternating courses of megestrol acetate and tamoxifen in advanced endometrial carcinoma: a Gynecologic Oncology Group study. *Gynecol Oncol.* 2004;92(1):10–14.

45. Rose PG, Brunetto VL, VanLe L, Bell J, Walker JL, Lee RB. A phase II trial of anastrozole in advanced recurrent or persistent endometrial carcinoma: a Gynecologic Oncology Group study. *Gynecol Oncol.* 2000;78(2):212–216.

46. Thangavelu A, Hewitt MJ, Quinton ND, Duffy SR. Neoadjuvant treatment of endometrial cancer using anastrozole: a randomised pilot study. *Gynecol Oncol.* 2013;131(3):613–618.

47. Calle EE, Thun MJ, Petrelli JM, Rodriguez C, Heath CW Jr. Body-mass index and mortality in a prospective cohort of US adults. *N Engl J Med.* 1999;341(15):1097–1105.

48. Renehan AG, Crosbie EJ, Campbell PT. Re: prediagnosis body mass index, physical activity, and mortality in endometrial cancer patients. *J Natl Cancer Inst.* 2014;106(2):djt375.

49. Crosbie EJ, Roberts C, Qian W, Swart AM, Kitchener HC, Renehan AG. Body mass index does not influence post-treatment survival in early stage endometrial cancer: results from the MRC ASTEC trial. *Eur J Cancer.* 2012;48(6):853–864.

50. Morrow CP, Bundy BN, Kurman RJ, et al. Relationship between surgical-pathological risk factors and outcome in clinical stage I and II carcinoma of the endometrium: a Gynecologic Oncology Group study. *Gynecol Oncol.* 1991;40(1):55–65.

51. Doll KM, Kalinowski AK, Snavely AC, et al. Obesity is associated with worse quality of life in women with gynecologic malignancies: an opportunity to improve patient-centered outcomes. *Cancer.* 2015;121(3): 395–402.

52. Smits A, Lopes A, Das N, Bekkers R, Galaal K. Quality of life in ovarian cancer survivors: the influence of obesity. *Int J Gynecol Cancer.* 2015;25(4):616–621.

53. Rouanet P, Dubois JB, Gely S, Pourquier H. Exclusive radiation therapy in endometrial carcinoma. *Int J Radiat Oncol Biol Phys.* 1993;26(2):223–228.

54. McCarroll ML, Armbruster S, Frasure HE, et al. Self-efficacy, quality of life, and weight loss in overweight/obese endometrial cancer survivors (SUCCEED): a randomized controlled trial. *Gynecol Oncol.* 2014; 132(2):397–402.

55. Nock NL, Dimitropolous A, Tkach J, Frasure H, von Gruenigen V. Reduction in neural activation to high-calorie food cues in obese endometrial cancer survivors after a behavioral lifestyle intervention: a pilot study. *BMC Neurosci.* 2012;13:74.doi:10.1186/ 1471-2202-13-74.

56. Nock NL, Dimitropoulos A, Rao SM, et al. Rationale and design of REWARD (revving-up exercise for sustained weight loss by altering neurological reward and drive): a randomized trial in obese endometrial cancer survivors. *Contemp Clin Trials.* 2014;39(2): 236–245.

57. Grigsby PW, Kuske RR, Perez CA, et al. Medically inoperable stage I adenocarcinoma of the endometrium treated with radiotherapy alone. *Int J Radiat Oncol Biol Phys.* 1987;13(4):483–488.

58. Taghian A, Pernot M, Hoffstetter S, Luporsi E, Bey P. Radiation therapy alone for medically inoperable patients with adenocarcinoma of the endometrium. *Int J Radiat Oncol Biol Phys.* 1988;15(5): 1135–1140.

59. Rose PG, Baker S, Kern M, et al. Primary radiation therapy for endometrial carcinoma: a case controlled study. *Int J Radiat Oncol Biol Phys.* 1993;27(3):585–590.

60. Chao CK, Grigsby PW, Perez CA, Mutch DG, Herzog T, Camel HM. Medically inoperable stage I endometrial carcinoma: a few dilemmas in radiotherapeutic management. *Int J Radiat Oncol Biol Phys.* 1996;34(1):27–31.

61. Fishman DA, Roberts KB, Chambers JT, Kohorn EI, Schwartz PE, Chambers SK. Radiation therapy as exclusive treatment for medically inoperable patients with stage I and II endometrioid carcinoma with endometrium. *Gynecol Oncol.* 1996;61(2):189–196.

62. Chao CK, Grigsby PW, Perez CA, et al. Brachytherapy-related complications for medically inoperable stage I endometrial carcinoma. *Int J Radiat Oncol Biol Phys.* 1995;31(1):37–42.

63. Niazi TM, Souhami L, Portelance L, Bahoric B, Gilbert L, Stanimir G. Long-term results of high-dose-rate brachytherapy in the primary treatment of medically inoperable stage I-II endometrial carcinoma. *Int J Radiat Oncol Biol Phys.* 2005;63(4):1108–1113.

64. Kupelian PA, Eifel PJ, Tornos C, Burke TW, Delclos L, Oswald MJ. Treatment of endometrial carcinoma with radiation therapy alone. *Int J Radiat Oncol Biol Phys.* 1993;27(4):817–824.

Urinary Incontinence

Eddie H. M. Sze, MD

INTRODUCTION

Urinary incontinence is a common and potentially debilitating condition. It affects about 10%–40% of adult women and is considered severe in approximately 3%–17%.[1] The true magnitude of this problem is unknown due to underreporting. About 60%–75% of incontinent patients do not seek treatment for their condition because of embarrassment, the belief that incontinence is a normal condition of aging, fear of needing surgery, the lack of knowledge about the treatments available, and skepticism about the effectiveness of the available therapies.[2–7] The World Health Organization has identified urinary incontinence as an important global health issue.

Although urinary incontinence usually does not affect a woman's physical well-being, it creates a significant social problem. Urinary incontinence has been found to reduce social interactions and physical activities and is associated with poor health, impaired emotional and psychological well-being, and interference with sexual relations.[8–11] In older patients, urinary incontinence doubles the risk of injury and bone fracture from falling and being admitted to a nursing home.[12,13] Because of these reasons, clinicians should routinely screen all their female patients for this prevalent condition.

Urinary incontinence in overweight and obese patients is evaluated and managed in a similar fashion as their normal-weight counterparts.[14–18] The efficacy of available treatments for urinary incontinence is determined almost exclusively from randomized controlled trials (RCTs) that included patients from all weight classes. The evaluation and treatment presented are based on findings from these trials with minor modifications for overweight and obese patients. Emphasis is on these modifications when applicable.

EVALUATION

Although urinary incontinence may be caused by numerous conditions, almost all incontinent patients seen by clinicians have either stress urinary incontinence (SUI), overactive bladder (OAB), or both, which account for about 50%, 25%, and 25% of the incontinent cases, respectively.[19] The initial evaluation of an incontinent patient is relatively straightforward. In addition to the standard history and physical examination used to evaluate any new gynecologic patient, we also assess the impact of urinary incontinence on the patient's quality of life (QoL); determine whether the patient has SUI, OAB, or both; and inquire about previous treatments.

Impact of Urinary Incontinence on Quality of Life

Urinary incontinence frequently has a negative effect on the patient's QoL, which is the major factor that determines whether she seeks care for her condition and the intensity of evaluation and treatment. Consequently, QoL assessment is an important part of evaluating urinary incontinence. For busy clinicians, the most convenient method to perform this assessment is to use one of the validated questionnaires designed to evaluate the impact of incontinence symptoms on a patient's QoL. At my facility, we use the International Consultation on Incontinence Modular Questionnaire—Urinary Incontinence Short Form, which consists of 4 questions related to the incontinence (Table 35-1). Clinicians can request permission to use this copyrighted questionnaire by writing to the Bristol Urological Institute (nikki.cotterill@bui.ac.uk).

Determine Whether the Patient Has SUI, OAB, or Both

Stress Urinary Incontinence

The International Continence Society (ICS) defined SUI as involuntary urine loss that occurs during periods of intra-abdominal pressure increase, such as when coughing, sneezing, and jumping.[20] If our initial evaluation identifies a patient with an uncomplicated problem (i.e., does not have pain, hematuria, recurrent infections, suspected or proven voiding problems, significant pelvic organ prolapse, persistent or recurrent

TABLE 35-1 International Consultation on Incontinence Modular Questionnaire: Urinary Incontinence (ICIQ-UI) Short Form[a]

ICIQ-UI Short Form (US English)

CONFIDENTIAL

Subject number　　Subject initial

D D　M M M　Y Y
Today's date

Many people leak urine some of the time. We are trying to find out how many people leak urine, and how much this bothers them. We would be grateful if you could answer the following questions, thinking about how you have been, on average, over the PAST FOUR WEEKS.

1　**Please write in your date of birth:**

DAY　MONTH　YEAR

2　**Are you** (Check one): Female ☐　Male ☐

3　**How often do you leak urine?** (Check one box)

never ☐	0
about once a week or less often ☐	1
two or three times a week ☐	2
about once a day ☐	3
several times a day ☐	4
all the time ☐	5

4　**We would like to know how much urine <u>you think</u> leaks. How much urine do you <u>usually</u> leak (whether you wear protection or not)?** (Check one box)

none ☐	0
a small amount ☐	2
a moderate amount ☐	4
a large amount ☐	6

5　**Overall, how much does leaking urine interfere with your everyday life?**
Please circle a number between 0 (not at all) and 10 (a great deal)

0 1 2 3 4 5 6 7 8 9 **10**
not at all　　　　　　　　　　　　　a great deal

ICIQ score: sum scores 3+4+5 ☐ ☐

6　**When does urine leak?** (Please check all that apply to you)

never – urine does not leak	☐
leaks before you can get to the bathroom	☐
leaks when you cough or sneeze	☐
leaks when you are asleep	☐
leaks when you are physically active/exercising	☐
leaks when you have finished urinating and are dressed	☐
leaks for no obvious reason	☐
leaks all the time	☐

Thank you very much for answering these questions.

[a]Copyright © ICIQ Group. Please contact www.iciq.net for permission to use ICIQ modules.

incontinence after pelvic irradiation, prior radical pelvic surgery, previous incontinence surgery, and suspected fistula) and produces a reasonably certain diagnosis of SUI, we routinely perform a urine analysis and possible culture and provide instructions on how to perform pelvic floor muscle exercises (PFMEs) prior to prescribing nonsurgical treatment.

We always perform a cough stress test and assess for postvoid residual (PVR) and the degree of urethral support when a patient with uncomplicated SUI is considering invasive, potentially morbid, or irreversible treatments or when a patient with a complicated presentation is considering nonsurgical or surgical treatment for her SUI.

We perform 3 tests in the following order:

1. Perform a cough stress test immediately after the patient has voided and evaluate the degree of her urethral support. A positive cough stress test objectively demonstrates that the patient has SUI, while a positive test in the supine position immediately after voiding indicates severe SUI and may require urodynamic studies (UDS) preoperatively to diagnose an associated intrinsic sphincter deficiency (ISD) because some procedures may be less effective in SUI associated with ISD.[21-23.] The degree of urethral support is often assessed by the Q-tip test. We rarely use this test because inserting a cotton swab into the urethra is painful, and urethral hypermobility can be similarly diagnosed by observing the distal anterior vaginal wall descended close to the hymen with Valsalva or cough.[24,25]

2. If the postvoid cough stress test is positive, we conclude the evaluation by measuring the PVR using a bladder scanner or a red rubber catheter. The exact definition of an elevated PVR volume that is clinically relevant remains unclear. One frequently mentioned guideline considers a PVR less than 100 mL as normal and more than 200 mL as abnormal, while a volume between 100 mL and 200 mL requires clinical correlation to determine its significance. A single elevated PVR should always be confirmed with a second measurement. Patients with elevated PVR may be at increased risk for transient or permanent postoperative voiding difficulty after a continence procedure.

3. If the postvoid cough stress test is negative, we insert a red rubber catheter to measure the PVR and then attach the catheter to a 60-mL catheter tip syringe and fill the bladder in a retrograde fashion with room temperature saline. At maximum bladder capacity, we remove the catheter and repeat the cough stress test with the patient in the supine and standing position, if indicated. The cough stress test is reliable when it is performed at a bladder volume of 300 mL or symptomatic fullness. A negative cough stress test after bladder filling usually indicates that the patient does not have SUI, while a negative test without bladder filling may misdiagnose SUI in up to 80% of patients.[26-30]

Bladder filling may occasionally trigger detrusor overactivity, which manifests as a sudden rise in the meniscus in the syringe while the patient experiences urgency or urgency incontinence. If detrusor overactivity occurs prior to a positive cough stress test, the patient needs to be evaluated with a UDS.[26,30] Similarly, if the incontinence continues after the cough or Valsalva, the patient may have stress-induced detrusor overactivity, which also requires further testing with a UDS.

TABLE 35-2 Definition of Overactive Bladder

Presence of urinary urgency with or without urgency incontinence usually with frequency and nocturia in the absence of infection, metabolic disturbances, or obvious pathologic conditions that could account for these symptoms.
a. Infection: cystitis
b. Neurological disorders:
    1. Suprapontine cerebral lesion: Alzheimer disease, multiple sclerosis, Parkinson disease, cerebrovascular accident, traumatic brain injury, brain tumor
    2. Suprasacral infrapontine spinal cord lesion: spinal cord injury, myelomeningocele, spinal cord tumor, transverse myelitis, multiple sclerosis
    3. Peripheral nerve lesion: herniated disk, caudal equine syndrome, peripheral nerve injury, diabetes mellitus, chronic alcohol use, AIDs, vitamin B_{12} deficiency, radical pelvic surgery
c. Metabolic disturbances: diabetes mellitus and insipidus, pregnancy, atrophy
d. Physiologic causes: excessive fluid, alcohol, and caffeine intake
e. Pelvic malignancy and radiation: bladder and ovarian cancer
f. Gastrointestinal disorder: constipation
g. Mobility disorder

Overactive Bladder

Overactive bladder is defined as the presence of urinary urgency with or without urgency incontinence, usually with frequency and nocturia in the absence of infection or obvious pathologic conditions that could account for these symptoms (Table 35-2).[20] The first step in diagnosing OAB is to determine whether the patient has the characteristic symptoms of urinary urgency, frequency, nocturia, and urgency incontinence. The diagnosis of OAB requires the presence of urinary urgency, its hallmark symptom, plus 1 of the other 3 symptoms.[20]

Urinary urgency is defined as complaint of a sudden compelling desire to pass urine that is difficult to defer.[20] Increased daytime urinary frequency is defined as the complaint that micturition occurs more frequently during waking hours than previously deemed normal by the patient.[20] Frequency associated with OAB is typically characterized by small-volume voids.[18] Nocturia is defined as the complaint of interruption of sleep 1 or more times because of the need to micturate.[20] Each void is preceded and followed by sleep. Urgency incontinence is involuntary leakage from the urethra synchronous with the sensation of a sudden, compelling desire to void that is difficult to defer.[20]

The second part of diagnosing an OAB is to determine whether the patient's symptoms are precipitated or exacerbated by the following pathologic conditions:

CYSTITIS—Cystitis may cause OAB symptoms and SUI, especially in older patients.

NEUROGENIC BLADDER—When a neurologic disease disturbs the normal bladder function, the patient is considered to have a neurogenic bladder (NGB). Neurologic diseases that more commonly affect the lower urinary tract function are listed in Table 35-2. Bladder dysfunction may occur early in the course of the disease or as it progresses, either abruptly or gradually. NGB is extremely rare in patients who have no history of neurologic disease, are fluent in their speech, can give organized and appropriate responses to questions about past medical and family history, and have demonstrated normal mobility. These patients may be screened with a focused neurologic examination that evaluates sacral spinal cord segments 2 to 4 by testing the perineal sensation and sacral reflexes. If the history or general assessment suggests a neurologic disorder, the patient should be referred for a thorough evaluation.

METABOLIC DISTURBANCES—Metabolic conditions that may cause lower urinary tract symptoms include poorly controlled diabetes mellitus (DM), pregnancy, atrophic changes in the urogenital tract, and rarely, diabetes insipidus. Because DM is prevalent and often undiagnosed, all patients who present with OAB, especially if they are overweight or obese, should be screened for glycosuria and, if indicated, a random plasma glucose level.[31] Glycosuria and the associated osmotic diuresis often cause urinary frequency, urgency, and nocturia. The presence of these symptoms and a random plasma glucose level of 200 mg/dL or greater is one criterion used to diagnose DM.

PHYSIOLOGIC CAUSES—The evaluation of OAB (and SUI) should include an inquiry into the type and amount of fluid intake each day because increased fluid, caffeine, and alcohol intake may precipitate or exacerbate an OAB (and SUI).[32-34] Patients who are uncertain or unable to provide such information accurately should be asked to fill out a 3-day bladder dairy, which records the type and amount of fluid intake and measures urine output. Patients with polydipsia and the resulting polyuria have frequent normal or large-volume voids and a closely matched intake and output, while those with OAB have frequent small-volume voids. These two conditions can be distinguished by a bladder diary.

PELVIC MALIGNANCY—Ovarian and bladder malignancy and pelvic radiation may cause OAB symptoms or SUI. Patients who present with OAB should always have an abdominal and pelvic examination, and, if needed, a pelvic ultrasound, to screen for ovarian malignancy. Similarly, they should have a urine dipstick test or analysis to screen for bladder cancer, which most frequently manifests as painless hematuria and second most commonly with urinary urgency and frequency. Hematuria diagnosed by a urine dipstick test should always be confirmed or refuted by a microscopic examination.[35]

GASTROINTESTINAL CONDITION—Constipation has frequently been cited as a transient cause of urinary incontinence, especially in older patients. Although it is significantly more prevalent among patients who have OAB than asymptomatic controls, we are uncertain whether relieving constipation would improve OAB symptoms.[36] Because it may cause abdominal and pelvic pain and discomfort, fecal incontinence, anal fissure, rectal and pelvic organ prolapse from prolonged straining, and possibly exacerbated OAB symptoms, we routinely screen for constipation using the Rome III criteria (Table 35-3) and treat this prevalent gastrointestinal condition when present.[37,38]

MOBILITY DISORDER—Frequently, OAB coexists with other disorders, such as dementia, severe arthritis, morbid obesity, or hemiplegia, that severely restrict a patient's mobility and exacerbates her urinary incontinence because she cannot get to the bathroom after experiencing an urge to void. Clinicians should recognize that these patients may need other measures, such portable commodes and assistance to get to a toileting facility in addition to the standard therapy to manage their OAB.

Previous Treatments for Urinary Incontinence

Clinicians should inquire about previous therapies, duration of treatment, outcome, associated adverse events, and the reason for discontinuing each therapy.

TABLE 35-3 Rome III Criteria[a]

For Constipation

Presence of symptoms at least 25% of the time during the past 3 months Need 2 of the 6 symptoms plus the absence of irritable bowel syndrome
1. Have 0–2 (<3) bowel movements a week
2. Have hard or lumpy stools
3. Straining during a bowel movement
4. Incomplete bowel movement
5. Feels like there is a blockage in the rectum
6. Have to press around your bottom or vagina

For Irritable Bowel Syndrome Module

Diagnosis requires the presence of 1 plus 2 of the other 3:
1. In the last 3 months, did you often have discomfort or pain in your abdomen?
2. Does your pain or discomfort get better or stop after you have a bowel movement?
3. When the pain or discomfort starts, do you have a change in your usual number of bowel movements?
4. When the pain or discomfort starts, do you have either softer or harder stools than usual?

[a]From Cammu H, Van Nylen M, Blockeel C, et al. Who will benefit from pelvic floor muscle training for stress urinary incontinence? *Am J Obstet Gynecol.* 2004;191:1152–1157.

INITIAL TREATMENT FOR STRESS URINARY INCONTINENCE: NONSURGICAL VERSUS SURGICAL OPTION

Pelvic floor muscle exercises, which have a reported subjective cure rate of 53%–97% and an objective cure rate of 5%–49%, are widely accepted as the first-line treatment for SUI.[15,16,38,39] However, PFMEs are less effective in patients with more severe SUI (more than 1–2 leaks per day), and their efficacy is infrequently maintained long term.[38-42] The only sustained benefit of PFME was attributed largely to knack, which is contraction of the pelvic floor muscles before coughing, sneezing, and other similar activities to prevent involuntary urine loss.[41,42]

In many patients, PFMEs in the long run just postponed the surgery. After 3 to 15 years, 25%–50% of patients initially treated with PFMEs have proceeded to surgery.[41-43] Patients who did not respond to PFMEs initially had incontinence surgery sooner than those who responded well.[41]

The minimally invasive synthetic midurethral sling is widely regarded as an effective treatment for SUI, with subjective and objective cure rates between 57% and 92%. It is often performed in an ambulatory setting with minimal complications.[44-46]

This difference in the reported frequencies of a successful outcome between these two treatments raises the question whether all patients, especially those with more severe SUI, should be initially treated with PFMEs or the minimally invasive sling.

In a large, multicenter, prospective, randomized Dutch trial, which involved 460 patients with moderate-to-severe SUI, 49% assigned to PFMEs crossed over to the surgical option within 12 months, while 11% assigned to the surgical group crossed over to the PFME group.[40] Intent-to-treat analysis at 12 months showed that the surgery group had significantly higher subjective and objective cure rates and greater improvement in urogenital distress inventory scores than the PFME group. The authors concluded that patients with moderate-to-severe SUI should be counseled regarding both PFME and surgery as initial treatment options.

Given the variability in a patient's tolerance for incontinence and moderate at best correlation among various severity of incontinence measures, we routinely offer all patients who present with bothersome SUI both PFMEs and surgery as initial treatment options.[47]

OUR FIRST-LINE NONSURGICAL TREATMENT FOR SUI: PFME WITH BEHAVIORAL THERAPIES

We usually prescribe PFME with behavioral therapies, which include bladder retraining, weight loss, avoidance of bladder stimulants, and fluid reduction and constipation treatment, if indicated, as the first-line nonsurgical treatment for SUI. PFMEs are significantly more effective than placebo and topical estrogen and are either superior or similar to vaginal cone and pelvic floor electrical stimulation in managing SUI.[48-51]

A 2011 Cochrane review concluded that contracting the correct muscles at the right time and performing a sufficient number of PFMEs were important for successful treatment, but there were insufficient data to determine the best approach (such as frequency of training, type of contraction) to train the pelvic floor muscles.[52] Its only recommendation is to offer patients reasonably frequent follow-ups during the training period because such follow-ups improved the efficacy of PFMEs.[53] One or 2 additional sessions may be just as or more effective than more numerous follow-up visits. We recommend that clinicians follow the National Institute for Health and Care Excellence and American Urogynecologic Society guidelines, which recommend 10 PFMEs 3 times each day with frequent follow-up visits as suggested by the Cochrane review.[17,53,54]

Modifying caffeine and fluid intake has a significant beneficial effect on SUI. A 4-week prospective study found that by eliminating caffeine and limiting fluid intake to no more than 750 mL daily reduced the incontinence episodes by 65% among 39 subjects with mild-to-moderate SUI.[32]

Weight loss, which includes massive loss in obese women after bariatric surgery and more modest loss in overweight and obese subjects with nonsurgical treatments, is an effective treatment for SUI.[55,56] We rarely recommend weight loss as the initial treatment for SUI because most, if not all, overweight and obese patients had already attempted to lose weight numerous times using different methods and failed. Also, we do not recommend or encourage bariatric surgery or pharmacologically induced weight loss for urinary incontinence because both are associated with significant morbidity, while involuntary urine loss rarely affects patients' physical health. We do inform them that a moderate amount of weight loss (about 15 pounds) would improve their QoL by significantly lessening their chances of experiencing incontinence.[56]

For patients actively trying to lose weight, we rarely prescribe time-consuming and labor-intensive bladder retraining because managing several treatments that require significant time and effort simultaneously may exceed their ability to incorporate each into their daily activities and cause them to abandon their treatments. We do, however, take time during each office visit to recognize their effort to lose weight and encourage them to persist in their endeavor.

Combining PFMEs with other nonsurgical treatments for SUI, such as the continence ring and vaginal cone, have not been shown to increase its efficacy.[57-60]

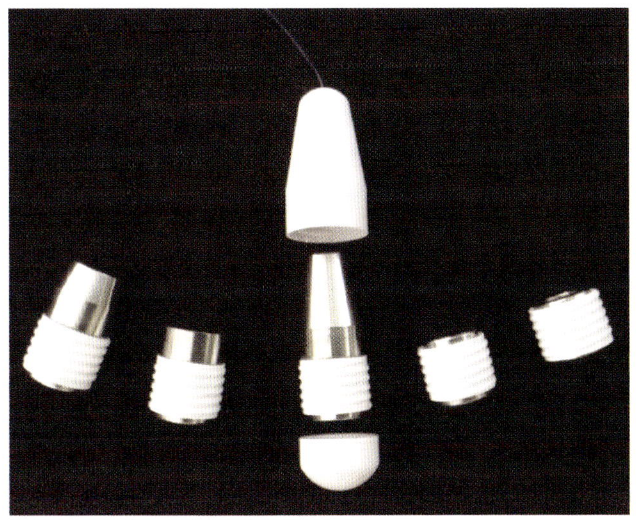

FIGURE 35-1. Vaginal cones.

SECOND-LINE NONSURGICAL TREATMENT FOR SUI: VAGINAL CONES OR CONTINENCE RING WITH TOPICAL ESTROGEN

For approximately 8% of patients who are unable to perform PFMEs, a vaginal cone is an alternative approach to exercise the pelvic floor muscles (Figure 35-1).[61] A 2013 Cochrane review found that the subjective and objective cure or improvement rates were similar between vaginal cone and PFMEs.[62] However, vaginal cones had a significantly lower compliance rate than PFMEs because they are uncomfortable and patients do not like to use them.[63,64]

The continence ring may be used to treat SUI even if patients do not have concomitant pelvic organ prolapse and is as effective as PFMEs. In a large, well-designed, multicenter, randomized trial, PFMEs, pessary, and the combination of both therapies were equally efficacious in managing SUI.[65] The continence ring is useful in about 25% of women with SUI, and its long-term efficacy is uncertain. In a prospective study, 239 women with SUI were offered pessary; 119 (50%) accepted the offered therapy, 106 (44%) were successfully fitted, and 55 (23%) used the pessary for at least 6 months.[66]

Topical estrogen may be used with the continence ring to minimize the risk of vaginal erosion in women who have a severely atrophic vagina and reduce the frequency and severity of SUI in postmenopausal women.[49,67]

SURGICAL TREATMENT FOR STRESS URINARY INCONTINENCE

- Our surgical treatment of choice for SUI is tension-free vaginal tape (TVT).
- Our second surgical choice for SUI is an autologous fascial lata sling.
- Our third surgical choice for SUI is open retropubic colposuspension (Burch).

For overweight and obese patients who did not respond to nonsurgical treatment, we routinely recommend weight loss as an effective and less-morbid option to surgical intervention for their SUI. For those who choose the surgical option, we use the TVT (Gynecare, Ethicon, Inc., Somerville NJ) as our surgical procedure of choice.

Minimally invasive midurethral synthetic slings have been described as an ideal surgical treatment for SUI in obese patients because they have a short operating time and a low rate of complications and are probably as effective in obese as in normal-weight patients.[44,68–70] Two possible drawbacks are that the prepackaged trocars and slings may not have sufficient length to reach the abdominal incision in a small number of morbidly obese patients, and a very thick vulva may push the trocar cephalad during its insertion into the retropubic space and increase the risk of bladder perforation and possibly bowel and vascular injuries. Clinicians should carefully assess each patient carefully during the preoperative examination and determine whether the sling can be placed safely.

The TVT is the most frequently used retropubic midurethral sling and the most common surgical option for SUI at present. We choose TVT because it is as effective as open retropubic colposuspension (Burch) and an autologous fascial sling and more effective than laparoscopic colposuspension (Burch) and transobturator tape (TOT) midurethral synthetic sling, especially in patients with ISD and recurrent SUI, and TVT has excellent long-term outcome.[44,71–79]

For patients who have mesh complications, erosions, and allergy or do not want a foreign material in their body, we use an autologous fascial sling to treat their SUI because it is more efficacious than traditional slings that used xenograft or allograft graft and open Burch and is as effective as TVT.[79–82] If the patient is also scheduled to undergo a laparotomy, we use open Burch and place two sutures on each side.[83–85]

MIXED URINARY INCONTINENCE

For patients who have mixed urinary incontinence, we routinely treat their OAB first. Although a substantial portion of mixed urinary incontinence resolves after midurethral synthetic slings, their cure rates are often lower than for pure SUI and tend to progressively deteriorate as urgency incontinence gradually increases with time.[73–75] This seems to occurs more frequently with retropubic than transobturator slings.

When surgical treatment for mixed urinary incontinence is indicated, we repeatedly counsel each patient about choosing between retropubic and transobturator slings and inform her in person and with printed information that urgency incontinence often persists or recurs years after the sling placement. This repeat counseling is paramount because patient satisfaction is related directly to her expectation of treatment outcome.[86,87] Despite this intensive preoperative counseling, clinicians can still anticipate that many of their patients will expect surgery to provide near or complete relief of their urgency and urgency incontinence.[88]

MANAGING OVERACTIVE BLADDER

There are several options for managing overactive bladder:

- Selecting a treatment
- First-line treatment for OAB: behavioral therapies
- Second-line treatment for OAB: ring pessary with topical estrogen
- Third-line treatment for OAB: percutaneous tibial nerve stimulation
- Fourth-line treatment for OAB: antimuscarinic and mirabegron

Selecting a Treatment

The first step in selecting a treatment is to educate patients that OAB is a chronic condition, which often waxes and wanes, with good days and bad days, and needs to be managed over time. Although a proportion of OAB remits during a given year, symptoms usually persist for years and exacerbate with age.[89]

Patients should also be informed that OAB does not have an ideal treatment, and whether it will respond to a particular therapy and the degree of response are difficult to predict. Most available therapies can improve but infrequently cure its symptoms.[18]

Patients often have to try several different treatments before they can find one that would adequately control their symptoms. In addition, these treatments often have adverse side effects.

Having realistic expectations, a clear understanding of the OAB's chronic course, the adverse side effects, and the amount of required effort associated with a particular treatment and the necessity of a trial-and-error approach in selecting a therapy are paramount because they can ultimately influence the patient's satisfaction with the treatment process and outcomes.[86] Clinicians can facilitate this process by considering each patient's preferences when selecting a treatment.

Our First-Line Treatment for OAB: Behavioral Therapies

Behavioral therapies are widely recommended as the first-line treatment for OAB because they are just as effective as or maybe more effective than an antimuscarinic; are noninvasive and inexpensive; have minimal adverse effects; and may be combined with other treatments.[14-18] We usually prescribe bladder retraining, urge suppression using PFMEs, avoiding bladder stimulants, and if indicated, fluid reduction, treatment for constipation, and weight loss. If the OAB is severe, we usually prescribe behavioral therapies with an antimuscarinic medication.

We believe that behavioral therapy is an ideal treatment for overweight and obese patients because their active participation in improving bladder control promotes self-confidence that they can improve their QoL, which in turn may motivate them to lose weight.

Bladder Retraining

Table 35-4 contains a bladder retraining and urge suppression instruction sheet for a patient who normally voids every hour during the day. The choice of the initial voiding interval should be similar to how often the patient normally voids and is gradually increased at 15- or 30-minute increments until she is voiding every 3 hours.

TABLE 35-4 Bladder-Retraining Instructions

The goal of this training program is to regain control of your bladder:
1. Go to the bathroom and empty your bladder every hour on the hour during the day or waking hours.
2. Do not empty your bladder between the scheduled voiding times. Do your best to control your urge to void. If you have an accident, do not become discouraged. Continue to follow the voiding schedule.
3. When you are sleeping at night, empty your bladder only as needed. Do not get up every hour to void when you are sleeping.
4. When you wake up next morning, empty your bladder and then follow the voiding schedule again.
5. You may skip one or more scheduled voidings if you do not feel the urge to void.
6. After the first week, increase the time interval between voiding by **15** minutes.
    First week: Void every **1** hour.
    Second week: Void every **1** hour and **15** minutes.
    Third week: Void every **1** hour and **30** minutes.
7. Increase the time interval between emptying your bladder by **15** minutes every week until you are voiding every **3** hours.
8. To avoid losing control of your bladder between the scheduled voiding:
    a. As soon as you feel **any** urgency (no matter how little) to void, stop what you are doing and stay still.
    b. Perform **4** Kegel exercises as hard as you can and keep repeating 4 Kegel exercises as many times as you need to make the urgency go away.

Most patients treated with bladder retraining and PFMEs experience a 50%–80% reduction in the frequency of urgency incontinence, with significant improvement in QoL, but this combination of therapies infrequently provides complete symptom relief.[18] The combination of bladder retraining and PFMEs produces symptomatic relief and improves QoL faster than either treatment alone.[90]

Clinicians should schedule frequent follow-up visits during the treatment to promote patient compliance and enhance patients' satisfaction and treatment outcome.[91] If bladder retraining does not achieve the desired outcome, adding an antimuscarinic may further improve symptom control and QoL.[18]

Pelvic Floor Muscle Exercises

The PFMEs augment bladder retraining and are just as effective in managing OAB by inhibiting detrusor contractions and increasing the strength and tone of the pelvic floor muscle to enhance the patient's ability to hold urine.[91-93] Most patients are unable to learn to perform PFMEs correctly from verbal or written instructions alone.[94] We usually teach PFMEs during pelvic examination and confirm that the patient is performing the exercises correctly by detecting a palpable increase in the firmness of the levator ani and watching her external anus drawing inward and upward.

We do not use biofeedback to teach PFMEs because the two commonly employed biofeedback techniques, which utilize perineal electrocardiographic (ECG) surface pads and a vaginal probe to measure the electromyographic activities and vaginal pressure increase, respectively, frequently cannot distinguish between Valsalva maneuver and PFMEs. If we are unable to teach PFMEs, our preference is to refer these patients to a physical therapist who specializes in treating pelvic floor disorders.

Avoiding Bladder Stimulants and Fluid Reduction

Table 35-5 contains a sample instruction on fluid and caffeine intake. The optimal daily fluid intake has not been determined by clinical studies. In 2004, the Institute of Medicine reported that most people meet their daily hydration needs by letting their thirst be their guide.[95] Unless the patient is exercising heavily or works in hot conditions, she can drink less than the frequently recommended 64 ounces each day. However, clinicians may not want to prescribe fluid reduction for OAB unless a voiding diary showed that their patient's daily fluid intake is significantly more than 64 ounces a day without a valid indication and she has polyuria, which is defined as more than 40 mL/kg body weight during a 24-hour period.[20] For patients who are drinking large amounts of water to lose weight, we usually ask them to decrease their intake by an amount that they do not feel would interfere with their endeavor.

Weight Loss

Weight loss is a highly effective therapy for OAB.[55,56] As with patients with SUI, we rarely recommend this treatment to overweight and obese patients who are already participating in time-consuming and labor-intensive bladder retraining. In addition, other therapies regain bladder control faster than weight loss. We usually prescribe weight loss when other therapies had either failed or did not provide sufficient relief of OAB.

Placebo Effect

An important but rarely mentioned benefit of choosing an inexpensive and safe treatment as the first-line therapy for OAB is that some patients will experience spontaneous remission over time and respond regardless of which treatment is prescribed, as evidenced by the 20%–60% placebo response rate in RCTs.[50,56]

TABLE 35-5 Lifestyle Changes to Improve Your Bladder Function

1. Avoid excessive fluid intake.
   Most people can meet their daily fluid needs by letting their thirst determine how much to drink. You do not need to drink the frequently recommended 64 ounces each day unless you are exercising heavily or working in a hot environment.
   Suggestions to avoid excessive fluid intake:
   Do not carry a bottle of water with you.
   a. Use a smaller cup or glass.
   b. If your mouth is dry, try sugar-free gum or candy, ice chips, small sips of water, oral lubricants.
   You should not avoid drinking fluids because you are afraid of having an accident.
2. The following products may irritate your bladder; avoid or modify their intake as much as possible:
   Caffeine: Coffee, tea, green tea, cola, diet cola, Pepsi, and Mountain Dew, as well as many other sodas, chocolate, and energy drinks, contain caffeine. Caffeine may irritate your bladder and is also a diuretic.
   Artificial sweeteners: Beverages that contain artificial sweeteners such as aspartame or saccharin *may* also irritate your bladder.
   Diet Pepsi, Diet Coke, and Diet Mountain Dew contain not only artificial sweeteners but also caffeine.
   Citrus juice: Sometimes orange or grapefruit juice can irritate your bladder.
   Alcohol *may* irritate your bladder.
3. Weight loss: If you are overweight, weight loss will relieve some of the pressure on your bladder and help you regain your bladder control.
4. Stopping cigarette smoking will not only improve your health but also *may* improve your bladder control.

Our Second-Line Treatment for OAB: Ring Pessary and Topical Estrogen

There are few data that demonstrate the efficacy of a ring pessary in managing OAB.[96-99] Despite this paucity of data, we choose the ring pessary with topical estrogen as the second-line treatment for patients with OAB who have any degree of anterior vaginal wall prolapse because it is widely applicable, inexpensive, and easily managed and has minimal, if any, adverse effects. Topical estrogen minimizes the risk of vaginal erosion in patients who have severe genital atrophy and may improve OAB symptoms.[100]

Our Third-Line Treatment for OAB: Percutaneous Tibial Nerve Stimulation

Percutaneous tibial nerve stimulation (PTNS) frequently reduces OAB symptoms and improves QoL; it is more effective than placebo, immediate-release (IR) oxybutynin, and extended-release (ER) tolterodine.[18,101] The treatment benefits are retained for 4 to 6 months once the treatment ceases but may be extended for at least 3 more years (probably much more, but this has not been studied) by maintenance therapy in which an additional PTNS session is prescribed when the patient starts to experience a recurrence of OAB symptoms. The effectiveness of PTNS may be increased by combining it with an antimuscarinic.[18]

The most frequently utilized treatment protocol involves one 30-minute stimulation session once a week for 12 weeks.[18] Adverse events are relatively uncommon and mild. The most frequently reported complications were painful sensation during stimulation that did not interrupt the treatment and minor bleeding at the insertion site.

Our Fourth-Line Treatment for OAB: Antimuscarinic and Mirabegron

Overactive bladder is a chronic condition that requires long-term treatment with an antimuscarinic medication. However, medical claim studies reported that about 43%–83% of patients discontinued their antimuscarinic within the first 30 days, while 37%–68% did not refill their prescription during the study period.[102-104] The discontinuation rate increased to 70%–95% within 12 months. In addition, patients usually discontinued their initially prescribed antimuscarinic without switching to a second formulation. The persistence rate for an antimuscarinic was equally dismal in Canada, the United Kingdom, Norway, Denmark, and Sweden. The most frequently cited reasons for the discontinuation were that the medication did not work as expected (35%–45%) and the presence of adverse side effects (35%).

To increase persistence, clinicians should educate their patients about the effectiveness of antimuscarinic medications and set realistic expectations. Studies found that the degree of 24-hour urinary frequency and urgency incontinence reduction was closely related to the baseline symptom levels for each antimuscarinic.[18] Specifically, patients with more severe symptoms, on average, experienced greater symptom reductions. However, only patients with relatively low baseline levels of incontinence were likely to experience complete symptom relief. In contrast, the degree of reduction in urinary urgency and nocturia was not related to the severity of baseline symptoms.

Also, patients should be informed that if they experience inadequate symptom control or unacceptable adverse side effects with one antimuscarinic, adjusting the dose, combining dose reduction with another therapy, or changing to a newer antimuscarinic may improve efficacy or adverse event profiles.[18]

Ideally, clinicians should be able to prescribe an antimuscarinic that is effective and has a low rate of adverse side effects. Unfortunately, this is not always possible. Our choice of antimuscarinic is usually dictated by the insurers' formularies, which frequently only include IR oral oxybutynin and tolterodine, while ER and newer formulations are only available to patients who have failed another antimuscarinic and receive preapproval by the insurer. Because the vast majority of the patients discontinued their first antimuscarinic without switching to a second formulation, clinicians have to find a balance between efficacy and side effects that is acceptable to the patients with the antimuscarinic(s) that is on the insurer's formulary to maintain persistence of treatment.

Our preference is to use flexible dosing, which allows patients to increase and decrease their dose of antimuscarinic within a time frame and dose range predetermined with their clinicians. This allows each patient to determine the optimal balance between efficacy and adverse side effects for herself. RCTs have shown that flexible dosing of IR oxybutynin was able to achieve an impressive 75%–80% mean reduction in urgency incontinence episodes and continence in 40% of patients.[105,106] The rate of moderate-to-severe xerostomia was less than 25%, suggesting that a dose increase was not consistently associated with a corresponding increase in the rate of adverse side effects.

Our starting dose for oxybutynin IR is 5 mg or 10 mg twice daily depending on the baseline frequency of urgency incontinence. Each patient is instructed to increase the dose by 5 mg each week until she experiences an 80% reduction in her urgency incontinence episodes, reaches a maximum dose of 40 mg daily, or has significant side effects, which she can relieve by a 5-mg dose reduction every 3 days until the adverse events are tolerable or relieved by other prophylactic methods. After 4 weeks, we reevaluate each patient to determine the treatment outcome and discuss whether she would like to increase or continue the present dose or change to another antimuscarinic or treatment. Whether flexible dosing increases patient persistence has not been adequately evaluated.

Our starting dose for solifenacin is 5 mg, which is increased to 10 mg if needed after 2 weeks. The starting dose for tolterodine is 1 mg, which is increased weekly to a maximum dose of 8 mg daily.

Overweight and obese patients do not need a higher dose of antimuscarinic. The only precaution is to prescribe IR and avoid ER formulations for patients who had bariatric surgery (malabsorption type) because of gastric dumping.

An antimuscarinic should be prescribed with extreme caution for patients who are already using other anticholinergic medications; who are frail and elderly; who have cognitive deficits, especially memory difficulties; who have impaired gastric emptying; or who have a history of urinary retention. Because of their potentially serious adverse effects, the American Geriatrics Society recommends that all 6 antimuscarinics currently approved for OAB treatment in the United States should be avoided in older adults.[107]

Mirabegron

Mirabegron is a β_3-adrenoceptor agonist that was approved in 2012 by the Food and Drug Administration (FDA) to treat OAB. The 2014 American Urological Association/ Society of Urodynamics, Female Pelvic Medicine, and Urogenital Reconstruction (AUA/SUFU) literature review concluded that mirabegron produced relatively modest symptom reduction and appeared to have similar efficacy as an antimuscarinic, but has a significantly lower rate of xerostomia that is similar to placebo.[18] Its long-term outcome and efficacy on more severe OAB has not been adequately evaluated.

We use mirabegron in patients who have very good OAB control with an antimuscarinic but are unable to tolerate xerostomia and had failed or are not interested in other therapies.

No Treatment

Clinicians should inform patients that they may opt for no treatment at any time with a minimal adverse effect on their health or impact on the success of later management should they decide to pursue treatment again in the future.

Indication for Referral

For patients whose OAB did not respond to behavioral therapies, the ring pessary, PTNS, and antimuscarinics, we recommend referral to a specialist for further evaluation and treatment.

SUMMARY

The most important aspect of treating urinary incontinence in overweight and obese women is to routinely screen them for this prevalent condition. Those who have bothersome incontinence should be evaluated and treated like their normal-weight counterparts. Clinicians should not assume or suggest that their urinary incontinence is caused by excessive body weight or prescribe weight reduction as the primary or only treatment for their involuntary urine loss.

REFERENCES

1. Hunskaar S, Burgio K, Diokono et al. Epidemiology and natural history of urinary incontinence (UI). In: Abrams P, Cardozo L, Khoury S, eds. *Incontinence.* 2nd ed. Plymouth, UK: Health Publication; 2002;165–201.
2. Burgio KL, Matthews KA, Engel BT. Prevalence, incidence, correlates of urinary incontinence in healthy, middle-aged women. *J Urol.* 1991;146:1255–1259.
3. Holst K, Wilson PD. The prevalence of female urinary incontinence and reasons for not seeking treatment. *N Z Med J.* 1988;101:756–758.
4. Burgio KL, Ives DG, Locher JL, et al. Treatment seeking for urinary incontinence in older adults. *J Am Geriatr Soc.* 1994;42:208–212.
5. Goldstein M, Hawthorne ME, Engeberg S, et al. Urinary incontinence: why people do not seek help. *J Gerontol Nurs.* 1992;18:15–20.
6. Norton PA, MacDonald LD, Sedgwick FM, et al. Distress and delay associated with urinary incontinence, frequency, and urgency in women. *BMJ.* 1988;297:1187–1189.
7. Branch LG, Walker LA, Wetle TT, et al. Urinary incontinence knowledge among community-dwelling people 65 years of age and older. *J Am Geriatr Soc.* 1994;42:1257–1262.
8. Resnick NM, Yalla SV, Laurino E. The pathophysiology of urinary incontinence among institutionalized elderly persons. *N Engl J Med.* 1989;320:1–7.
9. Hunskaar S, Vinsnes A. The quality of life in women with urinary incontinence as measured by the sickness impact profile. *J Am Geriatr Soc.* 1991;39:378–382.
10. Johnson TM, Kincade JE, Bernard SL. The association of urinary incontinence with poor self-rated health. *J Am Geriatr Soc.* 1998;46:238–248.
11. Temmel C, Haidinger G, Schmidbauer J. Urinary incontinence in both sexes: prevalence rates and impact on quality of life and sexual life. *Neurourol Urodyn.* 2001;19:259–271.
12. Brown JS, Vittinghoff E, Wyman J, et al. Urinary incontinence: does it increase risk for falls and fractures? *J Am Geriatr Soc.* 2000;48:721–725.
13. Wagner TH, Hu TW, Bentkover J, et al. Health-related consequences of overactive bladder. *Am J Manag Care.* 2002;8(19S):S598–S607.
14. Qaseem A, Dallas P, Forciea MA, et al. Nonsurgical management of urinary incontinence in women: a clinical practice guideline from the American College of Physicians. *Ann Intern Med.* 2014;161:429–440.
15. Thuroff JW, Abrams P, Andersson K-E, et al. EAU guidelines on urinary incontinence. *Eur Urol.* 2011;59:387–400.
16. Bettez M, Tu LM, Carlson K, et al. 2012 update: guidelines for adult urinary incontinence collaborative consensus document for the Canadian Urological Association. *Can Urol Assoc J.* 2012;6:354–363.
17. National Institute for Health and Care Excellence. Urinary incontinence in women: the management of urinary incontinence in women. http://guidance.nice.org.uk/CG 171. Clinical guideline 171. Accessed 2015.
18. Gormley EA, Lightner DJ, Burgio K, et al. Diagnosis and treatment of overactive bladder (non-neurogenic) in adults: AUA/SUFU guideline. http://www.auanet.org/education/guidelines/overactive-bladder.cfm. Accessed 2015.
19. Milsom I, Altman D, Cartwright R, et al. Epidemiology of urinary incontinence (UI) and other lower urinary tract symptoms (LUTS), pelvic organ prolapse (POP) and anal incontinence (AI). In: Abrams P, Cardozo L, Khoury S, Wein A, eds. *Incontinence.* Fifth International Consultation on Incontinence Recommendations of the International Scientific Committee: evaluation and treatment of urinary incontinence, pelvic organ prolapse and faecal incontinence; February 23–25, 2012; Paris. Brussels, Belgium: International Consultation of Urological Diseases (ICUD); 2013:28.
20. Haylen BT, de Ridder D, Freeman RM, et al. An International Urogynecological Association (IUGA)/International Continence Society (ICS) joint report on the terminology of female pelvic floor dysfunction. *Neurourol Urodyn.* 2010;29:4–20.
21. McClennan MT, Bent AE. Supine empty stress test as a predictor of low Valsalva leak point pressure. *Neurourol Urodyn.* 1998;17:121–127.
22. Hsu TH, Rackley RR, Appell RA. The supine stress test: a simple method to detect intrinsic urethral sphincter function. *J Urol.* 1999;162:460–463.
23. Schierlitz L, Dwyer PL, Rosamilia A, et al. Three-year follow-up of tension-free vaginal tape compared with transobturator tape in women with stress urinary incontinence and intrinsic sphincter deficiency. *Obstet Gynecol.* 2012;112:1253–1261.
24. Caputo RM, Benson JT. The Q-tip test and urethrovesical junction mobility. *Obstet Gynecol.* 1993;82:892–896.
25. Cogan SL, Weber AM, Hummel JP. Is urethral mobility really being assessed by the pelvic organ prolapse quantification (POP-Q) system? *Obstet Gynecol.* 2002;99:473–476.
26. Swift SE, Yoon EA. The test-retest reliability of the cough stress test in women with urinary incontinence. *Obstet Gynecol.* 1999;94:99–102.

27. Kadar N. The value of bladder filling in the clinical detection of urine loss and selection of patients for urodynamic testing. *BJOG*. 1998;95:698–704.

28. Scotti RJ, Myers DL. A comparison of the cough stress test and single-channel cystometry with multichannel urodynamic evaluation in genuine stress incontinence. *Obstet Gynecol*. 1993;81:430–433.

29. Summitt RL, Stovall TG, Bent AE, et al. Urinary incontinence: correlation of history and brief office evaluation with multichannel urodynamic testing. *Am J Obstet Gynecol*. 1992;166:1835–1844.

30. Weidner AC, Meyer ER, Visco AG, et al. Which women with stress incontinence require urodynamic evaluation? *Am J Obstet Gynecol*. 2001;184:20–27.

31. McGill JB. Diabetes mellitus and related disorders. In: Foster C, Mistry NF, Peddi PF, Sharma S, eds. *The Washington Manual of Medical Therapeutics*. 33rd ed. Philadelphia: Wolters Kluwer/Lippincott Williams & Wilkins; 2010;793-826.

32. Hashim H, Abrams P. How should patients with an overactive bladder manipulate their fluid intake? *BJU Int*. 2008;102:62–66.

33. Bryant CM, Dowell CJ, Fairbrother G. Caffeine reduction to improve urinary symptoms. *Br J Nurs*. 2002;11:560–565.

34. Swithinbank L, Hashim H, Abrams P. The effect of fluid intake on urinary symptoms in women. *J Urol*. 2005;174:187–189.

35. Davis R, Jones JS, Barocas DA, et al. Diagnosis, evaluation and follow-up of asymptomatic microhematuria (AMH) in adults: AUA guideline. https://www.auanet.org/education/guidelines/asymptomatic-microhematuria.cfm. Accessed 2015.

36. Coyne KS, Cash B, Kopp Z, et al. The prevalence of chronic constipation and faecal incontinence among men and women with symptoms of overactive bladder. *BJU Int*. 2011;107:254–261.

37. Longstreth GP, Thompson WG, Chey WD, et al. Functional bowel disorders. *Gastroenterology*. 2006;130:1480–91.

38. Cammu H, Van Nylen M, Blockeel C, et al. Who will benefit from pelvic floor muscle training for stress urinary incontinence? *Am J Obstet Gynecol*. 2004;191:1152–1157.

39. Inamura M, Abrams P, Bain C, et al. Systemic review and economic modeling of the effectiveness and cost-effectiveness of non-surgical treatments for women with stress urinary incontinence. *Health Technol Assess*. 2010;14:1–188.

40. Labrie J, Berghman BLCM, Fischer K, et al. Surgery versus physiotherapy for stress urinary incontinence. *N Engl J Med*. 2013;369:1124–1133.

41. Bo K, Kvarstein B, Nygaard I. Lower urinary tract symptoms and pelvic floor muscle exercise adherence after 15 years. *Obstet Gynecol*. 2005;105:999–1005.

42. Cammu H, Van Nylen M, Amy JJ. A 10-year follow-up after Kegel pelvic floor muscle exercises for genuine stress incontinence. *BJU Int*. 2000;85:655–658.

43. Lamers BHC, van der Vaart CH. Medium term efficacy of pelvic floor muscle training for female urinary incontinence in daily practice. *Int Urogyn J*. 2007;18:301–307.

44. Ogah J, Cody JD, Rogerson L. Minimally invasive synthetic suburethral sling operations for stress urinary incontinence in women [Review]. *Cochrane Database Syst Rev*. 2009;(4):CD006375. doi:10.1002/14651858.CD006375.pub2.

45. Novara G, Artibani W, Barber MD, et al. Updated systemic review and meta-analysis of the comparative data on colposuspensions, pubovaginal slings, and midurethral tapes in the surgical treatment of female stress urinary incontinence. *Eur Urol*. 2010;58:218–238.

46. Lathe PM, Foon R, Toozs-Hobson P. Transobturator and retropubic tape procedures in stress urinary incontinence: a systemic review and meta-analysis of effectiveness and complications. *BJOG*. 2007;114:522–531.

47. Albo M, Wruck L, Baker J, et al. The relationships among measures of incontinence severity in women undergoing surgery for stress urinary incontinence. *J Urol*. 2007;177:1810–1824.

48. Bo K, Talseth T, Holme I. Single blind, randomized controlled trial of pelvic floor exercises, electrical stimulation, vaginal cone, and no treatment in management of genuine stress incontinence in women. *BMJ*. 1999;318:487–493.

49. Henalla SM, Hutchins CJ, Robinson P, et al. Non-operative methods in the treatment of female genuine stress incontinence of urine. *J Obstet Gynecol*. 1989;9:222–225.

50. Castro RA, Arruda RM, Zanetti MRD, et al. Single blind, randomized, controlled trial of pelvic floor muscle training, electrical stimulation, and no active treatment in the management of stress urinary incontinence. *Clinics (San Paulo, Brazil)*. 2008;64:465–472.

51. Dumoulin C, Hay-Smith EJC, Mac Habee-Seguin G. Pelvic floor muscle training versus no treatment, or inactive control treatments, for urinary incontinence in women [Review]. *Cochrane Database Syst Rev*. 2014;(5):CD005654. doi:10.1002/14651858.CD005654.pub3.

52. Hay-Smith EJC, Herdercshee R, Dumoulin C, et al. Comparisons of approaches to pelvic floor muscle training for urinary incontinence in women [Review]. *Cochrane Database Syst Rev*. 2011, issue 12, Art No.: CD009508. doi: 10.1002/14651858. CD009508.

53. Herderschee R, Hay-Smith EJC, Herbison GP, et al. Feedback or biofeedback to augment pelvic floor muscle training for urinary incontinence

in women (Review). *Cochrane Database Syst Rev.* 2011;(7):CD009252. doi:10.1002/14651858.CD009252.

54. American Urogynecologic Society. Lifestyle and behavioral changes, improving urinary urgency, frequency and urge incontinence. voicesforPFD.org/p/cm/ld/FID=170. http://www.augs.org/d/do/37. Accessed 2016.

55. Burgio KL, Richter HE, Clements RH, et al. Changes in urinary and fecal incontinence symptoms with weight loss surgery in morbidly obese women. *Obstet Gynecol.* 2007;110:1034–1040.

56. Subak LL, Wing R, West DS, et al. Weight loss to treat urinary incontinence in overweight and obese women. *N Engl J Med.* 2009;360:481–490.

57. Wilson PD, Herbison GP. A randomized controlled trial of pelvic floor muscle exercises to treat postnatal urinary incontinence. *Int Urogyn J.* 1998;9:257–264.

58. Goode PS, Burgio KL, Locher JL, et al. Effect of behavioral training with or without pelvic floor electrical stimulation on stress incontinence in women. *JAMA.* 2003;290:345–352.

59. Pieber D, Zivkovic F, Tamussino K, et al. Pelvic floor exercises alone or with vaginal cones for the treatment of mild to moderate stress urinary incontinence in premenopausal women. *Int Urogyn J.* 1995;6:14–17.

60. Williams KS, Coleby D, Abrams K, et al. Randomised controlled trials of the effectiveness of pelvic floor therapies for urodynamic stress and mixed incontinence. *BJU Int.* 2006;98:1043–1050.

61. Bo K, Hagen RH, Kvarstein B, et al. Pelvic floor muscle exercises for the treatment of female stress urinary incontinence: III. Effect of two different degrees of pelvic floor muscle exercises. *Neurourol Urodyn.* 1990;9:458–502.

62. Herbison GP, Dean N. Weighted vaginal cones for urinary incontinence. *Cochrane Database Syst Rev.* 2013;(7):CD002114. doi:10.1002/14651858.CD002114.pub2.

63. Cammu H, Van Nylen M. Pelvic floor exercises versus vaginal weight cones in genuine stress incontinence. *Eur J Obstet Gynecol Reprod Biol.* 1998;77:89–93.

64. Olah KS, Bridges N, Denning J, et al. The conservative management of patients with symptoms of stress incontinence: a randomized prospective study comparing weighted vaginal cones interferential therapy. *Am J Obstet Gynecol.* 1990;126:87–92.

65. Richter HE, Burgio KL, Brubaker L, et al. Continence pessary compared with behavioral therapy or combined therapy for stress incontinence: a randomized controlled trial. *Obstet Gynecol.* 2010;115:609–617.

66. Donnelly MJ, Powell-Morgan S, Olsen AL, et al. Vaginal pessaries for the management of stress and mixed urinary incontinence. *Int Urogyn J.* 2004;15:302–307.

67. Zullo MA, Plotti F, Calcagno M, et al. Vaginal estrogen therapy and overactive bladder symptoms in postmenopausal patients after a tension-free vaginal tape procedure: a randomized clinical trial. *Menopause.* 2005;12:421–427.

68. Ku JH, Oh JG, Shin JW, et al. Outcome of mid-urethral sling procedures in Korean women with stress urinary incontinence according to body mass index. *Int J Urol.* 2006;13:379–384.

69. Mukherjee K, Constantine G. Urinary stress incontinence in obese women: tension-free vaginal tape is the answer. *BJU Int.* 2001;88:881–883.

70. Skriapas K, Poulakis V, Dillenburg W, et al. Tension-free vaginal tape (TVT) in morbidly obese patients with severe urodynamic stress urinary incontinence as last option treatment. *Eur Urol.* 2006;49:544–550.

71. Paraiso MF, Walters MD, Karram MM, et al. Laparoscopic Burch colposuspension versus tension-free vaginal tape: a randomized trial. *Obstet Gynecol.* 2004;104:1249–1258.

72. Persson J, Teleman P, Eten-Bergquist C, et al. Cost-analysis based on a prospective, randomized study comparing laparoscopic colposuspension with tension-free vaginal tape procedure. *Acta Obstet Gynecol Scand.* 2002;81:1066–1073.

73. Richter HE, Albo ME, Zyczynski HM, et al. Retropubic versus transobturator midurethral sling s for stress incontinence. *N Engl J Med.* 2010;362:2066–2076.

74. Albo ME, Litman HJ, Richter HE, et al. Treatment success of retropubic and transobturator mid urethral slings at 24 months. *J Urol.* 2012;188:2281–2287.

75. Kenton K, Stoddard AM, Zyczynski H, et al. 5-year longitudinal follow-up after retropubic and transobturator mid urethral slings. *J Urol.* 2015;193:203–210.

76. Pradhan A, Jain P, Latthe PM. Effectiveness of midurethral slings in recurrent stress urinary incontinence: a systemic review and meta-analysis. *Int Urogyn J.* 2012;23:831–841.

77. Aigmueller T, Trutnovsky G, Tamussino K, et al. Ten-year follow-up after the tension-free vaginal tape procedure. *Am J Obstet Gynecol.* 2011;205:496:e1–e5.

78. Nilsson CG, Plava K, Rezapour M, et al. Eleven years prospective follow-up of the tension-free vaginal tape procedure for the treatment of stress urinary incontinence. *Int Urogyn J.* 2008;19:1043–1047.

79. Svenningsen R, Staff AC, Schiotz HA, et al. Long-term follow-up of the retropubic tension-free vaginal tape procedure. *Int Urogyn J.* 2013;24:1271–1278.

80. Albo ME, Richter HE, Brubaker L, et al. Burch colposuspension versus fascial sling to reduce urinary stress incontinence. *N Engl J Med.* 2007;356:2143–2155.

81. Brubaker L, Richter HE, Norton PA, et al. 5-year continence rates, satisfaction and adverse events of Burch urethropexy and fascial sling surgery for urinary incontinence. *J Urol.* 2012;187:12324–12330.

82. Guerrero KL, Emery SJ, Wareham K, et al. A randomized controlled trial comparing TVT,

Pelvicol, and autologous fascial slings for the treatment of stress urinary incontinence in women. *BJOG.* 2010;117:1493–1503.

83. Ward K, Hilton P, on behalf of the UK & Ireland TVT trial group. Prospective multicenter randomized trial of tension-free vaginal tape and colposuspension as primary treatment for stress incontinence. *BMJ.* 2002;325:67–73.

84. Ward K, Hilton P, UK & Ireland TVT trial group. A prospective multicenter randomized trial of tension-free vaginal tape and colposuspension as primary urodynamic stress incontinence: two-year follow-up. *Am J Obstet Gynecol.* 2004;190:324–331.

85. Ward K, Hilton P, on behalf of the UK & Ireland TVT trial group. Tension-free vaginal tape versus colposuspension for primary urinary stress incontinence. *BJOG.* 2008;115:226–233.

86. Kenton K, Pham T, Mueller E, et al. Patient preparedness: an important predictor of surgical outcome. *Am J Obstet Gynecol.* 2007;197:654.e7–654.e6.

87. Teleman PM, Lidfeldt J, Nerbrand C, et al. Overactive bladder: prevalence, risk factors and relation to stress incontinence in middle-aged women. *BJOG.* 2004;111:600–604.

88. Mallett VT, Brubaker L, Stoddard AM, et al. The expectations of patients who undergo surgery for stress incontinence. *Am J Obstet Gynecol.* 2008;198:308.e1–308.e6.

89. Wennberg A-L, Molander U, Fall M, et al. A longitudinal population based survey of urinary incontinence, overactive bladder, and other lower urinary tract symptoms in women. *Eur Urol.* 2009;55:783–791.

90. Wyman J, Fantl JA, McClish DK, et al. Comparetive efficacy of behavioral interventions in the management of female stress urinary incontinence. *Am J Obstet Gynecol.* 1998;179:999–1007.

91. Burgio KL, Locher JL, Goode PS, et al. Behavioral therapy vs drug treatment for urge urinary incontinence in older women. A randomized controlled trial. *JAMA.* 1998;280:1995–2000.

92. Burgio KL, Goode PS, Locher JL, et al. Behavioral training with and without biofeedback in the treatment of urge incontinence in older women. A randomized controlled trial. *JAMA.* 2002;288:2293–2299.

93. Burgio KL, Kraus SR, Menefee S, et al. Behavioral therapy to enable women with urge incontinence to discontinue drug treatment. *Ann Intern Med.* 2008;149:161–169.

94. Bump RC, Hurt WG, Fantl JA, et al. Assessment of Kegel pelvic muscle exercise performance after brief verbal instruction. *Am J Obstet Gynecol.* 1991;165:322–9.

95. Institute of Medicine of the National Academies. Dietary reference intake: water, potassium, sodium, chloride, and sulfate. Iom.edu/Reports/2004/Dietary-Reference-Intake-Water-Potassium-Sodium-Chloride-Sulfate. https://fnic.nal.usda.gov/sites/fnic.nal.usda.gov/files/uploads/73-185.pdf. Accessed 2015.

96. Clemons JL, Aguilar VC, Tillinghast TA, et al. Patient satisfaction and changes in prolapse and urinary symptoms in women who were fitted successfully with a pessary for pelvic organ prolapse. *Am J Obstet Gynecol.* 2004;190:1025–1029.

97. Fernando R, Thakar R, Sultan AH, et al. Effect of vaginal pessary on symptoms associated with pelvic organ prolapse. *Obstet Gynecol.* 2006;108:93–99.

98. Hanson LA, Schulz JA, Flood CG, et al. Vaginal pessaries in managing women with pelvic organ prolapse and urinary incontinence: Patient characteristics and factors contributing to success. *Int Urogyn J.* 2006;17:155–159.

99. Sze EHM, Hobbs G. A retrospective comparison of ring pessary and multicomponent behavioral therapy in managing overactive bladder. *Int Urogyn J.* 2014;25:1583–1588.

100. Cody JD, Jacobs ML, Richardson K, et al. Oestrogen therapy for urinary incontinence in postmenopausal women. *Cochrane Database Syst Rev.* 2012;(10):CD001405. doi:10.1002/14651858. CD001405.pub3.

101. Peters KM, Carrico DJ, Woolridge LS, et al. Percutaneous tibial nerve stimulation for the long-term treatment of overactive bladder: 3-year results of the STEP study. *J Urol.* 2013;189:2194–2201.

102. Shaya FT, Blume S, Gu A, et al. Persistence with overactive bladder pharmacotherapy in a Medicaid population. *Am J Manag Care.* 2005;11(4 Suppl):S121–S129.

103. Varadharajan S, Jumadilova Z, Girase P, et al. Economic impact of extended-release tolterodine versus immediate- and extended-release oxybutynin among commercially insured persons with overactive bladder. *Am J Manag Care.* 2005;11(4 Suppl):S140–S149.

104. Malone DC, Okano GJ. Treatment of urge incontinence in Veterans Affairs Medical Centers. *Clin Ther.* 1999;21:867–877.

105. Anderson RU, Mobley D, Blank B, et al. Once daily controlled versus immediate release oxybutynin chloride for urge incontinence. *J Urol.* 1999;161:1809–1812.

106. Versi E, Appell R, Mobley D, et al. Dry mouth with conventional and controlled-release oxybutynin in urinary incontinence. *Obstet Gynecol.* 2000;95:718–721.

107. The American Geriatrics Society 2012 Beers Criteria Update Expert Panel. American Geriatrics Society updated Beers criteria for potentially inappropriate medication use in older adults. *J Am Geriatr Soc.* 2012;60:616–631.

Index

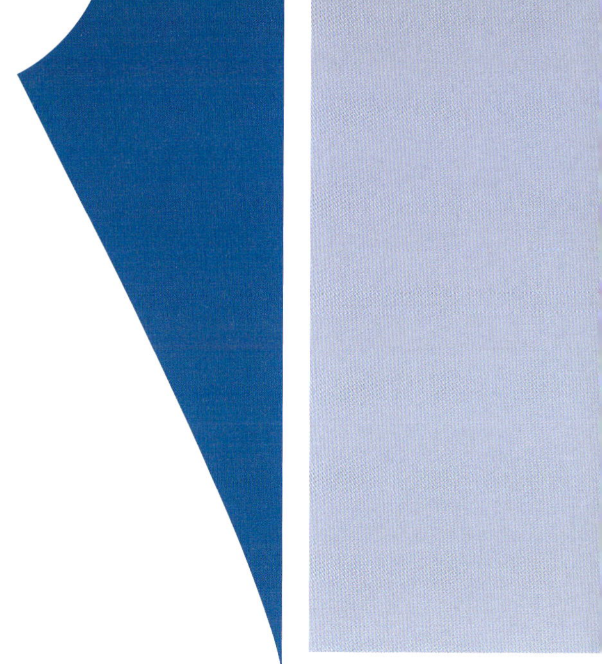

Note: Page numbers followed by *f* indicate figures, and those followed by *t* indicate tables.